Current Topics in Medical Mycology 2

Michael R. McGinnis
Editor

Current Topics in Medical Mycology

VOLUME 2

With 92 Illustrations

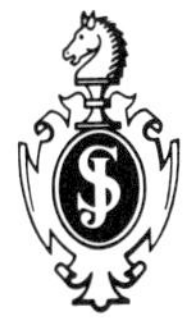

Springer-Verlag
New York Berlin Heidelberg
London Paris Tokyo

Series Editor
Michael R. McGinnis, Ph.D.
Department of Microbiology and Immunology
University of North Carolina at Chapel Hill
Chapel Hill, North Carolina 27514, USA

ISSN 0177-4204

Typeset by Asco Trade Typesetting Ltd., Hong Kong.
Printed and bound by Arcata Graphics/Halliday, West Hanover, Massachusetts.
Printed in the United States of America.

9 8 7 6 5 4 3 2 1

ISBN 0-387-96543-2 Springer-Verlag New York Berlin Heidelberg
ISBN 3-540-96543-2 Springer-Verlag Berlin Heidelberg New York

Series Preface

Current Topics in Medical Mycology, is intended to summarize current research areas in medical mycology for medical mycologists and other scientists who are working in microbiology and immunology. Topics to be included in each volume will serve as contemporary reviews, summaries of current advancements and future directions, and mechanisms to enhance the interdisciplinary use of medically important fungi in understanding pathogenesis, epidemiology, mycotoxins, taxonomy, and other areas where basic, applied, and clinical sciences are used.

Michael R. McGinnis

Contents

Contributors

Jeffrey M. Becker, Ph.D.
Professor, Department of Microbiology and Program in Cellular, Molecular, and Developmental Biology, University of Tennessee, Knoxville, Tennessee, USA

Alois A. Bell, Ph.D.
U.S. Department of Agriculture, Agricultural Research Service, Cotton Pathology Research Unit, College Station, Texas, USA

Marcel Borgers, Ph.D.
Department of Life Sciences, Janssen Pharmaceutica, Beerse, Belgium

Robert Cherniak, Ph.D.
Professor, Department of Chemistry and Laboratory of Microbial Biochemical Sciences, Georgia State University, Atlanta, Georgia, USA

Roderick J. Hay, D.M., M.R.C.P.
Senior Lecturer in Clinical Mycology, Department of Medical Microbiology, London School of Hygiene and Tropical Medicine, London, England

Michael J. Kennedy, Ph.D.
Microbiology and Nutrition Research Unit, The Upjohn Company, Kalamazoo, Michigan, USA

Fred Naider, Ph.D.
Professor, Department of Chemistry, College of Staten Island, City University of New York, Staten Island, New York, USA

DEMOSTHENES PAPPAGIANIS, M.D., Ph.D.
Professor, Department of Medical Microbiology and Immunology, University of California, Davis, California, USA

ANGELA RESTREPO M, Ph.D.
Corporación de Investigaciones Biológicas, Hospital Pablo Tobón Uribe, Medellín, Colombia, South America

WILLIAM A. RUTALA, Ph.D., M.P.H.
Research Associate Professor, Department of Medicine, University of North Carolina at Chapel Hill, Chapel Hill, North Carolina, USA

MAXWELL G. SHEPHERD, Ph.D.
Professor, Department of Experimental Oral Biology and Oral Pathology, School of Dentistry, University of Otago, Dunedin, New Zealand

DAVID J. WEBER, M.D., M.P.H.
Assistant Professor, Departments of Medicine, Pediatrics, and Epidemiology, University of North Carolina at Chapel Hill, Chapel Hill, North Carolina, USA

MICHAEL H. WHEELER, Ph.D.
U.S. Department of Agriculture, Agricultural Research Service, Cotton Pathology Research Unit, College Station, Texas, USA

YUZO YOSHIDA, Ph.D.
Associate Professor, Department of Biochemistry, Faculty of Pharmaceutical Sciences, Mukogawa Women's University, Nishinomiya, Hyogo, Japan

1—Ultrastructural Correlates of Antimycotic Treatment

MARCEL BORGERS

The descriptive ultrastructure of a large variety of fungal species either grown under in vitro culture conditions or in situ during infection of the host has been reported in detail. Morphologic characterization of yeasts, dimorphic fungi, and filamentous fungi has been done using scanning electron microscopy to elaborate the surface structure, transmission electron microscopy to reveal the internal subcellular organelles, and freeze-fracture electron microscopy to display some intramembranous molecular structures (2, 3, 5, 6, 12, 17, 28, 31, 45, 50, 61, 64, 66, 70, 75, 83, 85, 112, 113, 124). For a long time the detailed description of fungal substructure has been hampered by the lack of adequate methodology. From the early days of explorative research, especially the field of transmission electron microscopy has been encumbered with difficulties of clear-cut visualization, hence obscuring the interpretation of the observations (17).

Auxiliary techniques to fill morphologic "lacunes," such as ultrastructural cytochemistry of enzymes; microanalysis of elements; autoradiography; specific and/or selective stains for carbohydrates, lipids, proteins, RNA, and DNA; and, last but not least, immunocytochemistry, have been more than complementary to elucidate many basic questions and problems related to the structural identification and the interrelationships of subcellular entities (31, 41, 43, 44, 45, 50, 70, 79, 85, 102).

To interpret the physiopathologic changes in subcellular structures brought about by antimycotic treatment, a clear picture of the normal structure is an absolute requirement. During the past two decades an important number of methodologic breakthroughs have been realized so that the cytologic and cytochemical correlates of antifungal action could be approached in great detail, at least for some drugs and against some fungal species.

Combined biochemical and cytologic studies supported by cytochemical assays have led to the elucidation of the mechanism of action of several antimycotics. Individual compounds for which effects on fungal structure are well documented are amphotericin B and nystatin (polyene antimicrobic), griseofulvin (antimicrobic), 5-fluorocytosine (antimetabolite); miconazole, clotrimazole, econazole, ketoconazole, and itraconazole (azole-derivatives); and naftifine and lamisil (allylamines). Scanty reports are available describing the ultrastructural changes induced by other antifungals such as pyrazolylalkyl sulfides, isoconazole, bifonazole, fenticonazole, tioconazole, povidone-iodine, pentachloronitrobenzene, echinocandin, levorin, amphoglucamin, mepartricin, diamidine compounds, radicicolin, aculeacin A, papulacandin B, and potassium iodide.

The aim of this chapter is to summarize the ultrastructural correlates of antimycotic treatment in relation to the current knowledge of the molecular mechanism of action of these various antimycotic drugs.

Polyene Antimicrobics

Polyenes are widely used agents for the treatment of fungal disease. Amphotericin B and nystatin are the most prominent members of this group of antimicrobics, which chemically differ in the lactone ring structure and number of double-bonded carbon atoms (54).

The mechanism of action of polyene antifungal agents is based on a specific interaction with membrane sterols, resulting in a changed permeability (51, 77). The nature of the sterol is of primary importance for membrane susceptibility. The specificity of interaction also depends on the polyene structure itself. Amphotericin B is bound more tightly to ergosterol than to cholesterol, desmosterol, lanosterol, β-sitosterol, and stigmasterol (104).

One of the earliest detectable effects of treatment with a polyene antimicrobic is the release of potassium ions from sensitive cells. That the loss of potassium and the associated uptake of protons might be responsible for the fungicidal effects is supported by the finding that *Candida albicans* cells can be protected against the effects of amphotericin B methyl ester by the addition of potassium to the culture medium (68). However, the studies of Palacios and Serrano (92) indicate that the induced potassium loss in not the primary effect of the tetraene nystatin and of the heptaene, amphotericin B. These authors have tested the effects of low concentrations of amphotericin B on the proton permeability of yeast cells. An increased influx was observed resembling that found with the proton conductor, 2, 4-dinitrophenol. The increased proton permeability collapses the proton gradient. The latter plays an important role in the functioning of the yeast plasma membrane, generating an electrochemical gradient required for active transport (48) and the maintenance of the intracellular potassium pool (93). Based on these studies it is now accepted that the primary effect of amphotericin B is the dissipation of the proton gradient. Dissipation of the proton gradient would explain the effects of amphotericin B on potassium release, active transport of nutrients, fermentation, and growth.

It is well known that membrane sterols play a key role in controlling fluidity of the lipid bilayer. Binding of amphotericin B and other polyene molecules with ergosterol will interfere with the interactions of this sterol with the acyl side chains of the phospholipids and thus alter membrane fluidity. Therefore, Kerridge and Whelan (67) suggest that the enhanced permeability to protons results from the localized effect of the polyene antimicrobic on the physical state of the lipids within the bilayer.

Because ergosterol is its primary molecular target, the morphologist's attention has been focused to the substructure of cell membranes and the cell wall (29, 89).

As for most other antifungal molecules, the activity of amphotericin B, including its methyl ester, nystatin, mepartricin, levorin, and amphoglucamin has been investigated in *Candida* species, especially *C. albicans.* The ultrastructure of *C. albicans* is shown in Fig. 1-1.

In vitro exposure of *C. albicans* cells to 10^{-4}M of amphotericin B induces necrosis of the entire population (15). All subcellular membrane systems deteriorate with only remnants of barely recognizable organelles left behind. The cell wall retains its usual structure (Fig. 1-2). The degree of destruction appears to be correlated with the concentration of the drug and to the incubation time.

In a freeze-fracture electron microscopy study comparing the effects of amphotericin B and its methyl ester on plasma membranes of *C. albicans* and red blood cells, Sekiya et al (109) showed marked changes in aggregation and density intramembranous particles in *C. albicans*, whereas red blood cell membranes were only marginally affected by the same treatment. The effects in *C. albicans* were less pronounced with amphotericin B than with its methyl ester. These results suggest that amphotericin B methyl ester affects the ergosterol-containing membranes more than amphotericin B, and that ergosterol from the yeast cell has a higher sensitivity for these polyene antimicrobics than cholesterol from the red blood cell.

Aggregation of intramembrane particles has been found also as a correlate of sensitivity of some strains of *C. albicans* to nystatin. Nonsensitive mutant strains apparently did not show any modification in size and distribution of intramembrane particles (94). Studies by Bastide et al (9, 10, 11), comparing different azoles with amphotericin B and nystatin, have shown that in contrast to some azoles, the polyenes easily pass through the cell wall of *C. albicans* and interact with the cytoplasmic membrane. Similar observations have been reported recently by Petrou and Rogers (96) showing the cell membrane to be the primary target site of mepartricin and amphotericin action. In addition, mepartricin caused a delayed separation of dividing cells and damaged both sides of the septum, which lead the authors to suggest an interference of the latter compound with enzymatic mechanisms of septum formation through inhibition of chitin synthesis.

Strains of *C. tropicalis* resistant to nystatin revealed marked ultrastructural

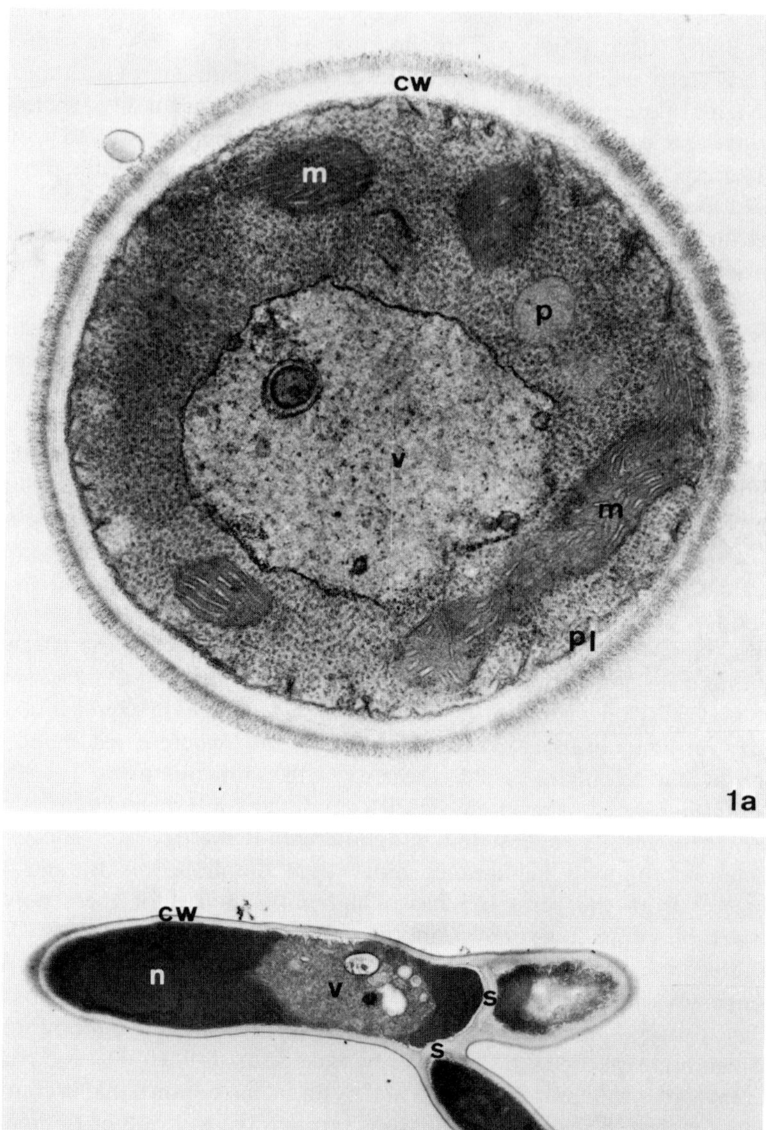

FIG. 1-1. Normal cultures of *C. albicans* (transmission electron microscopy). (a) Yeast cell: cross section showing thick cell wall (cw), undulated plasma membrane (pl), vacuole (v), mitochondria (m), and peroxisome (p) (× 34,500; reduced by 9%). (b) Mycelial form: cell wall is thinner than in yeast cell, all other organelles are identical. Septum (s); nucleus (n) (× 8,200; reduced by 9%).

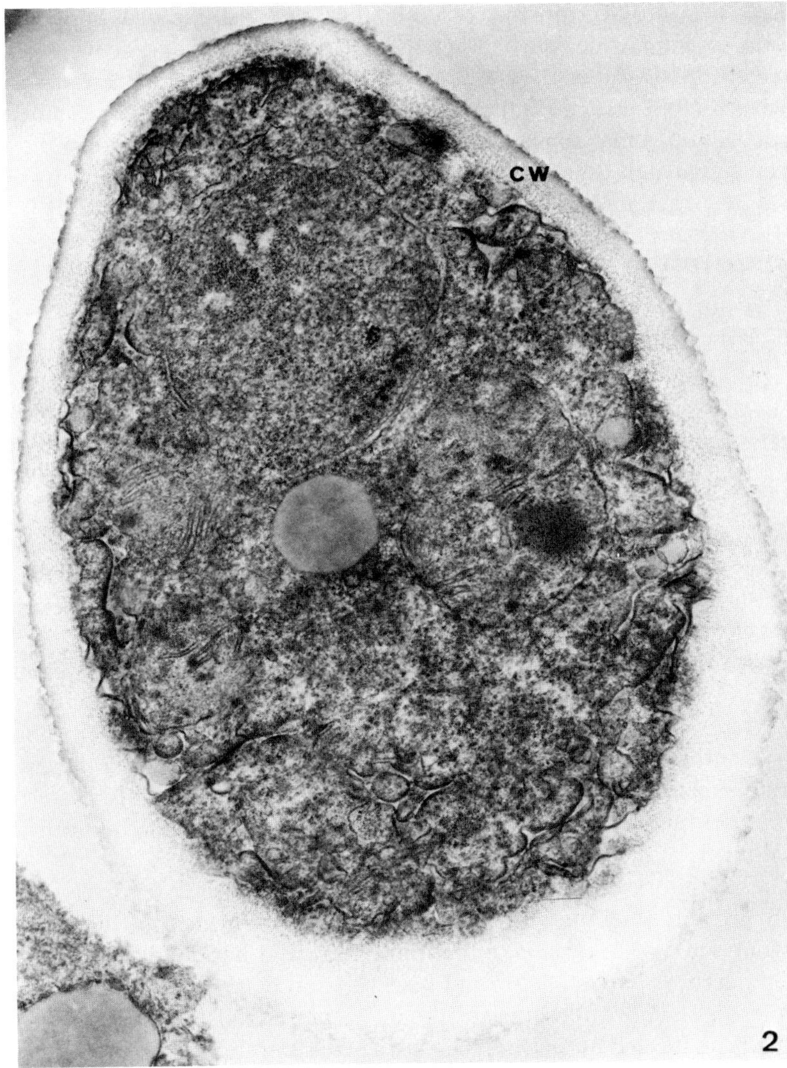

FIG. 1-2. Transmission electron micrograph of *C. albicans* yeast form treated with 10^{-4} M amphotericin B for 24 hours. All internal organelles are fully necrotized. The origin of the membranous elements is no longer recognizable. The cell wall (cw) appears unaltered (×38,000; reduced by 9%).

differences such as abnormal thickening of the cell wall, formation of invaginations into the cytoplasm, formation of microbodies and large vacuoles, and reduction in the number of mitochondrial cristae. These changes have been mainly attributed to altered steroid content and changes in other lipid classes (34).

Transmission electron microscopy of *C. albicans* exposed to nystatin, levorin, or amphoglucamin has demonstrated that early changes concerned an enlargement of the central vacuole in which cytoplasmic organelles were discarded (105). Fragmentation of the cytoplasmic membrane, plasmolysis, vacuolization, and cytoplasmic necrosis were considered as progressive signs of cell destruction. Again no obvious changes were seen in the cell wall (105).

Griseofulvin

Only few reports deal with the effects of griseofulvin on the ultrastructure of susceptible fungi. Griseofulvin, an antimicrobic isolated from *Penicillium griseofulvum* is active only against dermatophytes. Over the years a variety of effects at different subcellular sites have been proposed to account for its antifungal activity. These include inhibition of the synthesis of hyphal cell wall material (13, 47), binding to RNA (13), interference with nucleic acid synthesis and mitosis (13, 71, 123), and inhibition of microtubules (71, 88). In view of the fact that griseofulvin is only active on growing cells, the hypothesis on the primary interaction with mirotubules is very attractive for it may explain some of the previously formulated proposals, that is, as a blocker of mitosis (spindle microtubules) or lack of adequate renewal of cell wall material (cytoplasmic microtubules). Indeed, there is evidence that griseofulvin not only acts as a spindle poison but also interferes with cytoplasmic microtubules (71). Considering the role of microtubules in the cytoplasmic transport of secretory material toward the cell periphery (22), one might speculate that after microtubule destruction the processing of newly synthetized cell wall constituents at the growing hyphal tips is impaired.

The inhibitory effects of this drug are limited almost exclusively to actively growing fungi in which chitin is a major constituent of the cell wall (Zygomycetes, Ascomycetes, Fungi Imperfecti, and Basidiomycetes). Single-celled microorganisms (yeasts and bacteria) and filamentous fungi in which cellulose is a major structural constituent of the cell wall (Oomycetes) remain virtually unaffected by relatively high drug concentrations. In dermatophytes griseofulvin induced swelling and ballooning of the hyphae, the cell wall thickened, and the cytoplasm desintegrated (14).

The cell wall of fungal hyphae laid down in the presence of radicicolin and griseofulvin is thicker and stronger than in normal hyphae. In *Aspergillus niger* radicicolin and griseofulvin induced the formation of swollen and misshapen cells that differed from normal cells only in size and thickness of the cell wall (47). Electron micrographs revealed no abnormalities in orientation or thickness of the structural microfibrils in the walls of the swollen and misshaped cells. Hyphal septa were similar in structural detail to the rest of the cell wall and consequently may become thickened and malformed in the presence of these antifungals. These results are in support of the idea that radicicolin and griseofulvin act in the region of the cell wall bound on the inner surface by the plasma membrane, to disrupt the normal process of hyphal extension at the cell tip. The deposition of additional cell wall material on swollen hyphae is seen as a response on the part of the fungus to maintain the integrity of these wider malformed cells (47).

5-Fluorocytosine

5-Fluorocytosine (5-FC) is a fluorinated pyrimidine that was initially developed as an antimetabolic drug for use in cancer chemotherapy. This drug has a narrow spectrum of antifungal activity; its activity appears to be limited to yeast-like fungi (110), although successful treatment of pulmonary aspergillosis has been reported (35).

The mechanism of action of 5-FC has been investigated in *Saccharomyces carlsbergensis*, *S. cerevisiae*, *C. albicans*, *Cryptococcus neoformans*, *Aspergillus fumigatus*, and *Wangiella dermatitidis* (67, 107). The drug is taken up by sensitive cells via a transport system similar to the energy-dependent transport of the purine bases adenine, guanine, hypoxanthine and of the pyrimidine base, cytosine (99). Inside the cell 5-FC is deaminated to the antineoplastic compound 5-fluorouracil (5-FU) by cytosine deaminase. The fact that this key enzyme in the metabolism of 5-FC is absent or has only weak activity in mammalian cells is held responsible for the low toxicity of 5-FC in the mammalian host. Once formed, 5-FU is then further metabolized by uridine monophosphate pyrophosphorylase to 5-fluorouridine monophosphate and to 5-fluorouridine-diphosphate and -triphosphate, which is incorporated into RNA resulting in the production of aberrant RNA and inhibition of ribosomal protein synthesis. 5-Fluorouracil is also metabolized to 5-fluorodeoxyuridine monophosphate, a potent inhibitor of the thymidylate synthetase and hence of DNA synthesis. Either the effect of RNA or on DNA can be responsible for the observed growth inhibition of sensitive fungal organisms.

Detailed ultrastructural changes after 5-FC exposure of *C. albicans* and *S. cerevisiae* cultures have been reported by Arai et al (4). Shortly after drug contact the cells displayed a marked enlargement of their volume. This effect was most pronounced with *C. albicans*. Characteristic changes consisted of an enlarged nucleus and a thinned cell wall (Fig. 1-3). The latter change was considered the result of the marked increase in cell volume together with the impairment of cell wall synthesis. Germ tube formation in *C. albicans* apparently was not affected by 5-FC. In another study the effects of 5-FC have been shown in *A. fumigatus* (43). They consisted in slight alterations of the cell wall, the formation of lipid globules and typical nuclear changes. Most of the nuclei showed granular heterochromatin, which took up a very large part of the nucleoplasm. A few nuclei showed blebbing and partial disintegration of their

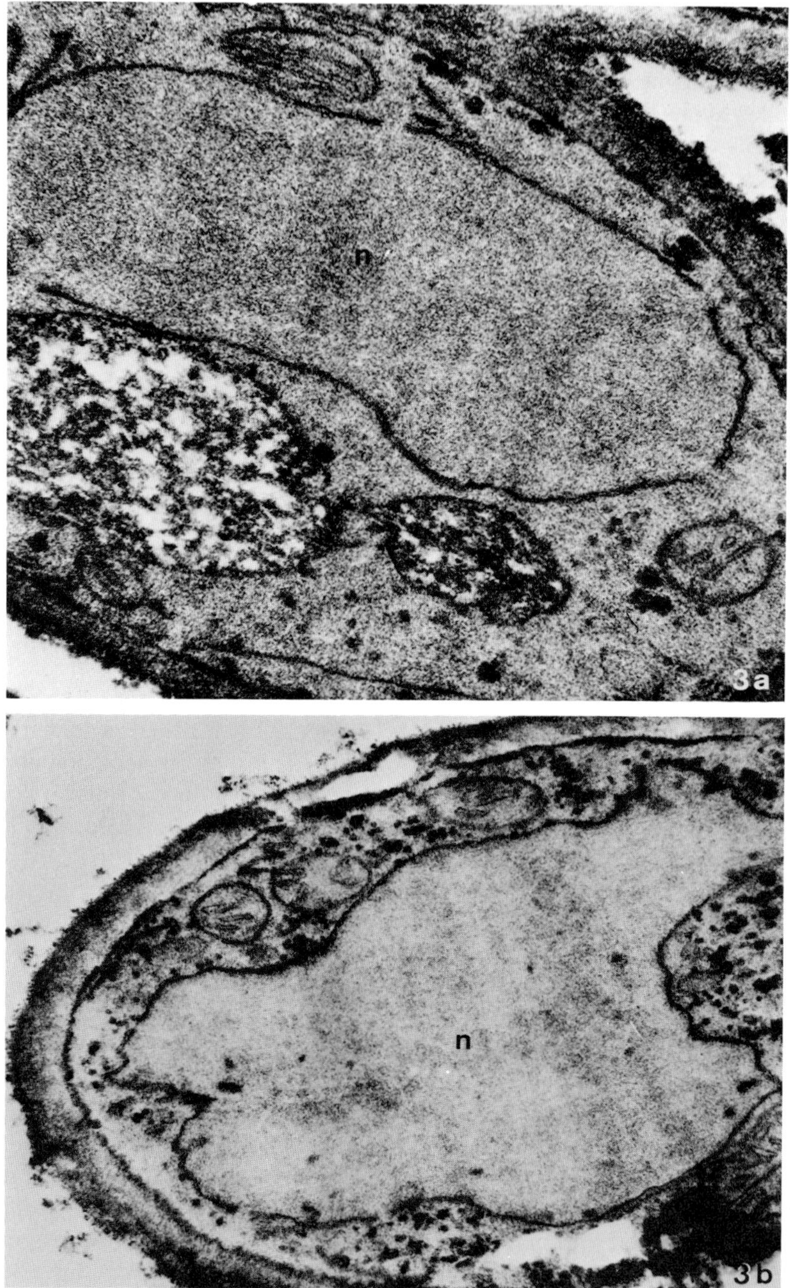

FIG. 1-3. Transmission electron micrograph of *C. albicans* yeast cell treated with 5-fluorocytosine. (a) After a 2-hour contact with 10 μg/ml. Except for an enlargement of the nucleus (n), no alterations are obvious ($\times$ 36,000; reduced by 9%). (b) After a 12-hour contact with 10 μg/ml. Note the enlarged nucleus (n) in this voluminous yeast cell ($\times$ 25,800; reduced by 9%). (Courtesy of Prof. Dr. T. Arai, Research Institute for Chemobiodynamics, Chiba University, Chiba, Japan.)

membrane. The appearance of small vesicles in the nucleoplasm and a patchy distribution of the heterochromatin also was seen. Moreover, densely stained material, abundantly present in cells altered as such, was thought to be derived from pyknotic nuclei or from fused vacuoles with nuclei. These typical morphologic changes are displayed in Fig. 1-4. Elemental analysis by laser microprobe mass analysis showed an increased calcium load after 5-FC treatment of *A. fumigatus* (43). Deteriorative changes in the structure of *Cryptococcus neoformans* after treatment of patients with 5-FC have been documented (59). However, a direct cause-effect relationship between the observed changes and the applied treatment could not be ascertained.

Azole Derivatives

The ultrastructural changes after azole treatment have been the subject of many research reports. This relatively new family of broad-spectrum antimycotics can already be subdivided into three generations of antifungal drugs. Although the effects of the first antifungal azole, benzimidazole, were described in 1944 (125), active development of azole antifungal chemotherapeutic agents started some 18 years ago with the introduction of clotrimazole and miconazole (52, 97). The most attractive aspects of these antifungal agents are: the spectrum of activity against yeasts, dimorphic and filamentous fungi, virtual absence of primary and secondary resistance, and limited toxicity. In the years after the introduction of clotrimazole and miconazole, two chemical analogues of the latter, econazole and isoconazole, were developed (52, 55, 69). Bifonazole (98), tioconazole (63), oxiconazole (82), fenticonazole (32, 33), butoconazole (122), and sulconazole (114) recently have been introduced. With the exception of miconazole, for which an intravenous preparation is also available, all these azoles are used solely for topical application.

Ketoconazole is the first of a generation of orally active imidazole compounds (56) and the most widely studied antifungal as far as molecular and structural mode of action is concerned. Triazole derivatives such as itraconazole (58), terconazole (57, 116), vibunazole (49, 127), and fluconazole (60) are the most recently synthetized antifungal azoles that are currently under clinical investigation. All these derivatives most probably share the same molecular mechanism of action. The current ideas on this mechanism are comprehensively reviewed by Vanden Bossche and co-workers (118, 119, 120).

In view of this activity against most yeast, pleomorphic and filamentous fungal species, the reported ultrastructural alterations as studied by transmission and/or scanning electron microscopy bear on a large number of organisms including *C. albicans* (7, 8, 24, 38, 39, 40, 46, 62, 95, 101, 102, 106), *Coccidioides immitis* (25), *Histoplasma capsulatum* (19, 86), *Paracoccidioides brasiliensis* (21, 86), *Trichophyton rubrum* (26, 37, 100, 102), *T. mentagrophytes*

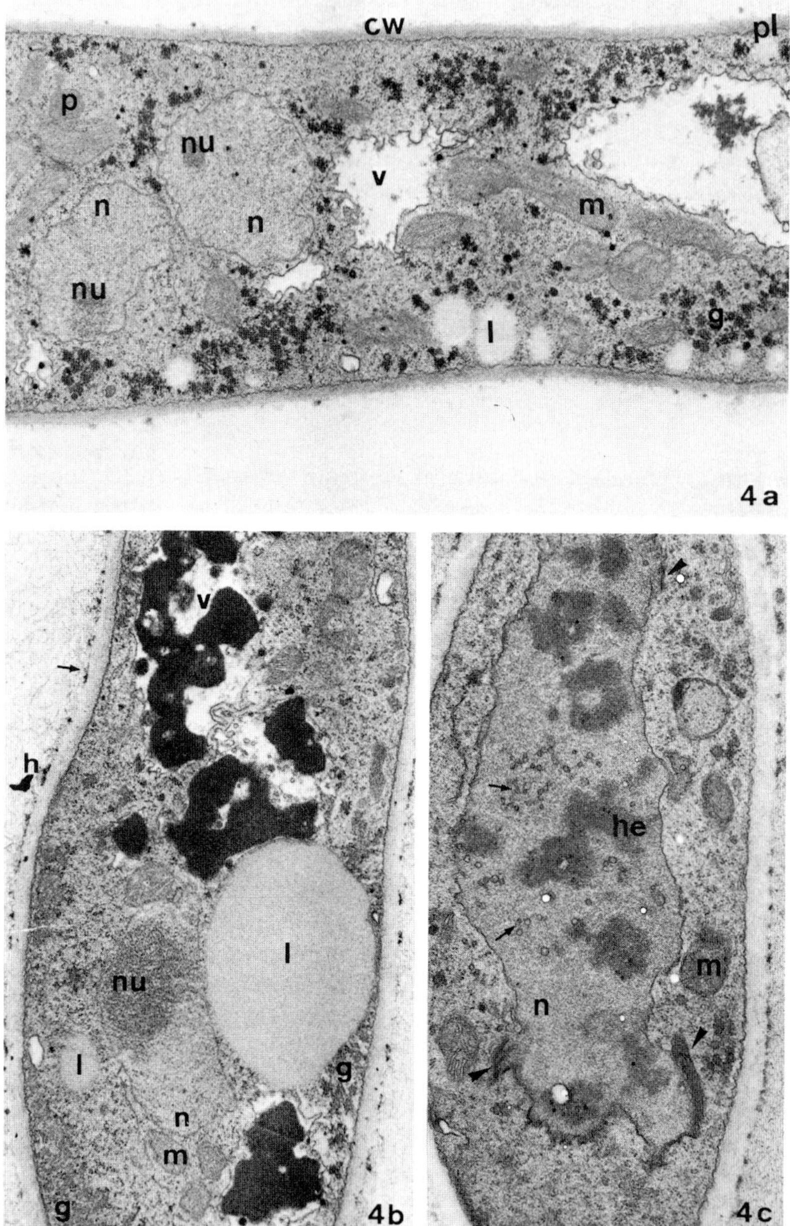

FIG. 1-4. Transmission electron micrograph of *A. fumigatus* after exposure to 5-fluorocytosine. (a) Control cell showing well-preserved subcellular organelles. Cell wall (cw); plasma membrane (pl); nucleus (n); nucleolus (nu); mitochondria (m); vacuole (v); lipid globules (l); glycogen (g); and peroxisome (p) (× 18,000; reduced by 9%). (b) After treatment with 100 μg/ml for 24 hours. Note the cell wall (*arrows*). The cell is

(74, 90, 91, 108), *Microsporum canis* (76), *Sporothrix schenckii* (87), *Cryptococcus neoformans* (21, 87), *Aspergillus fumigatus* (117), *A. nidulans* (15), *Malassezia furfur* (18), *Torulopsis glabrata* (7, 8), and *Saccharomyces cerevisiae* (126).

The organism that is studied in greatest detail is *C. albicans*. Descriptive fungal cytology has for many years struggled with the problem of adequate permeation of chemical fixatives through the cell wall and plasmalemma. This is especially true for *C. albicans* (50).

The slow permeation of chemical fixatives into the cytoplasm poses a serious problem in the morphologic identification of the organelles of *C. albicans*. The fact that no adequately preserved untreated control cells could be obtained made the interpretation of drug-induced morphologic alterations very difficult.

Potassium permanganate, the commonly used fixative for *C. albicans*, revealed fairly well the membranous components but failed to display ribosomes and the various nuclear and nucleolar substructures (84). Moreover, this fixative cannot be used for the preservation of cells for enzyme cytochemistry. Using a modification of the conventional preparation procedures (17), this problem has been largely solved in the sense that all subcellular organelles were made fairly visible and enzymes retained their activity after glutaraldehyde fixation. As far as the degree of preservation of subcellular organelles obtained with this procedure is concerned, the results are quite comparable to those for *Cr. neoformans* (3). With this yeast there is apparently no major problem of permeation of chemical fixatives, because all cytoplasmic organelles were nicely demonstrated without the aid of freeze-sectioning.

Enzyme cytochemistry through the display of specific marker enzymes for well-known subcellular organelles was revealed to be very useful in studying the nature and the possible functional significance of the substructures in *C. albicans*. Some of the cytoplasmic substructures of *C. albicans*, although clearly visible, remained difficult to interpret in terms of their nature and origin. The ovoid or round bodies limited by a single membrane could represent lysosomal structure as reported by Günther et al (53) in *S. cerevisiae*, and by Montes et al (84) in *C. albicans*, or peroxisome-like particles as found by Avers and Federman (5) in *S. cerevisiae*. Whether the short membrane fragments found in variable amounts from one cell to another are strands of smooth endoplasmic reticulum, or represent, in fact, flattened sacs of the

---

◁ surrounded by a halo (h) of detached cell wall material filling most of the intracellular space. Many lipid globules (l) are seen, surrounded by accumulated glycogen (g) (×17,000; reduced by 9%). (c) Same as (b) A drastic change in nuclear content is obvious. Abnormal distribution of heterochromatin (he), vacuolizations (*arrows*), blebbing and proliferation of the nuclear envelope (*arrowhead*) (×21,000; reduced by 9%). (Courtesy of Dr. S. De Nollin, Department of Medicine, University of Antwerp, Antwerp, Belgium.)

vacuolar apparatus remains unsettled. Moreover, the possible intermembranous connections between the plasmalemmal protrusions and the vacuolar membranes are difficult to elucidate by morphologic observation alone.

Azole derivatives such as miconazole, econazole, and clotrimazole have been studied in detail as to their effects on ultrastructure (38, 62, 102, 103). For miconazole, in addition, a detailed analysis has been done on enzyme composition of different subcellular compartments (23, 41, 42). Observations in *C. albicans* after clotrimazole treatment on vacuole enlargement, membrane proliferation, and plasmolysis were reported first by Iwata et al (62).

From ultrastructural observations made on *C. albicans* after exposure to low doses of miconazole, it appears that this drug exerts its primary effect on the plasmalemma and the cell wall, involving other cell constituents later or with higher doses. The excessive accumulation of membranous material along the plasmalemma and more particularly at sites of bud formation, as seen after low-dose treatment, has been given special attention. According to Matille et al (75), a budding process involves proliferation of smooth membranes and synthesis of degradative as well as synthetizing enzymes. The presence of the abnormal membranous components both in the plasmalemma and cell wall interspace as in the cell wall itself and this over the whole length of the wall could be interpreted as the morphologic expression of drug interaction with these proliferative processes. More recent work of Marichal et al (73) has shown that the changes that involve the whole contour of the cell coincide with the random production of chitin subsequent to a P450-dependent α-demethylase block and chitin synthase activation.

The abnormal membrane-bound structures consisted of highly osmiophilic vesicles (membranous bodies), which most probably represent altered membrane constituents that are sequestrated in the cell wall and in the central vacuole. At the same time a large increase in cell volume took place and abnormalities of cell division occurred (Fig. 1-5). The presence of randomly distributed bud scars together with abnormal deposition of phospholipidic vesicles is suggestive for uncontrolled attempts to divide. The latter is even more strongly supported by ad random the presence of chitin (73). Exposure to higher concentrations of azoles reportedly results in a series of alterations, varying from early cytoplasmic breakdown to complete cell death (Fig. 1-6). As Gale (50) pointed out, cytologic response toward drugs appears to be a function primarily of exposure time and individual variations within the cell population. Progressive sequestration of altered cytoplasmic parts and their subsequent extrusion into the central vacuole where this material can be digested by the present hydrolases (41, 42) are very likely part of the defense

---

FIG. 1-5. Transmission electron micrograph of *C. albicans* after exposure to 10^{-6} M ▷ itraconazole for 24 hours. Cross section shows enlarged vacuoles (v), filled with cytoplasmic debris. The thickened cell wall contains numerous membranous bodies (*arrows*) (× 15,150; reduced by 9%). Inset: scanning electron micrograph (SEM) showing the surface of cells, which remain attached to each other (× 4,050; reduced by 9%).

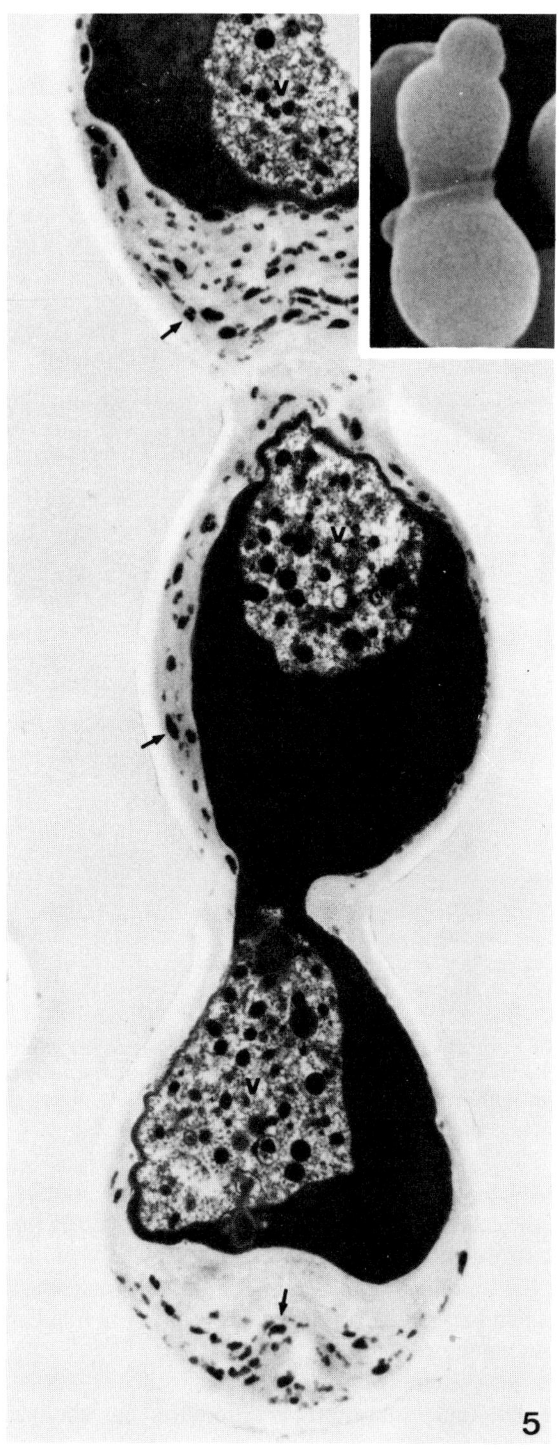
V
V
V
5

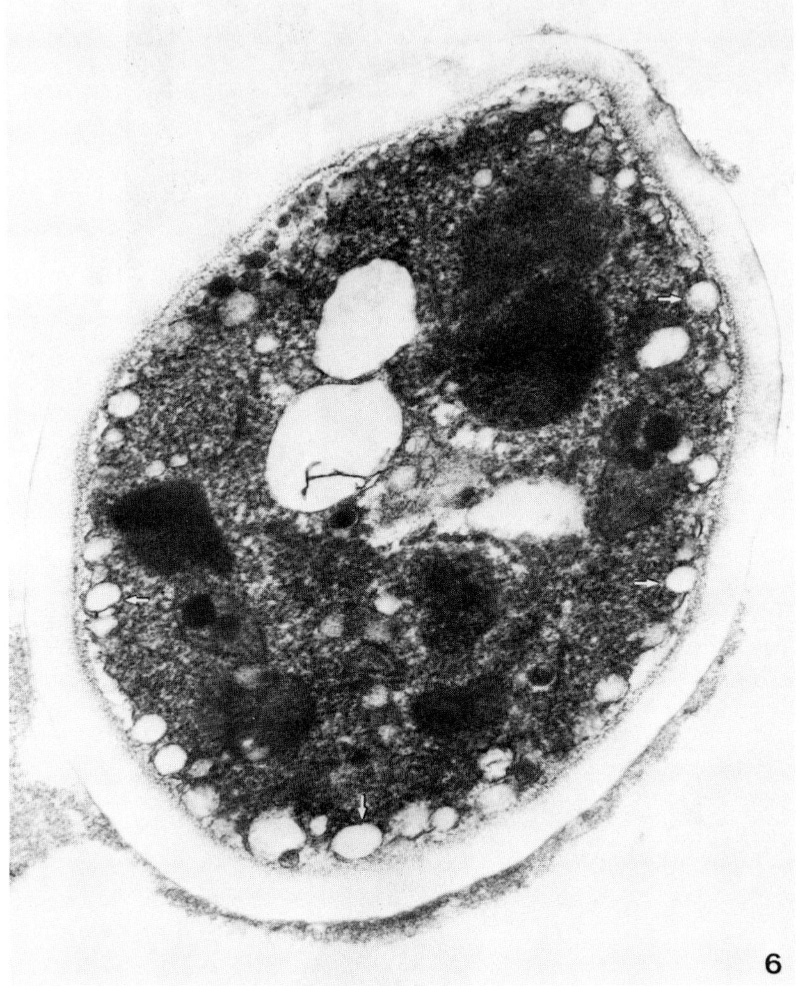

FIG. 1-6. Transmission electron micrograph of *C. albicans* after exposure to 10^{-4} M miconazole for 24 hours. Numerous lipid droplets (*arrows*) assemble at the periphery of the cytoplasm. Other organelles are barely recognizable. The cell wall remains structurally intact (× 30,250; reduced by 9%).

mechanism of the cell. The excessive accumulation inside the vacuole and the extrusion of cytoplasmic remnants through the plasmalemma are probably indicative for the inability of the cell to eliminate such an amout of lytic material. Cytochemistry of hydrolytic enzymes have provided interesting data in regard to these lytic processes (42).

Similar morphologic changes in *C. albicans* as those described earlier have been reported with only quantitative differences for econazole, a closely related chemical analogue of miconazole (100, 101, 102); clotrimazole, with the exception of effects seen in the high-dose range (40); ketoconazole (15, 16, 19, 24); terconazole (116); bifonazole (7, 8); fenticonazole (33); and itraconazole (21, 117).

During the evaluation of the antifungal profile of ketoconazole, it was noted that when *C. albicans* was cultured in its mycelial form (for some strains pseudomycelium) the effect of the drug on the structural changes was different. The medium used to promote the outgrowth of mycelium from inoculated yeast cells was Eagle's minimum essential medium (EMEM) supplemented with nonessential amino acids and 10% fetal calf serum. Long-lasting hyphal growth was obtained when cultures were grown in a humidified atmosphere of 5% CO_2 at 36°C (24, 36). The azole derivatives inhibited the transformation from yeast into mycelium in concentrations ranging between 0.005 and 0.5 μg/ml (Fig. 1-7). These low doses, however, permitted a limited outgrowth of clustered yeast cells. Higher concentrations of miconazole and ketoconazole (50 μg/ml) caused massive necrosis of the inoculated cells, again with fatty overload (15, 26). The complete inhibition of transformation with ketoconazole and itraconazole can be obtained at 10- to 100-fold lower concentrations than with miconazole, econazole, isoconazole, and clotrimazole (21, 26).

Experiments with mixed cultures of *C. albicans* and leukocytes revealed a synergistic action between host defense cells and imidazole antifungals (36). The EMEM used to culture *C. albicans* mycelial phase cells is a medium originally used for culturing mammalian cells and lends itself extremely well to mixed culture experiments, thereby mimicking to some degree a host-pathogen situation. In such a system, polymorphonuclear leukocytes and macrophages avidly engulf the yeast phase cells. However, they are unable to eradicate *C. albicans* completely. This is due to the decline in functional capacity of the host cells in culture on the one hand and to the morphogenetic transformation of ingested *C. albicans* cells to hyphae on the other. Surviving yeast cells germinate and grow out of the host cells developing into long branching hyphae, which are too large to be handled further by the leukocytes. Moreover, leukocytes degenerate through their interactions with mycelial cells. Addition of ketoconazole in concentrations as low as 0.1 μg/ml (a concentration that inhibits the outgrowth of hyphae from yeast phase cells and suppresses the growth of the remaining yeast cells) leads to complete elimination of the fungus. Recently a similar study has been reported using leukocytes and *A. fumigatus* in co-culture showing a clear cooperative action between the host cells and itraconazole (1).

Another type of investigation initiated to verify the mode by which fungi are inhibited in their growth at low doses and killed at high doses of azoles has been the application of cytochemistry of hydrolytic, oxidative, and peroxidative enzymes (23, 42). Yeast cells exposed to different doses of the antimycotic agent miconazole revealed important cytochemical changes in the topographic distribution of the phosphatases. Possible "dormant" phosphatases became active after low-dose treatment with miconazole (42). A

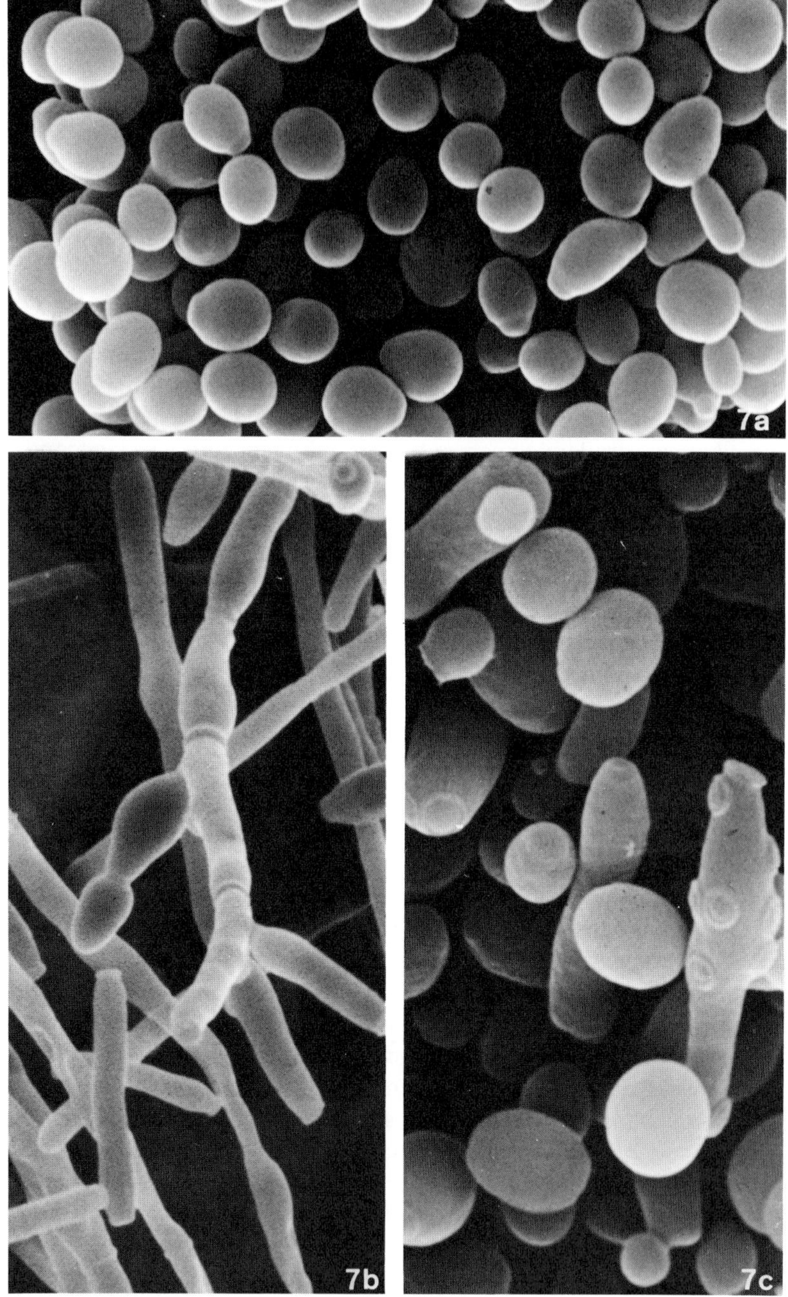

FIG. 1-7. Scanning electron micrograph of *C. albicans*. (a) Yeast inoculum (× 2,700; reduced by 9%). (b) Normally grown cells after 24 hours in a mycelium-promoting Eagle's medium (× 2,700; reduced by 9%). (c) Same as (b), but in the presence of 10^{-8} M ketoconazole. Note a complete inhibition of mycelium outgrowth. Swollen yeast cells and abnormally shaped short germ tubes are formed instead (× 3,300; reduced by 9%).

strong effect of miconazole also was observed on the behavior of oxidative and peroxidative enzymes. Decreased cytochrome c-oxidase and -peroxidase activity and increased catalase activity were seen after treatment with a fungistatic drug concentration, whereas a complete disappearance of these enzymes was observed after treatment with a minimal fungicidal dose of miconazole. This was in complete agreement with the quantitative biochemical assessments (42).

Furthermore, exposure of *C. albicans* cells to the antimycotic miconazole resulted in a strong increase in reduced nicotinamide adenine dinucleotide (NADH) oxidase activity. A hypothesis has been forwarded that this enzyme, together with peroxidative and catalytic enzymes, may be implicated in the mechanism by which miconazole exerts its lethal effect on *C. albicans*. The marked inhibition of cytochrome c-peroxidase activity after fungistatic doses of miconazole and the simultaneous increase of catalase activity (suggesting a rescue response) while NADH oxidase is stimulated, strongly points in the direction of peroxide accumulation. After exposure to the minimal fungicidal dose of miconazole, the activities of cytochrome c-peroxidase and catalase disappear completely. Under these conditions NADH oxidase is still very active, which indicates that peroxide production goes on. In this situation the intracellular peroxide concentration may reach levels that are incompatible with the viability of the cell (23, 42).

The ultrastructural and cytochemical results largely support the biochemical findings (118) which proposed the following three different molecular targets to explain the dose-related degenerative changes in *C. albicans* after azole treatment:

1. Drug concentrations greater than or equal to 0.1 nmol/l: interference with the microsomal lanosterol 14α-demethylase system (which is cytochrome P-450 dependent; see below), resulting in the accumulation of 14α-methyl sterols and decreased availability of ergosterol.
2. Drug concentrations greater than or equal to 10 nmol/l: interference with the fatty acid desaturase system, resulting in an enrichment in saturated fatty acids (mainly palmitic acid).
3. Drug concentrations greater than or equal to 10 μmol/l: direct interaction of some of these antifungal compounds (for instance, miconazole) with lipid constituents, resulting in a change in lipid organization in the membranes.

Whether one or more of these targets are directly or indirectly the cause of the observed enzymatic changes in *C. albicans* is presently not elucidated. With most other species such as *Co. immitis* (25), *T. mentagrophytes* (74), *T. rubrum* (18), *Cr. neoformans* (87), and *A. fumigatus* (117) the same subcellular changes have been found. With other species the characteristic alterations at the cell periphery and central vacuole are only present occasionally such as in *P. brasiliensis* (86) (Fig. 1-8) or not present at all such as in *M. furfur* (18) (Fig. 1-9). In the latter two species, a direct necrotizing effect has been obtained

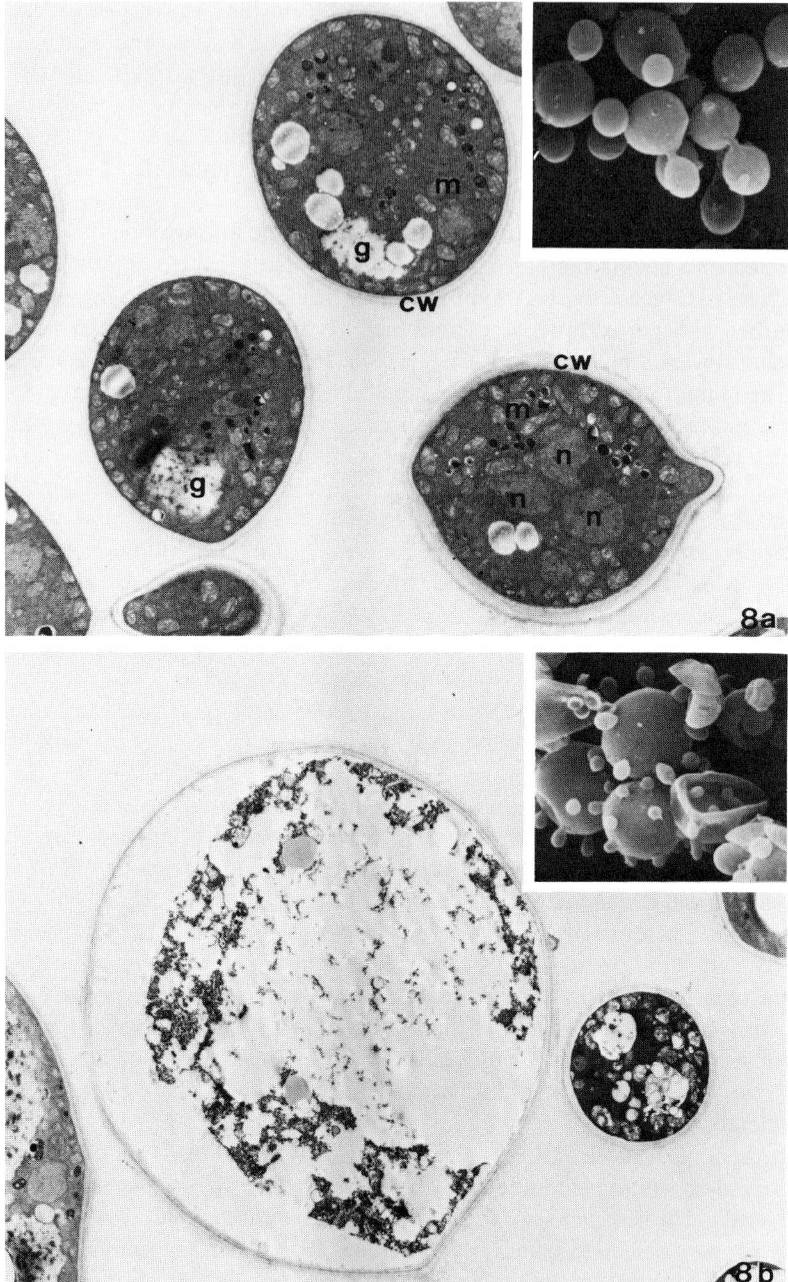

FIG. 1-8. Transmission and scanning electron micrographs of *P. brasiliensis.* (a) Large yeast cells in control culture showing multinuclei (n), relatively thin wall (cw), glycogen areas (g), and mitochondria (m) (× 6,050; reduced by 9%). Inset: SEM of surface structure (× 900; reduced by 9%). (b) After treatment with 10^{-7} M ketoconazole. Complete destruction of internal organelles is seen (× 5,500; reduced by 9%). Inset: SEM showing the collapsed state of some cells (× 900; reduced by 9%).

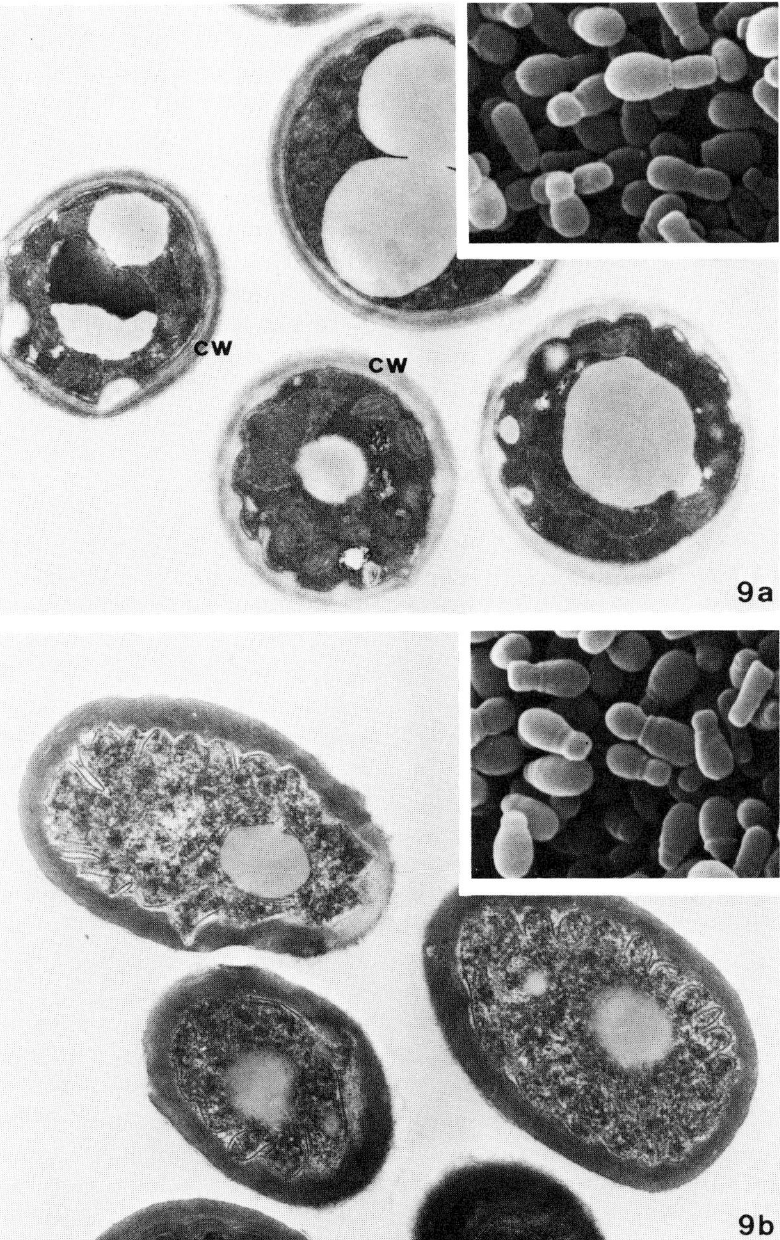

FIG. 1-9. Transmission and scanning electron micrographs of *M. furfur* in culture. (a) Control cells showing the compact cytoplasm surrounded by a densely stained, thick cell wall (cw) (× 24,800; reduced by 9%). Inset: SEM of the surface structure (× 2,700; reduced by 9%). (b) After exposure to 10^{-7} M itraconazole. Although the cytoplasm is fully necrotized, the cell wall appears unaltered (× 31,000; reduced by 9%). Inset: SEM demonstrating further the "mummifying" effect of the drug (× 2,700; reduced by 9%).

showing complete degeneration of internal organelles, however, without obviously altering the cell periphery. Such a "mummifying" effect of azoles may foster confusion about therapeutic outcome when therapy is verified by whole mount inspection of the fungus as usually done in pityriasis versicolor.

An interesting view on the deteriorative changes in *T. mentagrophytes* after miconazole treatment has been published by Masperi et al (74). As observed by many others, they located the initial changes in the growing hyphal elements and not in the parts distant from the apex. The latter parts were considered as being involved in restoring new growth after drug withdrawal. The authors thus concluded that fungicidal effects are attained only when the drugs' concentration is high enough to provoke lytic phenomena in both young and old cells. This view touches on the complex and in my opinion unraveled problem of what is meant by static and cidal effects after host treatment (see below).

Aspergillus fumigatus strains are not very sensitive to azole treatment, with the exception of itraconazole. Exposure to concentrations as low as 10^{-7} M exerts a complete necrotization of the hyphae, conidiophores, and phialides and, in addition, a partial killing of conidia (117). Fig. 1-10 demonstrates the changes after itraconazole exposure. Ketoconazole (21) at concentrations of 100–1000 times higher did not succeed in necrotization of the various elements of *A. fumigatus*.

Laser microprobe mass analysis of cytochemically localized calcium has been done after exposure of *A. fumigatus* to high doses of econazole (43) and ketoconazole (44). Using the combined oxalate pyroantimonate method (43), calcium was detected as an electron-dense precipitate. In the control cells, deposition of precipitate was found on the limiting membranes of the vacuoles. Treatment with azoles resulted in a substantial increase of the vacuolar Ca^{2+} precipitate as compared with the control cultures (Fig. 1-11). Parts of the plasmalemma, inclusions in the cell wall, glycogen, and, sometimes, the whole cytoplasm contained the precipitate. Mitochondria, showing vesiculization or even complete deterioration were heavily loaded with calcium deposits. Quantification of calcium with laser microprobe mass analysis matched completely the cytochemical findings. The authors proposed that elemental analysis and cytochemical localization, which demonstrated cellular calcium overload, may be an important factor in the antimycotic activity of these azoles.

Although the basic mechanism of action appears to be the same, considerable differences are sometimes noted in comparative studies between the various azole derivatives, for example, miconazole versus clotrimazole in the high-dose range in *C. albicans* cultures (40), miconazole versus ketoconazole in *T. mentagrophytes* (108), and itraconazole versus ketoconazole in *A. fumigatus* (117). These differences apply not only to the induction of the changes but also to the reversibility of the morphologic changes. Different pharmacokinetics may be at the basis of their variant behavior.

Freeze-fracture electron microscopy of the effects of econazole on *S. cerevisiae* (126) revealed that this drug caused profound structural alterations

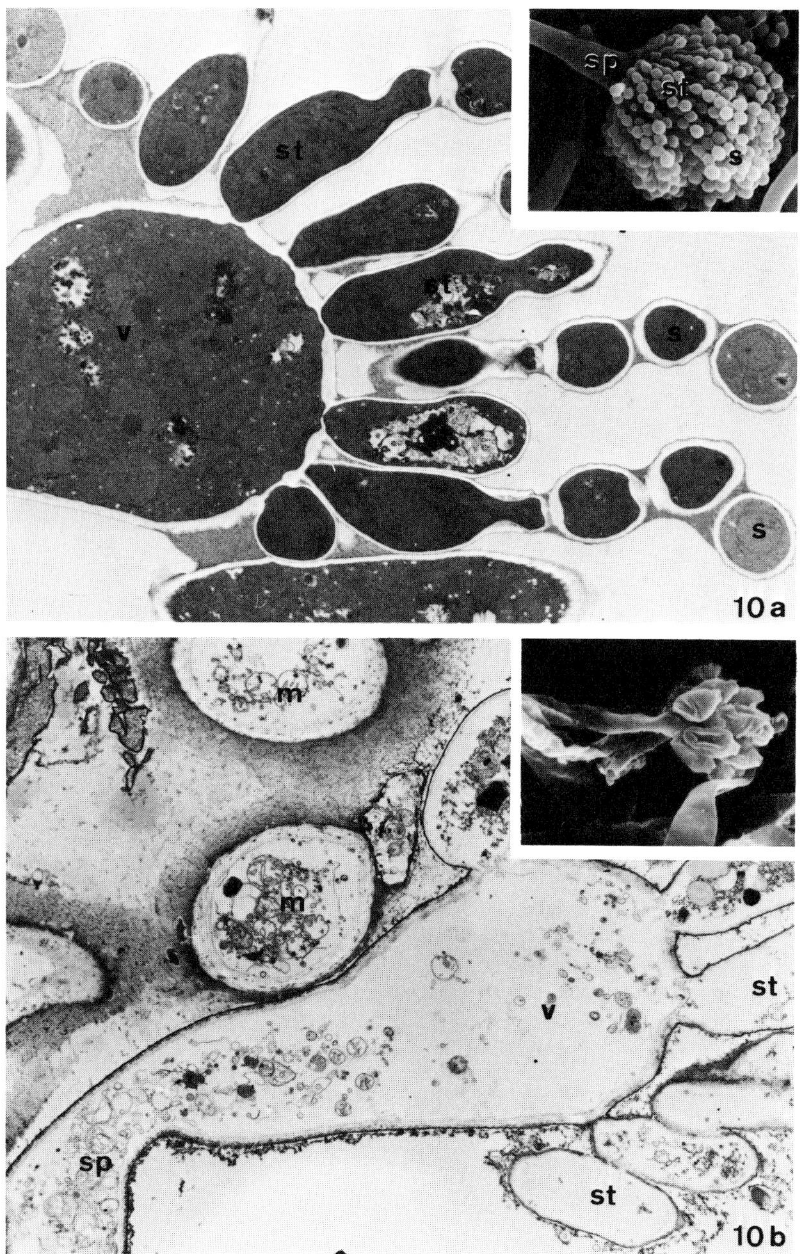

FIG. 1-10. Transmission and scanning electron micrographs of *A. fumigatus*. (a) Control culture 7 days after inoculation and growth at 25°C. Different subcellular organelles are shown. Vesicle (v), phialides (st), and conidia (s) (× 6,600; reduced by 9%). Inset: SEM picture of the surface of a conidiophore (sp), phialides (st), and conidia (s) (× 750; reduced by 9%). (b) After exposure for 7 days to 2.10^{-7} M itraconazole. The degenerative effects are seen in the conidiophore (sp), vesicle (v), phialides (st), and hyphae (m). A number of conidia (not present in this picture) remain structurally unaltered (× 7,500; reduced by 9%). Inset: collapsed structures as seen with SEM (× 750; reduced by 9%).

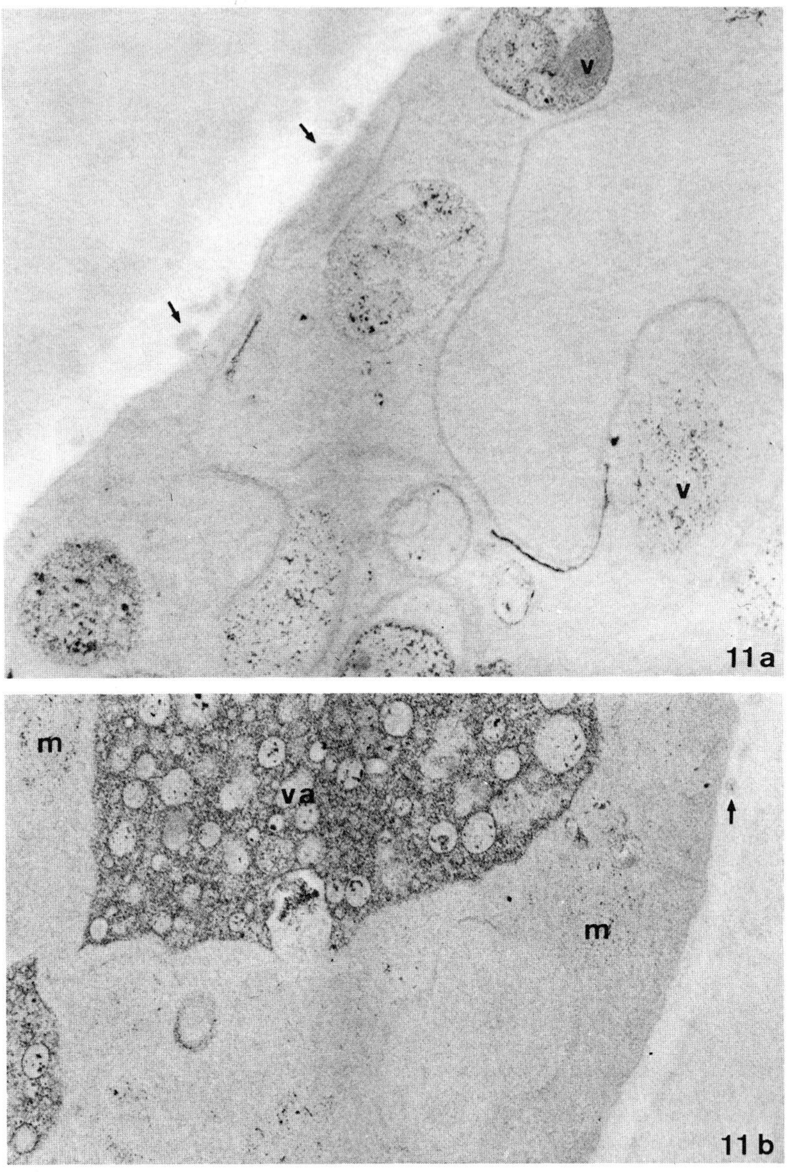

FIG. 1-11. Transmission electron microscopy. Ca^{2+} localization in *A. fumigatus* exposed to 50 μg/ml econazole for 24 hours. Several mitochondria (m), small vacuoles (v), as well as large vacuoles (va) present Ca^{2+} precipitates. The membranous bodies (*arrows*) in the cell wall are devoid of deposits (a: × 74,000; b: × 29,250; reduced by 9%). (Courtesy of Dr. S. De Nollin, Department of Medicine, University of Antwerp, Antwerp, Belgium).

in both fracture faces of the cell membrane which were characterized by a decrease in compactness of intramembranous particles, emergence of large smooth areas encircling particle islands, and formation of depressions over the entire surface. Cross-fractured specimens of the econazole-treated cells exhibited marked changes of contour and texture of the boundary membrane of cytoplasmic organelles such as mitochondria and nuclei. The results of these electron microscopic studies reportedly correspond to biochemical studies indicating that fungicidal concentrations of econazole severely damage fungal membranes through interaction with membrane phospholipids.

Exposure of *C. albicans* cells to bifonazole (7) resulted in similar alterations, for example, deformation and decrease in number of invaginations in the protoplasmic fracture face and corresponding ridges on the exoplasmic fracture face, and in separation of the plasma membrane from the cell wall, leaving a gap that frequently contained small vesicles. Moreover, parts of the inner half of the plasma membrane of *C. albicans* cells had been torn off and adhered to the exoplasmic fracture face. Cross-fracture specimens of bifonazole-treated cells of *C. albicans* showed swollen mitochondria and cytoplasmic lipid globules. These observations are in agreement with the changes oberved by conventional electron microscopy as described earlier.

The morphologic counterpart of in vivo azole treatment of patients and animals infected with *C. albicans*, *T. rubrum*, *T. mentagrophytes*, *T. verrucosum*, and *M. furfur* closely resembled that seen after in vitro exposure to these drugs (Fig. 1-12) (19, 20, 37, 84, 111, 115). Fortunately, azoles provoke unique alterations at the cell periphery that never occur in "spontaneously" degenerating cells. If it were not for this characteristic peculiarity it would be almost impossible to judge the outcome of antifungal treatment on an individual basis with morphologic criteria. But even with this fortunate coincidence only semiquantitative data on response to treatment can be generated from in vivo studies, and this mainly due to limited sample size of the infected area under investigation and the phenomenon of changes occurring "spontaneously" or to undetermined host factors.

Ultrastructural studies on the interference of drugs with host-fungus interrelationships are of great importance to complement the knowledge on the mechanism of drug action or to explain some of the apparent discrepancies between in vitro sensitivity of a given fungal organism for a drug and its in vivo potency to eradicate fungal disease.

In vaginal candidiasis it has been observed that symptomatology goes along with the presence of *C. albicans*, predominantly in its hyphal form, and that invasiveness critically depends on the yeast-hyphae transformation (20, 111). However, in the deeper layers of the flattened keratinocytes, a mixture of hyphae and yeast cells is usually present. Yeast form cells are regularly seen within the keratinocytes. These were found to be less responsive to treatment than the more superficially located hyphae. It may be speculated that such cells are metabolically inactive or less active ("dormant cells"), hence less

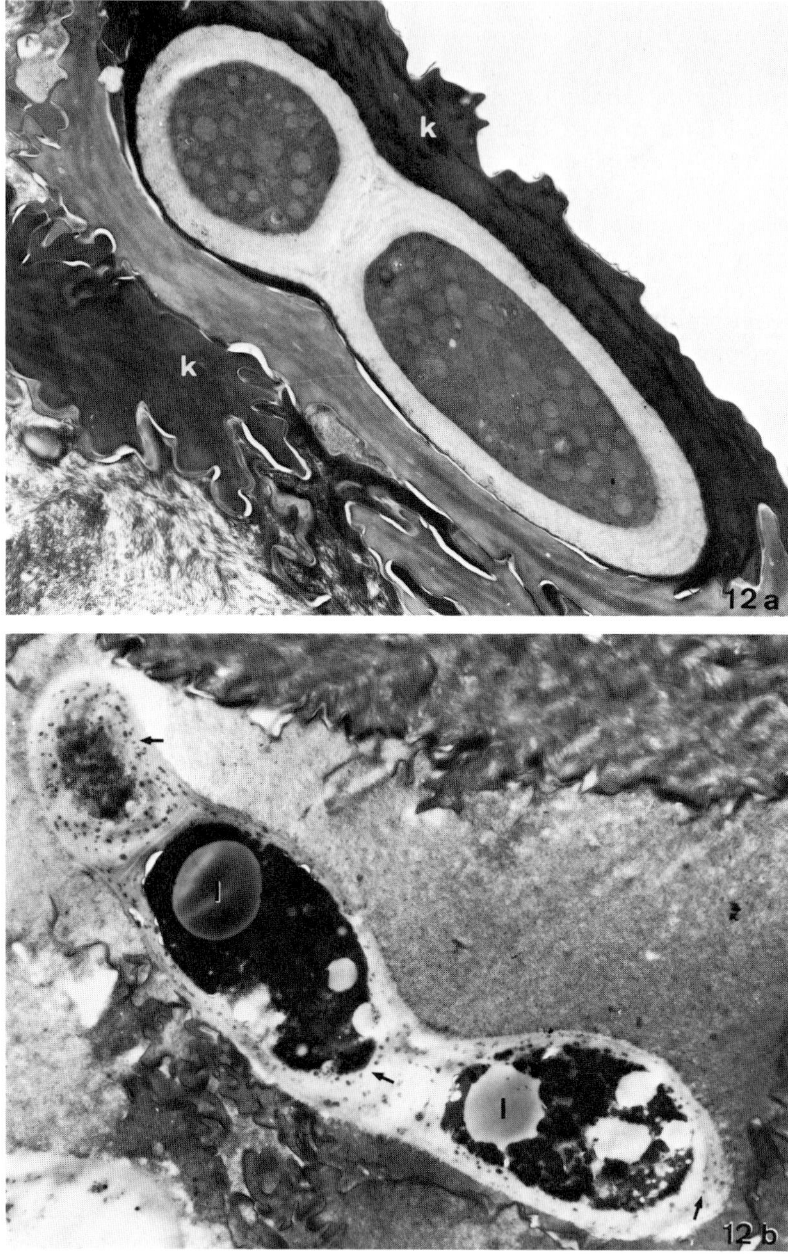

FIG. 1-12. Transmission electron micrograph of *T. rubrum* in stratum corneum of an infected patient. (a) Before treatment. Two thick-walled hyphal parts are surrounded by densely stained keratinocytes (k) (× 10,700; reduced by 9%). (b) After 9 days of treatment with 200 mg o.d. ketoconazole. Destructive changes typical for azole treatment, such as the formation of membranous bodies (*arrows*) in the cell wall and lipidification (l) of the cytoplasm, are seen (× 9,300; reduced by 9%).

influenced by treatment that causes inhibition of some vital biosynthetic pathways. Another possibility is that the antifungals do not easily penetrate the keratinous cells, making it difficult for effective concentrations to reach the yeast. Moreover, inactivation to some extent of the drug by binding to host cell proteins and in lipids cannot be ruled out to explain the lower sensitivity of the intracellularly located yeast organisms. These observations may be closely linked to the occurrence of relapse. When keratinocytes, which harbor dormant yeast cells, reach the more superficial layers after the normal differentiation process, the dormant yeast cells may be activated, sprout germ tubes, and develop into branching hyphae giving rise to the usual clinical symptoms. If at the time of "awakening" an azole derivative is present in amounts sufficient to inhibit the morphogenetic transformation into mycelium, the keratinocytes with the noninvasive yeast cell desquamates, hence preventing relapse. If not, yeast cell transformation into mycelium takes place and relapse evolves. This idea is in agreement with the fact that too short treatment regimens generally result in a higher relapse rate. Complete eradication of infections caused by *C. albicans* can be achieved by treatment with concentrations that are merely growth and morphogenetic transformation inhibitory. So direct fungicidal concentrations are not a prerequisite to obtain a complete cure.

Another fungal species that has been located frequently inside skin corneocytes is *M. furfur*. A remarkable change takes place during invasion of *M. furfur* (mostly hyphae) of the uppermost cell layer of the skin. Before as well as after therapy, variously sized spherical structures are observed on the surface of the keratinocytes (Fig. 1-13). Transmission electron microscopic examinations revealed *M. furfur*, predominantly in its mycelial phase, inside keratinocytes. Other structures, as observed by scanning electron microscopy, appeared to be amorphous lipid-like droplets, originating from bursted keratinocytes. The cytoplasm of the keratinocytes was, at least partly, occupied by the same amorphous material. It is therefore suggested that *M. furfur* penetrates the keratinocytes where degradation of the normal keratinous content to amorphous material takes place. This newly formed lipidic substrate may be an essential nutritive factor (Borgers et al, unpublished). It is speculated that the presence of large quantities of this lipid-like material might be the possible cause for hypopigmentation because it may constitute an ultraviolet light block. Whereas itraconazole completely eradicated the fungus after a 1-week treatment, the lipidification of the stratum corneum persisted for at least another 3 weeks.

Allylamines

Naftifine and its recently developed derivative lamisil (SF 86-327) belong to a new class of synthetic antifungals, the allylamines. The antifungal activity of

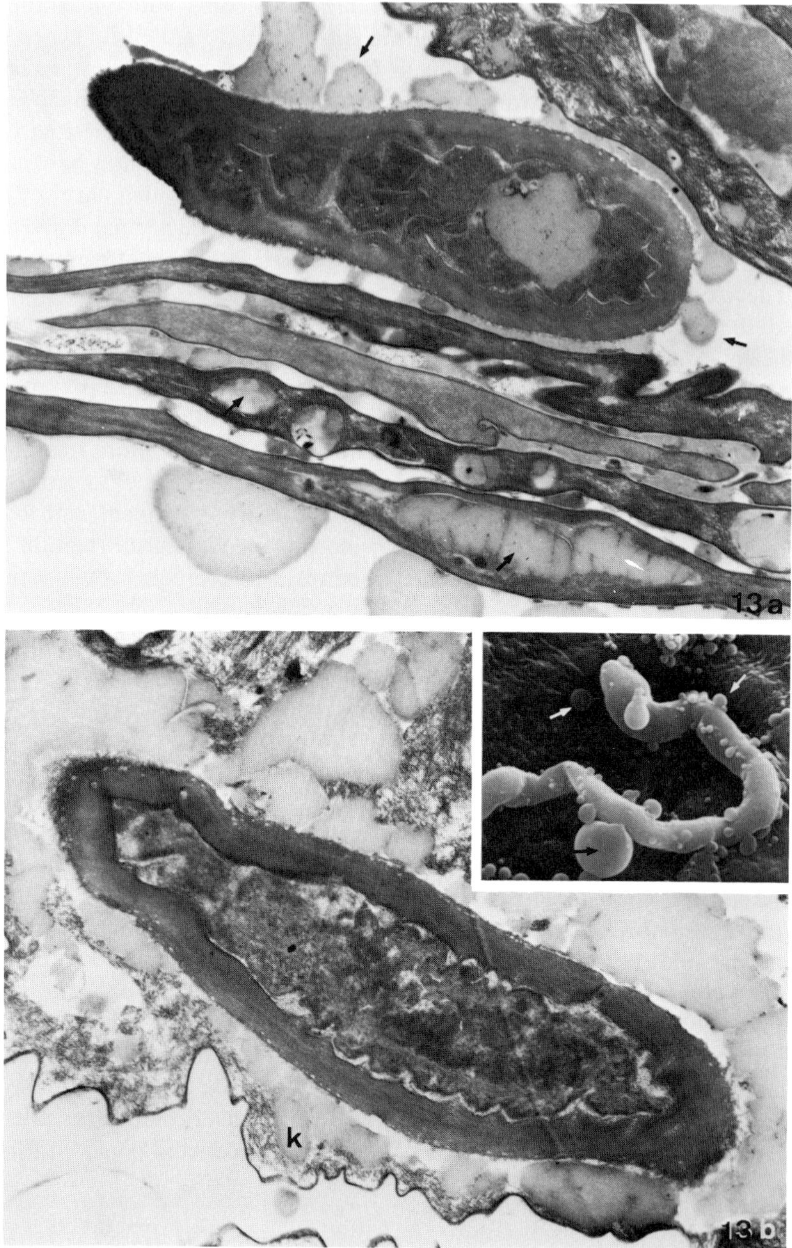

FIG. 1-13. Transmission and scanning electron micrographs of pityriasis versicolor in patients. (a) Untreated. An intact hyphal element of *M. furfur* embedded in a lipid-laden stratum corneum. Lipidic structures are also present between the keratinocytes (*arrows*) (× 18,150; reduced by 9%). (b) After treatment for 7 days with 100 mg o.d. itraconazole. A necrotic hyphal element is seen within a lipidified keratinocyte (k) (× 12,600; reduced by 9%). Inset: SEM showing the lipid-like globules (*arrows*) on the surface of keratinocytes and the *M. furfur* (× 1,500; reduced by 9%).

these drugs is based on the inhibition of ergosterol biosynthesis and concomitant accumulation of squalene (78, 80). In contrast to azole derivatives, which inhibit sterol biosynthesis at the lanosterol 14α-demethylation step, these compounds inhibit the enzyme squalene epoxidase. The main difference, therefore, is that in the latter no 14α-methylsterols accumulate.

The effects of naftifine and lamisil on the fine structure of *C. albicans* and *T. mentagrophytes* has been studied by transmission electron microscopy of thin sections as well as cross-fracture preparations (Fig. 1-14 and 1-15) and scanning electron microscopy (78, 79, 80, 81). The allylamine-induced changes are, at least some of them, similar to those observed after azole treatment.

In *T. mentagrophytes* the most striking changes observed after treatment were bulb-shaped thickenings at the hyphal tips and dose-dependent, spherical or drop-shaped depositions of varying size within the cells. The abnormal formations were not only visible in the cytoplasm (discrete or aggregated in vacuoles), but also in the region of the cell membrane, in all layers of the cell wall, and on the cell surface. Their lipid nature can be deduced from several significant characteristics including osmiophily, the conchoidal fracture surface observed in freeze-fracture replicas, and their extractability with acetone (79).

In cultures treated for 39 hours with 5 mg/l, cultures contained only autolysed germinated microconidia. The cell wall was thickened, and round osmiophilic particles were observed in all layers and at the surface of the cell wall. Similar particles were present between the cell wall and the cell membrane, which was deeply folded and fragmented. No organelles were perceptible in the interior. Round osmiophilic particles and remnants of membranous structures were only seen (Fig. 1-14). Freeze-etch preparations revealed cells filled with irregularly shaped lipid bodies (Fig. 1-14).

Freeze-fracture preparations of *C. albicans* exposed to lamisil (81) and *C. parapsilosis* exposed to naftifine (78) revealed accumulation of lipid particles in the cytoplasm, thickening of the cell wall, and alterations of the plasma membrane by the occurrence of vesicular structures (Fig. 1-15). Vesicular inclusions also have been observed in the cell wall.

In addition, nuclei were irregularly shaped, sometimes lobed with irregularly distributed nuclear pores as described previously. Globular lipid inclusions within those cells also were noted. The majority of cells treated with 5.0 mg/l lamisil exhibited radical changes in the cell membrane. Irregular invaginations and the formation of bulges caused loss of the normal membrane structure. The rod-like invaginations disappeared. Many flat vesicles were present between the cell membrane and the thickened cell wall, which contained only few globular structures. The autolyzed cells contained numerous oviform or globular lipid particles. These destructive changes of the cell architecture are presumed to result from interaction of the allylamine derivatives with fungal sterol biosynthesis.

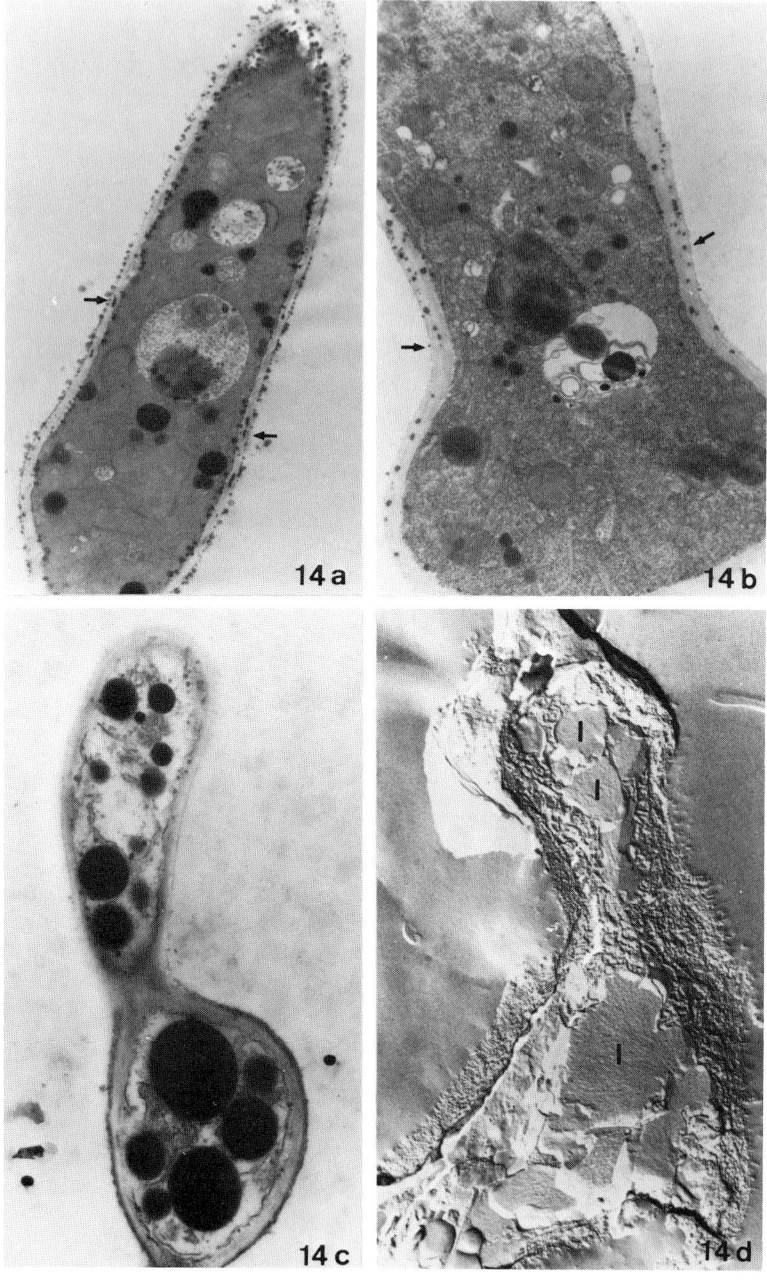

FIG. 1-14. *T. mentagrophytes* after exposure to allylamines. (a) Transmission electron micrograph (TEM) showing hyphal part exposed to 0.5 μg/ml naftifine for 24 hours. Membranous bodies (*arrows*) are present in the cell wall (× 10,000; reduced by 9%). (b) TEM showing a hypha exposed to 0.01 μg/ml lamisil for 24 hours. Similar changes as in (a) are seen (× 16,000; reduced by 9%). (c) TEM of germinated microconidium exposed to 0.003 μg/ml lamisil for 39 hours. Necrosis of the cell interior is obvious (× 15,000;

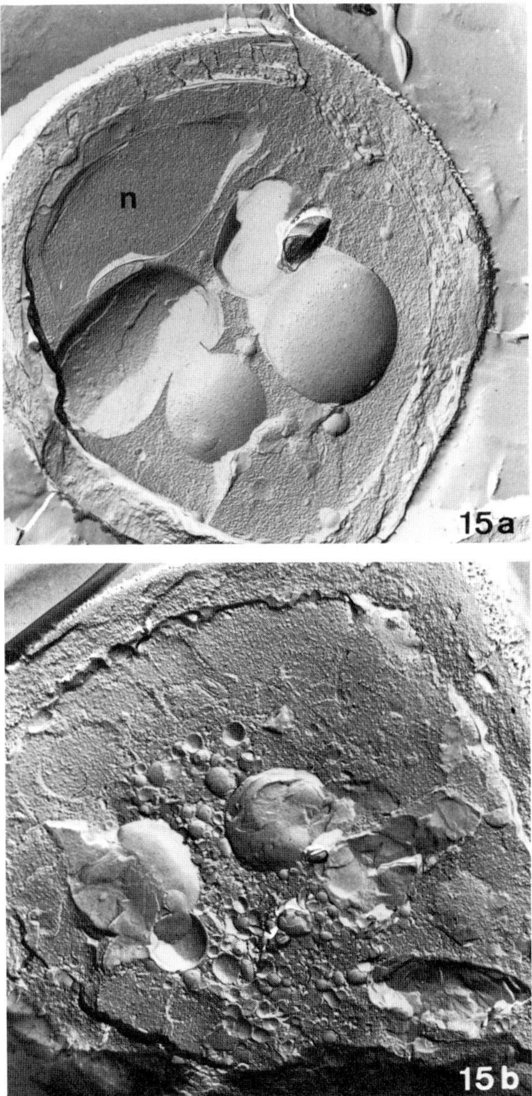

FIG. 1-15. Freeze-etch preparation of *C. albicans* after exposure to lamisil. (a) Yeast cells exposed to 0.5 μg/ml lamisil for 24 hours showing irregularly shaped nuclei (n) with irregularly distributed pores (× 12,000; reduced by 9%). (b) Yeast cell exposed to 10 μg/ml lamisil for 24 hours showing a partially autolysed cell (× 20,800; reduced by 9%). (Courtesy of Dr. J. Meingassner, Sandoz Forschungsinstitut, Vienna, Austria.)

◁ reduced by 9%). (d) Freeze-etch preparation of germinated microconidium exposed to 0.03 μg/ml lamisil for 39 hours. The cell is filled with irregularly shaped lipid bodies (l) (× 15,000; reduced by 9%). (Courtesy of Dr. J. Meingassner, Sandoz Forschungsinstitut, Vienna, Austria.)

Miscellaneous

Echinocandin is a new antimicrobic produced by strains of *A. nidulans* described to have potent antiyeast activity. A study by Cassone et al (30) showed that echinocandin provoked the lysis of exponentially growing cells, whereas stationary phase cells were not affected. A cytologic study of the effects of echinocandin at lytic doses on osmotically protected yeast cells revealed a substantial thinning of the cell wall at the budding site and derangement of its constitutive layers within 5–10 minutes, showing that the balance of wall growth was quickly and critically affected by the drug. Associated with this effect, a number of membranous bodies of myelin-like appearance were often seen in close proximity to the plasma membrane of the emerging bud. From 15 minutes after treatment onward, convoluted bodies were detected in the nuclear and other intracytoplasmic membranes. Subsequent events eventually resulted in complete lysis of the cell cytoplasmic structure, at least in part of the cell population. These results suggest that echinocandin may block a biosynthetic step during wall construction, or that it could alter wall metabolism as a result of a primary interaction with membranes.

Much less dramatic changes have been reported in *C. albicans* cultures treated with aculeacin A and papulacandin B, two closely related antimycotics which reportedly interfere with the synthesis of alkali-insoluble cell wall constituent β-1, 3-glucan (27). The periphery of the treated cells was highly distorted and wrinkled, and cells often collapsed. Defective separation of dividing cells was frequently observed. Approximately 20% of the cells demonstrated complete cell necrosis accompanied by cytoplasmic deterioration, layered and distorted walls, and improperly formed buds and scars.

The morphologic counterpart of the antifungal effects a pyrazolyl-alkyl sulfide derivative that has been demonstrated in *C. albicans*, *M. cookei*, and *T. mentagrophytes* (121). In the yeast, mitochondria were the only cell targets affected, whereas in the dermatophytes cell wall, plasmalemma and the main cytoplasmic organelles were damaged to various degrees. As the most remarkable alterations were connected with membrane abnormalities, the cytologic changes observed were tentatively interpreted as a consequence of the compounds' intrusion into the lipid bilayer of the membranes, because the drug is lipophilic in nature.

The changes related to the plasma membrane were particularly remarkable. The occurrence of membranous bodies were interpreted as the counterpart of an oversynthesis of membrane components, probably because the hyphal cells, under the influence of the drug, became stimulated to repair the membrane damage. Presumably, due to the absence of the hyphal polar growth, the newly formed membranous materials can not be transported and inserted regularly, and therefore formed random aggregates. The vesicles near the plasmalemma may be interpreted as a means to exclude more or less large portions of damaged membrane and/or as an attempt to segregate the toxicant that reached the cell membrane. Because endocytosis is an exceptional event in wall-bound cells, an alternative interpretation may suggest that vesiculation is of secretory nature, and is probably related to membrane-repairing mechanisms. As the membranous bodies in the cell wall strongly resemble those seen after azole and allylamine treatment, a tempting hypothesis is that ergosterol synthesis is inhibited also by this type of drug.

Povidone-iodine preparations are reported to be efficacious in pityriasis versicolor and ringworm infection. A scanning electron microscopic study revealed swelling of fungal elements; however, a direct relation between the observed changes and mode of action of the treatment has not been shown (72).

The effects of 4, bis-(m,m′-amidinophenoxy methyl)-cyclohexane dilactate (MAC), a diamidine compound, against *C. albicans* have been studied by freeze-fracture electron microscopy (65). MAC caused aggregation of membrane particles and patch formation on the P face, which suggest that the drug causes membrane disruption. The cell wall was not affected, nor did any cell lysis occur. Kanazawa (65) suggested that MAC, by interacting with membrane phospholipids altered by permeability of the membrane, hence induced leakage of intracellular components. Although binding to another membrane constituent as the polyene antibiotics do, the effect on permeability might be similar. Interestingly, Ca^{2+} and Mg^{2+} counteracted the effects of this drug. Such an effect of divalent cations has been reported for other antifungal agents as well. It has been suggested that cations protect the membrane from attack by membrane-disrupting agents (65).

Conclusion

The knowledge acquired during the past two decades on the ultrastructural correlates of antifungal action has contributed in a considerable way to the understanding of the mode of action of the principal antimycotic drugs. The main classes of antifungals comprising the polyene antimicrobics amphotericin B and nystatin, griseofulvin, 5-fluorocytosine, the azole derivatives, and the allylamines vary greatly from each other as far as their spectrum of activity, potency, and safety margin is concerned. These properties are largely determined by their particular mode of action and pharmacokinetics. Depending on the nature and the function of the attained target a drug exerts fungicidal effects, morphologically expressed by subcellular necrosis and plasmalemmal breakdown or will be merely fungistatic and acts preferentially or uniquely against certain species. The morphologic counterpart of a fungistatic effect is complex and varies from slight mitochondrial swelling, vacuolar extention, plasmalemmal proliferation, cell wall thickening, and deposition of abnormal membranous bodies in the cell wall to a huge increase in cell volume with formation of numerous peroxisomes, lipid globules, and lysosome-like bodies. The cooperative action between drug and host defense cells which have been recently reported for some antifungals is of considerable interest, especially in the treatment of deep mycoses.

Antimycotic drugs interfere with the normal life cycle of fungi by inhibiting normal functioning of one or several vital cellular entities. The effects of these agents are reflected in altered patterns of growth, differentiation, transformation, ultrastructure, and viability of the fungus. Subcellular entities that may be injured reversibly or irreversibly are the cell wall, plasma membrane, nucleus, mitochondria, microtubules, ribosomes, intracellular membranes, and peroxisomes. Damage to any of these organelles may affect cellular function in general.

The molecular target sites and subcellular target organelles for antimycotic action have been established for most antifungal drugs. Polyenes bind irreversibly to cell membranes. Alteration of the permeability of these structures precedes metabolic disruption and cell death. Griseofulvin deteriorates spindle and cytoplasmic microtubules, influencing cell division and outgrowth of hyphal tips. 5-Fluorocytosine, once deaminated and phosphorylated, incorporates in RNA which impairs protein synthesis. Another metabolite of 5-FC inhibits DNA synthesis. Azole derivatives through their interaction with cytochrome P450-dependent 14α-demethylase inhibit the biosynthesis of ergosterol, and hence methylated sterols accumulate. Moreover, azoles affect the synthesis of triglycerides and phospholipids. Changes in oxidative and peroxidative enzyme activities, as shown after exposure to miconazole, lead to an intracellular buildup of toxic concentrations of hydrogen peroxide and may contribute to the observed deterioration of subcellular organelles and to cell necrosis. Allylamines affect sterol synthesis in a manner similar to the azoles, although through interference with another enzymatic event. Morphologically, the early changes to be observed at the cell periphery and the central vacuolar system are very similar. The ability to induce cell necrosis after short exposure periods is, however, dissimilar between these antifungal compounds.

Acknowledgments

I would like to thank Dr. Paul Janssen for his continuous support and guidance during the many years of research devoted to fungal structure and function. My sincere thanks go also to my co-workers M. Van de Ven, F. Thoné, L. Leijssen, and K. Donné.

References

1. Aerts F, Van Cutsem J, De Brabander M: The activity of ketoconazole and itraconazole against *Aspergillus fumigatus* in mixed cultures with macrophages or leukocytes. *Mykosen* 29:165–176, 1986.

2. Agar HD, Douglas HD: Studies on the cytological structure of yeast: Electron microscopy of thin section. *J Bacteriol* 73:365–375, 1957.
3. Al-Doory Y: The ultrastructure of *Cryptococcus neoformans*. *Sabouraudia* 9:113–120, 1971.
4. Arai T, Mikami Y, Yokoyama K, Kawata T, Masuda K: Morphological changes in yeasts as a result of the action of 5-fluorocytosine. *Antimicrob Agents Chemother* 12:255–260, 1977.
5. Avers CJ, Federman M: The occurrence in yeast of cytoplasmic granules which resemble microbodies. *J Cell Biol* 37:555–560, 1968.
6. Bakerspigel A: Some observations on the cytology of *Candida albicans*. *J. Bacteriol* 87:228–237, 1964.
7. Barug D, de Groot C: Microscopic studies of *Candida albicans* and *Torulopsis glabrata* after in vitro treatment with bifonazole. *Arzneim Forsch Drug Res* 33:538–545, 1983.
8. Barug D, Samson RA, Kerkenaar A: Microscopic studies of *Candida albicans* and *Torulopsis glabrata* after in vitro treatment with bifonazole. *Arzneim Forsch Drug Res* 33:528–537, 1983.
9. Bastide M. Jouvert S, Bastide JM: Action des antifongiques sur la paroi et la membrane cytoplasmique de *Candida albicans* revelée par microscopie électronique a balayage. I. Amphotericine B et nystatine. *Bull Soc Mycol Med* 10:113–118, 1981.
10. Bastide M, Jouvert S, Bastide JM: A comparison of the effects of several antifungal imidazole derivatives and polyenes on *Candida albicans*: An ultrastructural study by scanning electron microscopy. *Can J Microbiol* 28:1119–1126, 1982.
11. Bastide M, Jouvert S, Bastide JM: Etude cytologique de l'action des imidazoles sur *Candida albicans*. *Pathol Biol* 30:458–462, 1982.
12. Beckett A, Heath IB, McLaughlin DJ: *An Atlas of Fungal Ultrastructure*. London, Longman, 1972, pp 1–221.
13. Bent KJ, Moore RH: The mode of action of griseofulvin, in *Biochemical Studies of Antimicrobial Drugs*. 16th Symposium of Society of General Microbiology. London, Cambridge University Press, 1966, pp 82–110.
14. Blank H, Taplin D, Roth FJ: Electron microscopic observations of the effects of griseofulvin on dermatophytes. *Arch Dermatol* 81:667–680, 1960.
15. Borgers M: Mechanism of action of antifungal drugs, with special reference to the imidazole derivatives. *Rev Infect Dis* 2:520–534, 1980.
16. Borgers M: *Antifungal Azole Derivatives*. Symposium of the Society for General Microbiology. Scientific Basis of Antimicrobial Chemotherapy, Greenwood D. O'Grady F (eds). London, Cambridge University Press, 1985, pp 133–153.
17. Borgers M, De Nollin S: The preservation of subcellular organelles of *Candida albicans* with conventional fixatives. *J Cell Biol* 62:574–581, 1974.
18. Borgers M, Van Cutsem J: Ketoconazole induced morphological changes in yeasts and dermatophytes, in Meinhof W (ed): *Oral Therapy in Dermatomycoses: A Step Forward*. The Medicine Publishing Foundation, 1985, pp 51–60.
19. Borgers M, Vanden Bossche H: The mode of action of antifungal drugs, in Levine HB (ed): *Ketoconazole in the Management of Fungal Disease*. New York, Adis Press, 1982, pp 25–27.
20. Borgers M, Van de Ven M: Sensitivity testing and morphological changes in *Candida albicans* after ketoconazole treatment. *The Cervix* 2:149–158, 1984.
21. Borgers M, Van de Ven MA: Degenerative changes in fungi after itraconazole treatment. *Rev Infect Dis*, 9 (suppl. 1):S33–S42, 1987.
22. Borgers M, De Nollin S, Verheyen A, De Brabander M, Thienpont D: Effects of new anthelmintics on the microtubular system of parasites, in Borgers M and De

Brabander M (eds): *Microtubules and Microtubule Inhibitors*. Amsterdam, North Holland, 1975, pp 497–508.
23. Borgers M, De Nollin S, Thoné F, Van Belle H: Cytochemical localization of NADH oxidase in *Candida albicans*. *J Histochem Cytochem* 25:193–199, 1977.
24. Borgers M, Vanden Bossche H, De Brabander M, Van Cutsem J: Promotion of pseudomycelium formation of *Candida albicans* in culture: A morphological study of the effects of miconazole and ketoconazole. *Postgrad Med J* 55: 687–691, 1979.
25. Borgers M, Levine HB, Cobb JM: Ultrastructure of *Coccidioides immitis* after exposure to the imidazole antifungals miconazole and ketoconazole. *Sabouraudia* 19:27–38, 1981.
26. Borgers M, Vanden Bossche H, De Brabander M: The mechanism of action of the new antimycotic ketoconazole. *Am J Med* 74:2–7, 1983.
27. Bozzola JJ, Mehta RJ, Nisbet LJ, Valenta JR: The effect of aculeacin A and papulacandin B on morphology and cell wall ultrastructure in *Candida albicans*. *Can J Microbiol* 30:857–863, 1984.
28. Breslau A, Hensley T, Erickson J: Electron microscopy of cultured spherules of *Coccidioides immitis*. *J Biophys Biochem Cytol* 9:627–637, 1961.
29. Cassone A, Kerridge D, Gale EF: Ultrastructural changes in the cell wall of *Candida albicans* following cessation of growth and their possible relationship to the development of polyene resistance. *J Gen Microbiol* 110:339–349, 1979.
30. Cassone A, Mason RE, Kerridge D: Lysis of growing yeast-form cells of *Candida albicans* and by echinocandin: A cytological study. *Sabouraudia* 19:97–110, 1981.
31. Catterall MD, Ward ME, Jacobs P: A reappraisal of the role of *Pityrosporum orbiculare* in pityriasis versicolor and the significance of extracellular lipase. *J Invest Dermatol* 71:398–401, 1978.
32. Costa AL: In vitro antimycotic activity of fenticonazole. *Mykosen* 25:47–52, 1981.
33. Costa AL, Valenti A, Veronese M: Study of the morphofunctional alterations produced by fenticonazole on strains of *Candida albicans*, using the scanning electron microscope (S.E.M.). *Mykosen* 27:29–35, 1983.
34. Danilenko II, Stepanyuk VV: Ultrastructure, composition of neutral lipids and their fatty acids of *Candida tropicalis* strain D-2 mutants resistant to the polyene antibiotic nystatin. *BBA* 691:201–210, 1982.
35. D'Arcy PF, Scott EM: Antifungal agents, in E Jucker (ed): *Progress in Drug Research*. Basel, Birkhäuser Verlag, 1978, pp 93–147.
36. De Brabander M, Aerts F, Van Cutsem J, Vanden Bossche H, Borgers M: The activity of ketoconazole in mixed cultures of leukocytes and *Candida albicans*. *Sabouraudia* 18:197–210, 1980.
37. Degreef H, Van De Kerckhove M, Gevers D, Van Cutsem J, Vanden Bossche H, Borgers M: Ketoconazole (R 41 400) in the treatment of dermatophyte infections. *Int J Dermatol* 20:662–669, 1981.
38. De Nollin S, Borgers M: The ultrastructure of *Candida albicans* after in vitro treatment with miconazole. *Sabouraudia* 12:341–351, 1974.
39. De Nollin S, Borgers M: Scanning electron microscopy of *Candida albicans* after in vitro treatment with miconazole. *Antimicrob Agents Chemother* 7:704–711, 1975.
40. De Nollin S, Borgers M: An ultrastructural and cytochemical study of *Candida albicans* after in vitro treatment with imidazoles. *Mykosen* 19:317–328, 1976.
41. De Nollin S, Thoné F, Borgers M: Enzyme cytochemistry of *Candida albicans*. *J Histochem Cytochem* 23:758–765, 1975.
42. De Nollin S, Van Belle H, Goossens F, Thoné F, Borgers M: Cytochemical and

biochemical studies of yeasts after in vitro exposure to miconazole. *Antimicrob Agents Chemother* 11:500–513, 1977.
43. De Nollin S, Jacob W, Garrevoet T, Van Daele A, Dockx P: Influence of econazole and 5-fluorocytosine on the ultrastructure of *Aspergillus fumigatus* and the cytochemical localization of calcium ions as measured by laser microprobe mass analysis. *Sabouraudia* 21:287–302, 1983.
44. De Nollin S, Jacob W, Dockx P: Laser microprobe mass analysis (LAMMA) of cytochemically localized calcium on *Aspergillus fumigatus* after exposure to ketoconazole. *Abstr 4133, IIIth Int Congress on Cell Biology*, Tokyo, p. 464, 1984.
45. Djaczenko W, Cassone A: Visualization of new ultrastructural components in the cell wall of *Candida albicans* with fixatives containing Tapo. *J Cell Biol* 52:186–192, 1971.
46. Dockx P: In vitro microscopic study of fungus cells treated with econazole. *Mykosen* 24:218–223, 1980.
47. Evans G, White NH: Effect of the antibiotics radicicolin and griseofulvin on the fine structure of fungi. *J Exp Bot* 18:465–470, 1967.
48. Foury F, Goffeau A: Stimulation of active uptake of nucleosides and amino acids by cyclic adenosine 3′:5′-monophosphate in the yeast *Schizosaccharomyces pombe*. *J Biol Chem* 250:2354–2362, 1975.
49. Fromtling RA, Yu HP, Shadomy S: In vitro inhibitory activities of 2 new orally absorbable imidazole derivatives: Bay n7133 and Bay L 9139. *Sabouraudia* 21:179–184, 1983.
50. Gale GR: Cytology of *Candida albicans* as influenced by drugs acting on the cytoplasmic membrane. *J Bacteriol* 86:151–157, 1963.
51. Gale EF, Cundliffe E, Reynolds PE, Richmond MH, Waring MJ: *The Molecular Basis of Antibiotic Action*. London, Wiley & Sons, 1982, pp 201–219.
52. Godefroi EF, Heeres J, Van Cutsem J, Janssen PAJ: The preparation and antimycotic properties of derivatives of 1-phenethylimidazole. *J Med Chem* 12:784–791, 1969.
53. Günther TH, Kattner W, Mesher HJ: Über das Verhalten und die Lokalisation der sauren Phosphatase von Hefezellen bei Repression und Derepression. *Exp Cell Res* 45:133–138, 1966.
54. Hamilton-Miller JMT: Chemistry and biology of the polyene macrolide antibiotics. *Bacteriol Rev* 37:166–196, 1973.
55. Heel RC, Brogden RN, Speight TM, Avery GS: Econazole: A review of its antifungal activity and therapeutic efficacy. *Drugs* 16:177–201, 1978.
56. Heeres J, Backx LJJ, Mostmans JH, Van Cutsem J: The synthesis and antifungal activity of ketoconazole, a new potent orally active broad-spectrum antifungal agent. *J Med Chem* 22:1003–1007, 1979.
57. Heeres J, Hendrickx R, Van Cutsem J: Antimycotic azoles. Part 6. Synthesis and antifungal properties of terconazole, a novel triazole ketal. *J Med Chem* 26: 611–613, 1983.
58. Heeres J. Backx LJJ, Van Cutsem J: Antimycotic azoles. Part 7. Synthesis and antimycotic properties of a series of novel triazol-3-ones. *J Med Chem* 27: 894–900, 1984.
59. Hino H, Takizawa K, Asboe-Hansen G: Ultrastructure of *Cryptococcus neoformans*. *Acta Dermatovener* 62:113–117, 1982.
60. Humphrey MJ, Jevons S, Tarbit MH: Pharmacokinetic evaluation of UK-49858, a metabolically stable triazole antifungal drug, in animals and humans. *Antimicrob Agents Chemother* 28:648–653, 1985.
61. Ito S: Fine structure of *Cryptococcus neoformans*. An electron microscopic study. *Jpn J Dermatol* 76:65, 1966.
62. Iwata K, Kanda Y, Yamaguchi H, Osumi M: Electron microscopic studies on the

mechanisms of action of clotrimazole on *Candida albicans*. *Sabouraudia* 11:205–209, 1973.

63. Jevans S, Gymer GE, Brammer KW, Cox DA, Lemming MRG: Antifungal activity of tioconazole (UK-20.349), a new imidazole derivative. *Antimicrob Agents Chemother* 15:597–602, 1979.
64. Karaoui R, Bou-Resli M, Al-Zaid NS, Mousa A: Tinea versicolor: Ultrastructural studies on hypopigmented and hyperpigmented skin. *Dermatologica* 162: 69–85, 1981.
65. Kanazawa T: Antimycotic action of A diamidine compound, 1, 4-bis-(M,M'-amidinophenoxymethyl)-cyclohexane dilactate on *Candida albicans*. *Acta Med Okayama* 35:327–341, 1981.
66. Keddie FM: Electron microscopy of *Malassezia furfur* in tinea versicolor. *Sabouraudia* 5:134–137, 1966.
67. Kerridge D, Whelan WL: The polyene macrolide antibiotics and 5-fluorocytosine: Molecular actions and interactions, in APJ Trinci, JE Ryley (eds): *Mode of Action of Antifungal Agents*. London, Cambridge University Press, 1984, pp 343–375.
68. Kerridge D, Koh TY, Johnson AM: The interaction of amphotericin B methyl ester with protoplasm of *Candida albicans*. *J Gen Microbiol* 96:117–123, 1976.
69. Kessler HJ: Mikrobiologische Untersuchungen mit Isoconazolnitrat, einem Breitspektrum-Antimykotikum aus der Gruppe der Imidazol-Derivate. *Arzneim Forsch* 29:1344–1351, 1979.
70. Kitajima Y, Sekiya T, Nozawa Y: Freeze fracture ultrastructural alterations induced by filipin, pimaricin, nystatin and amphotericin B in the plasma membrane of *Epidermophyton*, *Saccharomyces* and red blood cells. A proposal of models for polyene ergosterol complex-induced membrane lesions. *BBA* 445: 452–465, 1976.
71. Malawista SE: Microtubules and the movement of melanin granules in frog dermal melanocytes. *Ann NY Acad Sci* 253:702–710, 1975.
72. Manna VK, Pearse AD, Marks R: The effect of Povidone-Iodine paint on fungal infection. *J Int Med Res* 12:121–123, 1984.
73. Marichal P, Gorrens J, Vanden Bossche H: The action of itraconazole and ketoconazole on growth and sterol synthesis in *Aspergillus fumigatus* and *Aspergillus niger*. *Sabouraudia: J Med Vet Mycol* 22:13–21, 1984.
74. Masperi P, Dall'olio G, Calefano A, Vannini GL: Autophagic vacuole development in *Trichophyton mentagrophytes* exposed in vitro to miconazole. *Sabouraudia: J Med Vet Mycol* 22:27–35, 1984.
75. Matille PH, Moor H, Robinow C: Biology of yeast, in A Rose, J Harrison (eds): *Yeast Cytology*, Vol. 1. London and New York, Academic Press, 1969, pp 219–302.
76. Mazabrey D, Nadal J, Seguela JP, Linas MD: Scanning and transmission electron microscopy: Study of effects of econazole on *Microsporum canis*. *Mycopathologia* 91:151–157, 1985.
77. Medoff G, Kobayashi GA: The polyenes, in DEC Speller (ed): *Antifungal Chemotherapy*. London, Wiley & Sons, 1980, pp 3–33.
78. Meingassner JG, Sleytr UB: The effects of naftifine on the ultrastructure of *Candida parapsilosis*: A freeze fracture study. *Sabouraudia* 20:199–207, 1982.
79. Meingassner JG, Sleytr U, Petranyi G: Morphological changes induced by naftifine, a new antifungal agent, in *Trichophyton mentagrophytes*. *J Invest Dermatol* 77:444–451, 1981.
80. Meingassner JG, Sleytr UB, Petranyi G: SF 86-327: Effects on the ultrastructure of *Trichophyton mentagrophytes* in vitro. *13th Int Congress of Chemotherapy*, Vienna PS 4.8/4.7, 1983.
81. Meingassner JG, Müller M. Sleytr UB: SF-86-327: Effects on the ultrastructure

of *Candida albicans* in vitro. *13th Int Congress of Chemotherapy*, Vienna, 1983, PS 4.8/4-8.
82. Mixich G, Thiele K: Ein Beitrag zur stereospezifischen Synthese von antimykotisch wirksamen Imidazolyloximäthern. Oxiconazole-nitrat (Sgd 301–76), ein neues Breitbandantimykotikum. *Arzneim Forsch* 29:1510–1513, 1979.
83. Montes LF: Systemic abnormalities and the intracellular site of infections of the stratum corneum. *JAMA* 213:1469–1472, 1970.
84. Montes LF, Patrick TA, Martin SA, Smith M: Ultrastructure of blastospores of *Candida albicans* after permanganate fixation. *J Invest Dermatol* 45:227, 1965.
85. Moor H, Mühlethaler K: Fine structure in frozen-etched yeast cells. *J Cell Biol* 17:609–628, 1963.
86. Negroni de Bonvehi MB, Borgers M, Negroni R: Ultrastructural changes produced by ketoconazole in the yeast-like phase of *Paracoccidioides brasiliensis* and *Histoplasma capsulatum. Mycopathologia* 74:113–118, 1981.
87. Negroni de Bonvehi MB, Van de Ven M, Borgers M, Negroni R: Ultrastructural changes produced by ketoconazole in *Cryptococcus neoformans* and *Sporothrix schenckii. Clin Res Rev* 3:5–11, 1983.
88. Norberg B: Cytoplasmic microtubules and radial segmented nuclei (Rieder cells). Effects of osmolality, ionic strength, pH, penetrating non-electrolytes, griseofulvin and a podophyllin derivative. *Scand J Haematol* 7:445–454, 1970.
89. Nozawa Y, Kitajima Y, Sekiya T, Ito Y: Ultrastructural alterations induced by amphotericin B in the plasma membrane of *Epidermophyton floccosum* as revealed by freeze-etch electron microscopy. *BBA* 367:32–38, 1974.
90. Osumi M, Yamada N, Okada J, Yamaguchi H, Hiratani T, Plempel: The effect of bifonazole on the structure of *Trichophyton. Arzneim Forsch Drug Res* 33: 1484–1491, 1983.
91. Osumi M, Yamada N, Yamada Y, Yamaguchi H: The effect of bifonazole on the structure of *Trichophyton mentagrophytes. Dermatologica* 169:19–32, 1984.
92. Palacios J, Serrano R: Proton permeability induced by polyene antibiotics. A plausible mechanism for their inhibition of maltose fermentation in yeast. *FEBS Letters* 91:198–201, 1978.
93. Pena A: Studies on the mechanism of K^+ transport in yeast. *Arch Biochem Biophys* 167:397–419, 1975.
94. Pesti M, Novak EK, Ferenczy L, Svoboda A: Freeze fracture electron microscopical investigation of *Candida albicans* cells sensitive and resistant to nystatin. *Sabouraudia* 19:17–26, 1981.
95. Pesti M, Becher D, Bartsch G: The effect of miconazole on ergosterolless mutant of *Candida albicans. Acta Microbiol Hung* 30:25–29, 1983.
96. Petrou MA, Rogers TR: A comparison of the activity of mepartricin and amphotericin B against yeasts. *J Antimicrob Chemother* 16:169–178, 1985.
97. Plempel M, Bartmann K, Büchel KH, Regel E: Experimentelle Befunde über ein neues oral wirksames Antimykotikum mit breiten Wirkungsspecktrum. *Deutsche Med Wochenschr* 94:1356–1364, 1969.
98. Plempel M, Regel E, Büchel KH: Antimycotic efficacy of bifonazole in vitro and in vivo. *Arzneim Forsch* 33:517–524, 1982.
99. Polak A, Grenson M: Evidence for a common transport system for cytosine, adenine and hypoxanthine in *Saccharomyces cerevisiae* and *Candida albicans. Eur J Biochem* 32:276–282, 1973.
100. Preusser HJ: Die Wirkung von Econazol auf die Feinstruktur der Zellen von *Trichophyton rubrum. Mykosen* 18:453–465, 1975.
101. Preusser HJ: Effects of in vitro treatment with econazole on the ultrastructure of *Candida albicans. Mykosen* 19:304–316, 1976.
102. Preusser HJ: *Trichophyton rubrum/Candida albicans.* Stuttgart, Gustaf Fischer Verlag, 1982, pp 1–109.

103. Raab WPE: *The Treatment of Mycoses With Imidazole Derivatives.* Berlin, Springer-Verlag, 1980.
104. Readio JD, Bittman R: Equilibrium binding of amphotericin B and its methyl ester and borate complex to sterols. *BBA* 685:219–224, 1982.
105. Scheklakow ND, Delektorski WW, Golodova OA: Veränderungen der Ultrastruktur von *Candida albicans* unter der Einwirkung von Polyenantibiotika. *Mykosen* 24:140–152, 1981.
106. Scherwitz C: Ultrastrukturelle Untersuchungen zur Wirkung von Econazolnitrat auf die *Candida albicans* Mykose der menschlichen Haut. *Mykosen* 24: 244–247, 1980.
107. Scholer HJ: Flucytosine, in DCE Speller (ed): *Antifungal Chemotherapy.* London, Wiley & Sons, 1980, pp 35–106.
108. Scott EM, Gorman SP, McGrath SJ: Inhibition of hyphal development in *Trichophyton mentagrophytes* arthroconidia by ketoconazole and miconazole. *J Antimicrob Chemother* 15:405–415, 1985.
109. Sekiya T, Yano K, Nozawa Y: Effects of amphotericin B and its methyl ester on plasma membranes of *Candida albicans* and erythrocytes as examined by freeze-fracture electron microscopy. *Sabouraudia* 20:303–311, 1982.
110. Shadomy S: In vitro studies with 5-fluorocytosine. *Appl Microbiol* 17:871–877, 1969.
111. Sobel JD: Pathogenesis of vaginal candidosis, in BW Eliot (ed): *Oral Therapy in Vaginal Candidosis.* Oxford, Medicine Publishing Foundation, 1984, pp 1–13.
112. Sun SH, Huppert M: A cytological study of morphogenesis in *Coccidioides immitis. Sabouraudia* 14:184–198, 1976.
113. Sun SH, Sekhon SS, Huppert M: Electron microscopic studies of saprobic and parasitic forms of *Coccidioides immitis. Sabouraudia* 17:265–273, 1979.
114. Tanenbaum L, Anderson C, Chaplin M, Jones R, Matthews T, Walker K: Sulconazole nitrate 1% cream: Preclinical and clinical profile. *Abstr 11th Int Congr Chemother.* No. 148, Boston, 1979.
115. Thienpont D, Van Cutsem J, Borgers M: Ketoconazole in experimental candidosis. *Rev Infect Dis* 2:570–576, 1980.
116. Tolman EL, Isaacson DM, Rosenthale ME, McGuire JL, Van Cutsem J, Borgers M, Vanden Bossche H: Anticandidal activities of terconazole, a broad-spectrum antimycotic. *Antimicrob Agents Chemother* 29:986–991, 1986.
117. Van Cutsem J, Van Gerven F, Van de Ven MA, Borgers M, Janssen PAJ: Itraconazole, a new triazole that is orally active in aspergillosis. *Antimicrob Agents Chemother* 26:527–534, 1984.
118. Vanden Bossche H: Biochemical targets for antifungal azole-derivative. Hypothesis of the mode of action. *Curr Topics Med Mycol* 1:313–351, 1985.
119. Vanden Bossche H, Willemsens G, Cools W, Marichal P, Lauwers W: Hypothesis on the molecular basis for the antifungal activation of N-substituted imidazoles and triazoles. *Biochem Soc Trans* 11:665–667, 1983.
120. Vanden Bossche H, Lauwers, W, Willemsens G, Marichal P, Cornelissen F, Cools W: Molecular basis for antimycotic and antibacterial activity of N-substituted imidazoles and triazoles: The inhibition of isoprenoid biosynthesis. *Pest Sci* 15:188–198, 1984.
121. Vannini GL, Mares D, Giori P, Bonora A: Antifungal properties of some pyrazolyl-sulfides. *Mycopathologia* 74:7–14, 1981.
122. Walker KAM, Braemer AC, Hitt S, Jones RE, Matthews TR: 1-[4-(4-chlorophenyl)-2-(2, 6-dichlorophenylthio)-n-butyl]-1H-imidazole nitrate, a new potent antifungal agent. *J Med Chem* 21:840–843, 1978.
123. Weber K, Wehland J, Herzog W: Griseofulvin interacts with microtubules both in vivo and in vitro. *J Mol Biol* 102:817–830, 1976.

124. Wiemken A: Eigenschaften der Hefevacuole (thesis). Zürich, Eidgenössischen Technischen Hochschule, 1969.
125. Wooley DW: Some biological effects produced by benzimidazole and their reversal by purines. *J Biol Chem* 152:225–232, 1944.
126. Yamaguchi H, Iwata K, Nagano M, Osumi M: Ultrastructure of *Saccharomyces cerevisiae* treated with econazole. *J Electron Microsc* 30:305–314, 1981.
127. Yamaguchi H, Hiratani R, Plempel M: In vitro studies of a new oral azole antimycotic, BAY n7133. *J Antimicrob Chem* 11:135–149, 1983.

2—Soluble Polysaccharides of *Cryptococcus neoformans*

Robert Cherniak

The cell envelope of *Cryptococcus neoformans* is composed of a rigid wall constituted mainly of complex glucans (37); an acidic heteropolysaccharide principal antigen composed of mannose, xylose, and glucuronic acid; and at least two minor polysaccharide antigens (55). The relationship of the principal capsular antigens of *C. neoformans* to pathogenicity has been demonstrated, and it is considered to be a major virulence factor (12, 30, 39). The cryptococcal capsule is antiphagocytic (11, 13, 22, 41, 42, 52) and enables the yeast to avoid immune surveillance, cross the blood-brain barrier, and proliferate in the central nervous system by a mechanism reminiscent of bacterial agents of meningitis (57). The capsular polysaccharide persists in body fluids and invokes tolerance (1, 43, 51). Cryptococcal meningitis has been encountered relatively infrequently, but with the increased occurrence of Acquired Immunodeficiency Syndrome (AIDS), a concomitant increase in cryptococcosis has resulted (16).

Purified high molecular weight polysaccharides (8, 55) have been obtained from the four recognized serotypes, A through D (65), and from the newly defined A-D serotype (35) of *C. neoformans*. A retrospective review of the soluble polysaccharides of *C. neoformans* is presented. For previous reviews the reader is directed to references 8, 29, 55, 59.

Cryptococcus neoformans was originally subdivided by Evans (23, 24) into three antigenic types that were designated A, B, and C. The proposed serologic classification was shown by Evans and Kessel (25) to be based on soluble capsular polysaccharides. The unfractionated capsular polysaccharides exhibited both type-specific and species-specific determinant groups (25). Wilson et al (65) identified a fourth serotype, D, and provided evidence for the existence of *C. neoformans* strains of mixed type, A-D. Strains possibly of the A-D type have been observed also by Mishra et al (47), Kaplan et al (38), and Ikeda et al (34, 35). Specific fluorescent antibody reagents were developed by Kaplan et al (38) and were used successfully for differentiating *C. neoformans* types. In a comprehensive study, Ikeda et al (34) delineated eight factors responsible for serologic classification of *C. neoformans* into types A, B, C,

D, and A-D. The chemical basis for the eight typing factors was not determined (34).

An attempt to characterize the immunodeterminants of *C. neoformans* was reported by Bhattacharjee et al (7). They obtained antibodies to the capsular polysaccharides of *C. neoformans* type D that appeared to be specific for the nonreducing residues of the immunizing antigens. However, all the antibody fractions precipitated purified type A polysaccharide as well as type D polysaccharide. A test for the possibility of cross-reactions with types B and C was not performed. Therefore, the antibodies could be either A and D specific or simply species specific. It has been stated that the acapsular mutant *C. neoformans* 602, originally derived from a serotype D parent, was nontypable (40). However, *C. neoformans* 602 produces minor polysaccharide components that are discrete from the major capsular polysaccharide (40). Antiserum to cells of *C. neoformans* 602 agglutinated sheep erythrocytes sensitized either with polysaccharides from the 602 mutant or those from a type D reference strain. Specific agglutination of erythrocytes sensitized with capsular polysaccharide obtained from serotypes A, B, and C was not observed. It is thus possible and certainly has not been ruled out that the type specificity observed in previous studies resides with a minor capsular component and that group specificity (A, D) and (B, C) and species specificity (antigen common to A, B, C, and D) resides with the major capsular polysaccharide. The preparation of antisera specific for eight antigenic factors of *C. neoformans* should allow the unequivocal determination of the chemical basis for the current serotyping scheme (34). The presence of more than one serologically active capsular antigen was demonstrated by Bennett and Hasenclever (1) by double diffusion in gel. The presence of several capsular antigens of *C. neoformans* is a general phenomenon observed by many, and galactose can be considered a marker of capsular heterogeneity (9, 19, 25, 27, 28, 34, 46, 53, 58) in view of findings by Cherniak et al (19) that two serologically distinct heteroglycans could be obtained by differential precipitation with cetyltrimethylammonium bromide (CTAB). The major capsular antigen, *C. neoformans* type A acidic glucuronoxylomannan (GXM-A), was precipitated, whereas a galactoxylomannan remained in solution. The galactoxylomannan (GalXM) was fractionated into two distinct entities, a galactoxylo-enriched component and a mannoprotein, by affinity chromatography on Concanavalin-A agarose (64). Reiss et al (54) have measured immunoglobulin M (IgM) levels to GalXM and its two components by indirect enzyme immunoassay in patients with cryptococcosis, in patients with other mycoses, and in normal individuals. Most of the demonstrable serologic activity of IgM was directed mainly against the mannoprotein.

The role, if any, that the minor capsular antigens play in determining the serotypes of *C. neoformans* has not been investigated. A comprehensive serologic comparison of purified antigens from several authentic strains representing all the serotypes should be made in order to determine the basis for the subdivision of *C. neoformans* into serotypes.

TABLE 2-1. Composition of the Glucuronoxylomannan of *Cryptococcus neoformans*

Serotype	Mannose	Xylose	Glucuronic Acid	*O*-Acetyl (%)	Reference
A	3	2	1	ND	46
A	5	2	1	6.5	18
A	3.3	1.5	1	ND	6
B	3	3	1	10.5	5
C	3	4	1	3.0	2, 4
D	3	1	1	10.3	3
D	4.4	1.6	1	ND	6
A-D	7	2	2	2.8	35

ND = Not determined.

The major capsular polysaccharide of *C. neoformans* inhibits phagocytosis (11, 13, 40, 41, 42, 52) and is considered a major virulence factor. This view is supported by the observation that, whereas the wild type strains of *C. neoformans* were 100% lethal for mice, acapsular mutants were not (30).

Purified high molecular weight (2, 3, 4, 5, 18, 46) polysaccharides have been obtained from the four recognized serotypes, A through D, and from the newly defined A-D serotype (35) of *C. neoformans*. All have been reported to be related, nonidentical, *O*-acetylated heteroglycans composed of mannose, xylose, and glucuronic acid (2, 3, 4, 5, 18, 46) (Table 2-1). It is convenient to refer to this family of antigens as glucuronoxylomannans. Structural models based on methylation-fragmentation analysis showed that the major capsular polysaccharides are composed of a linear backbone of (1→3)-linked D-mannopyranosyl (man*p*) residues substituted with D-xylopyranosyl (xyl*p*) and glucopyranosyluronic acid (glc*p*A) nonreducing termini (2, 3, 4, 5, 18, 46) (Scheme 2-1). Serotypes A and D (3, 6, 18, 46) are substituted at *O*-2 only, whereas serotypes B and C (2, 4, 5) are substituted with xyl*p* at *O*-4 as well as at *O*-2 (Scheme 2-1). The assignments of the respective α and β configurations of the mannan backbone and the nonreducing substituents were determined by chromium trioxide oxidation, enzymic digestion with β-glucuronidase, and optical rotation analysis of isolated oligosaccharides (5).

An early attempt to define the carbohydrate compositions of the soluble antigens was done by Evans and Mehl (26). The qualitative analysis by partition paper chromatography of the carbohydrate composition of *C. neoformans* serotypes A, B, and C polysaccharides identified xylose, mannose, glucuronic acid, and galactose.

Evans and Theriault (27) demonstrated the heterogeneity of the soluble capsular polysaccharides by differential precipitation with heavy metal salts. Lead acetate precipitated a fraction that was galactose free. This was perhaps the first chemical evidence for the composite nature of the capsular polysaccharide antigens. The effect of this method of separation was not confirmed or expanded since the original report. The capsular polysaccharide of *C. neofor-*

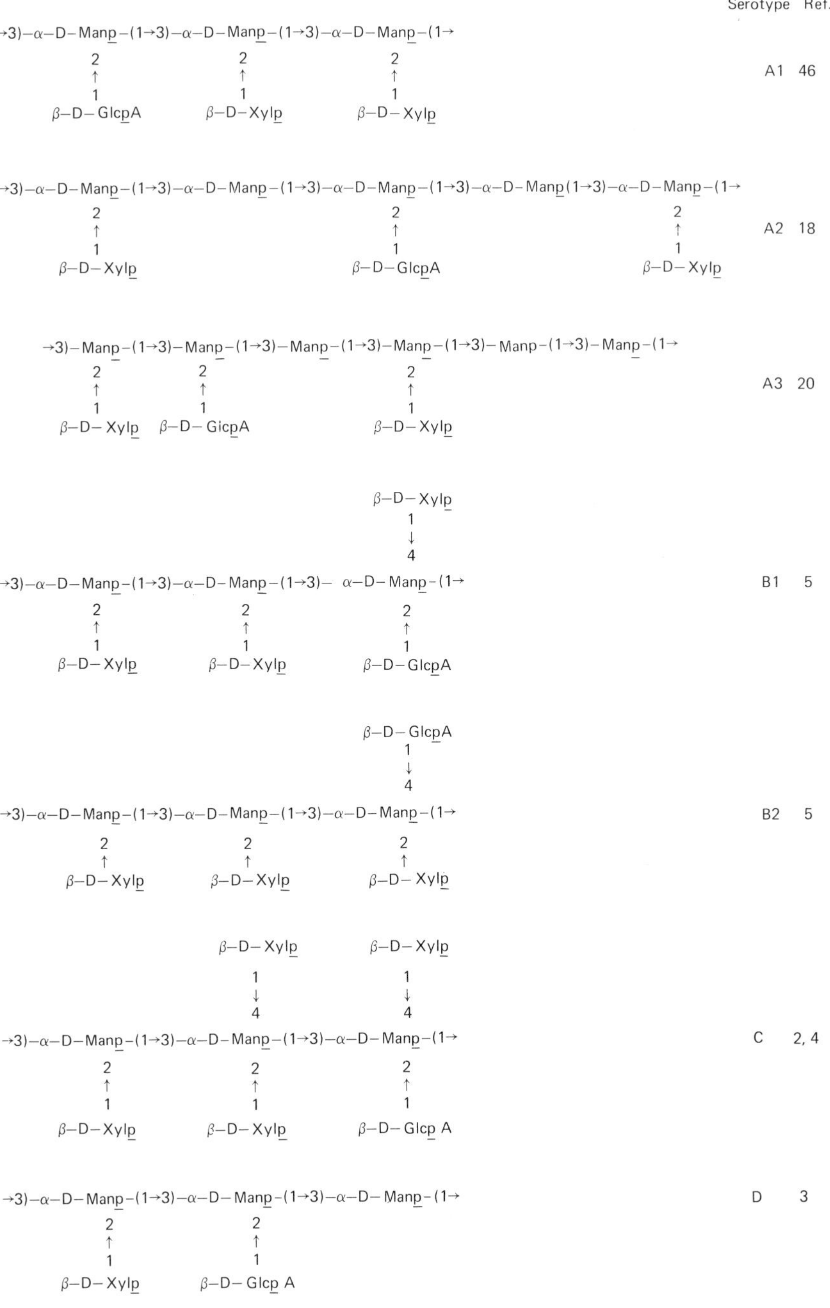

SCHEME 2-1. Structural models of the major capsular polysaccharides of *Cryptococcus neoformans*. These models represent idealized situations as presented in the literature. No attempt has been made to rationalize the variability of molar ratios of the component residues by the construction of alternate models.

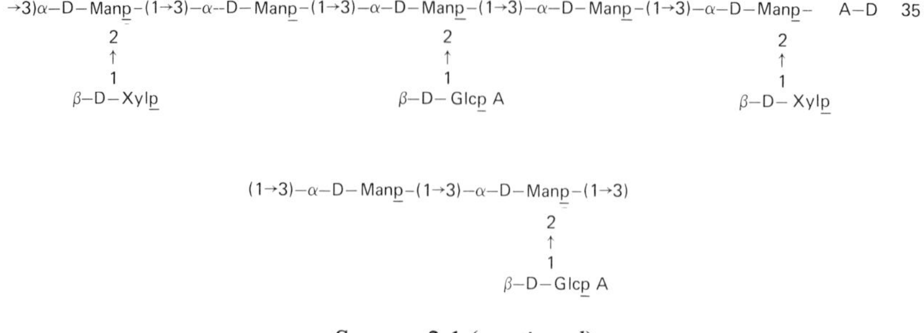

SCHEME 2-1 (*continued*)

mans type A was precipitated by treatment with CTAB by Rebers et al (53), and the precipitate was composed of xylose, mannose, galactose, and glucuronic acid as determined by partition paper chromatography. It was concluded that no fractionation had occurred because the composition of the precipitated polysaccharide paralleled that of the original material. However, it was observed that a portion of the polysaccharide was not precipitable with CTAB. Polysaccharides recovered from the CTAB precipitate and the CTAB supernate exhibited cross-reactivity with anti-*Streptococcus pneumoniae* type XIV serum. The specificity for this antiserum is dependent on the presence of galactose residues (45). The reaction of type XIV anti-*S. pneumoniae* serum and cryptococcal polysaccharides produced a precipitate enriched in galactose (53). Although complete separation was not achieved, this evidence supports the idea that the soluble capsular polysaccharides elaborated by *C. neoformans* are a composite of several discrete heteroglycans. The first attempt at detailed structural determination by methylation analysis was reported by Miyazaki (48, 49, 50). Miyazaki used purified polysaccharide extracted from whole cells grown on agar medium. The polysaccharide was a low molecular weight polymer composed of mannose/xylose/glucuronic acid in a molar ratio of 3 : 1 : 1; no galactose was reported. The proposed (1→2)-linkage of the backbone is at variance with all current data. The polysaccharide characterized by Miyazaki may reflect the isolation of a mixture of polysaccharides from a lightly encapsulated yeast. In particular the presence of (1→2)-linked man*p* residue may have been contributed by a surafce mannoprotein of *C. neoformans* that is known to possess the (1→2)-mannosyl linkage (19, 64). The preliminary reports of Miyazaki were not extended, and thus the significance of his findings cannot be assessed.

A soluble capsular polysaccharide obtained from the culture supernate of *C. neoformans* type B by Blandamer and Danishefsky (9) was partially purified by precipitation with ethanol. The chemical or serologic homogeneity of the polysaccharide preparation was not demonstrated, and additional physicochemical fractionation was not attempted. Mannose/xylose/glucuronic acid/galactose, in the molar ratio of 3 : 2 : 1 : 0.5, were the only carbohydrate constituents found. Partial acid hydrolysis produced a series of oligosaccharides composed of mannose, xylose, and glucuronic acid, and mannose was always on the reducing end. Galactose was present only as a monosaccharide. A trisaccharide substituted with xylose and glucuronic acid also was characterized. These data were consistent with a polysaccharide constructed of a mannan backbone bearing xylose and glucuronic acid nonreducing termini. Other oligosaccharides were composed of mannose and xylose only. Based on more recent knowledge, the galactose probably arises from a separate polysaccharide (19, 46, 64).

A soluble capsular polysaccharide from *C. neoformans* type A, strain CIA, was prepared by precipitation with ethanol from the culture supernatant followed by deproteinization using solvent denaturation (28). The molar ratio of mannose/xylose/glucuronic acid/galactose was 9 : 4 : 3.5 : 2. The molecular weight of the polysaccharide was reported to be 10,000–15,000 daltons, a value range at variance with the high molecular weights that have been consistently reported over the past few years. This discrepancy in values may be due to the shear force to which the sample was exposed during eight cycles of solvent denaturation. A decrease in viscosity and molecular weight of the polysaccharide occurs upon sonication of the native polysaccharide as reported by Cherniak et al (20, 21).

A significant advance in the knowledge of the composition and structure of the major capsular polysaccharides of *C. neoformans* was made by Bhattacharjee et al (2). The soluble capsular polysaccharide from a type C strain was obtained by precipitation with ethanol as in previous studies. But in this instance purification was extended by chromatographic fractionation of the soluble capsular polysaccharide on an anion exchange column of DEAE-cellulose. The major capsular polysaccharide antigen glucuronoxylomannan (GXM-C) exhibited a high molecular weight and was composed of mannose/xylose/glucuronic acid in the molar ratio of approximately 3 : 4 : 1 and was partially *O*-acetylated (3%). Galactose was not present in the major capsular polysaccharides. Bhattacharjee et al performed the first methylation analysis of a homogeneous *C. neoformans* capsular polysaccharide. The methylated monosaccharide derivatives showed that mannopyranosyl (man*p*) residues were 2,3,4-tri-*O*- and 2,3-di-*O*-substituted and that the xylopyranosyl (xyl*p*) and glucopyranosyluronic acid (glcA*p*) were linked as nonreducing termini to *O*-2 and *O*-4 of mannose (Scheme 2-1C). Oxidation of GXM-C with $NaIO_4$ destroyed all the xyl*p* and glc*p*A, leaving a (1→3)-linked water-insoluble mannan that was resistant to further oxidation. These data confirmed the assignments of xylose and glucuronic acid to the *O*-2 and *O*-4 positions of mannose. Methylation analysis of an aldobiuronic acid obtained by partial acid hydrolysis showed that glucuronic acid was in *O*-2-linkage. That glc*p*A was in *O*-2-linkage and xyl*p* residues were in 2-*O*- and 4-*O*-linkages were confirmed by alkaline degradation methylation because a new *O*-2 position was exposed for each glc*p*A degraded (2). A structural model for the type C polysaccharide was proposed (Scheme 2-1C). The anomeric configurations of the linkages shown in Scheme 2-1C were determined by chromium trioxide oxidation (80% loss of xyl*p* after 3 hours) and by optical rotation determination on appropriate derivatives [α-(1→3)-mannan $[\alpha]_D^{20}$ of +102°; β-(1→2)-aldobiuronic acid $[\alpha]_D^{20}$ of −20°].

The molar ratios of the various methylated derivatives did not exactly correspond to those obtained by gas-liquid chromatography for the alditol acetates of the free sugars. The discrepancy in values was explained as being due to the high volatility of several of the highly methylated monosaccharides. Quantitative aspects of methylation analysis are influenced by: 1) undermethylation, 2) incomplete hydrolysis, 3) degradation and demethylation during hydrolysis, 4) incomplete reduction and acetylation for the formation of alditol acetates, 5) selective loss of volatile components during evaporation of solvents, and 6) losses on glassware (33). The ramifications of these pitfalls were apparent in methylation data for GXM-C and in similar analyses done on other *C. neoformans* serotypes (see below). Therefore, current structural models based solely on methylation analysis must be accepted with reservations. Two additional carbohydrate peaks were eluted from the DEAE-cellulose column, but unfortunately no analytic data were presented to characterize these fractions. It is possible that one of these fractions may have contained the elusive galactose.

The major capsular antigen from *C. neoformans* serotype D, GXM-D, was prepared and analyzed by procedures analogous to those discussed earlier for serotype C (3). The experience gained in the previous study resulted in the improvement in the quality of subsequent methylation data. The mannose/xylose/glucuronic acid molar ratio of GXM-D was approximately 3 : 1 : 1, and the polymer was partially *O*-acetylated (10.3%). Methylation analysis (Table 2-2) partially supported the structure shown in Scheme 2-1D. The 6-*O*-methylmannose was purported to arise from tetra-*O*-substituted mannose that occurs at a point of dual branching. The detection of 4,6-di-*O*-methylmannose in the methylation analysis of the mannan produced by oxidation with $NaIO_4$ could also have come from a branched polysaccharide. However, comparison of the methylation data with analyses of unmethylated GXM-D reveals significant quantitative inconsistencies (Table 2-2). In view of this, and other supporting evidence (20, 21, 46), the man*p* residues in GXM-D are probably arrayed as a linear, unbranched backbone. It is possible that a portion of the methylation data (eg, 6-*O*-methylmannose) may be in error because of undermethylation or a similar experimental inadequacy alluded to earlier. The structural model proposed for GXM-D shows a linear backbone of α-(1→3)-linked D-man*p* residues 2-*O*-substituted by D-xyl*p* and D-glc*p*A as nonreducing end groups (Scheme 2-1D). As in the previous study, the analysis of the secondary polysaccharide was not pursued.

The analytic methods used by Bhattacharjee et al (2, 3, 4,) were extended to an investigation of *C. neoformans* type B (5). The purified capsular polysaccharide GXM-B was composed of mannose/xylose/glucuronic acid in the molar ratio of approximately 3 : 3 : 1 and was partially *O*-acetylated (10.4%).

A structural model for GXM-B shown in Scheme 2-1B1 was based on

TABLE 2-2. Variation in Molar Ratios—*Cryptococcus neoformans* Serotype D

Derivative (Ref.)	Native (5)	Reduced (5)	Reduced (8)	Alkaline Degradation (8)	Mannan Smith Degradation (5)	Mannan Smith Degradation (8)	Native (5)	Native (8)
2,3,4,6-Me_4-Glc		1.3	0.55					
2,3,4-Me_3-Xyl	1	1	1	1				
2,4,6-Me_3-Man	1	1.7	0.83	1.94	4.9	9.7		
4,6-Me_2-Man	1.5	2	1.1	1.6	0.36	0.3		
6-Me-Man	0.35	0.3	0.16	0				
Branch-Man	1	1	1		1	1		
Total Me-Man	8	13	12.7		15	33		
Man	2.9	4	2.1	3.54			3	2.75
Xyl	1	1	1	1			1	1
Mannose							3	4.4
Xylose							1	1.6
Glucuronic Acid							1	1

methylation analysis. In addition to some inconsistencies in the methylation data, two sets of data were presented concerning the alkaline elimination of the methylated GXM-B followed by remethylation (5). One set, delineated in tabular form, indicated glc*p*A residues in (1→4) linkage; this linkage was cited in the abstract to the paper (5). A second set of data, which were presented in the text, was consistent with glc*p*A in (1→2)-linkage and these data were consistent with the structural model presented in the body of the paper that is usually referred to by others (Scheme 2-1B1 and 2-1B2). This report is the sole source of structural data for serotype B, and the removal of the ambiguity concerning the linkage of glc*p*A will require additional investigation.

Studies of the *C. neoformans* type A polysaccharide were done concurrently by Cherniak et al (18) and by Merrifield and Stephen (46). Both groups used differential complexation with CTAB to obtain purified capsular antigens. The selective removal of galactose was demonstrated in each instance. As in previous studies the presence of mannose, xylose, and glucuronic acid was identified. The molar ratio for mannose/xylose/glucuronic acid was 3 : 2 : 1 (46) and 5 : 2 : 1 (18). Cherniak et al (18) reported that GXM-A was *O*-acetylated (6.5%). The structural models are shown in Scheme 2-1A-1 and 2-1A-2. A mannan exhibiting low water solubility was isolated as a result of Smith degradation by both groups (18, 46); this property was first reported for the Smith degradation product of GXM-C by Bhattacharjee et al (2). The usual methylation procedure was altered by Merrifield and Stephen (46) to accommodate the low solubility of the mannan. The singular detection of 2,4,6-tri-*O*-methylmannose is characteristic of a linear mannan in which all man*p* residues are (1→3)-linked.

The obvious differences in molar ratios reported by Cherniak et al (18) and Merrifield and Stephen (46) and the fact that Bhattacharjee et al supplied *C.*

neoformans 371 to Cherniak et al prompted Bhattacharjee et al (6) to investigate their stock culture of *C. neoformans* NIH 371. Clones corresponding to serotypes A and D were identified and a representative sample of each type was selected for analysis; 371-a (type D) and 371-3 (type A). Analysis of the capsular polysaccharide of 371-3 gave the molar ratio for mannose/xylose/glucuronic acid as approximately 3.3 : 1.5 : 1 (gas-liquid chromatography). These data correspond to yet a third set of molar ratios for serotype A and are at variance with the values reported previously for this serotype (mannose/xylose/glucuronic acid, 3 : 2 : 1) (Table 2-1) (46). The type D clone, 371-a, showed a molar ratio for mannose/xylose/glucuronic acid of approximately 4.4 : 1.6 : 1 (gas-liquid chromatography). The data obtained by methylation analysis were consistent with previously proposed models for A and D capsular polysaccharides; substitution with xyl*p* and glcA*p* as (1→2) nonreducing termini to a (1→3) mannan (Scheme 2-1). The molar ratios for mannose/xylose/glucuronic acid, based on the recovery of methylated sugars of the carboxyl-reduced polysaccharides of 371-a and 371-3 were 3.8 : 1.8 : 1 and 3.2 : 1.6 : 1, respectively. The most significant difference between the methylation data reported for the three studies of *C. neoformans* serotype A was that little or no 2,4,6-tri-*O*-methylmannose was reported by Bhattacharjee et al (6) and Merrifield and Stephen (46), whereas Cherniak et al (18) found substantial quantities of the derivative. Based on these differences in molar ratios, Bhattacharjee et al (6) suggested that the strain originally provided to and studied by Cherniak et al (18) was really a serotype D isolate. In view of the concern resulting from the report of Bhattacharjee et al (6) that their stock culture of NIH 371 was heterogeneous, containing both A and D types, Reiss and Cherniak reinvestigated the purity of their stock culture. Cultures were streaked on Sabouraud glucose agar and five isolated colonies were cloned, coded, and serotyped in blind fashion with the immunofluorescence method of Kaplan et al (38). The results showed that all colonies were of serotype A and no variants were detected (unpublished observations). Therefore, the variation in results obtained by Merrifield and Stephen (46), Cherniak et al (18), and Bhattacharjee et al (6) may reflect experimental variations due to culturing conditions or strain-to-strain differences (17, 61).

The proposed structures of the capsular polysaccharides can be used to differentiate A or D from B or C because A and D lack the large amounts of tetrasubstituted mannose reported in B and C. However, the differentiation between A and D or between B and C cannot be based on molar compositions in the GXMs because of the variability in the published data. Also, for several serotypes only data for a single isolate have been reported (2, 4, 5). Moreover, there is no formal proof that unequivocally defines GXM as being the type-specific antigen of *C. neoformans*. Preliminary data indicate that the factor sera prepared by Ikeda et al (35) will provide strong evidence for the participation of GXM in the serotyping scheme.

Methylation analysis alone cannot yield the exact disposition and config-

→3)–α–D–Man*p*–(1→3)–α–D–Man*p*–(1→3)–α–D–Man*p*–(1→3)–α–D–Man*p*–(1

SCHEME 2-2. Mannan.

uration of the nonreducing residues along the mannan backbone, nor can it differentiate blocks of sequences from a strict repeating sequence. Therefore, the previously published depictions for *C. neoformans* polysaccharides (Scheme 2-1) must be considered merely examples of several equally representative models. An alternative approach to specifying the structural details of *C. neoformans* polysaccharides is the application of ^{13}C-nuclear magnetic resonance (nmr) spectroscopy as applied by Gorin (31, 32). An attempt at applying ^{13}C-nmr spectroscopic analysis to serotype A polysaccharide gave spectra too complex to permit the assignment of specific resonances to particular structural elements (6). A footnote to the ^{13}C-nmr spectroscopy data suggested that some of the mannose residues were substituted at *O*-6 with acetyl (6).

The complexity and viscosity of the major GXM of *C. neoformans* in its native form posed an intractable analytic problem for ^{13}C-nmr spectroscopy. Therefore, a scheme of physical and chemical degradation was devised by Cherniak et al which yielded a series of polysaccharide derivatives suitable for analysis by ^{13}C-nmr spectroscopy (20, 21). The GXM (18) was treated with lithium in anhydrous ethylenediamine to selectively remove the glucuronic acid residues. The product was a xylomannan (XM) with an apparent molecular weight of 35,000 daltons. Smith degradation of XM yielded two mannan products (Ms and Mi) that differed in their water solubility, but both products were soluble in DMSO. The proton-decoupled and proton-coupled ^{13}C-nmr spectra of M in DMSO proved M to be a linear polysaccharide with man*p* residues linked entirely α-(1→3) (Scheme 2-2) (20, 21). Similar data showed the xylomannan to consist of the M backbone, with about 91% of the xyl*p* on nonadjacent man*p* residues as *O*-2-β-D-xyl*p* nonreducing termini and about 9% as *O*-4-D-xyl*p* nonreducing residues on other man*p* residues (20, 21).

Brief ultrasonic exposure of a GXM solution yielded a polysaccharide preparation of reduced molecular weight (300,000 daltons) and viscosity. The Sonicated GXM (GXMS) was further partially depolymerized by mild acid hydrolysis (PAHGXMS), and PAHGXMS was de-*O*-acetylated by treatment with ammonia (DPAHGXMS). The glucuronic acid residues of sonicated GXM were converted to glucose by reduction, and the *O*-acetyl groups were removed by treatment with ammonia (DRGXMS). Proton-decoupled spectra of DPAHGXMS and DRGXMS showed that glc*p*A residues were attached as β-(1→2) nonreducing termini and disposed along M as shown in Scheme 2-4. The comparison of DPAHGXMS and GXMS by ^{13}C-nmr permitted the assignment of the *O*-acetyl groups to the *O*-6 positions of M (Scheme 2-4). Block sequences are not possible, but minor areas with short strings of unsubstituted man*p* are probably present. The proposed structure in Scheme 2-4 approxi-

β-D-Xylp (1→2) at two positions

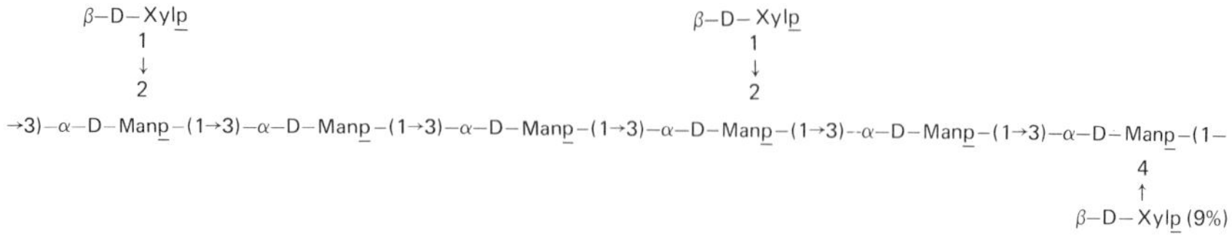

→3)-α-D-Manp-(1→3)-α-D-Manp-(1→3)-α-D-Manp-(1→3)-α-D-Manp-(1→3)-α-D-Manp-(1→3)-α-D-Manp-(1–

4 ↑ β-D-Xylp (9%)

SCHEME 2-3. Xylomannan.

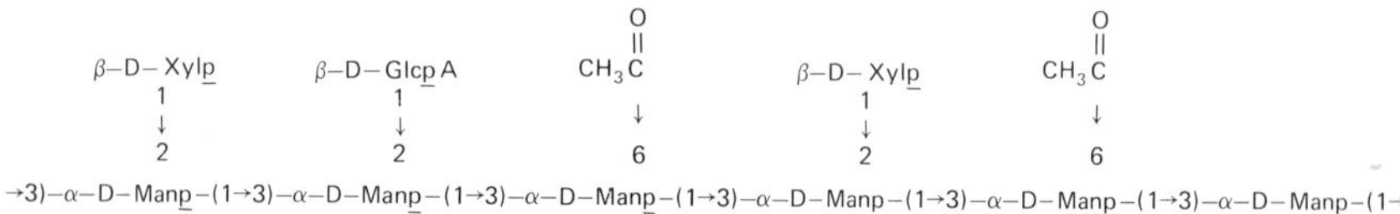

SCHEME 2-4. Glucuronoxylomannan. Man*p* residues to which the 6-*O*-acetyl groups are attached were randomly selected.

mates the carbohydrate stoichiometry of the serotype A polysaccharide of Cherniak et al (18) but differs from that of Bhattacharjee et al (6) and Merrifield and Stephen (46). The data obtained by ^{13}C-nmr spectroscopy resulted in the detailed structural elucidation of the major glucuronoxylomannan, residue disposition, linkage, and configuration, including that of the *O*-acetyl groups (20, 21). The presence of *O*-4-linked xyl*p* was observed for other serotype A strains (17).

Galactose as a constituent of the capsular polysaccharide of *C. neoformans* has been observed by numerous investigators in the past but was not detected in more recent reports (2, 3, 4, 5, 6), or its presence has been overlooked (46). CTAB precipitation of GXM of *C. neoformans* from the bulk polysaccharide, originally obtained by fractionation with ethanol, leaves a CTAB-nonprecipitable polysaccharide enriched in galactose (19, 46, 64). The polysaccharide was analyzed by Cherniak et al (19) and is characterized by 1) molar ratio of galactose/mannose/xylose/glucuronic acid (GalXM) of 1.9 : 1.8 : 1 : 0.2 and 2% *O*-acetyl; 2) a molecular weight of 275,000 $\pm$25,000 d; 3) extensive degradation by $NaIO_4$; 4) precipitation in gel by a lectin, Concanavalin A (ConA), indicating nonreducing mannosyl residues; and 5) a distinct immunoprecipitin arc in counterimmunoelectrophoresis.

The low glucuronic acid content probably accounts for its failure to form an insoluble CTAB complex. Turner et al (64) were able to fractionate GalXM, by differential affinity for ConA, into two discrete polymers: a galactoxylo-enriched polysaccharide (nonbound) and a mannoprotein (bound) component. The molar ratios for mannose/xylose/galactose for the mannoprotein and the galactoxylo-enriched polysaccharide were 7.6 : 1 : 0.8 and 1.5 : 1 : 1.8, respectively. The relative proportions of the three components of the soluble capsular polysaccharides of *C. neoformans*—GXM, GalXM, mannoprotein

—were 88%, 10%, and 2%, respectively. The mannoprotein was found to be 80 times more active serologically than GalXM as determined by enzyme immunoassay (54). Polysaccharides equivalent to GalXM and mannoprotein have been isolated by Turner et al (64) from acapsular mutants derived from *C. neoformans* serotype D by Jacobson et al (36). The primary structural elements of the mannoprotein appear to be man*p* residues linked (1→3) and (1→2) as determined by ^{13}C-nmr spectroscopy (64 and unpublished observation). In retrospect it is possible that the earlier methylation results by Miyazaki (50) reflected the presence of the unsuspected mannoprotein.

It is clear that the soluble capsular polysaccharide of *C. neoformans* is a composite of at least three distinct polymers. How these polysaccharides participate in the immune response to *C. neoformans* is unknown. Definitive serologic relationships using purified capsular polysaccharides (GXM, GalXM, and mannoprotein) have not been determined. A combination of chemical (methylation analysis), physical (^{13}C-nmr), and immunochemical (monoclonal antibodies and enzyme immunoassays) analyses must be used to delineate the nature of the type-specific and other immunodominant epitopes of *C. neoformans*. Use of several well-characterized strains representative of each serotype is mandatory to control for linkage variations among strains.

References

1. Bennett JE, Hasenclever HF: *Cryptococcus neoformans* polysaccharide: Studies of serologic properties and role in infection. *J Immunol* 94:916–920, 1965.
2. Bhattacharjee AK, Kwon-Chung KJ, Glaudemans CPJ: On the structure of the capsular polysaccharide from *Cryptococcus neoformans* serotype C. *Immunochemistry* 15:673–679, 1978.
3. Bhattacharjee AK, Kwon-Chung KJ, Glaudemans CPJ: The structure of the capsular polysaccharide from *Cryptococcus neoformans* serotype D. *Carbohydr Res* 73:183–192, 1979.
4. Bhattacharjee AK, Kwon-Chung KJ, Glaudemans CPJ: On the structure of the capsular polysaccharide from *Cryptococcus neoformans* serotype C-II. *Mol Immunol* 16:531–532, 1979.
5. Bhattacharjee AK, Kwon-Chung KJ, Glaudemans CPJ: Structural studies on the major capsular polysaccharide from *Cryptococcus bacillisporus* serotype B. *Carbohydr Res* 82:103–111, 1980.
6. Bhattacharjee AK, Kwon-Chung KJ, Glaudemans CPJ: Capsular polysaccharides from a parent strain and from a possible mutant strain of *Cryptococcus neoformans* serotype A. *Carbohydr Res* 95:237–247, 1981.
7. Bhattacharjee AK, Bennett JE, Bundle DR, Glaudemans CPJ: Anticryptococcal type D antibodies raised in rabbits. *Mol Immunol* 20:351–359, 1983.
8. Bhattacharjee AK, Bennett JE, Glaudemans CPJ: Capsular polysaccharides of *C. neoformans*. *Rev Infect Dis* 6:619–624, 1984.
9. Blandamer A, Danishefsky I: Investigations on the structure of the capsular polysaccharides from *Cryptococcus neoformans* type B. *Biochim Biophys Acta* 117:305–313, 1966.
10. Breen JF, Combee CL: Immunogenicity of cryptococcal capsular polysaccharide. *Abstr Ann Mtg Am Soc Microbiol*, 80th Annual Meeting. Abst F3:320, 1980.

11. Bulmer GS, Sans MD: *Cryptococcus neoformans* II. Phagocytosis by human leucocytes. *J Bacteriol* 94:1480–1483, 1967.
12. Bulmer GS, Sans MD, Gunn CM: *Cryptococcus neoformans* I. Nonencapsulated mutants. *J Bacteriol* 94:1475–1479, 1967.
13. Bulmer GS, Sans MD: *Cryptococcus neoformans* III. Inhibition of phagocytosis. *J Bacteriol* 95:5–8, 1968.
14. Cauley LK, Murphy JW: Response of congenitally athymic nude and phenotypically normal mice to *Cryptococcus neoformans* infection. *Infect Immun* 23:644–651, 1979
15. Chandler FW, Kaplan W, Ajello L: *A Colour Atlas and Textbook of Histopathology of Mycotic Diseases*. London, Wolfe Medical Publications, 1980.
16. Chandler FW: Pathology of the mycoses in patients with the acquired immunodeficiency syndrome (AIDS), in McGinnis MR (ed): *Current Topics in Medical Mycology*, Vol I. New York, Springer-Verlag, 1985, pp 1–23.
17. Cheeseman MM, Cherniak R, Jones RG, Reiss E: Structure heterogeneity in the capsular polysaccharides of *Cryptococcus neoformans* serotype A. *33rd Southwest/37th Southeast Regional ACS Meeting and Mid-South Chromatography Symposium*. Abst 118, 1985.
18. Cherniak R, Reiss E, Slodki ME, Plattner RD, Blumer SO: Structure and antigenic activity of the capsular polysaccharide from *Cryptococcus neoformans* serotype A. *Mol Immunol* 17:1025–1032, 1980.
19. Cherniak R, Reiss E, Turner SH: A galactoxylomannan antigen of *Cryptococcus neoformans* serotype A. *Carbohydr Res* 103:239–250, 1982.
20. Cherniak R, Jones RG, Reiss E: Structure elucidation of *Cryptococcus neoformans* serotype A glucuronoxylomannan by ^{13}C-nuclear magnetic resonance spectroscopy. *Abstr Ann Mtg Am Soc Microbiol*, 84th Annual Meeting. Abst F8:294, 1984.
21. Cherniak R, Jones RG, Reiss E: Structure determination of *Cryptococcus neoformans* serotype A-variant glucuronoxylomannan by ^{13}C-nmr spectroscopy. *Carbohydr Res* in press.
22. Diamond RD, Root RK, Bennett JE: Factors influencing killing of *Cryptococcus neoformans* by human leukocytes in vitro. *J Infect Dis* 125:367–376, 1972.
23. Evans EE: An immunologic comparison of twelve strains of *Cryptococcus neoformans* (*Torula histolytica*). *Proc Soc Exp Biol Med* 71:644–646, 1949.
24. Evans EE: The antigenic composition of *Cryptococcus neoformans*. I. A serologic classification by means of the capsular and agglutination reactions. *J Immunol* 64:423–430, 1950.
25. Evans EE, Kessel JF: The antigenic composition of *Cryptococcus neoformans*. II. Studies with capsular polysaccharide. *J Immunol* 67:109–114, 1951.
26. Evans EE, Mehl SW: A qualitative analysis of capsular polysaccharides from *Cryptococcus neoformans* by filter paper chromatography. *Science* 114:10–11, 1951.
27. Evans EE, Theriault RJ: The antigenic composition of *Cryptococcus neoformans*. IV. The use of paper chromatography for following purification of capsular polysaccharide. *J Bacteriol* 65:571–577, 1953.
28. Farhi F, Bulmer GS, Tacker JR: *Cryptococcus neoformans* IV. The not-so-encapsulated yeast. *Infect Immun* 1:526–531, 1970.
29. Fleet GH: Composition and structure of yeast cell walls, in McGinnis MR (ed): *Current Topics in Medical Mycology*, Vol I. New York, Springer-Verlag, 1985, pp 24–26.
30. Fromtling RA, Shadomy HJ, Jacobson ES: Decreased virulence in stable, acapsular mutants of *Cryptococcus neoformans*. *Mycopathologia* 79:23–29, 1982.
31. Gorin PAJ: Rationalization of carbon-13 magnetic resonance spectra of yeast mannans and structurally related oligosaccharides. *Can J Chem* 51:2325–2383, 1973.

32. Gorin PAJ: Carbon-13 nuclear magnetic resonance spectroscopy of polysaccharides. *Adv Carbohydr Chem Biochem* 38:13–104, 1981.
33. Harris PJ, Henry RJ, Blakeney AB, Stove BA: An improved procedure for the methylation analysis of oligosaccharides and polysaccharides. *Carbohydr Res* 127:59–73, 1984.
34. Ikeda R, Shinoda T, Fukazawa Y, Kaufman L: Antigenic characterization of *Cryptococcus neoformans* serotypes and its application to serotyping of clinical isolates. *J Clin Microbiol* 16:22–29, 1982.
35. Ikeda R, Nishikawa A, Shinoda T, Fukazawa Y: Chemical characterization of capsular polysaccharide from *Cryptococcus neoformans* serotype A-D. *Microbiol Immunol* 29:981–991, 1985.
36. Jacobson ES, Ayers DJ, Harrell AC, Nicholas CC: Genetic and phenotypic characterization of capsule mutants of *Cryptococcus neoformans*. *J Bacteriol* 150:1292–1296, 1982.
37. James PG, Cherniak R, Jones RG, Reiss E: Cell wall glucans of *Cryptococcus neoformans* cap 67. *XIII Int'l Carbohydr Symp Abstr* B57, 1986.
38. Kaplan W, Bragg SL, Crane S, Ahearn DG: Serotyping *Cryptococcus neoformans* by immunofluorescence. *J Clin Microbiol* 14:313–37, 1981.
39. Kozel TR, Cazin, Jr J: Nonencapsulated variant of *Cryptococcus neoformans*. I. Virulence studies and characterization of soluble polysaccharides. *Infect Immun* 3:287–294, 1971.
40. Kozel TR, Cazin, Jr J: Immune response to *Cryptococcus neoformans* soluble polysaccharide. I. Serological assay for antigen and antibody. *Infect Immun* 5:35–41, 1972.
41. Kozel TR, Mastroianni RP: Inhibition of phagocytosis by cryptococcal polysaccharide: Dissociation of the attachment and ingestion phases of phagocytosis. *Infect Immun* 14:62–67, 1976.
42. Kozel TR: Nonencapsulated variant of *Cryptococcus neoformans*. II. Surface receptors for cryptococcal polysaccharide and their role in inhibition of phagocytosis by polysaccharide. *Infect Immun* 16:99–106, 1977.
43. Kozel TR, Gulley WF, Cazin, Jr J: Immune response to *Cryptococcus neoformans* soluble polysaccharide: Immunological unresponsiveness. *Infect Immun* 18:701–707, 1977.
44. Kozel TR, McGaw TG: Opsonization of *Cryptococcus neoformans* by human immunoglobulin G: Role of immunoglobulin G in phagocytosis by macrophages. *Infect Immun* 25:255–261, 1979.
45. Lindberg B, Lonngren J, Powell DA: Structural studies on the specific type 14 pneumococcal polysaccharide. *Carbohydr Res* 58:177–186, 1977.
46. Merrifield EH, Stephen AM: Structural investigations of two capsular polysaccharides from *Cryptococcus neoformans*. *Carbohydr Res* 86:69–76, 1980.
47. Mishra SK, Staib F, Folkens U, Fromtling RA: Serotypes of *Cryptococcus neoformans* strains isolated in Germany. *J Clin Microbiol* 14:106–107, 1981.
48. Miyazaki T: Studies on fungal polysaccharides. I. On the isolation and chemical properties of the capsular polysaccharide from *Cryptococcus neoformans*. *Chem Pharm Bull* 9:715–718, 1961.
49. Miyazaki T: Studies on fungal polysaccharides. II. On the componential sugars and partial hydrolysis of the capsular polysaccharide from *Cryptococcus neoformans*. *Chem Pharm Bull* 9:826–829, 1961.
50. Miyazaki T: Studies on fungal polysaccharides. III. Chemical structure of the capsular polysaccharide from *Cryptococcus neoformans*. *Chem Pharm Bull* 9:829–833, 1961.
51. Murphy JW, Cozad GC: Immunological unresponsiveness induced by cryptococcal capsular polysaccharide assayed by the hemolytic plaque technique. *Infect Immun* 5:896–901, 1972.

52. Perfect JR, Lang SDR, Durak DT: Chronic cryptococcal meningitis. *Am J Pathol* 101:177–193, 1980.
53. Rebers PA, Barker SA, Heidelberger M, Dische Z, Evans EE: Precipitation of the specific polysaccharide of *Cryptococcus neoformans* A by types II and XIV antipneumococcal sera. *J Am Chem Soc* 80:1135–1137, 1958.
54. Reiss E, Cherniak R, Eby R, Kaufman L: Enzyme immunoassay detection of IgM to galactoxylomannan of *Cryptococcus neoformans*. *Diag Immunol* 2:109–115, 1984.
55. Reiss E: *Molecular Immunology of Mycotic and Actinomycotic Infections*. New York, Elsevier, 1986, pp 251–280.
56. Rhodes JC, Wicker LS, Urba WJ: Genetic control of susceptibility to *Cryptococcus neoformans* in mice. *Infect Immun* 29:494–499, 1980.
57. Robbins JB: Vaccines for the prevention of encapsulated bacterial diseases, current status, problems and prospects for the future. *Immunochemistry* 15:839–854, 1978.
58. Ross A, Taylor IEP: Extracellular glycoprotein from virulent and avirulent cryptococcus species. *Infect Immun* 31:911–918, 1981.
59. San-Blas G: The cell wall of fungal human pathogens: Its possible role in host-parasite relationships. *Mycopathologia* 79:159–184, 1982.
60. Shinoda T, Ikeda R, Nishikawa A, Fukazawa Y: The serological, chemical and physiochemical analyses of cryptococcal capsular polysaccharides. *Jpn J Med Mycol* 21:230–238, 1980.
61. Small JM, Mitchell TG, Wheat RW: Strain variation in composition and molecular size of the capsular polysaccharide of *Cryptococcus neoformans* serotype A. *Infect Immun* 54:735–741, 1986.
62. Staib F, Mishra SK, Grosse G, Abel R: Pathogenesis and therapy of cryptococcosis in animal experiments, in AM Beemer, A Ben-David, MA Klingberg, and ES Kuttin (eds): *Host-Parasite Relationships in Systemic Mycoses*. Part I. Proceedings of 21st Annual OHOLO Biological Conference. Ma'alot, Israel, March 1977. Basel, Karger, 1977, pp 48–59.
63. Tacker JR, Farhi F, Bulmer GS: Intracellular fate of *Cryptococcus neoformans*. *Infect Immun* 6:162–167, 1972.
64. Turner SH, Cherniak R, Reiss E: Fractionation and characterization of galactoxylomannan from *Cryptococcus neoformans*. *Carbohydr Res* 125:343–349, 1984.
65. Wilson DE, Bennett JE, Bailey JW: Serologic grouping of *Cryptococcus neoformans*. *Proc Soc Exp Biol Med* 127:820–832, 1968.

3—Tinea Imbricata

Roderick J. Hay

Tinea imbricata is the name given to infections caused by the dermatophytic fungus *Trichophyton concentricum*. The organism is an anthropophilic species and has no known natural reservoir other than humans. For a long time, tinea imbricata has captured the imagination of anthropologists, dermatologists, and medical mycologists because of its unusual geographic distribution and clinical appearances. The infection is found in endemic foci in the Far East, West Pacific, and parts of Central and South America. Infected individuals are frequently living in isolated and primitive conditions. The clinical features of tinea imbricata are dramatic. Many of those affected have more than half of their body surface area covered by loose or concentric rings of scales. From the large loose scales seen particularly on extensor surfaces of the arms the name imbricata (Latin, "tiled") is derived. The characteristic concentric rings of confluent scaling that cover the trunk and limbs with a bizarre pattern are used to describe the causative organism *T. concentricum*.

Tinea imbricata is not just a curiosity among dermatophyte infections. It has an important role to play in furthering our understanding of a number of factors concerned with the transmission of skin infections, susceptibility and resistance, as well as providing a challenge in therapy. This review is concerned with thc infcction itself as well as its relationship to other skin diseases that illustrate similar problems.

Epidemiology

The distribution of tinea imbricata is shown in Fig. 3-1. It is not clear where tinea imbricata originated in the Far East; travel and migration have obscured the picture. However, the disease has a scattered and patchy distribution throughout many of the islands of the West Pacific and Indonesia as well as the Philippines. The explorer William Dampier reported the characteristic appearances of the infection in the 17th Century on the island of Mindanao

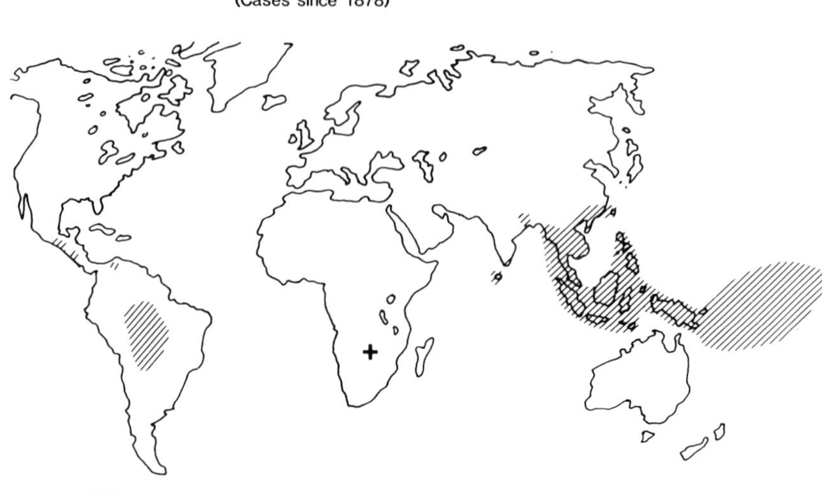

FIG. 3-1. Distribution map of endemic areas for reported cases of tinea imbricata.

in the Philippines. Sporadic reports of the disease were made subsequently, until 1878 when Manson described a case in Amoy, China, and wrote a full description with a report on experimental infection (33). Manson suggested that his patient had been infected in Malaya and had imported the infection into China. Subsequently the disease was reported sporadically in other parts of China (6) as well as Taiwan. The disease also has been described in Thailand (11), Vietnam, and Burma, although there are few recent reports from the latter areas. In Malaysia the disease is mainly confined to aboriginal populations (38). Dey and Maplestone (13) reported cases from Assam in northeastern India and cited examples of the disease in East Bengal and southern India. In the early part of this century, Castellani reported cases of tinea imbricata in Sri Lanka (9).

Pijper's (37) case from the Transvaal in South Africa was not supported by culture, and from the description the lesions might have been caused by another dermatophyte. The organism isolated was described as showing greenish pigmentation and was almost certainly a contaminant such as an *Aspergillus* species. No other confirmed cases have been reported from Africa. Tinea imbricata also has been described in South and Central America. Most cases have originated from Brazil. Roquette-Pinto (41) observed a persistent skin disease in the Indians of the Sierra do Norte in northwestern Brazil, but was unable to confirm the diagnosis. However, it seems likely that the disease observed was tinea imbricata. Da Fonseca (18) subsequently found cases of the infection in another part of western Brazil, and the disease is now known to exist among a number of tribes in central Brazil and the Amazon region.

The disease also is described in parts of Central America. In Guatemala, for instance, tinea imbricata has been described from a number of areas (17). There are also cases of the infection in Mexico, including the Sierra de Puebla (46) as well as zones near the Guatemalan border. In the former area the climate is only moderately humid and the mean altitude is approximately 2,500 m. The disease also shows some differences from those observed elsewhere. For instance many patients show spontaneous remission or cure with minimal therapy. In some cases improvement has been recorded in colder seasons with relapse occuring when the warm weather returns.

Cases also have been recorded from El Salvador and Colombia, but there have been no recent reports of the disease in these countries.

The distribution of tinea imbricata with two major foci of infection, occurring in the West Pacific region including many of the Polynesian islands and remote areas of South America has given rise to speculation on the relationship between the two communities. Tinea imbricata is an anthropophilic dermatophyte infection which is confined to isolated communities. Close contact with infected persons or fomites is required for spread. It seems likely from the reports of early European explorers that it was endemic in the Far East at least two centuries before its scientific "discovery." In consequence it has been suggested that the disease is of great antiquity and provides evidence for the colonization of South America by peoples originating from Polynesia lending credence to the reverse of the Kontiki legend (19). An alternative hypothesis, that it was already in existence when the original colonization of the Americas from Asia across a landbridge which previously joined the two sides of the Bering Straits, is equally fascinating as it would imply that tinea imbricata may be the forerunner of other dermatophyte infections. A further possibility, that it was transmitted with fomites from one area to another or with a single infected individual at a later event, is less exciting but equally plausible. At present there is no evidence that organisms isolated from the two geographic areas are different.

The reasons for the unusual geographic distribution of tinea imbricata still must remain speculative. However, subsequent experience would suggest that the infection is not easily transmitted to outsiders unless they share a close living or working environment with the indigenous population of an endemic area.

The Organism

The causative organism of tinea imbricata is the dermatophyte *Trichophyton concentricum*. The fungus had been assigned previously to other genera. The genus *Lepidophyton*, for instance was used but the organism described was almost certainly an *Aspergillus* species. Castellani described two organisms, *Endodermophyton tropicale* and *E. indicum* in classical cases of tinea imbricata (9, 10). Two other *Endodermophyton* species, *E. concentricum* and *E. mansonii*, were isolated from tinea intersecta, a more localized form of dermatophyte infection, whose relation to tinea imbricata is unclear. The species were separated by the intensity and speed of development of pigmentation. A further species, *E. roquettei*, was added later (18).

In a report of a case of tinea imbricata from Guatemala, Figueroa and Conant (17) discussed the classification of the organism and stated that there were insufficient grounds for distinguishing a number of different species. They also established that the name *Trichophyton concentricum* (4) should hold precedence. This view is upheld at present (40).

Trichophyton concentricum produces folded colonies on Sabouraud glucose agar. Young colonies are usually smooth, but later aerial mycelium may develop. Colonies are usually white to yellow with a fine powdery down prominent on the edges. The yellow pigment may diffuse into the medium. The under surface of the colony shows radiating folds and is dark yellow or tan in color. The pigmentation may be darker and approach a red or black color on 4% glucose agar (10). A substantial number of isolates of *T. concentricum* are stimulated by the presence of thiamine (16, 40).

The microscopic appearance of *T. concentricum* colonies is unexceptional. Irregular branching hyphae are seen. Microconidia are not present but rarely lateral macroconidia have been described (14), which may show blunt tips more suggestive of *Epidermophyton floccosum*. Such macroconidia are sparsely distributed in cultures.

Most authors have not experienced great difficulty in culturing the organism from skin scales, although Castellani and Chalmers (10) suggest softening scales in alcohol before inoculating material into glucose broth. A greater problem is secondary contamination of scales, particularly if these are held for any period of time, with environmental organisms such as aspergilli. The direct microscopy of skin scales is not typical, although there are usually large numbers of hyphae present.

Experimental Tinea Imbricata

A number of attempts have been made to establish experimental tinea imbricata infections in humans or animals. For instance, in one of the earliest reports of the disease, Manson (33) demonstrated transmission in humans. In a more detailed study (34), transmission of cultured organisms on wet gauze held against the skin was demonstrated in humans. Second infections could be established in humans, and weak positive 24-hour skin test responses were established after 6 weeks in some but not all subjects. In guinea pigs the same authors established more florid infections, some of which showed hair shaft invasion of both endo- and ectothrix types. In guinea pigs some protection was afforded by a previous infection. In a later study, guinea pigs sensitized by intradermal infections of *T. concentricum* cytoplasmic antigen in Freund's complete adjuvant were found to develop delayed type hypersensitivity to subsequent intradermal challenge with the same antigen as well as antigens from *T. rubrum*, *T. mentagrophytes* var. *interdigitale*, and, to a lesser extent, *T. verrucosum* (27).

These studies establish that tinea imbricata is not difficult to transmit in humans and that immunity, as indicated by skin test reactivity is variable in humans after experimental infection but can be established in guinea pigs. Cross-reactivity with other dermatophyte species is seen.

Clinical Features

The clinical appearances of tinea imbricata have been described by a number of authors (eg, 10, 19, 38). The most characteristic and well-described appearance is the development of confluent lesions with concentric rings of scales (Fig. 3-2), giving the appearance of sequential waves of scaling (Fig. 3-3) that may cover large areas of the body. In other cases the patterns are modified, consisting of diffuse scales or large areas of scaling.

In a recent survey of 102 patients in Papua New Guinea seven clinical patterns of tinea imbricata were distinguished (28) (Table 3-1). The concentric pattern was seen in 100 patients in at least one site and was the commonest and most extensive form. Individual plaques tended to coalesce to give a "rippled" pattern of scales over a wide area of the body. The concentric pattern was commonest over the trunk, face, and upper limbs (Fig. 3-4). Large scales, which were easily detached, were seen in 34 patients. Individual scales were between 1–2 cm long and usually irregular in shape. In eight patients lichenified lesions were seen (Fig. 3-5). All were older than 20 years of age, and the anterior cubital fossae were the commonest sites affected. These patients usually complained of severe pruritus. In three patients the lesions were annular but thickened and hyperpigmented. Clinically they were similar to the pattern of *T. rubrum* infection seen in the area. However, *T. concentricum* was isolated from these patients. This form of the disease was called annular or "ringworm-like." Two patients had solitary patches or plaques (plaque type) of scaling on the skin. In one of these the more typical pattern of concentric scaling was beginning at the edge and they may therefore represent early lesions (10). On the palms, scales were loose and irregularly distributed, particularly on the sides of the fingers. Scaling on the soles was less obvious, and a moccasin pattern typical of *T. rubrum* infections could not be distinguished. In only five cases was scaling of the sole accompanied by positive cultural isolation. Although onychomycosis has been described (19), a nail dystrophy compatible with fungal infection was only seen in four patients. In

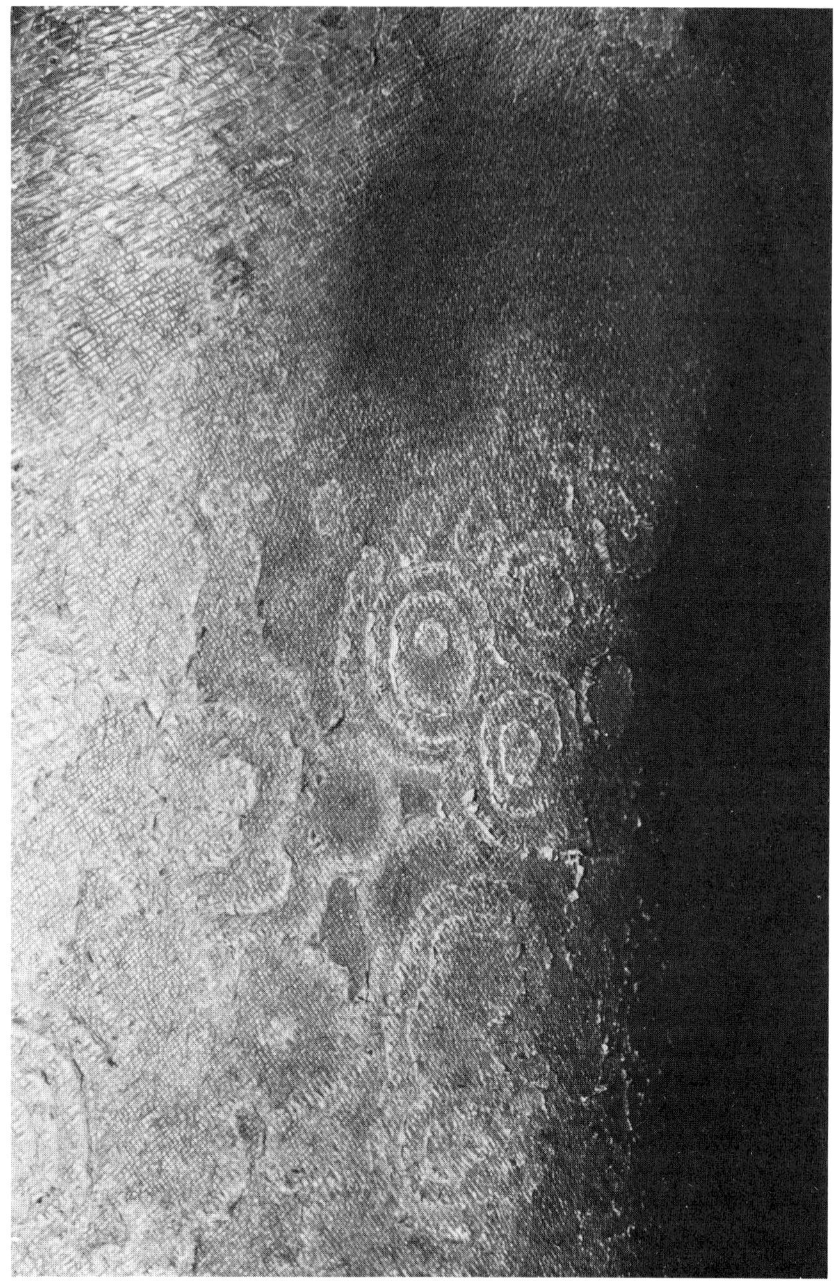

FIG. 3-2. Tinea imbricata—concentric pattern.

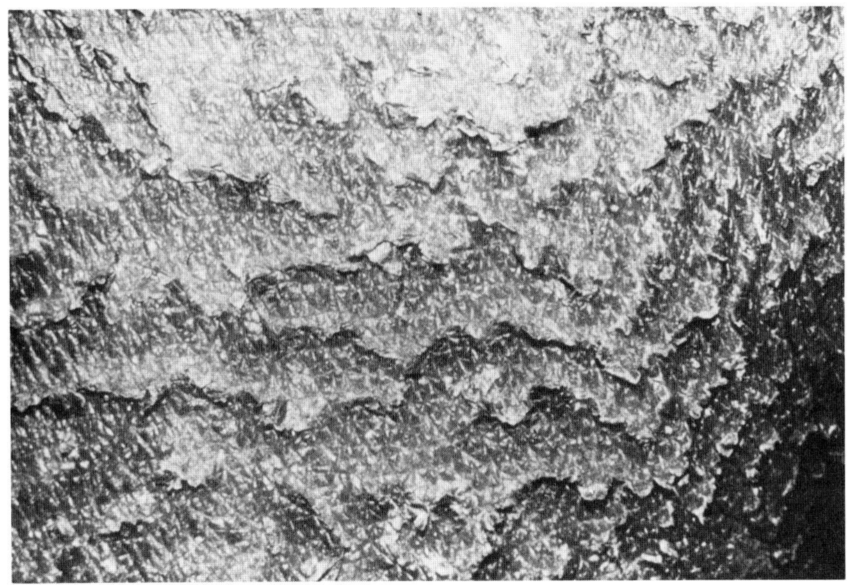

FIG. 3-3. Fusion of concentric scales of tinea imbricata.

TABLE 3-1. Clinical Pattern of Tinea Imbricata

1. Concentric		
2. Lamellar	—	Extensor surfaces, eg, forearms
3. Lichenified	—	In elbows, behind knees
4. Plaque-type	—	Common in relapsing disease
5. Annular (ringworm-like)		
6. Palmar/plantar		
7. Onychomycosis	—	Not supported by culture

only one patient with fingernail dystrophy did the affected nail contain hyphal elements on direct microscopy, but cultural studies were negative. The nail showed distal thickening and opacification but without significant onycholysis. It is therefore not possible from this study to comment on the existence of onychomycosis in tinea imbricata. Although suspected by a number of investigators, cultural confirmation is not available.

Most cases of tinea imbricata seen in this survey showed hypopigmentation. In some cases this was striking and may have led to sun-induced atrophic changes on the face of some patients. Hypopigmentation may be less common in other groups studied (19).

Polunin (38) found that in Malaysia the infection was of equal sex incidence, whereas Castellani reported more cases in males than females (9). In

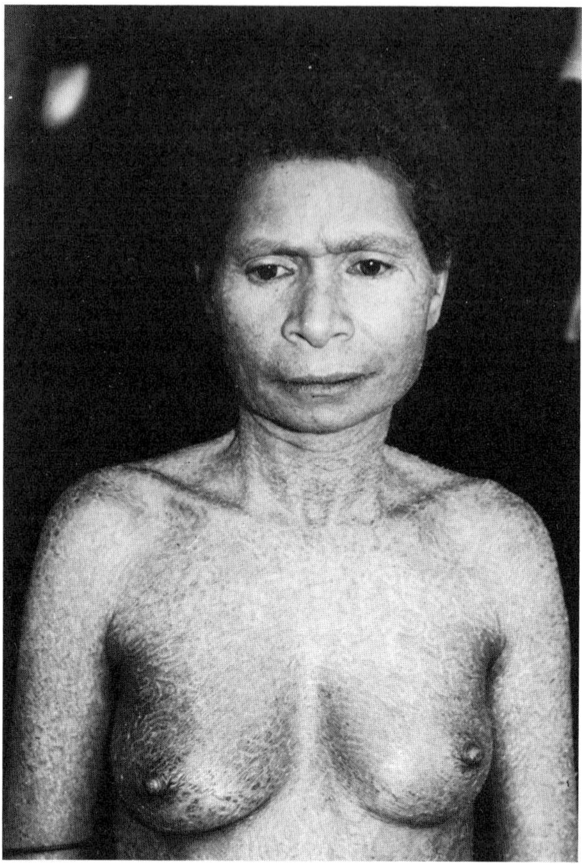

FIG. 3-4. Concentric tinea imbricata affecting upper trunk and face.

the study described previously (28), males predominated (56 versus 46); in children younger than 12 with the infection, 79% (26) were male and 12% (7) were female, whereas in older children and adults, females predominated 57% (39). Sex also appeared to have some effect on the distribution of the lesions. For instance, the face or ears were affected in 77% (30 of 59) of adult women and 65% (22 of 34) of children less than 12 years old compared with only 34% (10 of 28) of men. Although scalp involvement was seen, no examples of hair infection were recorded.

Some authors have recorded sparing of the groin and axillae (28, 38), although in individual cases these may be affected (6). It is possible that the local skin surface environment in these sites is not usually conducive to growth of the fungi. If this is so, *T. concentricum* would be quite different from other anthropophilic dermatophytes in this respect.

The symptoms of tinea imbricata are variable. Some patients appear to be

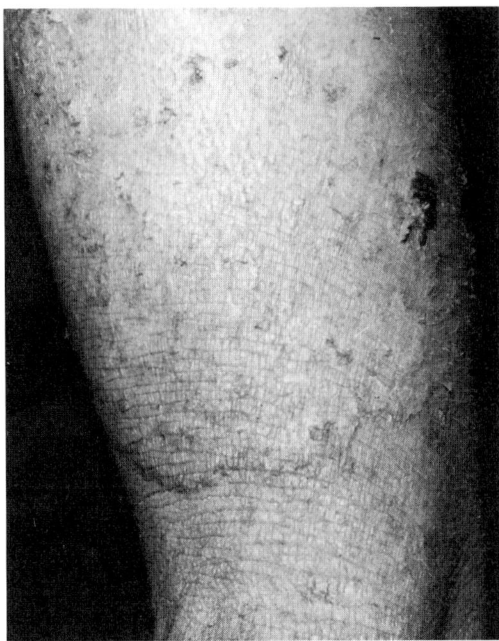

FIG. 3-5. Lichenified tinea imbricata on the arm. The patient is an albino.

little affected by the disease, whereas others are severely troubled by itching (10). Some degree of irritation is usual.

The clinical patterns of tinea imbricata change to some extent in different geographic or ethnic groups. For instance, the lamellar pattern where large numbers of loose scales are seen is the predominant form in some Brazilian Indians (41). The latter author also described the presence of vesicles in these patients. Although it is often stated that the pattern of disease is different in the nonindigenous population of an endemic area, this is not always the case. Certainly, fewer cases are described in this group (38), but there are a number of reports of very extensive tinea imbricata in Europeans infected in the Far East, which suggest that the ethnic origin of the patient is not a determinant of the extent of the infection (3, 12, 44).

Associated Conditions

Although there are individual case reports of tinea imbricata coexisting with other skin infections including other forms of dermatophytosis (44), there has been little to suggest that patients are unduly susceptible to skin infection (28). In the latter study the absence of pityriasis versicolor in the infected patients

was very common. Although the disease may coexist with tropical sore (47), there is nothing to suggest that patients with the latter are more susceptible to tinea imbricata. There is also no known association between other infections, including chest disease and malaria, and tinea imbricata.

In a study of climatic factors in tinea imbricata, MacLennan and O'Keefe (32) showed a negative correlation between altitude and tinea imbricata in the Asai valley of northern Papua New Guinea. They also noted that scaling was less profuse at higher altitudes. In a previous survey in a different area in New Guinea, Maprik, a correlation between failure to gain weight and tinea imbricata in infants was noted (42). Onset of the infection was common in infants who showed a transient slowing in the normal rate of weight gain. There was also less tinea imbricata in the heavier adults, although the authors pointed out that this could be accounted for by the fact that affected women tended to marry later and showed less weight gain than their uninfected contemporaries. There was no correlation between hemoglobin concentration or hepatomegaly and the disease, although patients sometimes developed tinea imbricata after an episode of bacillary dysentery or after pregnancy. The latter finding has not been a feature of surveys in other areas (28). Apart from the observations on poor weight gain and tinea imbricata described above (32), consistent differences in endemic areas between the disease and nutritional indexes have not been discovered (35,47).

A number of investigators have reported a high peripheral blood eosinophilia in patients with tinea imbricata. Castellani, working in Ceylon (9), described eosinophilia of 6–16% in infected individuals. Gomez (20) in Guatemala reports eosinophil counts of 12.0–17.6%. It is not possible to distinguish between eosinophilia due to tinea imbricata or a coexistent parasitic infection. For instance, in the latter survey most patients had intestinal infestations with either *Uncinaria*, *Ascaris*, or *Trichocephalus*.

Genetic Susceptibility

The prevalence of tinea imbricata in endemic areas and the tendency for several individuals of the same family to be affected have lent support to the possibility that susceptibility may be genetically determined. There are now a number of studies which throw light on this aspect of the disease.

In the first study patients with tinea imbricata in the Gogol Valley in northern Papua New Guinea were investigated (43). Detailed records were made of the prevalence of the disease within families. The technique for analysis used had originally been applied to the comparison of blood groups in a defined population. The method is based on the Hardy-Weinberg equilibrium, which allows the application of Mendelian genetic analyses to a large population assuming that the mutation rate is low and that the numbers of surviving progeny do not alter significantly from generation to generation. The actual and expected ratios of affected and nonaffected individuals within

TABLE 3-2. Tinea Imbricata on Goodenough Island—Test for Autosomal Recessive Inheritance*

Mating Type	No. of Families	No. of Families with Affected Child			No. of Affected Children		
		Observed	Expected	Variance	Observed	Expected	Variance
A Tl × Tl	35	35	13.2	8.1	78		
B Tl × ti	41	29			51	81	30.3
C ti × ti	51	47			70	97.6	29.4

* Gene frequency 0.57.
$\chi^2 = 59$ (A), 30 (B), 26 (C).

families are then compared assuming the different modes of inheritance. An equal or nearly equal sex incidence of the disease, for instance, tends to exclude a sex-linked recessive mode of transmission of susceptibility. Using these methods, Serjeantson and Lawrence (43) concluded that the pattern of distribution of tinea imbricata within the population studied was compatible with the transmission of an autosomal recessive susceptibility gene.

In a more detailed study of the disease in northern Papua New Guinea, a second group (39) reached similar conclusions. They pointed out that it was not possible to exclude the operation of an autosomal dominant gene showing incomplete penetration. This second study also took into account the possibility of individuals recovering from the infection, spontaneously or after treatment, who might otherwise be included as unaffected subjects.

In a third study carried out in Milne Bay Province, Papua New Guinea (Hay et al, unpublished data), a different conclusion was drawn. Included in the survey were 384 individuals from 127 families. An analysis (abbreviated) for autosomal recessive inheritance is shown in Table 3-2. The numbers of affected and unaffected children born to marriages between affected (homozygous) and unaffected (heterozygous or noncarriers) parents are shown. In this survey the results do not support a role for an autosomally recessive transmitted trait regulating susceptibility, although as with other surveys, an autosomal dominant gene with incomplete, but not complete, penetrance was a possibility (Table 3-3). In a few families the pattern of inheritance was compatible with an autosomal recessive mode of inheritance. Hence, the study does not completely exclude a genetic mechanism determining susceptibility. There are potentially important differences between the latter and previous investigations. Firstly, the disease was commoner in the general population affecting, for instance, 34% of the children at a local school, and the gene frequency, assuming a genetic mechanism, would be 0.57 compared with 0.43 or 0.49 in the other surveys. The groups studied also originated from two distinct areas, northwestern Papua New Guinea and an island off the eastern tip of the country.

TABLE 3-3. Tinea Imbricata on Goodenough Island—Test for Autosomal Dominant Inheritance

	Offspring of Parent with a Healthy Spouse		
Offspring	Normal	Affected	Total
Observed	119	53	172
Expected	86	86	172

$\chi^2 = 25.34$; $P < 0.001$.
Susceptibility is unlikely to be an autosomal dominant trait with complete penetrance, but incomplete penetrance is not excluded.

Immunity

There have been few studies of the host immune response in tinea imbricata. Observation of cases has suggested to many investigators that spontaneous resolution is rare and that relapse is common if patients are reexposed to disease. Both facts suggest that immunity is neither very effective nor long lived. Clinically the behavior of the disease is similar to that seen in "dry type" chronic *T. rubrum* infections (24, 25). However, there is an important difference in that tinea imbricata is usually very widespread, spares privileged sites such as nails and soles, but is associated with infiltration of skin with many hyphae presumably reflecting a high antigen load. Localization of dermatophyte infections in thickly keratinized sites affects the antibody and cell-mediated responses to the organisms (2). Tinea imbricata therefore is an infection in which the site of lesions should not compromise the host's immune response.

MacLennan (31) tested a group of patients with tinea imbricata using intradermal trichophytin (Hollister-Steir, USA). Although the antigen was not derived from the same species, a large proportion of patients showed immediate type hypersensitivity to the trichophytin (82% in males, 70% in females). Only 5% showed delayed type hypersensitivity. In a further study using a cytoplasmic antigen derived from *T. concentricum*, a second group showed similar responses (27), with 52 and 46% of patients (total 68) showing immediate type hypersensitivity (ITH) or negative responses to intradermal trichophytin. Only 9% (6) had delayed type (DTH) skin reactions over 5 mm in diameter, and of these four also showed ITH. There was no correlation between duration and extent of infection and ITH. Using a similar antigen the in vitro cell-mediated immune responses of patients and unaffected controls as assessed using the leukocyte migration inhibition test were not statistically different. It was noted that patients with less than 30% of the body surface area involved were significantly more likely to have migration indexes below as opposed to above 0.7 ($P < 0.5$, Fisher's test). Conversely 78% of 53 patients showed antibodies to *T. concentricum* using counterimmunoelectrophoresis. This suggests that although the formation of detectable antibody is a common feature of *T. concentricum* infections, specifically activated cell-mediated immune responses do not occur except in infections of limited extent. It is not clear whether this represents a primary defect in the initiation of a T-cell-mediated response or the intervention of a suppressor or blocking mechanism. There is no evidence at present that suppressor T-cells are recruited in tinea imbricata as they appear to be in other forms of chronic dermatophytosis (36). Other possibilities include a blocking mechanism involving antibody, circulating antigen, or immune complexes. It has been shown subsequently that although both infected and uninfected controls have elevated total serum IgE levels, only those with tinea imbricata have raised specific IgE antibody titers to *T. concentricum* (29). A further possibility is that histamine released from mast cells bearing specific IgE inhibits T-lymphocyte activation (5).

Treatment

In only a few patients is there a spontaneous remission, and therefore treatment is usually necessary. Unfortunately, if the patient remains in an endemic area, reinfection is highly likely in view of the absence of effective host resistance. The other problem is the extensive nature of the infection. This makes topical treatment very difficult to carry out effectively in view of the problems in covering all affected areas with medication. The most consistent results are obtained with oral griseofulvin.

The older forms of treatment which were reported to be effective included tincture of Benzoin, chrysarobin, iodine linament, and even 40% formalin. Whitfield's ointment is successful in some cases. In most areas local plants may be used as treatment. For instance in Papua New Guinea the leaves of *Cassia alata* are rubbed vigorously into skin lesions. Rapid cures for topically applied imidazole antifungals such as econazole have also been reported (15), although compliance is a problem in view of the extent of the lesions.

Griseofulvin in normal doses is rapidly effective in tinea imbricata, although some reports suggest that doses in adults need to be increased from 1.0–1.5 g daily. Remission is usually seen within 3–4 weeks of initiating treatment (12), although relapse can occur even if the patient does not return to an endemic area. The value of ketoconazole in tinea imbricata has not been fully evaluated. In one study (Reid, personal communication) less than 30% of those treated had responded within 1 month of therapy. In 28 isolates of *T. concentricum* from Papua New Guinea tested for in vitro sensitivity to ketoconazole, the mean inhibitory concentration was 22 mg/l (range, 1.8–50). This is much higher than for other dermatophytes and may explain the disappointing response seen in this area (Hay and Clayton, unpublished data).

Discussion

Tinea imbricata is therefore a distinctive disease because of its unusual clinical appearances, behavior, and geographic distribution. The development of concentric rings of scales is a unique feature for a dermatophyte infection. The appearance of the disease in small isolated communities is somewhat reminiscent of the spread of favus in some countries, and its prevalence in endemically affected villages suggests that it is easily transmitted to other humans. Despite this the infection characteristically involves large areas of the body surface with a heavy antigen load, but from the subsequent clinical behavior and the immunologic findings reported previously there would appear to be little or no effective resistance.

Resistance to dermatophyte infections depends on a number of factors which have been reviewed recently (1, 22, 26), and some of the conclusions are summarized below. Firstly, there is evidence of "innate" host resistance to dermatophytes which is not dependent on prior sensitization. For instance, nonimmune serum may inhibit the growth of dermatophytes and this effect is believed to be mediated, at least in part, by unsaturated transferrin. Other factors which have not been characterized as yet may also be involved. A second factor which has been implicated is the presence of certain unsaturated fatty acids in sebum. The appearance of inhibitory fatty acids in postpubertal sebaceous secretions is believed to be important in preventing scalp ringworm in older children. Other resistance mechanisms include increased epidermal cell turnover under the affected area of skin. The stimulus for this increased growth has not been categorized. In experimental candidosis in guinea pigs, maximum rates of increased turnover appear about 8 days after infection, suggesting that sensitization is required for this phenomenon (45). However, in dermatophyte infections of guinea pig skin grafted on nude athymic mice, which are defective in functional T-lymphocytes, increased epidermal replication also is seen (23). These apparently contradictory observations could be reconciled if it could be shown that increased basal cell replication in epidermis was triggered by tissue damage caused by the dermatophytes but that the response could be amplified by an immune mechanism possibly involving T-lymphocytes. The role of nonimmune phagocytosis in dermatophytosis is largely unexplored. However, certain dermatophytes are chemotactic for neutrophils and can activate the alternative complement pathway. This may contribute to the inflammatory response.

Although antibodies may be formed in the course of human and experimental dermatophytosis, their role in host resistance remains dubious (21). However, in human and animal infections the appearance of activated T-lymphocytes and delayed type hypersensitivity to trichophytin correlates with the onset of clinical recovery. In an experimental dermatophyte infection in mice, resistance could be transferred to recipient animals with T-lymphocytes from sensitized donor mice. These findings strongly support a central role for cell-mediated immune responses in host resistance to dermatophytes

(7). The mechanism by which the activation of T-lymphocytes influences recovery during a dermatophyte infection is not clear. However, in chronically infected patients poor cell-mediated immune responses as measured by negative trichophytin tests or poor lymphocyte transformation to dermatophyte antigens are frequently found (24). As most of the chronic infections studied have been sporadically occurring dermatophytosis caused by *T. rubrum* affecting peripheral sites such as the palms or soles, it has been suggested that the limited extent of the infection and its location may contribute to the poor immune response (30).

Tinea imbricata provides a useful comparison for these other studies. Firstly, its clinical behavior suggests that effective immunity as judged by resistance to infection, may not develop during the course of the illness despite the presence of widespread skin involvement. However, the infection is sufficient to stimulate the development of a vigorous antibody response. It is possible therefore that the poor cell-mediated responses are a primary cause of persistent infection. By this theory patients predisposed, possibly genetically, to develop poor cell-mediated immune responses to this infection would be susceptible to chronic disease. Against this view is the finding that most investigators have commented on the rarity of spontaneous recovery suggesting that persistence is the usual response. Also there is no evidence of underlying susceptibility to other infections and therefore the defect would have to be specific to *T. concentricum*. Therefore, an alternative hypothesis is that affected patients show defective responses either because of some idiosyncrasy in antigen presentation or an inherent inability of the organism to elicit adequate T-cell-mediated immunity or because of modulation of the immune response after infection. Although the former two possibilities cannot be excluded, the latter is more likely in view of the observation of adequate leukocyte migration inhibition in patients with limited or early disease. Patients with tinea imbricata show a high level of immediate type hypersensitivity responses and specific IgE antibody to *T. concentricum*. There have been similar findings in other dermatophyte infections (24), and it has been suggested that a similar ITH reaction occurring in the infected skin site could result in the liberation of histamine which, in turn, will inhibit T-cell-mediated responses. Unlike other dermatophyte infections there is no evidence that atopics, who have an inherent capacity for developing IgE responses to antigenic challenge, are more susceptible to tinea imbricata; in the absence of widespread respiratory allergy or eczema the diagnosis of atopy is difficult to make in areas endemic for tinea imbricata. High IgE levels formed in response to nematode infestation may precondition the patients B-lymphocyte regulatory mechanisms to allow the preferential synthesis of IgE to other antigens, including *T. concentricum*. Other possible mechanisms that could regulate the T-lymphocyte response to tinea imbricata include blocking antibody or the presence of circulating antigen. The latter can be shown to cause persistence of dermatophyte lesions in mice (7).

Both immunologic and other factors are closely interrelated in determining the course of infection. In tinea imbricata the prevalence of the disease in endemic areas suggests that irrespective of the subsequent immune response dependent on sensitization it is possible that patients may be particularly susceptible to the disease. Here genetic factors (39) may play a part in determining susceptibility.

The study of tinea imbricata is not therefore of purely academic interest but may have an important bearing on our understanding of the events which govern susceptibility to infections of the skin from the first moment of contact with the organism to the development and regulation of the subsequent immune response. To those who have the disease, tinea imbricata is a chronic, itchy dermatosis which affects both health and social existence. The difficulties of ensuring permanent cure in affected patients who remain in the endemic area have been discussed previously. The application of mass chemotherapy is only likely to be successful if the transmission cycle of the disease from infected to treated patients can be interrupted in view of the low level of resistance soon after an infection. It is possible that immunization might provide a solution if effective immunity can be stimulated by this mechanism. But whatever the method chosen, tinea imbricata represents an important challenge to the control of infection within the community.

Acknowledgments

Some of the work discussed here was carried out in Milne Bay Province, Papua New Guinea and was supported by a grant from the Wellcome Trust, whose help is gratefully acknowledged. I would also like to thank Drs. Sophie Reid and Ed Talwat as well as Kay MacNamara for their invaluable assistance and the Papua New Guinea Ministry of Health for facilitating this investigation.

References

1. Ahmed AR: Immunology of human dermatophyte infection. *Arch Dermatol* 118:521–525, 1982.
2. Attapattu MC: Investigation of the humoral antibody response in patients with *Trichophyton rubrum* infections. Doctoral thesis, University of London, 1977.
3. Belisario JC, Havyatt MT: A case of tinea imbricata in a white boy treated with griseofulvin. *Dermatologia* 119:158–164, 1959.
4. Blanchard R: Parasites vegetaux a l'excursion des bacteries. *Traite Pathol Gen* 2:916–917, 1896.
5. Brostoff J, Pack S, Lydyard PM: Histamine suppression of lymphocyte activation. *Clin Exp Immunol* 39:739–743, 1980.
6. Burkwall HF: Tinea imbricata in Hainan. *Chin Med J* 51:93, 1937.
7. Calderon RA, Hay RJ: Cell-mediated immunity in experimental murine dermatophytosis. II. Adoptive transfer of immunity to dermatophyte infection by lymphoid cells from donors with acute or chronic infections. *Immunology* 53:465–472, 1984.

8. Castellani A: Further researches on the hyphomycetes of tinea imbricata. *J Trop Med Hyg* 14:81–83, 1911.
9. Castellani A: Tinea imbricata (Tokelau). *Br J Dermatol* 25:377–401, 1913.
10. Castellani A, Chalmers AJ: Genus *Endodermophyton*, in *Manual of Tropical Medicine*. London, Bacilliere, Tindall and Cox, 1919, pp 1016–1023.
11. Chermsirivathana S, Bronsri P: A case of tinea imbricata (Hanumaru ringworm) treated with fulcin. *Aust J Dermatol* 6:63–64, 1961.
12. Church R, Sneddon I: Tinea imbricata—a report of two cases treated with griseofulvin. *Lancet* i:1215–1216, 1962.
13. Dey NC, Maplestone PA: Tinea imbricata in India. *Indian Med Gazette* 78:5–11, 1942.
14. Dompmartin D, Drouhet ME: Aspects cliniques et mycologiques de tinea imbricata (Tokelau). *Bull Soc France Dermatol Syph* 77:186–190, 1970.
15. Dompmartin D, Drouhet E, Moreau F: Nouvelle enquete sur tinea imbricata (tokelau) et autres epidermomycoses tropicales en Oceanie (iles Nouvelles—Hebrides et Banks). *Bull Soc France Dermatol Syph* 82:422–427, 1975.
16. Drouhet E, Mariat F: Recherches sur la nutrition des dermatophytes l. Etude des besoin vitaminiques. *Ann Inst Pasteur Paris* 82:337, 1952.
17. Figueroa H, Conant NF: The first case of tinea imbricata caused by *Trichophyton concentricum* (Blanchard 1896) reported from Guatemala. *Am J Trop Med* 20:287, 1940.
18. Da Fonseca O: Sur l'etologie du chimbere, nouveau type de dermatose endemique des indiens du fleuve S. Miguel, *Endodermophyton Roquettei*. *CR Soc Biol* (Paris) 92:305–310, 1925.
19. Da Fonseca O: The endodermophycae: Tinea imbricata (tokelau-Chimbere), in March J (ed): *Essays on Tropical Dermatology*. Amsterdam, Excerpta Medica, 1972, pp 339–355.
20. Gomez JE: Tokelau in Guatemala. *Arch Dermatol* 53:243–248, 1946.
21. Grappel SF, Blank F, Bishop F: Circulating antibodies in dermatophytosis. *Dermatologica* 144:1–11, 1972.
22. Grappel SF, Bishop CT, Blank F: Immunology of dermatophytes and dermatophytosis. *Bacteriol Rev* 38:220–250, 1974.
23. Green F, Lee KW, Balish E: Chronic *T. mentagrophytes* dermatophytosis of guinea pig skin grafts on nude mice. *J Invest Dermatol* 79:125–129, 1982.
24. Hanifin JM, Ray LF, Lobitz WC: Immunological reactivity in dermatophytosis. *Br J Dermatol* 90:1–8, 1974.
25. Hay RJ: Chronic dermatophyte infections. I. Clinical and mycological features. *Br J Dermatol* 106:1–7, 1982.
26. Hay RJ: Fungal infection, in Mackie RM (ed): *Immunodermatology*. Edinburgh, Churchill Livingstone, 1984.
27. Hay RJ, Reid S, Talwat E, Macnamara K: Immune responses of patients with tinea imbricata. *Br J Dermatol* 108:581–586, 1983.
28. Hay RJ, Reid S, Talwat E, Macnamara K: Endemic tinea imbricata—a study on Goodenough Island, Papua New Guinea. *Trans Roy Soc Trop Med Hyg* 78:246–251, 1984.
29. Hay RJ, Shennan G: Antibody responses in tinea imbricata: The role of IgE. *Trans Roy Soc Trop Med Hyg* 78:653–655, 1984.
30. Kaaman T: Cell mediated reactivity in dermatophytosis: Differences in skin responses to purified trichophytin in tinea pedis and tinea cruris. *Acta Dermatovenereologica* 61:119–123, 1981.
31. MacLennan R: The trichophytin test in tinea imbricata. *Papua New Guinea Med J* 15:201–202, 1972.
32. MacLennan R, O'Keefe: Altitude and prevalence of tinea imbricata in New Guinea. *Trans Roy Soc Trop Med Hyg* 69:91–93, 1975.

33. Manson P: Notes on tinea imbricata, an undescribed species of body ringworm. *Med Rep* (China) 16:1–11, 1878.
34. Ota M, Kawatsure S: Inoculabilite au cobaye et immunologie des champignons parasites du genre Endodermophyton castellani. *Ann Parasitol* IX:144–161, 1931.
35. Peters WE: Tinea imbricata and malnutrition. *Trans Roy Soc Trop Med Hyg* 51:197–198, 1960.
36. Petrini B, Kaaman T: T lymphocyte subpopulations in patients with chronic dermatophytosis. *Int Arch All Appl Immunol* 66:105–111, 1981.
37. Pijper A: Tinea imbricata in South Africa. *J Trop Med Hyg* 21:45–47, 1918.
38. Polunin I: Tinea imbricata in Malaya. *Br J Dermatol* 64:378–384, 1952.
39. Ravine D, Turner KJ, Alpers MP: Genetic inheritance of susceptibility to tinea imbricata. *J Med Genet* 17:342–348, 1980.
40. Rebell G, Taplin D: In *Dermatophytes, their recognition and Identification.* Miami, University of Miami Press, 1974, p 61.
41. Roquette-Pinto E: Rondonia, anthropologia, ethnographia. *Arch Mus Noc Rio J* 20:1–26, 1917.
42. Schofield FD, Parkinson AD, Jeffrey D: Observations on the epidemiology, effects and treatment of tinea imbricata. *Trans Roy Soc Trop Med Hyg* 57:214–227, 1963.
43. Serjeantson S, Lawrence G: Autosomal recessive inheritance of susceptibility of tinea imbricata. *Lancet* i:13–15, 1977.
44. Sharvill D: Tinea imbricata in a European: Double infection with *Trichophyton concentricum* and *Trichophyton rubrum. Br J Dermatol* 64:373–377, 1952.
45. Sohnle PG, Frank MM, Kirkpatrick CH: Mechanisms involved in elimination of organisms from experimental cutaneous *Candida albicans* infection in guinea pigs. *J Immunol* 117:523–527, 1976.
46. Velasco-Castrejon O, Gonzales-Ochoa A: La tinea imbricata en la sierra de Puebla, Mexico. *Rev Inv Salud Publ* (Mexico) 35:109–116, 1975.
47. Vines AP: An epidemiological sample survey of the Highlands, Mainland and Island Regions of the territory of Papua New Guinea. PNG Department of Public Health Publication, 1970, pp 394–414.

4—Adhesion and Association Mechanisms of *Candida albicans*

MICHAEL J. KENNEDY

Candida albicans is commonly found residing in the oral cavity, gastrointestinal (GI) tract, and female genital tract of humans (197). The yeast is usually commensal, but in predisposed persons clinical infection can occur as the result of its opportunistic nature. In patients who are compromised immunologically and undergoing prolonged antimicrobic therapy, *C. albicans* can reach high numbers in the GI tract and, subsequently, pass through the intestinal mucosa to initiate systemic infection by the hematogenous route (196).

Although the determinants of colonization and dissemination from the GI tract by *C. albicans* have not been completely defined, it is likely that association with intestinal mucosal surfaces may play an important role (140). Colonization of the small intestine, from which dissemination of *Candida* is thought to occur (312), could not take place in the face of the rapid passage of material through the small intestine due to peristalsis, unless these organisms could associate with the mucosa. Moreover, prevention of *Candida* mucosal association by bacterial antagonism reduced gut colonization and dissemination by this fungus (138). Considering further the sloughing of epithelial cells and the bathing actions of fluids over host mucosal surfaces and various tissues, and the fact that *Candida* lesions may arise in virtually any tissue of the body, suggests that adhesion is also an important determinant of thrush and denture stomatitis, vaginitis, endocarditis, keratitis, mucocutaneous candidiasis, and renal *Candida* infections (24, 25, 41, 104, 111, 112, 142, 144, 145, 159, 160, 172, 175, 179, 188, 191–193, 228, 246, 269, 276, 318).

This chapter presents an overview of the adhesion and association mechanisms of *C. albicans*, with particular reference to host colonization and pathogenesis. In addition, the cell wall and surface chemistry of *C. albicans* is briefly reviewed, and possible *Candida* adhesins and host surface receptors are discussed.

Definition of Terms

Current terminology regarding fungal "adherence" is not strictly defined. The term *adherence*, for instance, is less accurate than the terms *adhesion* and *adsorption* in describing the attachment of microorganisms to surfaces (178). The latter terms describe these interactions according to physiochemical principles defined by colloid scientists (178). For this reason, the term *adhesion* shall be used in this review to describe the relatively stable, essentially irreversible attachment of *C. albicans* to surfaces (117, 122), whereas *adsorption* denotes the accumulation of molecules at a fluid interface at a concentration exceeding that in the bulk fluid (243).

Adhesion involves macromolecules on the surface of the microorganism that interact with the surface of the substratum, macromolecules on that surface, or macromolecules adsorbed to that surface (243). The extent and strength of the adhesion, therefore, depends on the initial surface properties of both the organism and substratum involved, and can be influenced by several long-range, short-range, and hydrodynamic forces (243). For instance, during collision of an organism and substratum, the cell and substratum may become attached, due to several types of short-range attractive forces (eg, ionic, H-bonds, dipolar, hydrophobic interactions). This attachment is referred to as *nonspecific adhesion*. *Specific adhesion* requires "some form of stereochemical constraint which brings more than one (usually several) pair of neighboring, interacting groups on the microorganism and the substratum into contact" (243). Specific adhesion, therefore, is a "lock-and-key" type of mechanism that involves interactions between complementary molecular configurations on the substratum and cell surfaces. The term *adhesin* (117, 122) is used to describe any microbial surface macromolecule that mediates specific adhesion to a substratum surface receptor. *Receptors* are those components on substratum surfaces which bind specifically to "active sites" of microbial adhesins during specific adhesion (117, 122, 243).

Lectins are proteins that bind specifically to carbohydrate moieties without altering covalent structure, and which can specifically precipitate polysaccharides and glycoproteins (189). Because of this property, lectins (eg, Concanavalin A) have been frequently used in microbial adhesion research in attempts to identify microbial adhesins (57, 258, 259, 261, 264).

The term *association* is used to describe the interaction of a microorganism with a surface that causes an increased retention time of the microorganism or that allows the microorganism to resist physical removal (87). The term association does not specify the exact mechanism of interaction of the microorganism with a surface, and may be used to describe both adhesive (eg, adhesion to epithelial glycocalyx) and nonadhesive (eg, entrapment in the mucus gel) attachment mechanisms (87, 243). The term *association*, instead of adhesion, should be used until the specific mechanism of attachment by *C. albicans* to a substratum surface has been identified because there are at least five distinct mechanisms by which *C. albicans* can associate with intestinal, for example, mucosal surfaces (140).

Aggregation is a process leading to microbial aggregate formation (243). An *aggregate* has been defined to be a collection of microbial cells that are in intimate contact with one another (177). In this communication, the term aggregation will include intrageneric microbe-microbe and microbe-cell interactions leading to aggregate formation, and the term co-aggregation will be used to describe intergeneric microbial aggregate formation (177). The term *agglutination*, on the other hand, will be reserved for those reactions whereby various chemical substances are used to form aggregates (or *agglutinates*) of microbial cells in vitro. Examples of aggregation and co-aggregation would be colony formation and aggregate formation between *C. albicans* and *Escherichia coli* (190, 200), respectively.

Candida Cell Surface Composition, Ultrastructure, and Possible Adhesins

The cell wall of *C. albicans* is a complex structure approximately 100–300 nm thick in which at least five to eight distinct layers have been identifiied (26, 56, 69, 110, 220, 221, 260). Although little is known regarding the biosynthesis and architecture of the cell wall of *C. albicans*, the composition and appearance of these layers may vary according to morphologic form of the cell, age of the cells, environmental factors present during cell growth, and the fixation procedure used to visualize the structures (28, 30, 148). Because of the putative importance of cell wall structure and surface composition in *Candida* adhesion and pathogenesis, the chemical composition of the cell wall of *C. albicans* has been studied in great detail (22, 36, 100, 141, 218, 231). These studies have revealed that two polysaccharides, α-mannan and β-glucan, represent about 75–85% of the dry matter of *Candida* cell walls, and the remainder is composed of lesser amounts of chitin, protein, and lipid similar to that of *Saccharomyces cerevisiae* (7, 36, 141, 322, 323). The discussion to follow is not intended to be an exhaustive biochemical review of the cell wall composition of *C. albicans*, but instead to describe briefly the cell wall composition and ultrastructure as it relates to the adhesion process. In addition, those surface components that may serve as *Candida* adhesins will be discussed.

Cell Wall Composition

Chemical analyses of the cell wall composition of *C. albicans* have shown that mannan makes up nearly 35–40% of the total dry weight of the cell wall (12). *Candida* cell wall mannan is a highly branched polysaccharide that consists of a backbone of α-1, 6-linked mannose residues to which side chains attach via α-1,2- and rare α-1,3-bonds (293, 297). A large proportion of phosphate molecules linked together by phosphodiester bridges may also be contained in mannans (63). Analysis of mannans isolated from serotypes A and B of *C. albicans* has revealed differences between the mannans of these serotypes. These differences appear to be due to extent of branching, the length of the side chain (serotype A is thought to have longer side chains [202, 255]), and the proportion and position of α-1,2-linkages in the side chains (197, 293, 299). The impact these differences may have on *C. albicans* adhesion is presently unknown.

Glucan appears to be the most abundant polymer in the cell wall of *C. albicans* (14, 64, 101, 281, 296), and is considered to be the essential component of the "microfibrillar skeleton" (101, 218). Glucan is a highly branched polysaccharide that consists of a backbone of β-1,6-linked glucose residues to which side chains of β-1,3-linked glucose residues are attached (14, 322). Recent studies suggest that there may actually be two types of glucan found in the cell wall of *C. albicans*: either β-1,3-linkages or β-1,6-linkages, both of which are highly branched (101).

Glucoprotein, mannoprotein, and glucomannoprotein complexes have also been isolated from the cell wall of *C. albicans* (141, 149). These molecules are all more or less tightly associated with one another and with glucan and mannan (149), and may serve as necessary adhesive links between glucan and mannan (255). The proteins that are complexed with mannan and glucan, in yeast phase cells, are thought to be present as water-soluble proteins and water-insoluble glycopeptides (149). Mannan-protein complexes are thought to be linked through an N-acetylglucosamine residue and side chain amino groups (197). Glucan is also thought to be complexed to chitin (polymer of N-acetylglucosamine joined by β-1,4-linkages) adjacent to the plasma membrane (101). Although chitin helps to anchor glucan to the cell membrane, it comprises only a small part (< 1%) of the cell wall composition by dry weight (39, 218, 296). Most (approximately 90%) of the chitin has been shown to be associated with bud scars of yeast phase cells (3), and the remainder forms the link between the cell membrane and the innermost insoluble glucan possibly by a mixed β-1,3- β-1,6-linkage (101). All of these molecules are antigenic (115, 213, 218, 255, 286, 198), and some (eg, mannoproteins) may serve as *Candida* adhesins (181, 264).

The protein content of the cell wall of *C. albicans* has been studied less extensively than the polysaccharide content. Protein may, in some instances, make up to about 30% of the cell wall content (34, 36, 147). It had generally been thought that nearly all of the proteins found in the outer layers of the cell wall of *C. albicans* were associated with large mannan molecules (218). However, recent studies from several investigators do not support this view (212). Ponton and Jones (212) found that many proteins isolated from the cell wall of *C. albicans* had negligible mannose content. These authors further suggested that there may actually be a complex latticework of proteins situated in the outer layers of the cell wall of both yeast- and mycelial-phase organisms, and that inter- and intradisulfide bonds in these proteins are important in maintaining the structure of this latticework. This, coupled with fact that these proteins were secreted from the cell and were located in the outer layers of the cell wall (212, 218), allows one to speculate that proteins alone may serve as adhesins.

TABLE 4-1. Monosaccharide Composition of *C. albicans* Cell Wall*

	N-Acetylglucosamine	Glucose	Mannose	Galactose	Total Neutral Sugar	Growth Conditions
Yeast	1.5[†]	25.4	17.5	0	42.8	Starch medium 30°C
Yeast	1.7	29.5	15.2	0	44.8	Glucose medium 37°C
Mycelium	6.5	30.4	17.0	0	47.4	Starch medium 40°C
Mycelium	6.5	23.2	18.0	0	41.2	Ox serum 37°C

* Adapted from Bartnicki–Garcia (12).
[†] Values are expressed as % wall dry weight.

TABLE 4-2. Amino Acid Composition and Protein Content of *C. albicans* Cell Wall*

Form	Protein[†]	Ala[‡]	Arg	Asp	Cys	Glu	Gly	His	Ile	Leu	Lys	Met	Phe	Pro	Hyp	Ser	Thr	Tyr	Val	Other	% Recovery	Ratio Acidic to Basic Amino Acids
Yeast	25.6	8.9	0	6.5	?	6.6	6.9	1.2	5.3	6.3	2.6	7.9	?	6.3	0	5.6	6.1	5.1	5.1	2.8	98.4	3.4
Mycelial	15.7	10.7	5.3	6.5	?	9.1	7.4	0	5.9	7.5	0.8	2.2	?	3.7	3.1	5.6	7.4	3.6	9.4	4.3	89.9	2.6

* Adapted from Bartnicki–Garcia (11).
[†] Values expressed as % wall dry weight.
[‡] Values expressed as mole % of the sum total of amino acids.

TABLE 4-3. Comparisons of Lipids from Yeast and Mycelial Forms of *C. albicans* ATCC 10231*

Lipids	12 h Cultures		96 h Cultures	
	Yeast Forms	Mycelial Forms	Yeast Forms	Mycelial Forms
Apolar compounds				
Hydrocarbons	Tr[†]	Tr	Tr	Tr
Steryl esters	Tr	Tr	8.5	25.3
Alkyl esters	Tr	Tr	3.8	8.8
Triacylglycerols	Tr	Tr	6.4	16.5
Fatty acids	Tr	Tr	10.4	11.2
Sterols	14.8	Tr	9.3	Tr
Polar compounds				
Esterfied steryl glycosides	ND	ND	Tr	6.5
Monogalactosyldiacylglycerols	Tr	Tr	Tr	2.7
Steryl glycosides	Tr	16.5	Tr	9.1
Ceramide monohexosides	10.3	Tr	8.8	Tr
Phosphatidylethanolamines	11.4	12.7	9.6	Tr
Phosphatidylglycerols	9.2	Tr	7.3	Tr
Phosphatidylcholines	25.6	28.8	15.0	4.1
Digalactosyldiacylglycerols	Tr	10.2	Tr	6.2
Phosphatidylserines	8.8	9.9	6.9	ND
Phosphatidylinositols	10.9	11.4	8.9	ND
Phosphatidic acids	9.0	7.3	4.8	ND

* From Ghannoum et al. (95).
[†] Values are expressed as a percentage of the total lipids. Tr, traces; ND, not detected.

Analyses of the cell wall from *C. albicans* blastoconidia and mycelium indicate further that differences in cell wall composition between these two forms are primarily quantitative and not qualitative (13, 17, 31, 36, 37, 63; Tables 4-1 and 4-2). Chattaway et al. (36) found that chitin was present at levels three times higher and protein at levels nearly three times lower in the mycelial form. Bianchi (13) found twice as much lipid in hyphae as in blastoconidia, and three times as much carbohydrate has been found in hyphal membranes as in yeast membranes (272). Recent studies confirm this and found that mycelial forms were more active than yeast forms in the accumulation of steryl esters and triacylglycerols (95). Furthermore, it was shown that yeast lipids contained much larger proportions of free sterols than the mycelial lipids, whereas the mycelial lipids contained several times more sterols than the yeast forms (95). Other differences in lipid composition from yeast and mycelial forms are summarized in Tables 4-3, 4-4, and 4-5. Chemical analyses indicate further that there are quantitative differences in hexoses, hexosamines, and amino acids of purified cell wall preparations from blastoconidia and pseudohyphae (34, 35), which may be related to changes in the activities of glycolytic enzymes at the branch points for polysaccharide synthesis from hexoses in the glycolytic metabolic pathway (34, 35). Quantitative differences

TABLE 4-4. Identities and Relative Proportions (%) of Sterols in Total Lipids* from Yeast and Mycelial Forms†

Sterol	Yeast Forms	Mycelial Forms
Degradation product of ergosterol	4.5	ND
Cholesterol	ND†	37.8
Zymosterol	17.0	13.7
Ergosterol	14.6	5.6
24,28-Dehydroergosterol	42.7	18.8
3-β-Hydroxy-24-methyl cholesta-5,7-diene	11.7	22.2
4,4-Dimethylzymosterol	9.5	2.0

Cultures were 12 hours old.
* From Ghannoum et al. (95).
† Subjected to acid hydrolysis; ND, not detected.

TABLE 4-5. Fatty Acid Composition of Apolar and Polar Lipid Fractions from Yeast and Mycelial Forms*

	12 h Cultures				96 h Cultures			
	Yeast Forms		Mycelial Forms		Yeast Forms		Mycelial Forms	
Fatty Acid	Apolar Lipids (%)	Polar Lipids (%)	Apolar Lipids (%)	Polar Lipids (%)	Apolar Lipids (%)	Polar Lipids (%)	Apolar Lipids (%)	Polar Lipids (%)
14 : 0	4.3†	4.2	4.2	3.6	6.6	7.0	6.6	6.5
14 : 1	1.8	6.2	Tr	Tr	5.1	2.0	5.7	8.2
16 : 0	11.8	13.1	14.5	15.3	28.5	25.4	28.4	20.7
16 : 1	11.4	9.6	12.2	13.2	10.4	10.0	14.6	Tr
16 : 2	TR	Tr	Tr	Tr	8.7	3.1	6.0	9.9
18 : 0	14.0	10.3	16.7	15.2	14.5	7.4	10.4	12.1
18 : 1	37.6	41.5	26.7	26.7	14.7	22.4	15.9	8.2
18 : 2	12.0	10.7	16.3	13.5	5.5	18.8	2.7	Tr
18 : 3	7.5	4.4	9.4	12.5	5.7	3.9	9.3	33.7

* From Ghannoum et al. (95).
† Apolar lipid fractions cotained free fatty acids, triacyglycerols, and steryl esters; polar lipid fractions contained phospholipids and glycoplipids. Tr, traces.

of several hydrolytic and glycolytic enzymes between the two forms have also been reported (197, 273).

Cell Wall Ultrastructure

The ultrastructure of the cell wall of *C. albicans* has been examined by several investigators using a variety of procedures to reveal the precise location of the principle wall components (26, 29, 56, 221). Several cell wall layers have been identified for *C. albicans* (218). These layers (L0 to L8 [218]) have been

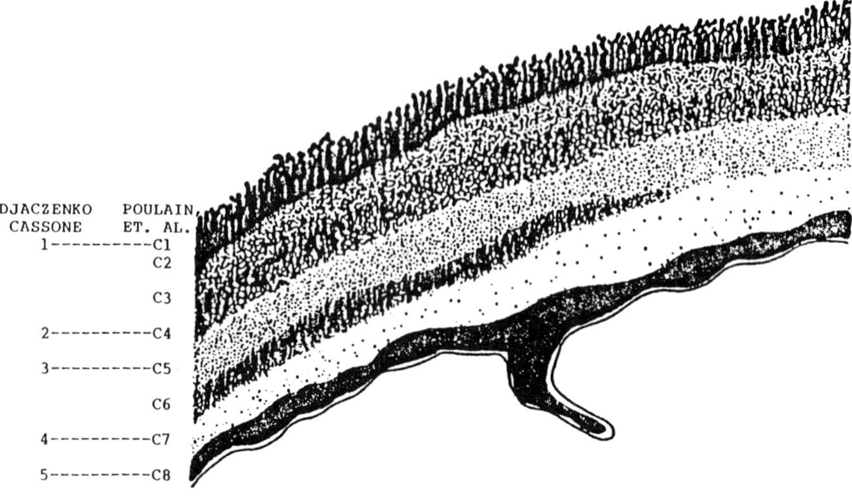

FIG. 4-1. The scheme of the cell wall of *C. albicans* yeast phase cells. Modified from Poulain et al. (218) to include layers corresponding to Djaczenko and Cassone (56). (Courtesy of D.M. Duberg and A.L. Rogers.)

illustrated schematically by Poulain et al. (218) as shown in Fig 4-1. Cytochemical staining (56, 221) revealed that each layer contains a dominant polysaccharide (218), and these have been described in detail elsewhere (218). The gross appearance of the cell wall as viewed by electron microscopy is that of a sandwich structure with an outermost set of layers of high electron density (L0 to L4), an inner layer of high electron density (L8), and an intermediate set of layers of lower electron density (L5 to L7) (218–221). It should be stressed that the gross appearance of the cell wall has been shown to be directly influenced by the growth parameters used for preparation of the test cells (30, 32, 56, 92, 194, 218–221, 260). Poulain and co-workers (218–221) found that both the growth medium and the age of the cells affected the number and appearance of layers in the cell wall. Recent studies have shown further that other growth parameters (eg, temperature) can also have significant effect on cell wall ultrastructure (179, 260). Moreover, some of these changes, particularly in the outermost layers, have been shown to correlate with the adhesiveness of *C. albicans* to both biological and nonbiological surfaces (59, 179, 180, 260).

Adhesins

Although there have been limited ultrastructural observations on the mechanisms of *C. albicans* adhesion, these studies do suggest that at least two morphologic classes of *Candida* adhesins exist: floccular and fibrillar. The

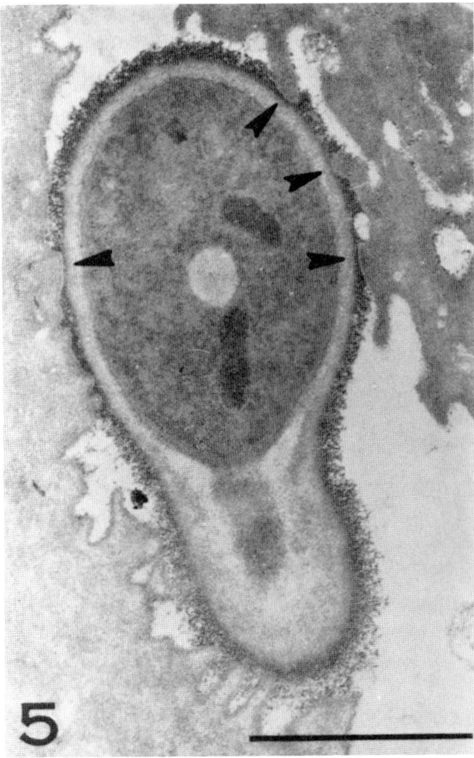

FIG. 4-2. Outer cell wall floccular layer of *C. albicans* apparently mediating adhesion between the fungus and oral epithelium (*arrows*). Bar = 1 μm. (From Howlett and Squier [113].)

floccular adhesins are present as a thick (approximately 100–400 nm) "fuzzy" cell wall coat and appear to be somewhat amorphous (260, 307). Occasionally, this material appeared to have an ordered alignment around the cell wall (307), whereas at other times it was unevenly distributed on the cell surface (179, 260) or localized only at an adhesive junction (113, 175). Ultrastructural studies of the adhesion of *C. albicans* to oral (25, 113, 175, 192, 307), urinary (175), and vaginal epithelium (25) showed the floccular structures to be present on yeast in infected tissues, and that they may indeed mediate *Candida* adhesion. Using tissue explants, for instance, Howlett and Squier (113) found that a floccular outer layer mediated the adhesion of *C. albicans* to oral mucosal cells (Fig. 4-2). *Candida* blastoconidia harvested from media with high concentrations of certain carbohydrates have been found to be highly adhesive, and contained an outermost floccular layer (Fig. 4-3a) that was absent from blastoconidia (Fig. 4-3b) that were significantly less adhesive which were cultivated in media without these carbohydrates (179).

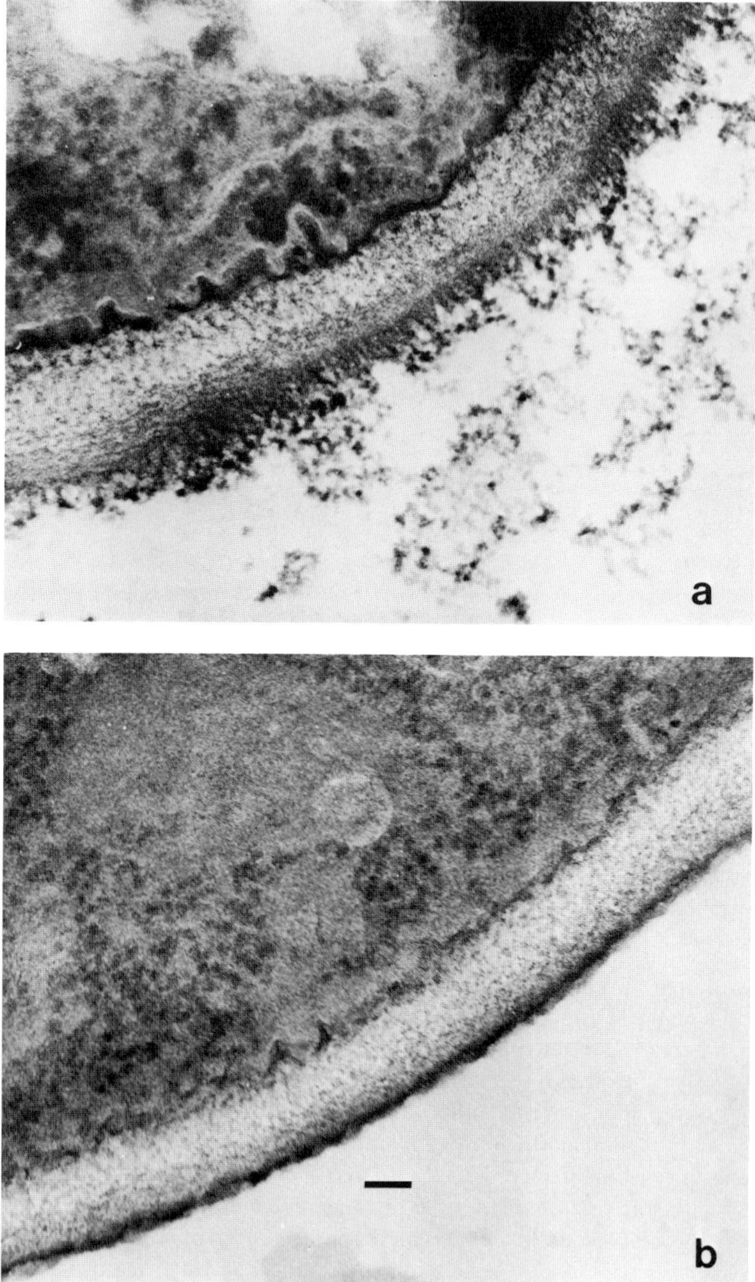

FIG. 4-3. Electron micrographs of thin sections of *C. albicans* MRL 3153 stained with ruthenium red. Cells were harvested in the stationary growth phase from yeast nitrogen base medium containing 500 mM sucrose (a) or 50 mM glucose (b). Bar = 0.1 μm; reduced by 10%. (From McCourtie and Douglas [179].)

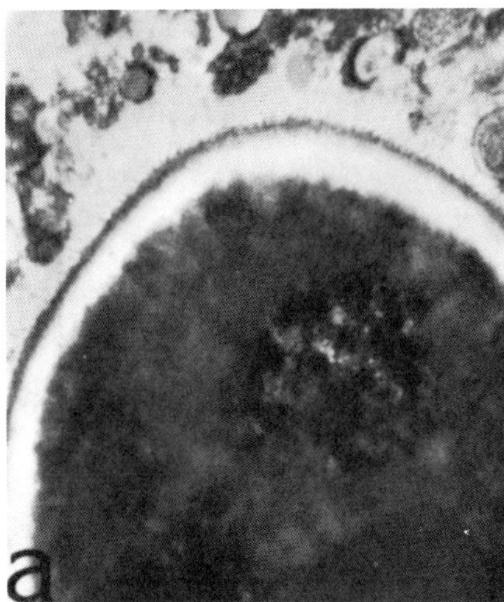

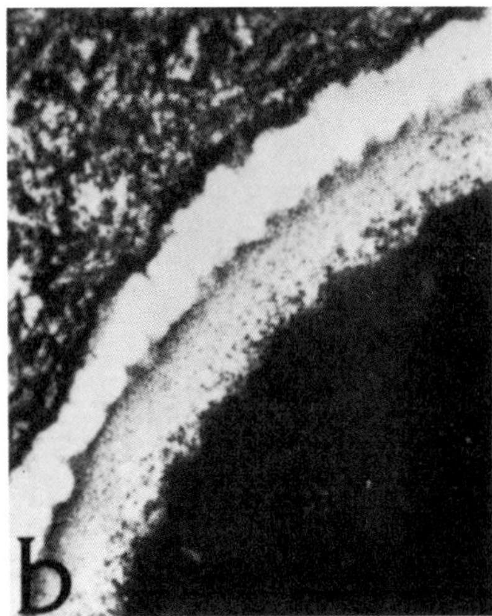

FIG. 4-4. *C. albicans* blastoconidia adherent to (a) a vaginal epithelial cell (× 50,000; reduced by 4%) and (b) an endothelial cell lining a renal peritubular capillary (× 113,500; reduced by 4%). Fibrils can be seen radiating from the blastoconidia. (From Lee and King [158].)

The fibrillar material (called elsewhere fimbriae [91]), in contrast, can be seen on the cell surface as thin filamentous structures arranged perpendicularly to the cell surface and evenly distributed around the entire cell (9, 158). Lee and King (158) viewed the fibrillar structures on the cell surface of *C. albicans* mediating adhesion to renal endothelium (Fig. 4-4a and b). The diameters of these structures have not been measured, but appear to be within the size range (2–10 nm) of fimbrial adhesins of bacteria (122). Likewise, the length of the fibrillar adhesins has not been accurately measured, but these appear to be less than 0.5 μm long (158), considerably shorter than bacterial fimbriae (122). Fibrillae also have been observed to mediate the adhesion of *C. albicans* to other surfaces (175, 236, 307). Both types of adhesins stain with ruthenium red (175), which has an affinity for anionic polymers such as polysaccharides (165).

The precise chemical and organizational nature of these two morphologic structures is not known. It is very likely, however, that these structures represent distinct adhesive entities. There is some evidence to suggest that *C. albicans* does produce more than one adhesin (57, 140, 258, 260). It should be noted that the presence of one or both types of structures on the cell surface of *C. albicans* does not, by itself, indicate that the structures play a role in adhesion (260). *Candida* cells devoid of floccular or fibrillar structures have been shown to be highly adhesive to buccal epithelial cells (BECs) (Fig. 4-5a and b). Furthermore, not all known microbial adhesins can be identifiable as discrete surface structures (122). This also implies that different adhesins may bind to a substratum in different ways. One adhesin may bind directly to a

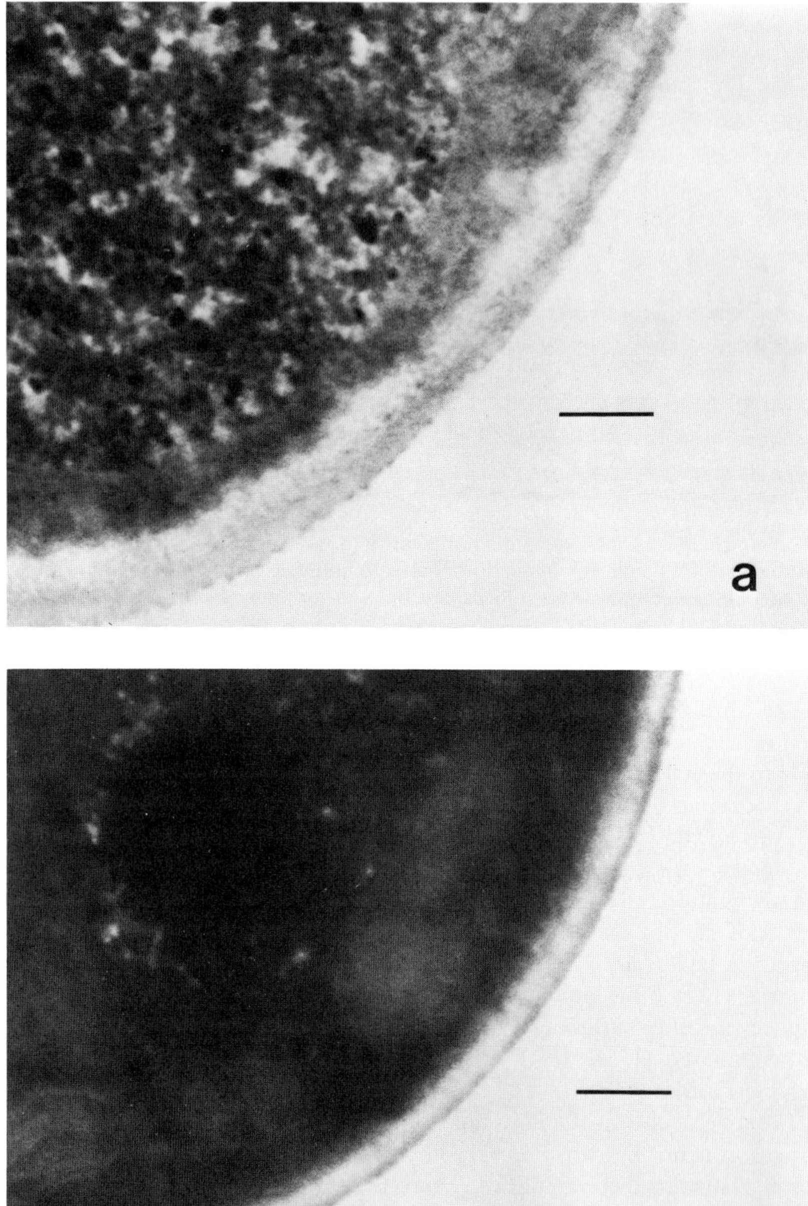

FIG. 4-5. Electron micrographs of thin sections of *C. albicans* AK785 stained by the "G-O-T-O-U" method (206). Cells were harvested from Sabouraud glucose agar after growth for 24 hours at 37°C (a) or from yeast extract medium (159) after growth to early stationary phase at 37°C (b). Both media were found to yield cells that were highly adhesive to buccal epithelial cells (see Table 4-18). Note the absence of extra cell wall "layers" or obvious adhesive appendages. Bar = 200 nm.

receptor, while another may require that divalent cations of appropriate ionic size act as a "bridge" between the surfaces (118, 119). Consequently, the use of several model systems may be necessary to characterize an adhesive activity, as well as to determine whether that activity plays a role in colonization, pathogenesis, or both.

Once an adhesive entity has been identified, it can be characterized by a number of methods. These have been reviewed by Freter and Jones (87) and are summarized in Table 4-6. Use of such methods has suggested that two cell wall components primarily act as adhesins for *C. albicans* (57, 58, 235). It has been suggested, for instance, that a mannose containing moiety, probably a mannoprotein (181), on the surface of *C. albicans* is the *Candida* adhesin (261, 264). However, analogous studies also have suggested a possible role for cell wall chitin as the adhesin (274). Lipids also have been suggested to play a role in adhesion to epithelial cells (93). Moreover, as mentioned earlier, other studies suggest that there may be more than one adhesin (57, 140, 258, 260), and at least one report suggests that *Candida* adhesion may not be mediated by a specific adhesin-receptor interaction but many instead be entirely nonspecific (230). Possible cell wall components that serve as *Candida* adhesins are listed in Table 4–7.

One explanation for these discrepancies is that major differences in various experimental parameters were used by investigators from different laboratories (25, 33, 44, 49, 59, 133, 143, 157, 179, 230, 264, 274, 289). Recent studies from our laboratory (260) showed that growth parameters, particularly growth medium, significantly modified *C. albicans* adhesion to BEGs. Therefore, it is of particular interest to note that no two investigators have used the same growth medium for *C. albicans* adhesion studies and that there are major differences between media used by those investigators proposing that different adhesins are responsible for adhesion to epithelial surfaces (230, 264, 274).

The majority of reports using lectin- and carbohydrate-blocking experiments have indicated that a mannoprotein on the surface of *C. albicans* probably serves as the adhesin in a number of adhesive reactions (57, 58, 235). Rossano and Tufano (234) and Sandin et al. (264), for instance, reported that pretreatment of *C. albicans* with Concanavalin A, a lectin which binds to α-D-mannosyl residues, inhibited adhesion of the yeast to human BECs. Adhesion could also be inhibited by adding mannose or α-D-methylmannopyranoside (a mannose derivative) to the adhesion assay medium during the incubation period (261, 264). Addition of tunicamycin, an antimicrobic which, in yeasts, specifically inhibits mannoprotein synthesis but not chitin or glucan synthesis (153), to cultures of *C. albicans* inhibited the formation of the floccular surface layer of *C. albicans* (60). Concurrently, there was a significant decrease in adhesion of *C. albicans* to BECs (59, 60). Moreover, Lee and King (157) found that extracted mannan-rich cell wall fragments of *C. albicans* attached to vaginal epithelial cells and that this attachment was abolished following treatment of the fragments with

TABLE 4-6. Methods for the Identification and Characterization of *C. albicans* Adhesion Mechanisms and Their Role in Human Disease*

Step	Purpose	Methodology
1.	Identify and describe adhesion mechanisms (and if there is more than one) that can be tested in simple in vitro systems.	Histological and ultramicroscopic examination of infected specimens followed by testing in simple in vitro adhesion assays (eg, exfoliated epithelial cell assays).
2.	Determine whether adhesion in simple in vitro assays is of the same nature as that of more complex models (that may more closely represent the situation in vivo)	Proceed to more complex in vitro models (eg, intestinal slices, tissue explants), and determine if the same inhibitors block adhesion.
3.	Attempt to describe the adhesion at the molecular level.	Alter physiochemical parameters of the adhesion assay, and isolate the adhesin and/or tissue receptor.
4.	Test whether inhibitors of adhesion that act in simple models also inhibit in vivo adhesion, and whether they affect the progress of colonization and/or experimental disease.	Proceed to animal model assay.
5.	Determine whether the adhesins discovered in step 3 are synthesized in vivo, and whether the natural host produces similar receptors.	Test whether mutants lacking a given cell surface component are avirulent or are unable to colonize in animal models. Determine whether revertants regain virulence or colonizing ability.
6.	Determine what factors modify adhesion or association in vivo.	Use a number of different animal models, or manipulate animals, and examine biochemical and physiochemical differences of the surrounding environment where differences are noted (eg, pH, eH, VFA, etc).
7.	Determine where in the body *Candida* cells are multiplying, dying, or both, what the population dynamics of association and disassociation are, and what the growth rate of the organism is in vivo.	Do quantitative counts on, for example, lumen contents and mucosal surface. Perform in vitro tests under parameters similar to that in vivo and determine binding kinetics and rates of disassociation.
8.	Determine the mechanisms of regulation and adhesin production.	Study the genetics of well characterized mutant strains.
9.	Determine what factors may prevent adhesion and association in humans (eg, antifungal drugs, immunization, etc)	After all the above parameters have been well characterized in experimental animals, studies in human volunteers with wild-type and mutant *C. albicans*.

*Adapted and modified from Freter and Jones (87).

TABLE 4-7. Possible Cell Surface Components Suggested to Serve as *Candida* Adhesins

Possible Adhesin Moieties	Examples of Inhibitors	References
Chitin	Glucosamine	274
	Chitin-soluble extract	274
	N-acetylglucosamine	274
	Mannosamine	274
Mannan/mannoprotein	Mannose	264
	α-mannosidase	264
	Tunicamycin	60
	α-methylmannosidase	157
	Conconavalin A	264
	D-methylmannopyranoside	264
Glucan	Glucose	
	Glucan	
Protein	Papain	157
	Pronase	157
	Pepsin	157
	Trypsin	157, 290
	Chymotrypsin	157, 290
Lipid	Sterols	93

α-mannosidase. This α-mannosidase selectively degraded mannan because it was free of proteases and did not contain glycosidic activity against p-nitrophenyl glucose or galactose substrate (157). McCourtie and Douglas (181) showed that a crude mannoprotein preparation obtained from culture supernatants of *C. albicans* also associated with BECs and inhibited subsequent yeast adhesion. This extracellular polymer of *C. albicans* was found to contain a high mannose content (65–82%), and lesser amounts of protein (7%), phosphorous (0.5%), and glucosamine (1.5%) (181).

The studies of Maisch and Calderone (173) suggest a role of α-mannan in the adhesion of *C. albicans* to fibrin-platelet clots formed in vitro (172). Sheep erythrocytes coated with an alkali-soluble cell wall extract attached to a fibrin-platelet matrix, whereas nonconjugated sheep erythrocytes did not attach. The adhesion-promoting effect was abolished by pretreating the alkali extract (72% polysaccharide and less than 1% protein) with α-mannosidase before conjugation to erythrocytes (173). Similarly, alkali extraction of *Candida* cells significantly inhibited C. *albicans* adhesion to human epithelial cells (258). Likewise, α-mannan or a mannan-associated cell wall constituent may also serve as an adhesin in attachment to vascular endothelium. Rotrosen et al. (236) showed that *Candida* immune serum significantly blocked adhesion to endothelial cells, but that this activity was abolished by immunoprecipitation of immune serum with *C. albicans* mannan but not by similar adsorption with particulate chitin.

There is also evidence to suggest that protein alone may serve as an adhesin, or that the protein portion of the mannoprotein complex is more important than the carbohydrate moiety in mediating attachment. Adhesion of *C. albicans* to epithelial cells has been shown to be decreased after exposure to heat or various proteolytic enzymes (157, 289). Pretreatment of *C. albicans* with trypsin, chymotrypsin or pronase reduced adhesion to fibrin-platelet clots (173). Likewise, Critchley and Douglas (57) found that pretreatment of an extracellular polymer (thought to serve as an adhesin) from *C. albicans* with heat, dithiothreitol or certain proteases, but not sodium metaperiodate or α-mannosidase, either partially or completely destroyed its ability to block *Candida* adhesion to BECs. Similarly, a protein component from *C. albicans* pseudohyphae also reduced the binding affinity of pseudohyphae for neutrophils (55). Studies on bacterial adhesion are consitent with this view as they have shown that most of the well characterized bacterial adhesins (with only two exceptions) are proteins (117, 122).

Other studies directed at identification of *Candida* adhesins using selective inhibitors of adhesion have suggested that cell wall chitin may be involved in *C. albicans* adhesion (274). Chitin, a hydrolysate derivative of chitin, and N-acetyl glucosamine all significantly inhibited attachment of *C. albicans* to vaginal epithelial cells (274). Moreover, it was also observed that the latter two substances also reduced the infection rate in a rat model of vaginitis (159). Other investigators have not been able to reproduce these results (264). Although it seems unlikely that such a small portion of the cell wall, which is localized only to inner layers of the cell wall or bud scars, could serve as an adhesin, it should again be noted that those investigators (264) did not use the same growth media as that used by Segal and coworkers (274). Further blocking experiments with chitin or "chitin-soluble extract" should be performed after growth of several strains of *C. albicans* on the yeast extract medium used by Segal et al. (274), compared with that after growth on other media (260), to determine more conclusively whether or not chitin plays a role in adhesion. Another approach to determine whether chitin or other cell wall components serve as adhesins would be to isolate and characterize nonadhesive mutants of *C. albicans*. It should be noted also that the preceding experiments do not rule out the possibility that chitin or its derivatives block adhesion by means of steric hindrance or that chitin can bind to the same receptor sites that mannoprotein adhesins bind to.

In another report, Sobel et al. (289) showed that D- and L-fucose inhibited the attachment of *C. albicans* to vaginal epithelial cells. However, in these experiments the fucose was allowed to react with the *Candida* cells first, suggesting not that a fucose-like component serves as an adhesin but that the receptor on the epithelial cell for *C. albicans* may also be a glycoprotein. Reinhart et al. (230) have also suggested that *Candida* adhesion to epithelial cells may be entirely nonspecific, and that such adhesion is mediated solely by hydrophobic properties (107). It seems unlikely, however, that a nonspecific phenomenon such as hydrophobicity could account for all of the distinct adhesive activities observed for *C. albicans* (140). Studies from our laboratory suggest that specific adhesion predominates over nonspecific adhesion (140). Therefore, the more likely explanation for *C. albicans* adhesion to various biological surfaces such as intestinal epithelial cells and other microorganisms is that adhesion is mediated by two or more distinct adhesive entities, in which nonspecific interactions (eg, hydrophobicity) may or may not play a role. There is already evidence to suggest that more than one adhesin may be involved in attachment to epithelial cells by *C. albicians*. However, the alternative proposition that many of the adhesive activities observed for *C. albicans* result from a single multifactoral adhesive cell wall component cannot be ruled out from studies to date.

Adhesion and Association Mechanisms

The association of *C. albicans* with both biological and nonbiological surfaces has been suggested to play an important role in host colonization and pathogenesis. Data has been presented on the adhesion and association of *C. albicans* with nearly every tissue of the body (9, 41, 71, 112, 139, 142, 192, 214, 215), as well as to a number of "plastic" surfaces that are used to make dental protheses, catheters, and prosthetic cardiac valves (146, 179, 236). In this section, a detailed discussion of the physiochemical factors involved in *C. albicans* adhesion to various surfaces is presented, and a number of adhesion and association mechanisms are described. These are summarized in Table 4-8.

TABLE 4-8. Adhesion and Association Mechanisms of *C. albicans*

	Nature of Mechanism			
Mechanism	Active or Passive	Specific or Nonspecific	Direct or Indirect	References
Adhesin-receptor interaction	A	S	D, I	24, 41, 140, 143, 157, 159, 160, 264, 274
Nonspecific adhesion	A, P	N	D, I	131, 140, 146, 187, 188, 191, 230
Coadhesion to adherent organisms	A	S, N	I	4, 33, 140, 260
Entrapment in tissue	P	N	D	23, 140, 216, 217
Germ tube penetration	A	N, S	D, I	113, 175, 236, 288

Physiochemical Considerations of Adhesion

The adhesion of *C. albicans* to any surface in vivo may vary considerably depending on host species, physiology, cell phenotype, and tissue involved (2, 246, 260, 276, 289). Likewise, the attachment of *C. albicans* to exfoliated epithelial cells, tissue explants, or various nonbiological surfaces, such as plastic or glass, can vary greatly in vitro depending on a number of experimental factors (eg, growth medium; see the discussion on adhesion models below). Moreover, a number of long-range, short-range, and hydrodynamic forces, only a few of which have been studied, may influence *C. albicans* adhesion ability (164, 176, 177, 244, 245, 285). Relatively little is known about the binding sites of *C. albicans* adhesins and even less is known about *Candida* binding kinetics. Because a complete physiochemical description of the adhesion of *C. albicans* to any one surface is not yet possible, the following discussion will present the fundamental physiochemical principles involved in *Candida*-substrum interactions.

In general, the cell surfaces to which *C. albicans* attaches, as well as the surfaces of *Candida* cells, have an overall negative surface charge (117). These negative potentials result from the ionization of various chemical groups (eg, sialic acid carboxyl groups of epithelial glycocalyces, acidic amino acid side chains, glycolipids and phospholipids, etc) of the cell surface. Likewise, glass and plastic surfaces may also possess a net negative surface charge, depending, of course, on the type and ionic strength of the surrounding milieu (176). These charged surface groups loosely attract oppositely charged ions (gegen- or counterions) from the surrounding solution to form a diffuse double layer of ions (176). The resulting electric double layer is considered to be a part of the cell surface, in that as the cell is caused to move (eg, due to brownian motion or with an electric field) the thin layer of fluid and the ions of the double layer move with the cell (117). Two models of the diffuse double layer have been proposed (164, 176). One concept, the Stern model, assumes that there is a one molecule thick layer of counterions held at the surface (the Stern layer) by electrostatic and London-van der Waals attraction forces which are sufficiently strong to overcome thermal agitation. The other concept, the Gouy-Champman model, describes that of a diffuse double layer without the Stern layer. These concepts have been described in detail elsewhere (164, 176) and will not be discussed further here. However, it should be noted that the ionic strength of the surrounding environment can greatly influence the dimensions of the dielectric layer, and, therefore, can also modify attractive and repulsive forces (117) because repulsion will occur when both the substratum and microorganism layers overlap (205). Not surprisingly, several studies have shown that *C. albicans* adhesion to epithelial cells varied according to selection of assay medium (142, 143, 179, 207).

The most useful descriptions of adhesive interactions between two negatively charged surfaces, which theoretically should repel one another, are those provided by the now classical lyophobic colloid theory of Derjaguin and

Landau (54) and of Verwey and Overbeek (313) (DLVO theory) and its many derivations (122). Briefly, the DLVO theory proposes that the forces of repulsion (electrostatic interactions in the overlapping double layers) and attraction (London-van der Waals forces) between two similarly charged surfaces are additive, but vary independently with the distance of separation between the bodies. There are two separation distances between cells at which attraction is greater than repulsion. These are called the primary minimum (at small distances of separation of <1 nm) where attraction forces are strong, and the secondary minimum (at relatively large distances of separation of >10 nm) where attraction forces are weaker and are easily reversible, for example, by mild fluid shear (122). Interposed between these two positions is a point at which repulsive forces predominate and the potential energy is maximized (122). The overall charge and shape of the bodies are important and contribute significantly to the net interaction (114). For example, repulsion forces decrease with bodies of decreasing radii of curvature (114, 122). Likewise, as ionic strength in an environment increases the energy maximum repulsion barrier decreases, and at high electrolyte concentrations the repulsion energy barrier may be eliminated altogether (122).

The DLVO theory describes long-range adhesive interactions (ie, those occurring at the secondary minimum) adequately where the bodies are held in a state of mutual attraction, but is inadequate in describing close-range interactions between adhesin and receptor, because bacteria and yeast do not possess sufficient kinetic energy to overcome the repulsion barrier (122, 244). Nevertheless, the DLVO theory remains valid to describe certain adhesive interactions (122, 245), but suggests that relatively irreversible adhesion (ie, binding at the primary minimum) may require adhesive appendages (ie, adhesins) that bridge the gap between cell surfaces to bind its complementary receptor (122, 177). Therefore, those interactions which occur at the secondary minimum are considered to be nonspecific and preliminary to irreversible adhesion (118). Both types of interactions may be necessary for adhesion to and colonization of host tissues. For instance, although curved bodies come closer together at the secondary minimum and require less kinetic energy to reach the primary minimum, and adhesion of yeast cells to cells with microvilli is energetically more favorable compared with other tissue of planar configuration, the effect of curvature may not decrease the repulsion sufficiently to permit *C. albicans* to reach the primary minimum. Thus, in a system such as the small intestine, the effect of fluid shear due to peristalsis and the bathing actions of mucosal secretions should dislodge *Candida* cells resulting in their removal from the tissue surface. Therefore, as *C. albicans* is known to bind essentially irreversibly to small intestinal microvilli (216, 217), it is likely that specific adhesin-receptor binding is involved (140). However, without the weak attraction at the secondary minimum it seems unlikely that the presumed stereochemical fit of adhesin with receptor could take place (74, 118). Marrie and Costerton (175) noted two types of *Candida*-epithelial cell interactions that preceded cell invasion. The first was a "loose" adhesion apparently mediated by a ruthenium red positive matrix, followed by a "tight" adhesion where no space could be seen between host and yeast cell.

Furthermore, it seems likely that adhesive appendages of very small radii of curvature relative to the yeast cell would favor contact with a tissue surface. Individual fibrillar adhesins, as those described earlier, with considerably smaller radii than the yeast cell could overcome repulsion due to the potential energy maximum required to bridge the gap between *C. albicans* and epithelium. Lee and King (157) found that "fibrils" from *C. albicans* blastoconidia mediated adhesion to vaginal epithelial cells and endothelial cells lining renal peritubular capillaries. It is also interesting to note that very small blastoconidia of *C. albicans*, as well as blastoconidia which possessed "tiny" (barely visible) germ tubes, were found to be significantly more adhesive to BECs than were "normal" size blastoconidia which did not possess germ tubes (260). It follows from the physiochemical principles described that the smaller radii of curvature of tiny germ tubes and smaller yeast cells may have facilitated adhesion. The alternative proposition that the increased adhesive activities for cells with germ tubes resulted from a concentration of adhesins, or the production of additional adhesins, cannot be ruled out at present. Nevertheless, the smaller radii of curvature of small blastoconidia and tiny germ tubes are more energetically favorable for adhesion.

At short distances several other interactions are important in adhesion. Such interactions include: dipole-dipole (Keesom) interactions, dipole-induced dipole (Debye) interactions, ion-dipole interactions, chemical bonds (eg, electrostatic, covalent, and hydrogen), and hydrophobic interactions (244, 245, 300). A number of these types of interactions have been shown to be important in bacterial adhesion (177). It should be noted, however, that short-range effects may be repulsive or attractive depending on the nature of the surfaces involved (245, 300), and are particularly important in aqueous systems (176, 244). The role most of these short-range forces may play in the adhesion of *C. albicans* to biological or nonbiological surfaces has not been examined. Another possibility that also has not been considered, is that the variability of the surface of *C. albicans* (eg, in charge, shape, appendages, etc) may lead to various types of synergistic interactions that take place simultaneously. In bacterial systems, hydrophobic interactions adjacent to ionic or hydrogen bonds have been shown to stabilize an otherwise energetically weak binding complex (61). Synergistic interactions can easily be imagined for *Candida* adhesion and should be investigated. Likewise, the effect surface topography (152) may have on *Candida* adhesion has only been examined in one study (260).

Only a limited number of physiochemical parameters have been studied in relation to *C. albicans* adhesion. Lee and King (157) examined the effect of certain physiochemical parameters on adhesion of *C. albicans* to human vaginal epithelial cells in vitro, and found that divalent cations, detergents, salts, and urea had no effect on adhesion. These findings suggest that hydrophobic, electrostatic, or ion-bridging bonds may be of little importance in adhesion to vaginal mucosal cells in this system. It should be emphasized that such results may be particular to the *C. albicans* strain and growth medium (and other assay parameters) used in that study. On the other hand, reducing agents (eg, β-mercaptoethanol and dithiothreitol) significantly diminished *C. albicans* adhesion, but did not effect viability (143, 157), suggesting that the structural integrity of the adhesive factor(s) is important.

In contrast to the study of Lee and King (157), Karaev et al. (131) showed that the introduction of Ca^{2+} and Mg^{2+} ions to in vitro assays led to a significant increase in *C. albicans* adhesion to BECs. Likewise, divalent cations were shown to promote the adhesion of *C. albicans* to acrylic, and at high concentrations these cations caused extensive coadhesion and aggregation of *C. albicans* (179). These studies indicate that ion-bridging mechanisms and electrostatic forces may be of primary importance in the adhesion of *C. albicans* to BECs, at least under some conditions, and acrylic surfaces in vitro.

Hydrophobic interactions also have been examined for their role in the adhesion of *C. albicans* to various denture base resin materials, plastics, and BECs (146, 187, 188, 191). Klotz et al. (146) found that the adhesion of *C. albicans* to plastic surfaces was predominantly controlled by hydrophobic forces, and that electrostatic forces also contributed to adhesion. This view is corroborated by the findings of Minagi et al. (187, 188), who showed that *C. albicans* could attach to denture materials in a similar manner. However, in the latter study *C. albicans* was significantly less hydrophobic, indicating that the surface free energy of the denture material itself greatly influenced *Candida* adhesion. Whereas hydrophobicity appeared to contribute to the adhesion of *C. albicans* to various plastics and denture materials, other nonspecific forces also probably contributed to the adhesion process. In contrast, recent studies from our laboratory showed that hydrophobicity may be little importance in association with intestinal mucosa (140) or BECs (260). However, hydrophobicity appeared to be important in yeast-to-yeast coadhesion, and may have indirectly influenced the total number of attached yeast by promoting coadhesion (260). The role cell surface hydrophobicity plays in *C. albicans* adhesion in vivo remains to be demonstrated.

The Oral Cavity

The adhesion and association of *C. albicans* with oral mucosal surfaces has been studied in a number of in vitro and in vivo systems. Such studies have included adhesion to exfoliated epithelial cells, colonization, and invasion of various tissue explants, as well as the ultrastructural characterization of attachment and penetration of *C. albicans* to oral epithelium obtained from infected patients or experimental animals. Some of these studies have focused on the nature of the adhesion, whereas others have focused primarily on tissue localization.

Howlett and Squire (113) examined the colonization and invasion of oral

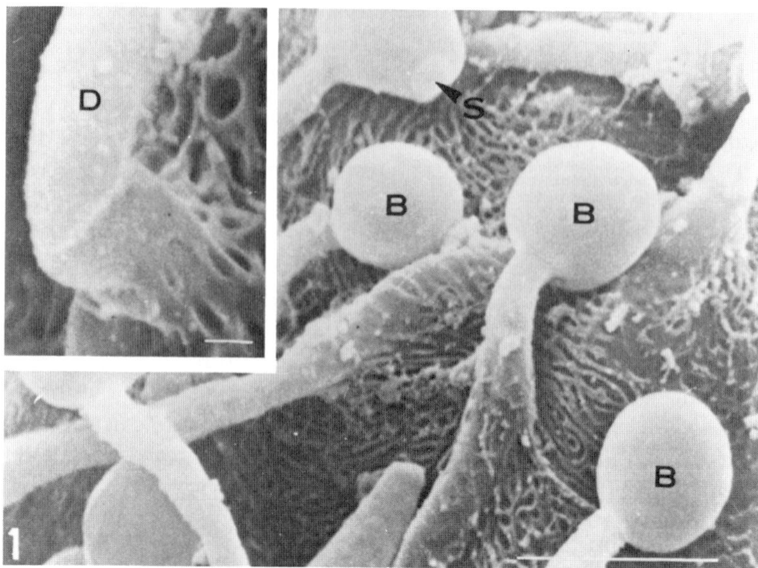

FIG. 4-6. Scanning electron micrograph showing *C. albicans* adhering to and penetrating keratinized rat tongue mucosa. The blastoconidia (B) have developed germ tubes and the extending hyphae are invading the superficial squames (S, bud scar). Bar = 1 μm ($\times$37,000; reduced by 26%). Inset: the junction between a hypha and the epithelial cell membrane. Irregular masses of material can be seen coating the fungal surface (D). Bar = 0.1 μm ($\times$84,000; reduced by 26%). (From Howlett and Squier [113].)

epithelium using tissue explants. Tissues were obtained from Sprague-Dawley rats and 4-day-old or younger New Zealand white rabbits, maintained in vitro in a chemically defined medium, and inoculated with *C. albicans*. Infected explants were maintained in vitro for 12 to 30 hours, and harvested at regular intervals to examine the various features of adhesion and association. Three types of interactions were noted. Blastoconidia of *C. albicans* were observed to be randomly adhering to the surface of the epithelium, and in many cases germ tubes were observed extending from the parent blastoconidia and penetrating into the tissue (Fig. 4-6). Adhesion of yeast cells to oral epithelium appeared to form an "intimate" contact between the cell surface and certain layers of the *Candida* cell wall. As shown in Fig. 4-7, the surface structure mediating attachment appears to be a floccular exterior layer. Five distinct layers in the cell wall of *C. albicans* could be observed in infected tissues. Moreover, the cell wall of *C. albicans* appeared to undergo ultrastructural changes during adhesion. This is similar to the observations of Tronchin et al. (307) who noted ultrastructural modifications of the fungal cell wall coat during the adhesion of *C. albicans* to BECs in vitro. In that study, various cytochemical staining techniques were used to visualize the adhesion process, and showed that *C. albicans* developed a fibrogranular surface layer that appeared to mediate

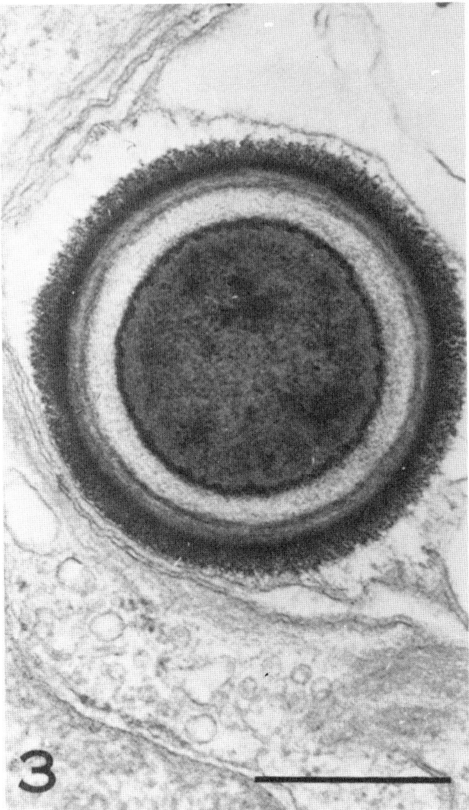

Fig. 4-7. Electron micrograph of thin section of oral epithelium infected with *C. albicans* showing five distinct layers in the fungal cell wall. Bar = 0.5 μm (× 54,000). (From Howlett and Squier [113].)

adhesion. Concanavalin A binding sites were increased after development of this material (307). Fig. 4-8 shows that at a putative germination site the outer layers appear to have merged to form a homogeneous electron-dense floccular layer.

The initiation of contact between *Candida* germ tubes and the epithelium may represent a distinct adhesive mechanism because no alteration of the epithelial cell surface was noted either at the point of entry or around the vicinity of *Candida* microcolonies. This was true for all types of epithelia examined. Studies by Sandin and coworkers (258) suggested that germ tubes may contain different adhesins, or concentrated amounts of adhesin (264). Others reported that germinated yeast cells were significantly more adhesive than their nongerminated counterparts (143). Within the epithelial cells of infected explants occasional loss of cytoplasmic components in the vicinity of the invading hyphae was noted (113). These findings indicate that if enzymatic

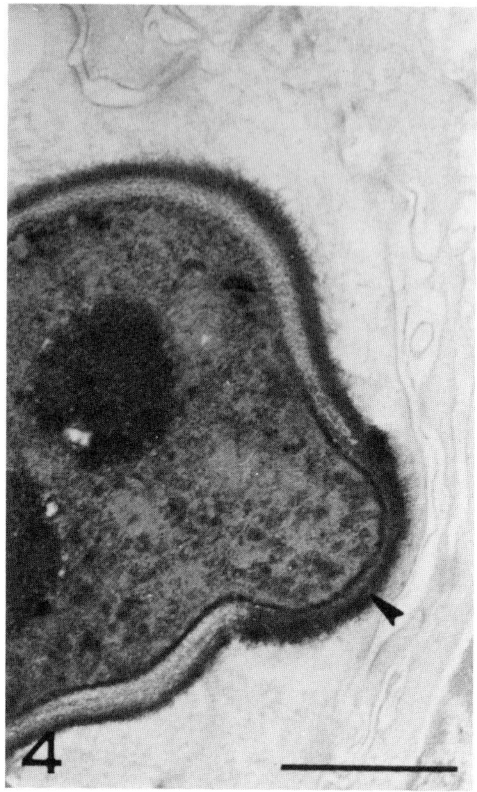

FIG. 4-8. Transmission electron micrograph of an ultrathin section of oral epithelium infected with *C. albicans*. Note where the fungal element appears to be germinating, changes are evident in the organization of the cell wall (*arrow*). Bar = 1 μm (×25,600). (From Howlett and Squier [113].)

lysis was associated with the invasive process it was localized, probably to the hyphal tips. Mechanical support provided by the adhesion of *Candida* cells to the epithelium may also facilitate growth and penetration into tissues (113). Other reports support the role of both hydrolytic enzyme activity (10, 37, 94, 224–227, 316) and mechanical force (65) in the invasion of animal cells by this fungus. There was no evidence that blastoconidia invaded the epithelium directly. In addition to yeast adhesion and germ tube penetration, it also was observed that long hyphae grew on and colonized the epithelial surface and penetrated deep into the tissue. Examination of the infected explants showed the hyphal form to predominate within the epithelium, especially at later times (112). Sequential characterization of hyphal penetration of the rat tongue showed further that penetration occurred in three stages: 1) penetration of the superficial keratin layer (at approximately 18 hours), 2) penetration of basal

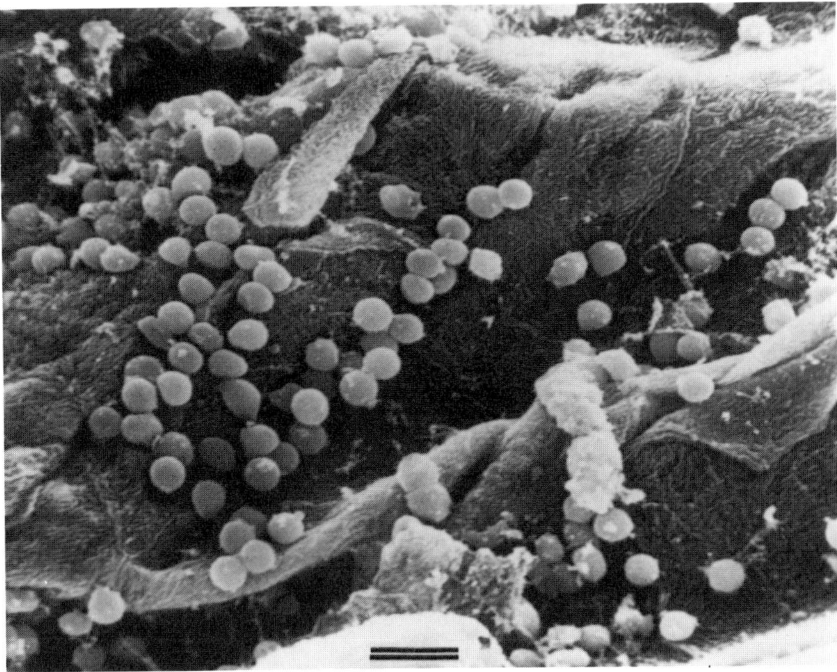

FIG. 4-9. Yeast cells adhering to the ventral tongue surface of an adult gnotobiotic mouse monoassociated with *C. albicans* B311 (type A). Bar = 10 μm. (From Balish et al. [5].)

epithelium and basement membranes (at approximately 28 hours), and 3) invasion of connective tissues (at approximately 35 hours) (112).

A number of studies examining infected tissues from patients and experimental animals have shown results similar to those described above. Fig. 4-9 and 4-10 show yeast cells of *C. albicans* adhering to the ventral tongue surface and cheek mucosal surface, respectively. Montes and Wilborn (192, 193) examined scrappings of plaque from the tongue of patients with chronic mucocutaneous candidiasis and found pseudohyphae of *C. albicans* growing profusely between epithelial cells and penetrating into them. In analogous studies these authors found that *Candida* pseudohyphae grew on and colonized the surface of the buccal mucosa, and pseudohyphae penetrated keratinized cells (318). Pseudohyphal forms were predominant in patients with chronic mucocutaneous candidiasis, although blastoconidia were often observed attached to and colonizing oral epithelium.

In another study (175), examination of plaques from the tongue and buccal mucosa of patients with oral candidiasis, revealed similar interactions between *C. albicans* and oral mucosa. These include a "loose" adhesion apparently mediated by a ruthenium red positive matrix (similar to floccular adhesins), a

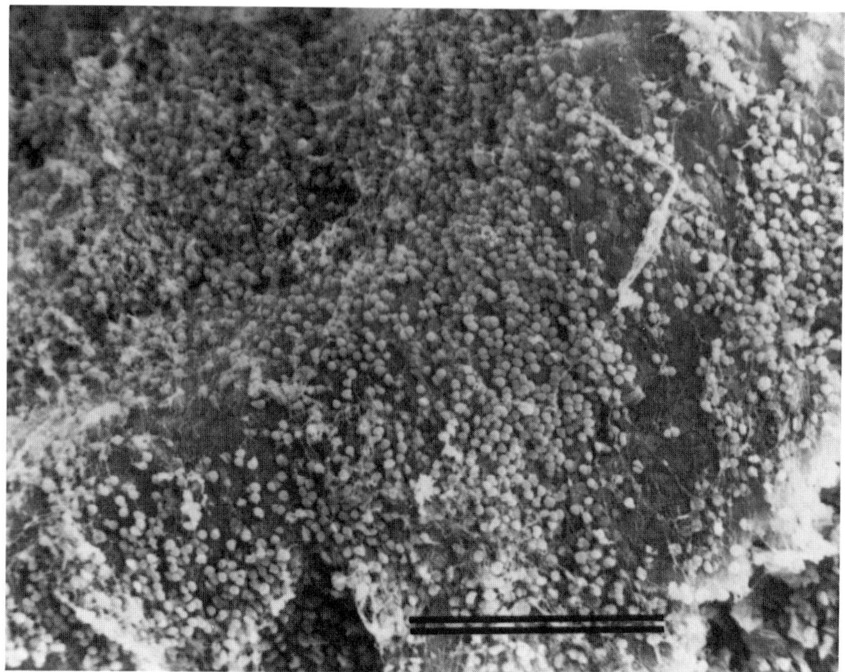

FIG. 4-10. Yeast cells adhering to the cheek mucosal surface of an adult gnotobiotic mouse monoassociated with *C. albicans*. Bar = 100 μm. (From Balish et al. [5].)

"tight" adhesion where no space could be seen between yeast and epithelium, and invasion of host cells by *C. albicans* hyphae. Coadhesion of *Candida* blastoconidia and indigenous bacteria to hyphal elements were also frequently noted (175). The adhesion of *C. albicans* to BECs in vitro was characterized by electron microscopy and appeared to proceed via similar mechanisms (25). Again, yeast adhesion appeared to be of both a tight and loose nature. In addition, yeast cells were often observed in phagocytic vacuoles of epithelial cells. From these and similar studies it is not clear whether these two ultrastructural forms represent distinct adhesive activities or phases of the same process. Although tight and loose adhesion of *C. albicans* could represent two different mechanisms of adhesion, they probably represent different stages of the same adhesion mechanism (259), similar to phases of reversible adhesion that precede irreversible adhesion in bacteria (123, 124). Studies using 0.4% formalin saline to kill *Candida* cells revealed that dead organisms formed a loose adhesion but that only viable cells bind irreversibly (314).

As noted earlier a number of studies have tried to characterize the nature of *Candida* adhesin(s), and to a much lesser extent epithelial cell receptor(s), by introducing various substances into an assay that might block adhesion or by pretreating host or yeast cells before preforming adhesion assays. Using the former approach it was found that *C. albicans* may bind reversibly for as long as 20 minutes, but thereafter the cells bind irreversibly (259). This suggests that the initial yeast-epithelium contact may be due to nonspecific adhesion, followed by specific adhesion, or that if the initial attachment is the result of specific adhesion, for example, "loose" binding via floccular adhesins, additional adhesion or association mechanisms may be required for irreversible binding (259). Modification of both host and yeast cells have been observed once *C. albicans* attaches (113, 307). It may be that as *Candida* cells "bump" into epithelial cells and bind reversibly, physiologic changes occur to both host and fungus that strengthen the adhesion. These changes could modify the epithelium to the extent that more or different receptors are exposed that, if bound to *Candida* cells, would stabilize and strengthen adhesion. Likewise, modifications of the cell wall of *C. albicans*, possibly causing an increase or concentration of adhesins, or an unmasking of different or more adhesins, have been noted at yeast-epithelial binding sites (see Fig. 4-8). Alternatively, the deposition of new cell wall material could occur after initial attachment. Tronchin et al. (307) have noted the reorganization and proliferation of an external cell wall layer of *C. albicans* during adhesion to BECs. Moreover, they noted an abundant extracellular material with numerous binding sites for Concanavalin A that appeared to be released from the yeast surface, leaving underlying cell wall layers exposed. Several descriptions of phases in *Candida* adhesion to epithelial cells exist (93), but further studies to characterize the affinity and number of binding sites will be necessary to present a more complete and accurate description.

It also has been suggested that the adhesion of *C. albicans* to buccal mucosal cells might entail ionic interactions involving divalent cations (131). The adsorption of macromolecules to epithelial cells is recognized to occur via electrostatic interactions involving calcium ions and other ionic groups. *Candida* cells could also attach by similar mechanisms. However, conflicting data do not permit definite conclusions to be drawn. For example, it was shown that at acidic and basic pHs *Candida* adhesion decreases (289). In another study (250), the opposite results were observed. These results, however, may be strain dependent (207). Also, cell surface hydrophobicity has been implicated in mediating *Candida* adhesion (107). In contrast, we have found that phenotypes of *C. albicans* showing significantly superior adhesion to BECs were significantly less hydrophobic than phenotypes with poor adhesion ability (Kennedy, unpublished data). One may speculate, therefore, that once long-range electrostatic forces are overcome, specific adhesin-receptor interactions become the important determinants of adhesion.

The Gastrointestinal Tract

Because of the possible ecologic and pathologic consequences of mucosal association by *Candida* in the GI tract (68,151), several methods have been used to examine the adhesion and association of *C. albicans* with gut mucosa. Most have involved removing infected tissues from animals and viewing the resulting association by scanning (SEM) or transmission (TEM) electron microscopy (5, 71, 138, 140, 214–217). Others have included examination of stained histologic sections or quantitative cultures to determine population levels of attached yeast in infected tissue (140, 216, 217). Tissue slices or isolated mucus gel have also been used to study mucosal association in vitro (138, 140, 275).

Animal models used to study colonization of the GI tract have included neonatal and adult conventional, specific pathogen-free, germ-free, antimicrobic-treated, and/or athymic gnotobiotic mice, hamsters, chickens, and rats (5, 6, 53, 71, 138, 140, 210, 214–217, 320, 321), and have revealed mucosal association by *C. albicans* in all regions of the GI tract (5, 71, 140, 216, 217). Different preferential sites of colonization, however, have been noted between various animal models. Pope et al. (71, 214–217), for instance, found that the stomach was the primary site of colonization in infant mice, whereas studies in antimicrobic-treated adult mice have revealed that the cecum was most heavily colonized by *C. albicans* (140, 309). It is also interesting to note that the GI tract of neonatal mice was not colonized as quickly with *C. albicans* as were adult mice (5). Nevertheless, the aforementioned studies have demonstrated

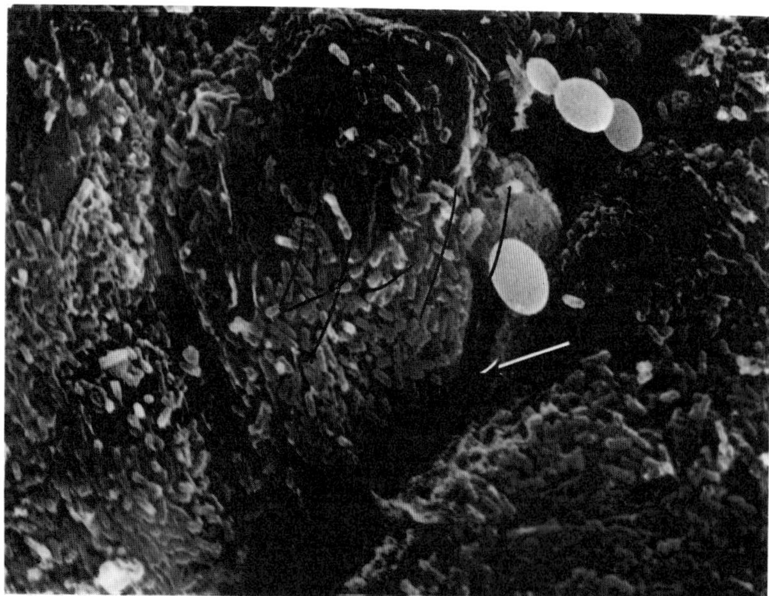

FIG. 4-11. Stomach epithelium from an infant mouse 30 minutes after intragastric inoculation with *C. albicans* CA30. Several yeast cells can be seen on the keratinized epithelium as well as a layer of rod-shaped bacteria. A yeast cell (*arrow*) is visible deep within a tissue fold (× 1,700). (From Pope and Cole [216].)

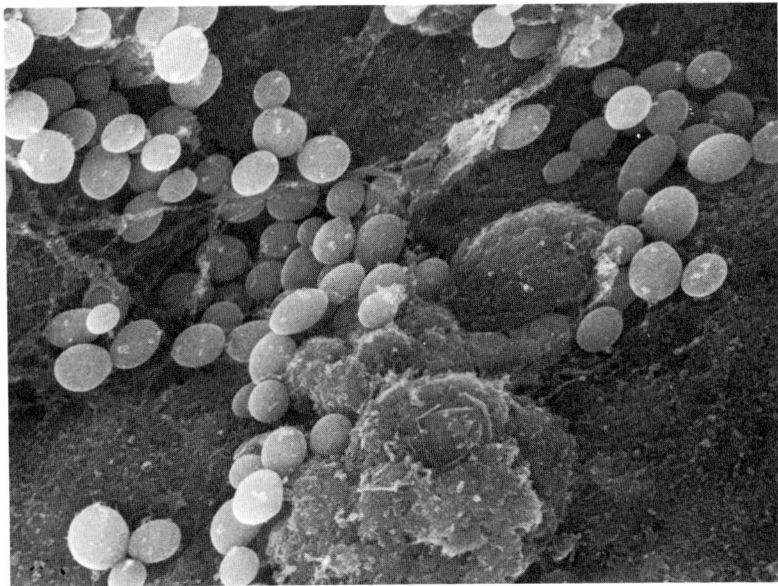

FIG. 4-12. Yeast on the secreting epithelium of the stomach from an infant mouse 30 minutes after oral innoculation with *C. albicans* CA30 (× 1,500). (From Pope and Cole [216].)

that *C. albicans* can associate with GI mucosa presumably by several different (distinct) mechanisms.

Examination of the stomach mucosa of infant mice revealed that at early times after *Candida* inoculation, yeast cells were attached to both keratinized squamous epithelia (Fig. 4-11) and columnar secreting epithelial (Fig. 4-12) surfaces. At later times, yeast were also seen attached to the secreting epithelium surrounded by and embedded in mucus (Fig. 4-13), and were observed to be associated with and attached to lactobacilli (Fig. 4-14) at the junction of the keratinized and secreting epithelium (5, 216, 217). Hyphal invasion of the keratinized region of the stomach has also been observed in both infant and adult mice (5, 216, 217). Fig. 4-15 shows yeast and hyphae in the cardial-atrium section of stomach from an adult gnotobiotic mouse which had been monoassociated with *C. albicans*. This site appears to be the preferential location in the stomach in some experimental animals (103), and in some studies it was observed to be the sole colonization and invasion site by *C. albicans* (5, 109, 216, 217). It may be that the cardial-atrium ridge contains an abundant number of receptors, which allow *C. albicans* to colonize this region of the stomach preferentially. These findings suggest that *C. albicans* can associate with stomach mucosa by a number of adhesion and association mechanisms. These include direct adhesion to the epithelium, indirect attachment to the epithelium by association with other microorganisms, and pene-

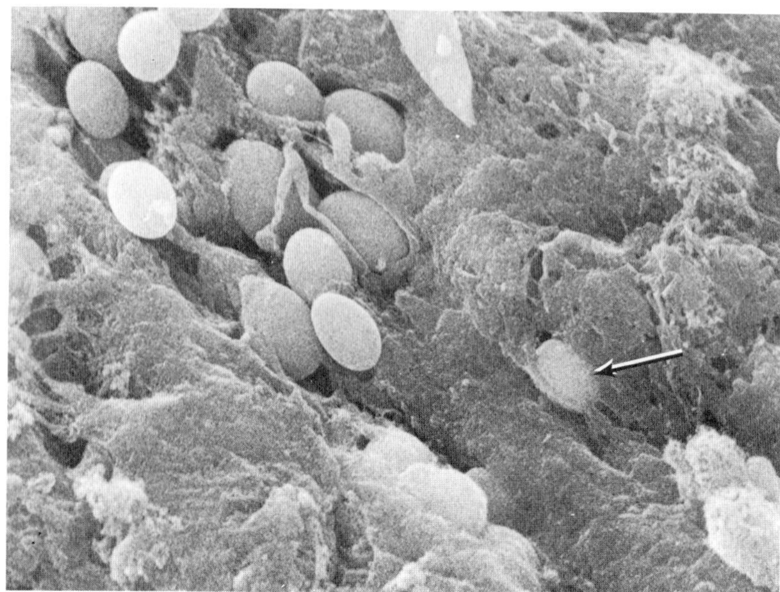

FIG. 4-13. *C. albicans* CA30 on the secreting epithelium of the infant mouse stomach 3 hours after intragastric inoculation. Yeast cells are surrounded by mucus, and one yeast cell is nearly covered by the mucus layer (*arrow*) (× 2,500). (From Pope and Cole [216].)

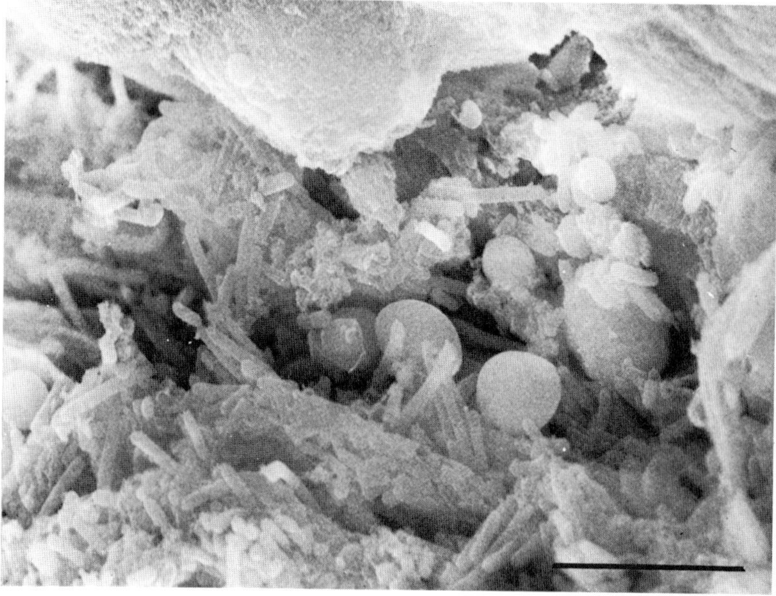

FIG. 4-14. Scanning electron micrograph of the junction of the keratinized epithelium of the stomach of an infant mouse 3 hours after inoculation with *C. albicans* CA30. Yeast cells appear to be attached to and associated with lactobacilli adherent to the keratinized epithelium (× 2,600). (From Pope and Cole [216].)

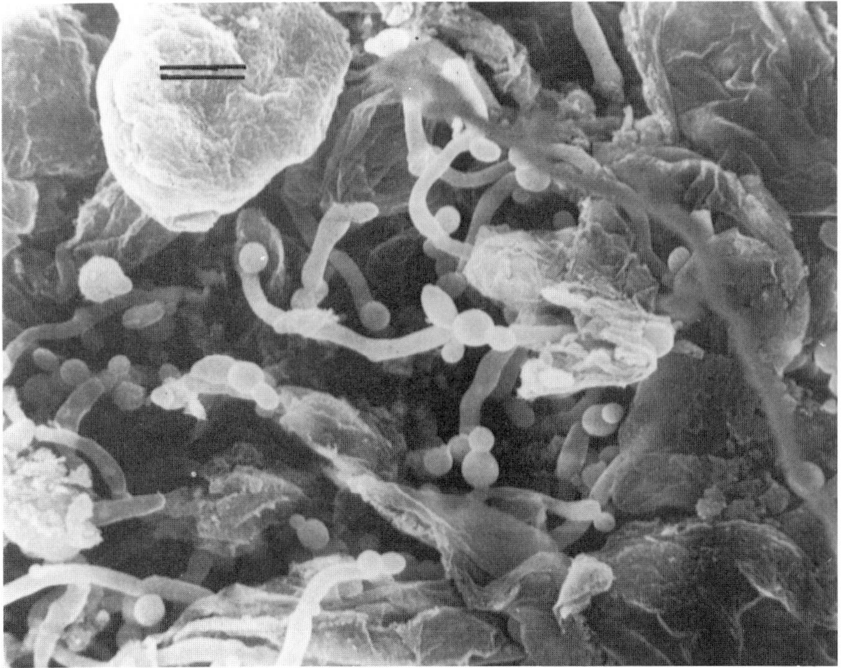

FIG. 4.15. Yeast and hyphae in the cardial-atrium section of the stomach of an adult gnotobiotic mouse monoassociated with *C. albicans* B311 (type A). Bar = 10 μm. (From Balish et al. [5].)

tration of the epithelium. At present, no attempt has been made to identify *Candida* adhesins or mucosal receptors that might be involved in gastric colonization by *C. albicans*.

The association of *Candida* with small intestinal mucosal surfaces has also been studied in infected animals. These studies have demonstrated that *C. albicans* can associate with intestinal mucosa by serveral different and distinct mechanisms (71, 216, 217). Using an infant mouse model Pope and Cole (71, 216, 217) reported that large numbers of *C. albicans* were clearly visible on the surface of villi (Fig. 4-16) in the small intestine within a short time after inoculation. A closer examination revealed that yeast adhered to all areas of the epithelium (Fig. 4-17). Fig. 4-18 and 4-19 show *C. albicans* on the surface of the villi at 6 h after intragastric inoculation. Many yeasts were also seen frequently in association with mucus, and appeared to be attached to, embedded in, and covered by a layer of mucus (Fig. 4-17 and 4-20). Histologic sections at 3 and 6 hours postchallenge also revealed cells embedded in the villus surface (Fig. 4-21), and that some yeasts were associating indirectly with the mucosa by attaching to adherent yeast (Fig. 4-22). Ultrathin sections from small intestinal mucosa showed that yeast cells did not attach to microvilli, but instead they attached to the epithelial glycocalyx (Fig. 4-23).

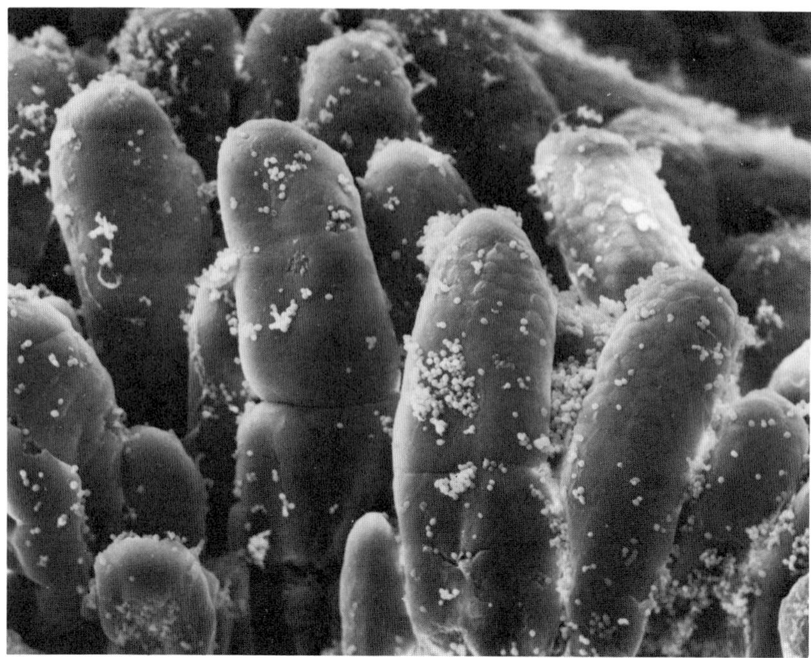

FIG. 4-16. Scanning electron micrograph of the small intestine of an infant mouse 6 hours after oral-intragastric inoculation with *C. albicans* CA30. A large number of yeast cells can be seen attached to intestinal villi (× 550). (From Pope and Cole [217].)

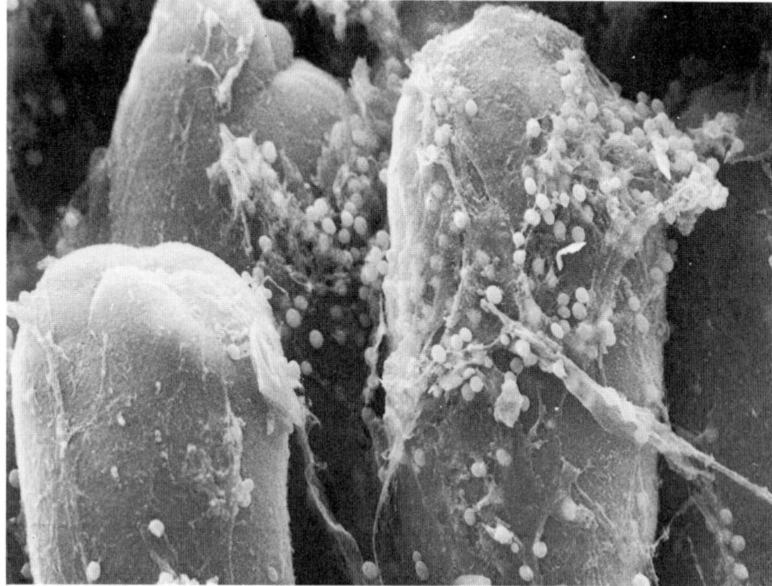

FIG. 4-17. Upper portion of the small intestine of an infant mouse 30 minutes after inoculation with *C. albicans* CA30. Many yeast cells can be seen adhering to all regions of the villus surface; some *Candida* cells are associated with and covered by a layer of mucus (× 520). (From Pope and Cole [216].)

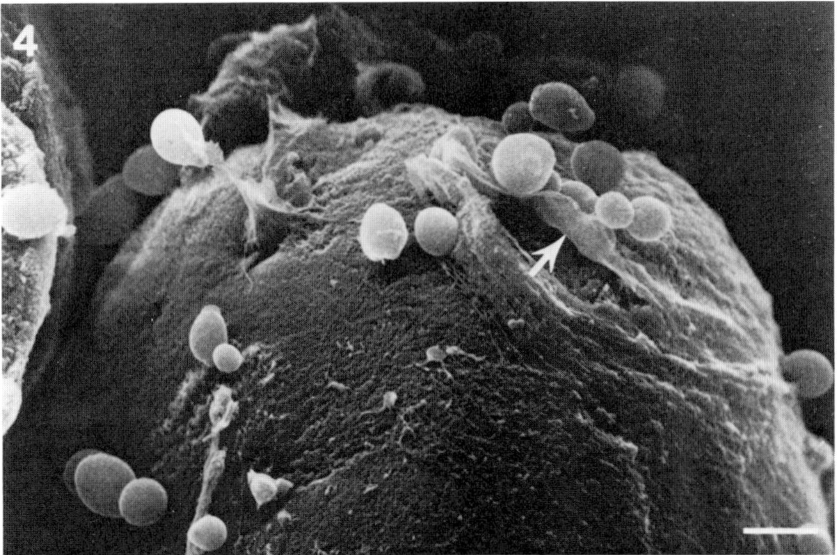

FIG. 4-18. Scanning electron micrograph of the tip of an ileal villus of an infant mouse at 6 hours after orogastric inoculation with *C. albicans* NS33. Yeast cells are attached to the villus and entangled in mucus (*arrow*). Bar = 5 μm; reduced by 15%. (From Pope et al. [215].)

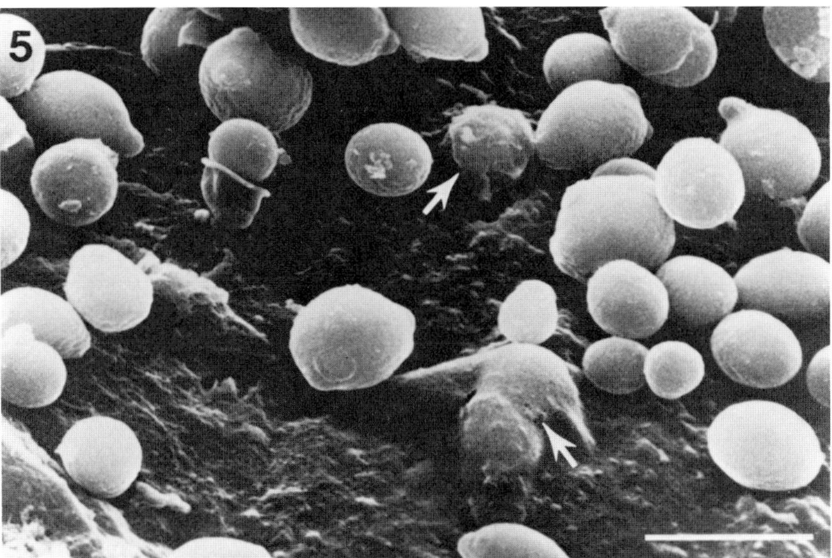

FIG. 4-19. Association of *C. albicans* NS33 with an ileal section of an infant mouse at 6 hours after inoculation. Note yeast cells beneath the mucus layer (*arrows*). Bar = 5 μm; reduced by 15%. (From Pope et al. [215].)

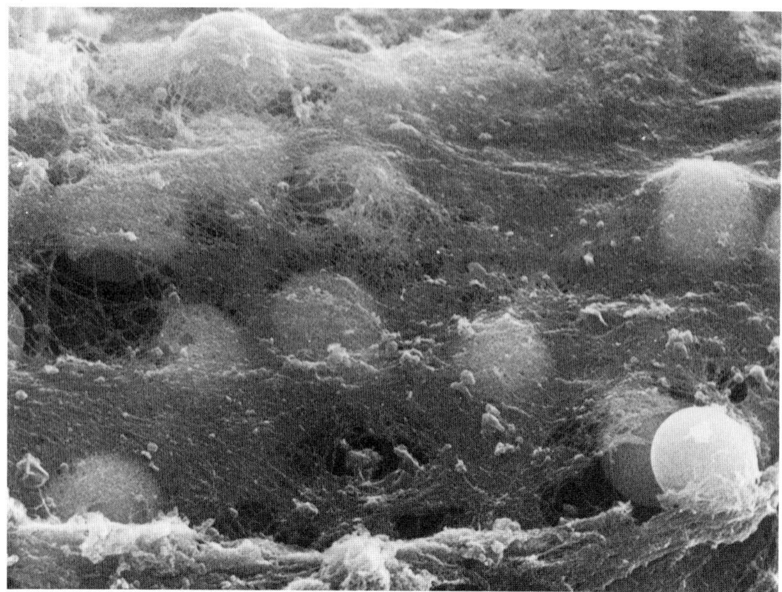

FIG. 4-20. Scanning electron micrograph of the upper intestine of an infant mouse 3 hours after intragastric inoculation with *C. albicans* CA30. Yeast cells attached to the epithelial surfaces are covered with a layer of mucus, which appears to be fibrous in some areas (× 2,800). (From Pope and Cole [216].)

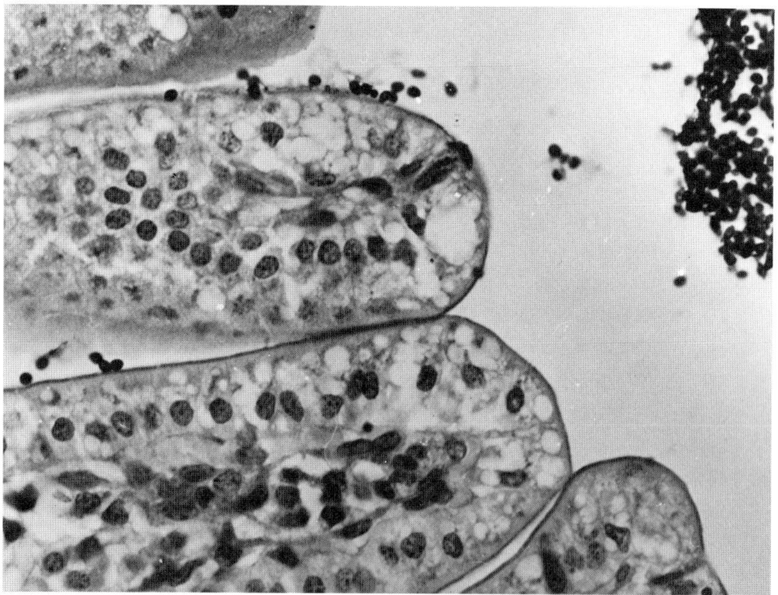

FIG. 4-21. Histologic section of the upper portion of the small intestine of an infant mouse 30 minutes after orogastric inoculation with *C. albicans* NS33. A yeast cell is embedded in the villus surface and other yeast cells appear to be attached to the surface. A bolus of yeast is visible in the lumen of the intestine (× 900). (From Pope and Cole [216].)

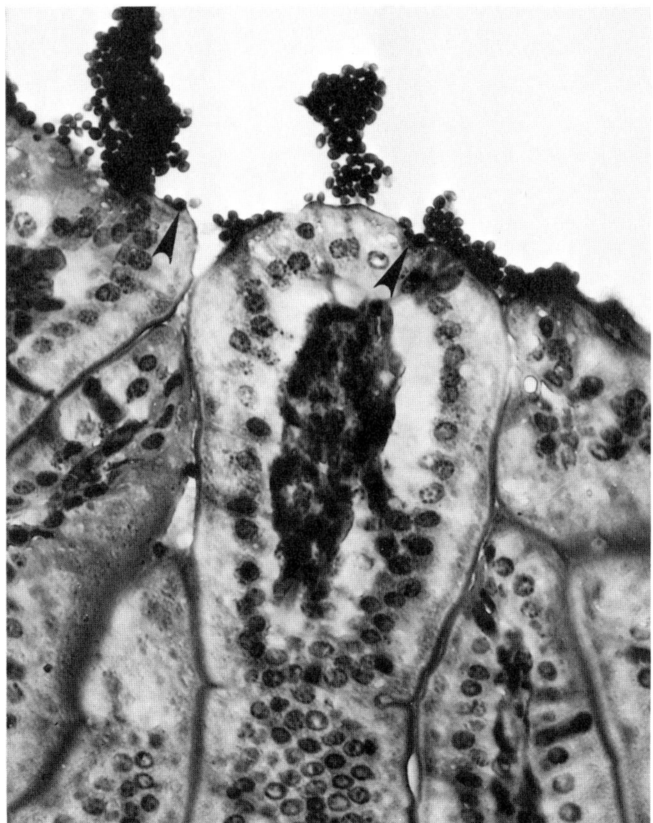

FIG. 4-22. Histologic section of tissue from the upper portion of the small intestine of a neonatal mouse 3 hours postchallenge with *C. albicans* NS33. Numerous yeast cells are attached to the epithelium en masse apparently due to coadhesion. Note individual yeast cells adherent to the villus tips associated with shallow depressions (*arrows*). Magnification × 1,100. (From Pope and Cole [217].)

Examination of large intestinal mucosal surfaces from adult animals revealed that *C. albicans* associated with these surfaces by similar mechanisms (138, 140). However, this was true only when the animals were given antimicrobics to disrupt the ecology of the indigenous bacterial flora (137, 139). SEM studies revealed that large numbers of *C. albicans* were present on the surface of the epithelium and mucus in antimicrobic-treated animals challenged with *C. albicans* (Fig. 4-24), whereas no yeast were observed associating with host mucosal surfaces of untreated animals similarly challenged. In the latter case, large numbers of indigenous bacteria were seen colonizing the mucosa (Fig. 4-25). In mice given antimicrobics, *C. albicans* could associate with the mucosa of all areas of the GI tract, but the cecum had the highest population levels.

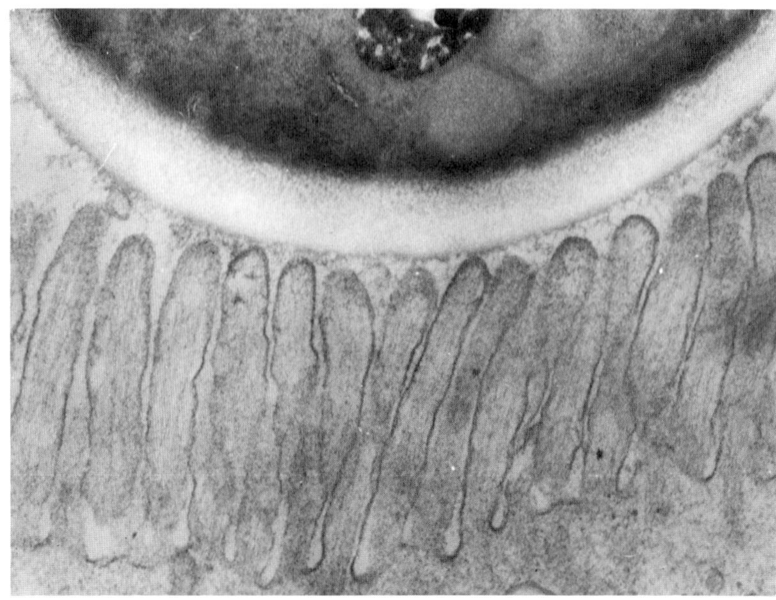

FIG. 4-23. An ultrathin section of the upper intestine of an infant mouse 3 hours after oral-intragastric inoculation with *C. albicans* NS33. A yeast cell has adhered to the villus surface without apparent damage to the microvilli. Note the dark fibrous material, which is probably the epithelial glycocalyx, at the yeast-microvillus junction. Magnification ×40,000. (From Pope and Cole [216].)

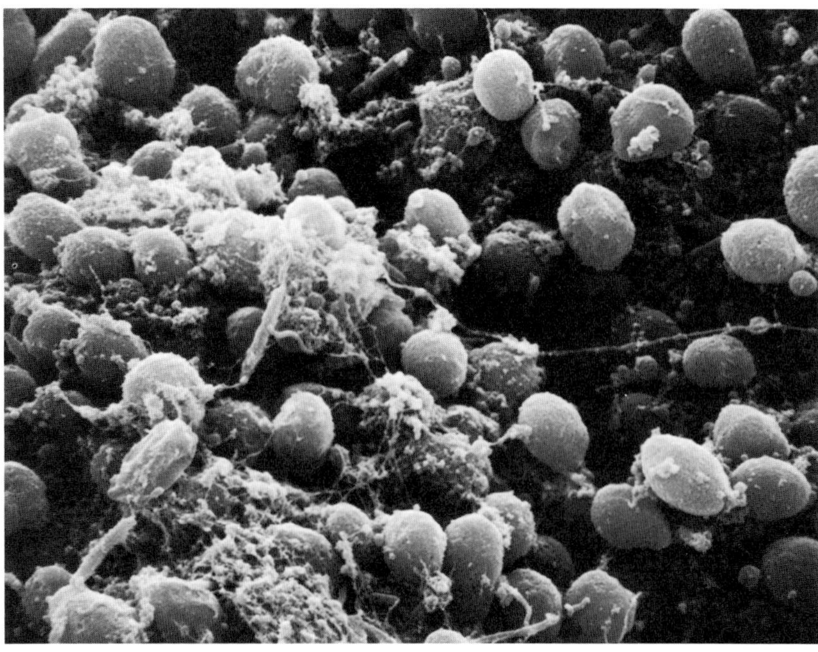

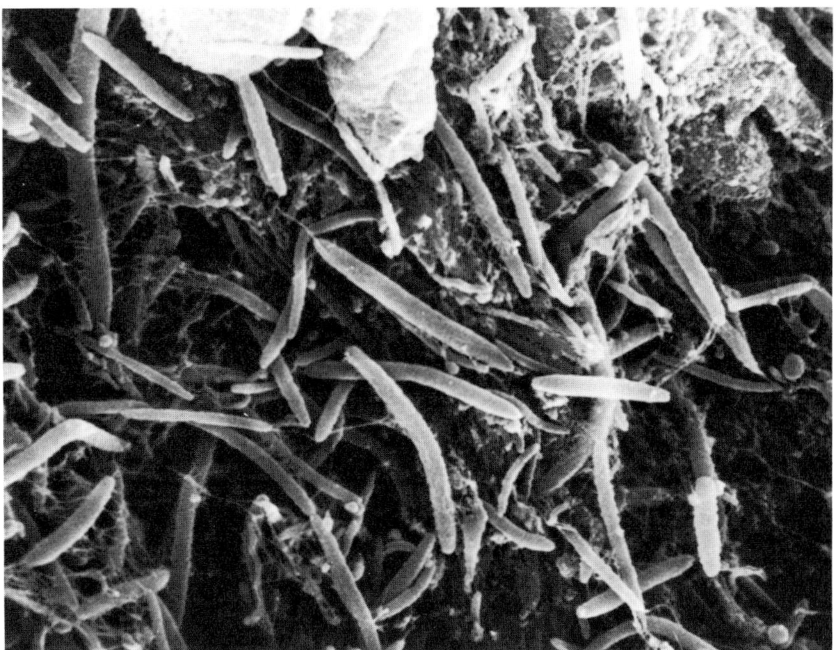

FIG. 4-25. Scanning electron micrograph of the cecum from an adult conventional mouse challenged with *C. albicans* CA34 72 hours after inoculation showing the surface-associated microbiota. The absence of large numbers of yeast as noted in Figure 4-24 is apparent. Magnification ×5,000. (From Kennedy et al. [140].)

Further examination of the cecal mucosa of antimicrobic-treated animals challenged with *C. albicans* revealed that *Candida* cells could attach to the epithelium (Fig. 4-26), possibly by adhesion to the epithelial glycocalyx (Fig. 4-27). In addition, yeast cells were observed to attach directly to or were seen embedded in mucus material (Fig. 4-28). It was also found that *C. albicans* could associate with the cecal mucosal surface indirectly by attaching to other adherent organisms. Fig. 4-29 shows *Candida* cells attached to adherent yeast cells, and Fig. 4-30 shows *Candida* cells attached to adherent bacteria. The possible importance of these interactions is apparent in Fig. 4-31 which shows a microcolony of *Candida* in the cecum at 72 hours after oral challenge, with some yeasts associated with the epithelium, and others attached to mucus material and other yeast cells. If these microcolonies are formed in intestinal mucosa in humans, this may explain the isolated plaques observed by certain

---

◁ FIG. 4-24. Scanning electron micrograph of the cecum from a penicillin-treated adult mouse 72 hours after orogastric inoculation with *C. albicans* CA34. Note the absence of indigenous mucosal-associated bacteria and the presence of adherent *Candida* cells. Magnification ×2,175. (From Kennedy et al. [140].)

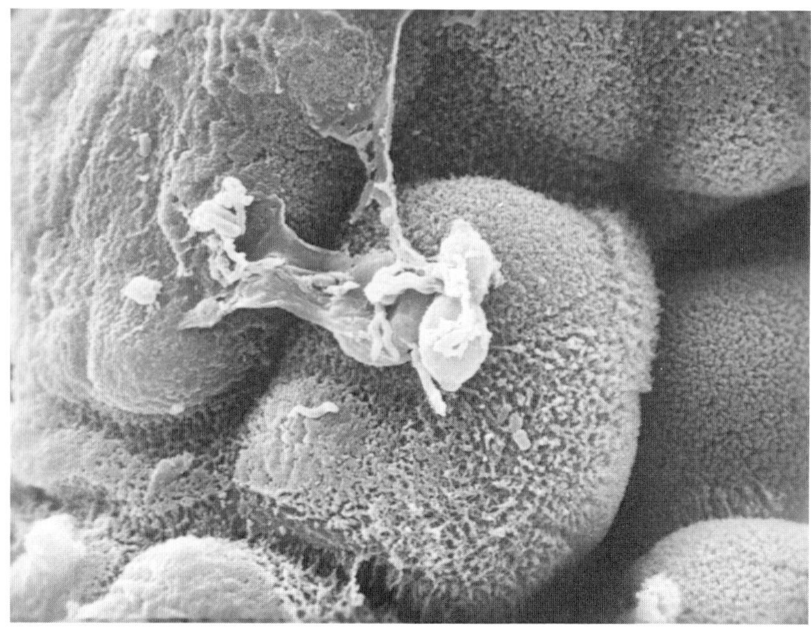

FIG. 4-26. Cecal mucosa from an adult mouse treated with vancomycin 72 hours after inoculation with *C. albicans* CA34 showing direct attachment to cecal epithelium. Magnification ×5,000. (From Kennedy et al. [140].)

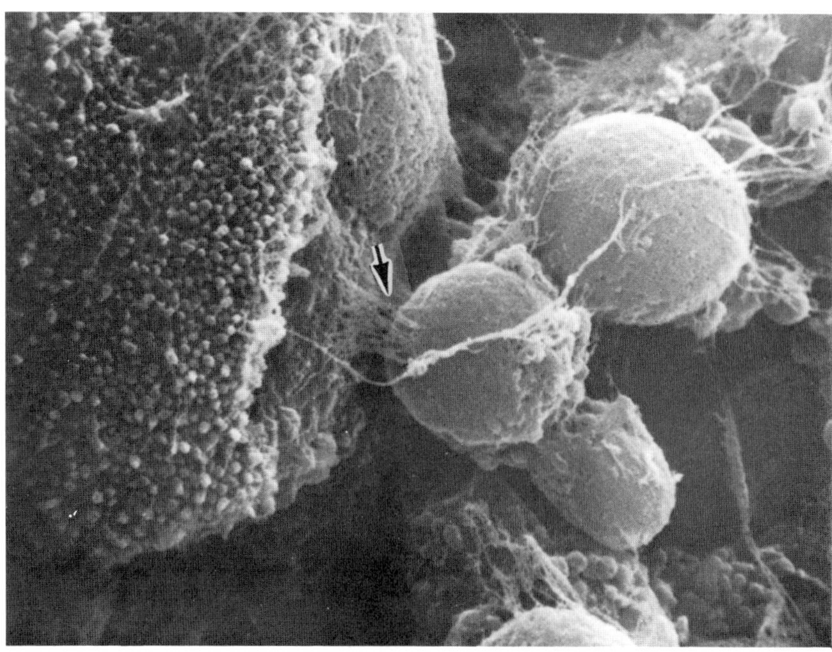

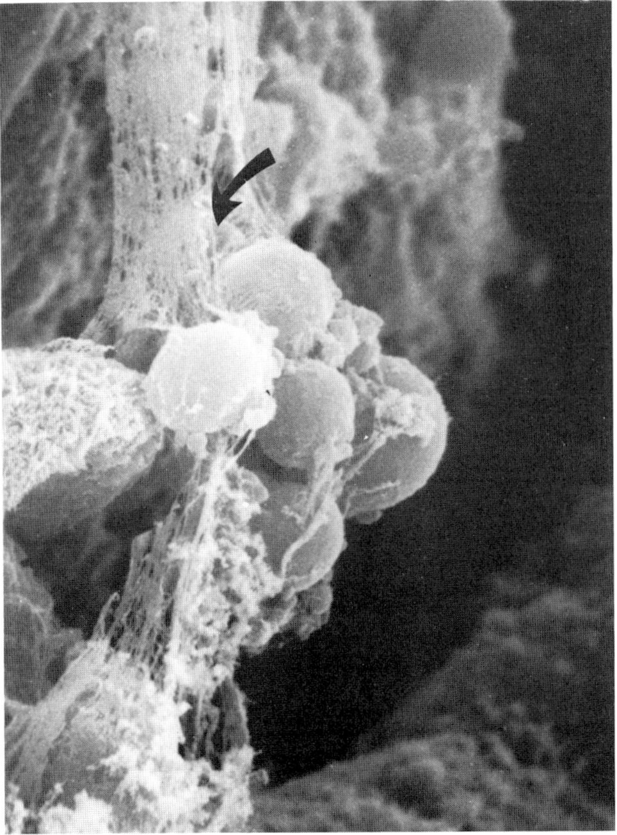

FIG. 4-28. Cecal mucosa from an adult penicillin-treated animal challenged by the oral-intragastric route with *C. albicans* CA34. Yeast cells can be seen attached to and embedded (*arrow*) in mucus. Magnification, × 7,000 (From Kennedy and Volz [138].)

workers on examination of intestinal mucosa infected with *C. albicans* (68, 129). Microcolony formation has been suggested to be of ecologic and pathologic importance in colonization of mucosal surfaces by other pathogens (38, 42, 43). Depressions in the epithelium also were observed under *Candida* cells, possibly due to enzymatic lysis which may expose underlying receptors and stabilize *C. albicans* to the epithelium after the initial adhesion. It is interesting to note that germ tubes or hyphae were not observed to penetrate the mucosa of the small or large intestine in these studies (138, 140).

◁ FIG. 4-27. Scanning electron micrograph of cecal mucosa from an adult penicillin-treated mouse 72 hours after oral intragastric inoculation with *C. albicans* CA34 showing yeast associated with the epithelium, possibly by adhesion to the epithelial glycocalyx (*arrow*). Magnification × 10,000. (From Kennedy et al. [140].)

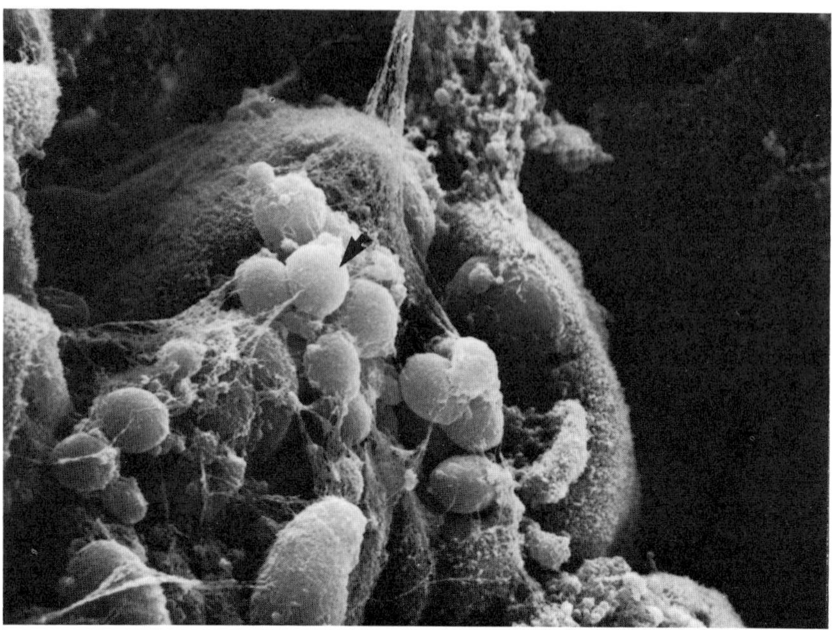

Fig. 4-29. Cecal mucosa from an adult conventional mouse treated with penicillin 72 hours after orogastric challenge with *C. albicans* CA34 showing yeast cells (*arrow*) indirectly associated with the mucus by attaching to other adherent yeast cells. Magnification ×3,000. (From Kennedy et al. [140].)

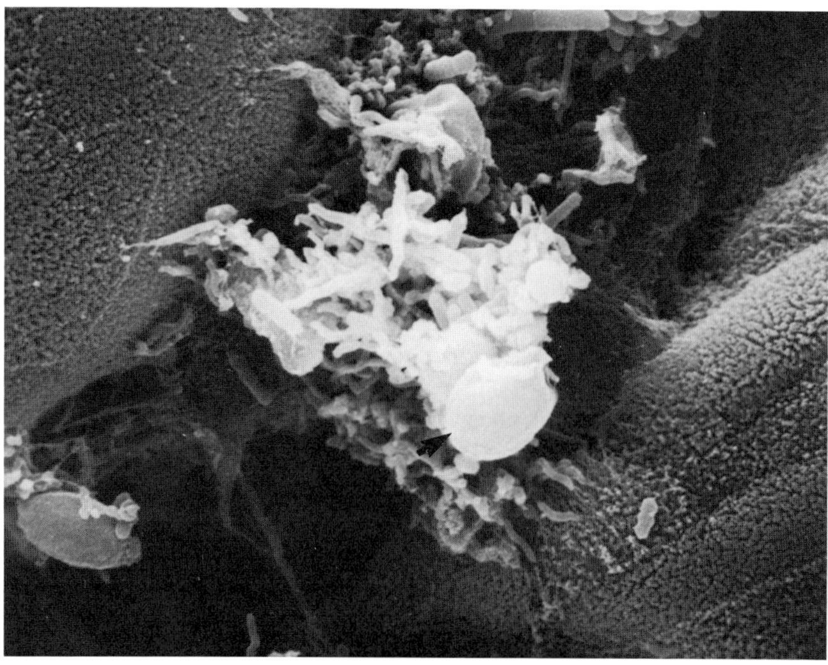

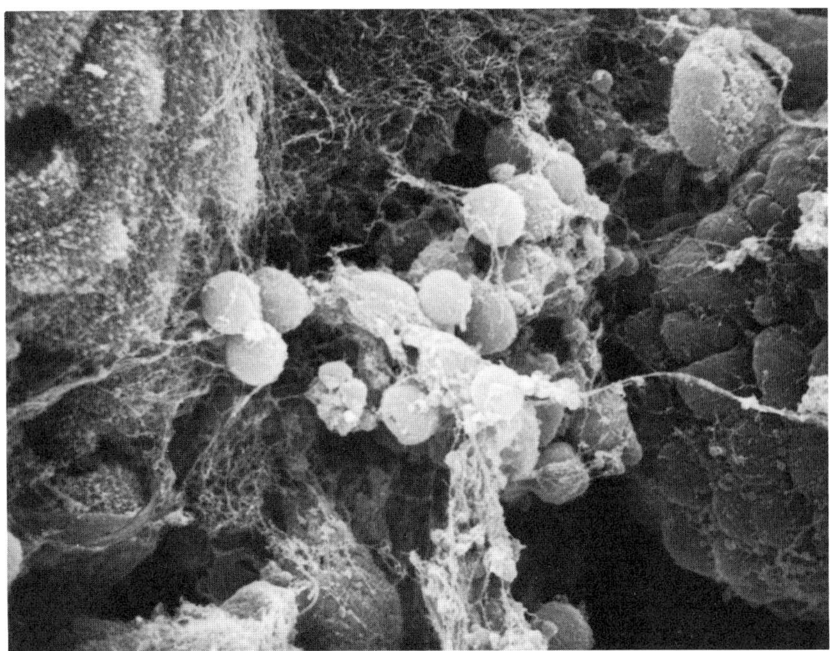

FIG. 4-31. Scanning electron microscopy of cecal mucosa from an adult penicillin-treated mouse showing a microcolony of *C. albicans* CA34 on the mucosal surface 72 hours after intragastric challenge. Note that some yeast cells are attached to the surface, while others are attached to adherent yeast. Magnification × 3,000. (From Kennedy et al. [140].)

Although *C. albicans* was observed to associate with, and appeared to attach to mucus in the specimens processed for electron microscopy described, the mucus gel was not maintained intact and appeared to be somewhat amorphous. Therefore, to determine more conclusively if *C. albicans* could associate with the mucus gel proper, and to insure that the apparent attachment to mucus was not due to specimen processing (which can cause mucus to shrink), *Candida* adhesion to mucus gel was tested in vitro (140). It was found that large numbers of *C. albicans* associated with intestinal mucus very rapidly (within 5 minutes) when mixed together in vitro, and that *Candida* organisms were attached to and embedded in the gel. Quantitative cultures of *Candida* in the mucosa of infected animals showed that approximately 20% of the associated *C. albicans* were present in the mucus gel (140).

The nature of the adhesive events between *C. albicans* and the intestinal mucosa, as well as between *Candida* and other adherent microorganisms,

---

◁ FIG. 4-30. *Candida* (CA34) cells (*arrow*) indirectly associated with the cecal mucosa of an adult mouse treated with vancomycin by attaching to adherent bacteria. Magnification × 5,000. (From Kennedy et al. [140].)

remains to be determined. It seems unlikely that nonspecific interactions, such as cell surface hydrophobicity, played a significant role in the adhesion of *Candida* to mucosa (135, 140). Studies with bacteria are consistent with this view, and suggest that specific adhesion predominates over nonspecific adhesion (119). Therefore, it seems likely that a complex adhesive system is involved in the attachment of *C. albicans* to various mucosal surfaces and other microorganisms, and may be mediated by two or more distinct adhesive entities in which nonsepcific interactions (eg, hydrophobicity) may or may not play a role (135, 140).

The Urogenital Tract

Examination of ultramicroscopic preparations of tissue from patients and experimental animals infected with *C. albicans*, and exfoliated epithelial cells mixed with *Candida* cells in vitro, have revealed that this fungus interacted with mucosal surfaces from urogenital systems by mechanisms similar to those described for oral and GI mucosa. Both yeast and hyphae have been observed to attach to vaginal mucosa in vitro and in vivo, and several adhesion and association mechanisms appeared to be involved. These include yeast and hyphal adhesion, hyphal penetration, and coadhesion to adherent organisms (5, 25, 175). Yeast cells were often seen partially enclosed in phagocytic-like invaginations of vaginal cells (25).

Two different mechanisms or phases of adhesion between *C. albicans* and vaginal epithelium also were noted (25, 175). Following inoculation with yeasts, experimental animals were sacrificed at various intervals thereafter and vaginal tissue examined by SEM, TEM, and light microscopy of histological sections. At early times after inoculation, yeast cells could be seen adhering to vaginal epithelial cells by both "loose" and "tight" adhesion (175). Again the former interaction was presumably mediated by a ruthenium red-staining matrix, whereas the latter association was not. In that instance, a close contact between the yeast and the host cell could be observed. Hyphal penetration of vaginal epithelial cell layers followed, and appeared to occur in a manner analogous to that observed in the penetration of oral and gastric epithelium. Fig. 4-32 shows yeast cells of *C. albicans* attaching to the mucosal surface from the vagina of an infected mouse.

Attempts to describe the physiochemical nature of adhesion of *Candida* to vaginal or urothelial cells have been few. Lee and King (157) studied *C. albicans* adhesion to vaginal epithelial cells and found that pretreatment of yeast cells with detergents, salts, or urea had little or no effect on adhesion. Furthermore, the addition of salts or divalent cations to the assay mixture had no effect on adhesion. On the other hand, pretreatment of *C. albicans* with β-mercaptoethanol and dithiothreitol reduced adhesion to vaginal epithelial cells by 55 and 51%, respectively. These studies suggest that the adhesion observed in this system was not solely mediated via hydrophobic, electrosta-

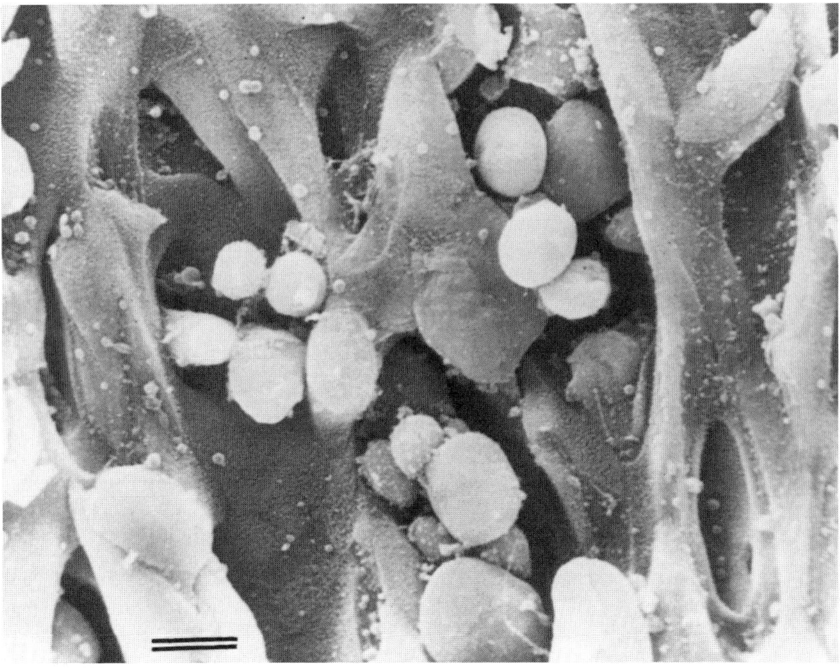

FIG. 4-32. Yeast cells adhering to the vaginal mucosal surface of an adult gnotobiotic mouse monoassociated with *C. albicans* B311 (type A). Bar = 10 μm. (From Balish et al. [5].)

tic, or ion-bridging bonds. The finding that reducing agents caused a reduction in adhesion, in contrast, may indicate that electrostatic interactions were important in adhesion, but it may also suggest that these treatments abolished the structural integrity of the adhesin(s) (157). Proof of the latter would indicate that specific adhesion was the critical step in attachment. The results of other studies are contradictory as to the role hydrophobic or electrostatic interactions may play in the adhesion of *C. albicans* to vaginal epithelial cells (207, 289, 290). All of these studies, however, used different *Candida* strains, environmental and assay parameters, and yeast growth media (157, 207, 289, 290). Moreover, only one of these studies used conditions that are similar to those found in the vagina (207). Therefore, it is difficult to compare these results, and it is even more difficult to determine which factors may be important in vivo.

Fibrin-Platelet Matrices and Endocardial Tissue

Candida endocarditis is characterized by the development of vegetations that form on the endothelium of damaged heart valves, to which *Candida* cells are readily attached and entrapped in (172, 173, 271, 284). These vegetations are composed primarily of fibrin, platelets, and erythrocytes, and enlarge due to the presence and influence of the yeast causing platelet aggregation (172, 284). Platelets also contribute to the pathogenesis of this infection by stimulating yeast germination, providing growth factors for the yeast and, possibly, by promoting the clotting cascade on the valve surface (172, 271, 284). From these studies it was suggested that circulating yeasts appear to selectively adhere to the fibrin-platelet network overlying the traumatized valvular leaflets.

Using a rabbit model of endocarditis, Calderone et al. (23) characterized the development of vegetation formation after intravenous injection of *C. albicans*. Within 30 to 90 minutes after infection, yeast cells were observed adhering to fibrin-platelet-erythrocyte deposits which formed preferentially in the left side of the heart. Previous studies by Freedman and Johnson (76) gave similar results and showed that populations of *Candida* cells in vegetations of the left side of the heart were always 2–3 logs higher than those in the right side (76). Nevertheless, as the infection progressed, vegetations near the aortic valve consisted of a dense layer of platelets and fibrin, and numerous macrophages were entrapped within the tight fibrin matrix. Forty-eight hours after inoculation, many macrophages within the vegetations contained phagocytized yeasts which had produced germ tubes. By 1 week, the mature vegetations were observed to contain a dense network of pseudohyphae, and apparently offered *Candida* cells a protective growth environment (23, 269).

These same authors have used fibrin-platelet matrices formed in vitro as a model to study early events of adhesion of *C. albicans* to damaged valvular endothelium and found these clots to closely resemble those formed in vivo (172). Moreover, the data obtained from using fibrin-platelet clots in in vitro adhesion assays correlate well with studies performed in the aforementioned rabbit model of endocarditis. Fig. 4-33 shows *C. albicans* cells attaching to a fibrin-platelet matrix in vitro in a manner similar to that seen on endocardial vegetations of infected rabbits (172).

From these and other studies (172, 284) it appears as though two association mechanisms are involved with the colonization of traumatized heart valves by *C. albicans*. The first mechanism appears to be the direct adhesion of *Candida* cells to the traumatized endocardium (172). Studies with two adhesion-negative mutants of *C. albicans* are consistent with this view, and suggest that adhesion is mediated by a specific adhesin-receptor interaction (24). Further studies are necessary, however, to determine the exact nature of adhesion, the surface factors that serve as the *Candida* adhesin and its corresponding fibrin-platelet surface receptor, and the number and affinity of binding sites. The second mechanism is the simple entrapment of *Candida* cells within the vegetation, which eventually gives rise to emboli (23, 132). Although the initial adhesion is probably the determinant of colonization in vivo, entrapment of *C. albicans* stabilizes colonization by preventing the *Candida* from being removed from the surface.

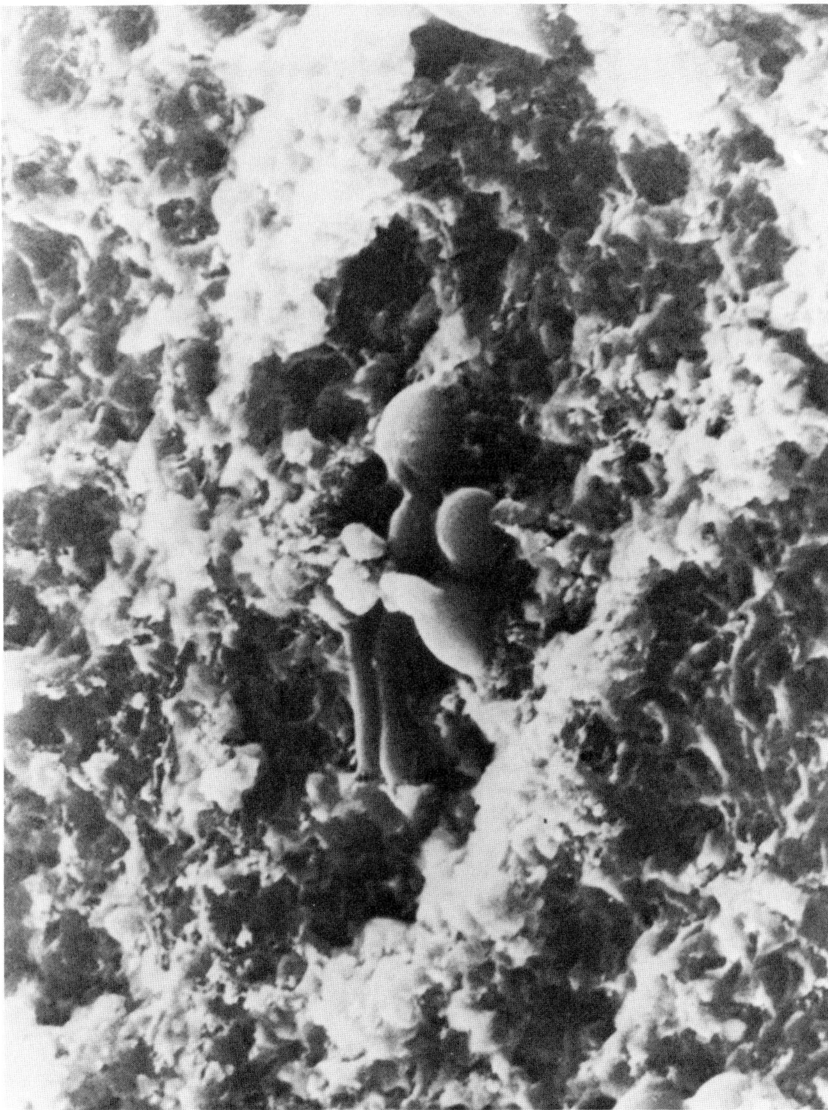

FIG. 4-33. Scanning electron micrograph showing *C. albicans* adherent to a fibrin-platelet clot formed in vitro (× 24,000; reduced by 3%). (From Maisch and Calderone [172].)

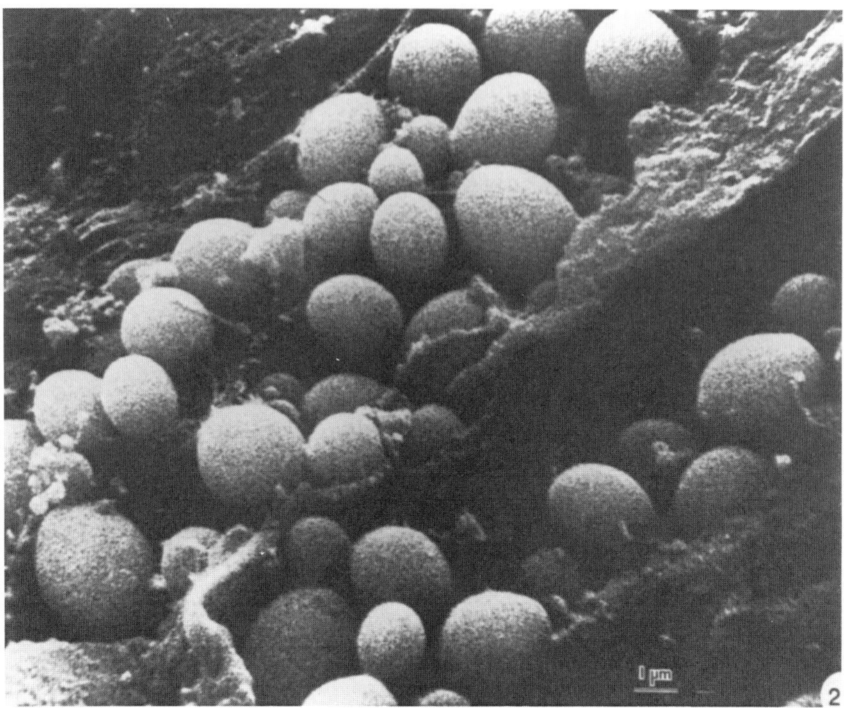

FIG. 4-34. Scanning electron micrograph of aortic endothelial tissue with adherent *C. albicans* 15 minutes after inoculation in vitro (× 6,300; reduced by 19%). (From Klotz et al. [145].)

Vascular Endothelium

Deep-seated infection after hematogenous dissemination of *C. albicans* is probably dependent on the fungus attaching to and traversing vascular endothelium (9, 146, 236). Several model systems have been used to study endothelial attachment and penetration by *Candida* in vitro and in vivo (146, 236). Klotz et al. (146) studied the adhesion and penetration of porcine vascular endothelium by *C. albicans* and followed the early progression of association and penetration ultrastructurally. Fig. 4-34 through 4-39 summarize these results. Fig. 4-34 shows the association of *C. albicans* to aortic endothelium at 15 minutes of incubation, and Fig. 4-35 shows the matching TEM photomicrograph obtained at the same time interval. As can be seen, within 15 minutes yeast attachment to the endothelium was apparently mediated by a tight adhesion, and a partial disruption of the endothelial surface. This was followed by a more severe damage to the endothelium at 30 minutes (Fig. 4-36 and 4-37), and by 60 minutes (Fig. 4-38 and 4-39) yeast cells had burrowed deeply into the aortic tissue. This penetration was apparently due to

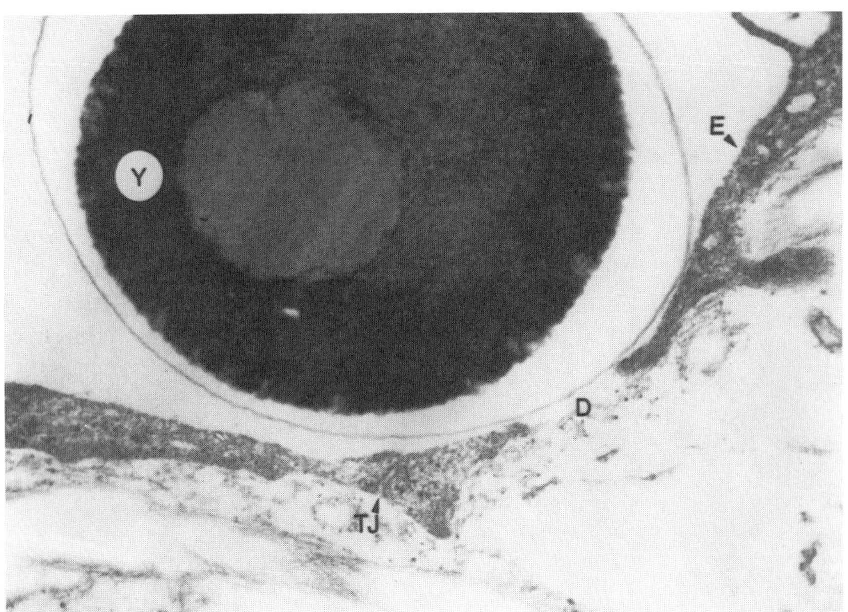

FIG. 4-35. An ultrathin section of aortic endothelial tissue (E) with an adherent *C. albicans* yeast (Y) cell after 15 minutes of incubation in vitro showing dissolution of endothelial cell continuity (D) near a tight junction (TJ) (× 41,000; reduced by 29%). (From Klotz et al. [145].)

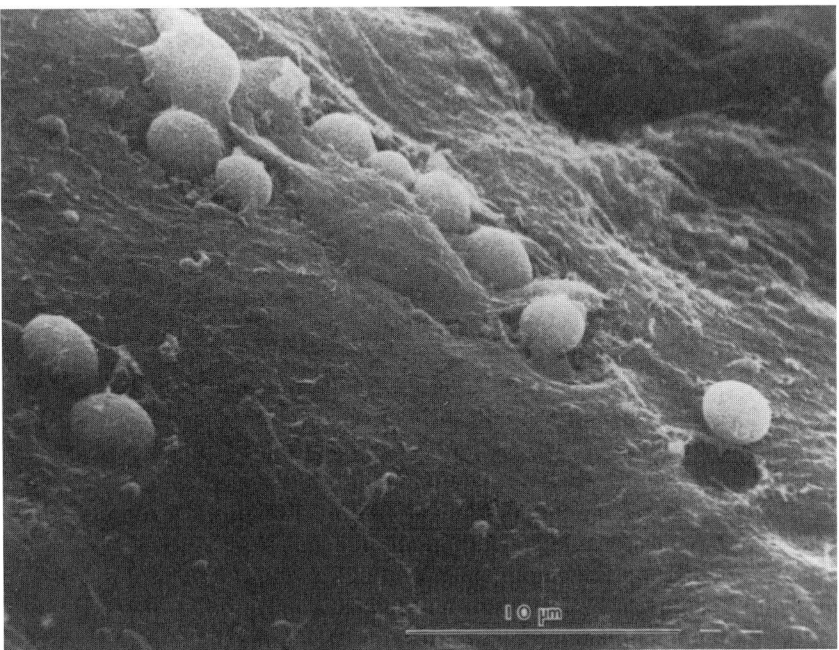

FIG. 4-36. Aortic endothelial tissue after 30 minutes of incubation with *C. albicans* yeast cells in vitro. Several yeast can be seen adherent to the tissue (× 4,000; reduced by 25%). (From Klotz et al. [145].)

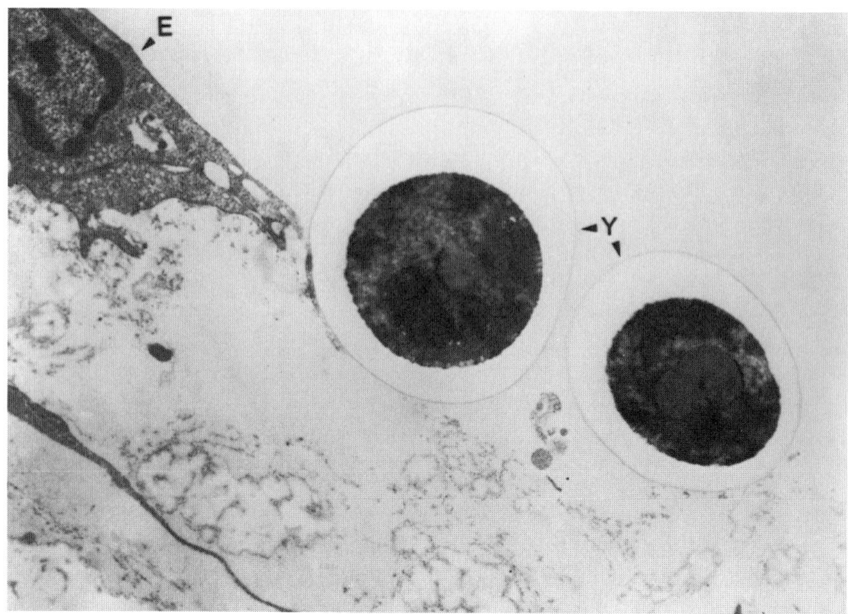

FIG. 4-37. Transmission electron micrograph of aortic endothelial tissue (E) with adherent *C. albicans* yeast cells (Y) after 30 minutes of incubation in vitro. Note the dissolution of the tissue (× 16,000; reduced by 29%). (From Klotz et al. [145].)

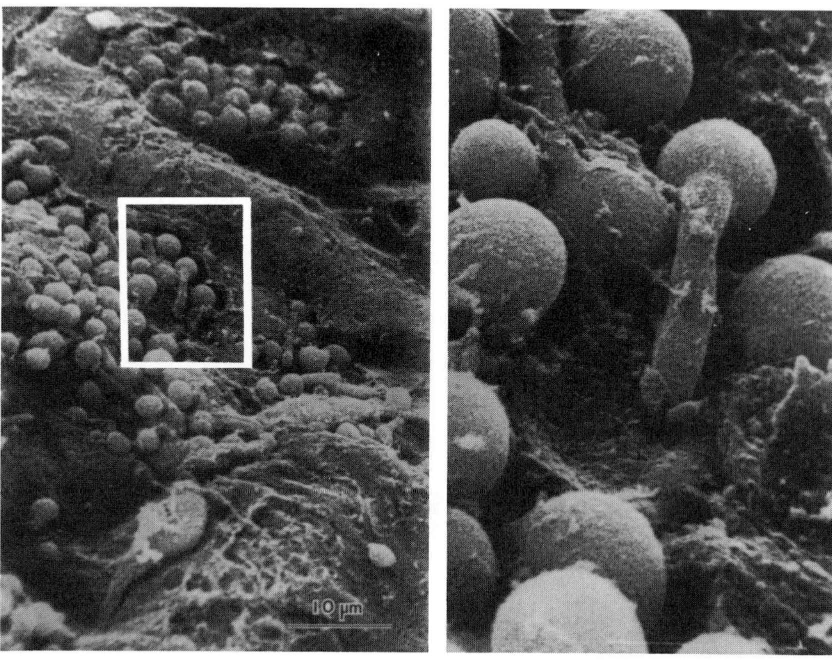

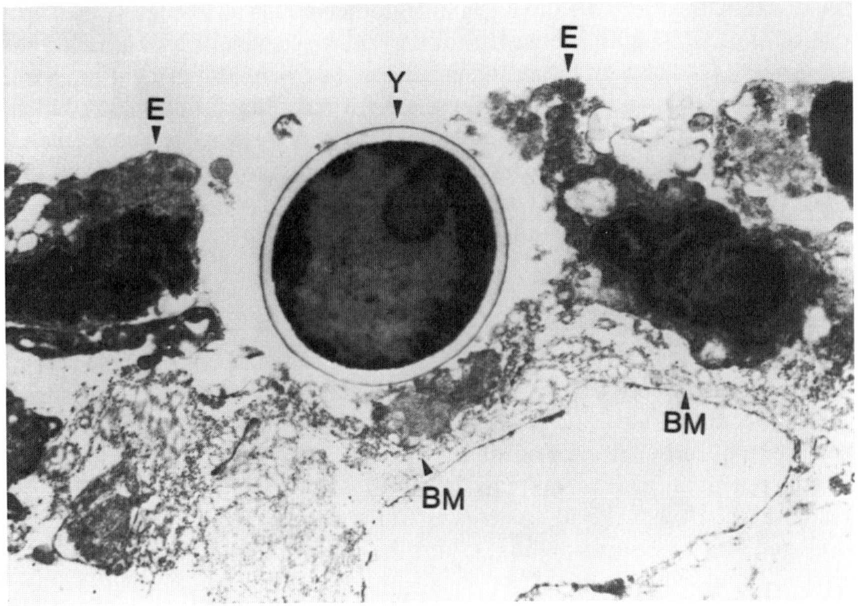

FIG. 4-39. Photomicrograph of *C. albicans* yeast (Y) interaction with porcine endothelial cells (E) after 60 minutes of incubation in vitro. Note the yeast cell has passed between two adjacent endothelial cells and is nearing the basement membrane (BM) (× 16,000; reduced by 29%). (From Klotz et al. [145].)

enzymatic activity by *C. albicans* because heat- or formalin-killed *C. albicans* failed to show evidence of penetration or burrowing, although they adhered to the tissue. Moreover, endothelial damage was limited strictly to yeast attachment sites.

Studies by Rotrosen et al. (236) showed a similar sequence of events in vascular colonization using monolayers of cultured human umbilical vein endothelial cells as the model. For instance, adhesion of *C. albicans* was noted as early as 10 minutes after inoculation to the assay system. This was then followed by invasion of the endothelial cells by the yeast. However, in this system both the mechanism of *Candida* adhesion and penetration of endothelial cells appeared to be different. Transmission electron microscopy of yeast attachment revealed that fungal cells were closely apposed to endothelial cells, but that this adhesion was apparently mediated by fibrillar surface

---

◁ FIG. 4-38. Scanning electron micrograph showing aortic endothelial tissue 60 minutes after inoculation with *C. albicans* in vitro. Note numerous yeast cells adherent to and penetrating the tissue (*inset*). The clustering of adherent yeasts may reflect the clustering of receptor sites on the endothelial tissue (× 1,600 and 81,000, respectively; reduced by 25%). (From Klotz et al. [145].)

appendages. Furthermore, invasion of endothelial cells proceeded via phagocytosis of *Candida* cells, in contrast to entry due to enzymatic lysis as noted by Klotz et al. (145). Germ tubes and pseudohyphae were also evident in endothelial cells in this study. Similarly, studies with experimental animals revealed that the initial penetration of endothelial tissues by *C. albicans* was preceded by adhesion to endothelial surfaces via fibrillar structures extending from the yeast cell, and penetration occured by active growth of germ tubes between or directly through cell bodies (145). Enzymatic lysis was not thought to accompany the initial penetration because germ tubes advanced through the tissue without apparent cellular damage (145).

All of these studies indicate the importance of the initial attachment in penetration of endothelial tissue, but present little data regarding the actual mechanism of adhesion. Lee and King (158) have suggested that attachment to renal endothelium is mediated by a specific adhesin factor, possibly cell surface fibrillae. Whether or not this is the same mechanism that was involved in attachment in the other systems described is not known. Furthermore, the penetration of endothelial tissue was found to proceed by at least three different mechanisms, including germ tube penetration, phagocytic invagination, and enzymatic lysis. Therefore, further studies will be needed to more clearly define the nature of these mechanisms.

Nonbiological Surfaces

The adhesion and association of *C. albicans* with a number of nonbiological surfaces can create a wide range of health problems for humans. Studies on the oral distribution of *Candida* in chronic atrophic candidiasis, a disease that is relatively common among elderly denture wearers (197), have shown that *C. albicans* was recovered more often and in higher numbers from the acrylic denture surface than from the palate (48). This suggests that colonization of the acrylic denture surface serves as a reservoir for infection, and that *Candida* adhesion to the denture surface may be prerequisite for colonization and infection of the palate (179). Likewise, the adhesion of *Candida* cells to various plastic surfaces that are used to make catheters and prosthetic cardiac valves, may also cause serious medical complications in a variety of patients. Relatively few studies on the adhesion of *C. albicans* to these surfaces, however, have been conducted.

The adhesion of *Candida* to acrylic has involved the majority of the studies (179, 183, 191, 248, 253), which have suggested that several factors are likely to be important in this association. Studies by McCourtie and Douglas (179) have shown that growth of *C. albicans* in a chemically defined medium supplemented with a variety of carbohydrates can greatly modify adhesion to acrylic surfaces. Growth of *Candida* in medium supplemented with 500 mM galactose, for instance, showed a significant increase in the amount and rate of adhesion and the production of an extra floccular surface layer (179). Production of this material, which may be a mannoprotein (181), has also been found to cause an increase in adhesion to BECs (59) and an increase in virulence in a systemic mouse model (180). These results have prompted some to suggest that dietary factors may have a profound influence on *Candida* adhesion in vivo (251, 252).

Nevertheless, studies aimed at characterizing the adhesive nature involved in the attachment of *C. albicans* to acrylic surfaces and denture base resins have suggested that cell surface hydrophobicity may mediate, or at least participate in adhesion (146, 187, 188, 191). Miyake et al. (191) found a strong correlation existed between the adhesion capacities of *Candida* species to acrylic surfaces and their cell surface hydrophobicities. It is interesting to note that in these studies *C. albicans* showed the lowest hydropobicity (187, 191, 260), which was probably due to the growth medium and environmental parameters used (260). We have found that growth of *C. albicans* in Sabouraud glucose broth at 37°C, as was used by Miyake et al. (191), produced cells that were only slightly hydrophobic (260). Therefore, it would be of interest to examine cell surface hydrophobicity and adhesion to acrylic after growth of *C. albicans* in a variety of media (260).

It is worth noting that four different methods have been used to determine the cell surface hydrophobicity of *C. albicans*. These included contact angle measurements, separation in water-hydrocarbon two-phase systems, plastic adhesion, and hydrophobic interaction chromatography (146, 187, 188, 191, 230). Comparison of the former two assays indicates that these methods gave similar results. Comparisons between hydrophobic interaction chromatography and the other two methods have not been conducted. All of these methods have certain drawbacks that may influence results. The currently described hydrophobic interaction chromatography method (287), for instance, has the drawback that *Candida* cells may be occluded in the gel, especially if they occur as pseudohyphae or aggregates. A modification of this producedure, where the sample is allowed to mix with the gel instead of passing through it, has been used to avoid this problem (Kennedy, unpublished data).

Ion-bridging bonds have also been suggested to play a role in the adhesion of *C. albicans* to acrylic (179). McCourtie and Douglas (179) found that the addition of divalent cations to assay mixtures caused an increase in *Candida* adhesion to acrylic. The addition of Ca^{2+} was shown to cause a greater increase in adhesion, than was the addition of Mn^{2+} or Mg^{2+}. Cations seemed to cause a slight decrease in adhesion, and EDTA had no effect on its own but abolished the adhesion promoting effect of Ca^{2+}. Cells grown in medium containing glucose, galactose, or sucrose were all found to have an increased adhesion due to Ca^{2+}, but this effect appeared to be greater with the latter sugar. $FeCl_2$ also promoted adhesion to acrylic, but at high concentrations it caused the yeast cells to aggregate and settle to the bottom of the assay wells (179). Thus ion-bridging mechanisms, in addition to cell surface hydrophobicity and other unknown factors (235), may play a role in the adhesion of *C. albicans* to acrylic surfaces.

Other nonbiological surfaces have been studied less extensively than acrylic in regard to *Candida* adhesion. In one study, *Candida* species were shown to attach to both polyvinyl chloride and Teflon catheters, although yeasts adhered more extensively to the former (237). Furthermore, it was also found that *C. tropicalis* adhered in greater numbers than *C. albicans*. In another study, the adhesion of *Candida* species was examined microscopically and revealed adherent *Candida* enmeshed in fibrin-like strands (163). Reinhart et al. (230) studied the adhesion of *C. albicans* to glass and concluded that adhesion was not due to cell surface hydrophobicity. Factors that may govern adhesion of *Candida* to a variety of plastic surfaces were investigated by Klotz et al. (146). These authors found that the adhesion of *C. albicans* to plastic was governed predominantely by hydrophobic properties of both the yeast and plastic surface. Kinetic analyses of the interaction between *C. albicans* and plastic also revealed negative cooperativity determined by Scatchard and Hill plots, due to electrostatic repulsion. This was determined by altering the surface charge of *Candida* cells by selectively blocking amino and carboxyl groups or increasing the ionic strength of the assay solution, and conducting adhesion assays. The more positively charged yeasts adhered in greater numbers, suggesting that the more negatively charged cells were more repulsive to the negatively charged plastic surface. Electrostatic forces were, therefore, deemed to be minor compared to the hydrophobic forces, as the adhesion of *C. albicans* to plastic occurred to a considerable extent.

The investigations of the adhesion of *C. albicans* to acrylic and various plastics described have provided some information that could be useful to prevent or reduce the adhesion of yeasts to these surfaces in vivo. However, further studies will need to be carried out to determine whether or not these in vitro phenomena are applicable to the situation in vivo. In the latter situation, numerous substances are adsorbed to these materials that probably alter their surface properties, and, therefore, the adhesion of yeast and bacteria to them. Saliva, which contains numerous components that adsorb to plastics and acrylic, has been shown to reduce *Candida* adhesion to acrylic when it was applied to acrylic before use in adhesion assays (179, 191, 253). The adsorption of these components may also suggest that specific adhesin-receptor interactions are involved in adhesion to molecules adsorbed to plastics in host tissue. Likewise, all of the previously described experiments have used different growth media and conditions which have been shown to influence *Candida* adhesion and hydrophobicity in vitro (107, 260). Therefore, although it is likely that these properties are important in the adhesion of *C. albicans* to various nonbiological surfaces, further studies are needed to determine the relevance of each in vivo.

Receptors

Jones (119) has described specific adhesion as a two-component system that depends as much on the number and distribution of host surface receptors as it

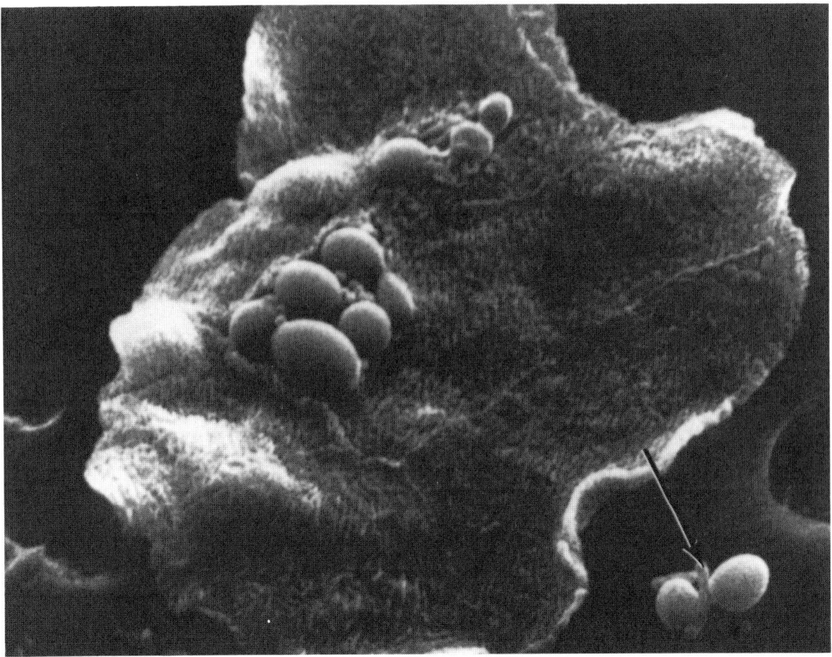

FIG. 4-40. A buccal epithelial cell showing *C. albicans* yeast cells adherent to one general area possibly due to a clustering of receptor sites. In the lower right portion of the micrograph, coaggregation of yeast and bacteria can be noted (*arrow*). Bar = 5 μm. (From Centeno et al. [33].)

does on the extent of adhesin production by the microorganism. Considering that adhesion is a highly selective process, it is reasonable to assume that a minimum number of adhesin-receptor interactions must be achieved before the irreversible adhesion of *C. albicans* to surfaces can occur. A binding site for *C. albicans*, therefore, exists on a surface where the receptor concentration is sufficient to allow adhesion (119). This may account for the differing receptivities of epithelial cells noted from donor to donor, age of donor, hormonal status of donor, body sites in the same donor and date of collection from the same donor (33, 44, 49, 263, 276). Furthermore, receptor concentration may in part account for the variation in the numbers of yeasts which can attach, the uneven distribution of attached yeasts on some surfaces, the preferential site of attachment (eg, microridges on vaginal epithelial cells), and the percentage of buccal cells with attached yeasts (207, 262). In Fig. 4-40, *Candida* cells can be observed adhering to one general area of a BEC, presumably due to a concentration of surface receptors.

Studies with bacteria suggest that most putative receptors on animal cell surfaces are carbohydrates in the D-configuration (with only one exception) (119). These can be associated with integral components of the cell surface such as glycoconjugates, or adsorbed films such as the "acquired pellicle" of tooth surfaces, and are likely to be very complex in nautre (118). Evidence in support of this has come from studies showing that carbohydrates, lectins, and selective enzyme treatments inhibited adhesion (122). Fibronectin, a major surface glycoprotein on animal cells (201), also has been shown to be a receptor for certain bacteria (40). Likewise, other constituents of mammalian cell membranes have been noted to serve as receptors for bacteria (117), but most have not been as well characterized as carbohydrate receptors.

The receptors on various tissues to which *C. albicans* attach are not well characterized. However, if the protein portion of the mannoprotein adhesin(s) of *C. albicans* is the principal attachment factor (57), then adhesion to animal cell receptors may be analogous to most bacterial adhesion mechanisms involving the interaction of a proteinaceous adhesin with a carbohydrate receptor of the animal cell surface (57). Consistent with this view is the finding that pretreatment of vaginal epithelial cells with L-fucose, a common monosaccharide constituent of epithelial cell membranes where it can function as a receptor for certain bacteria (122), inhibited *C. albicans* adhesion (289). Likewise, pretreatment of BECs with a lectin (from *Lotus tetragonolobus*) which is specific for L-fucose also significantly inhibited *Candida* adhesion (57). Conversely, pre-treatment of epithelial cells with these same inhibitors did not diminish adhesion of another strain of *C. albicans*, whereas pretreatment of epithelial cells with other lectins and sugars did block adhesion (57). This indicates that more than one surface component on epithelial cells may serve as receptors, and that adhesion to different sites may be strain specific. Fibronectin (285) and certain phospholipids (93) have also been suggested to serve as receptors for *C. albicans*. It should be noted, however, that most inhibition studies have been performed by placing the substance in question in the reaction mixture instead of pretreating the yeasts or epithelial surface under study. Consequently, the results obtained from such studies are difficult

TABLE 4-9. Possible Surface Receptors of *Candida* Adhesins

Possible Receptor Moieties	Epithelial Cell Type	Examples of Inhibitors	References
Fibronectin	Buccal	—	285
Fucose	Buccal	L-fucose Lectin from *Lotus tetragonolobus*	57
Lipids	Buccal	Phospholipids, sterols	93
Mannose	Buccal	Con A D-mannosc Methyl-α-D-mannoside	264
N-acetyl-D-glucosamine	Buccal	N-acetyl-D-glucosamine Wheat-germ agglutinin	57
Mucins	Intestinal	—	140
Fucose	Vaginal	L-fucose	290

to interpret. Nevertheless, these and other studies do indicate that there are differences in the receptivities of epithelial cells for *C. albicans* (44, 49, 133, 262, 263). Several experiments using potential inhibitors of adhesion suggest several possible surface components that may serve as receptors for *C. albicans* (Table 4-9).

Role of Adhesion in Colonization and Pathogenesis

Although Hippocrates is recognized as the first person to have described thrush in debilitated patients, and the association of *C. albicans* in plaques and lesions on mucosal surfaces has been noted for well over a century (232), the concept that mucosal attachment contributed to infectivity or colonizing ability of *C.albicans* remained virtually unexplored until only a few years ago. Howlett (112) and Kimura and Pearsall (142), in the late 1970s, were the first experimenters to describe the attachment of *C. albicans* to buccal cells using in vitro adhesion assays. Since then, numerous publications have described the adhesion and association of *Candida* with mammalian tissues as well as a number of nonbiological surfaces.

The current emphasis on *Candida* adhesion in infectious diseases research can be linked, at least in part, to the work cited above, and to a number of now classic publications on bacterial adhesion (77, 98, 99, 125). However, it should be noted that nearly all of the work in the area of fungal adhesion has focused on that of the adhesion process alone, whereas relatively little effort has been made toward understanding the role adhesion plays in colonization or pathogenesis. Several investigators have described and characterized *Candida* attachment mechanisms, for instance, but few have determined what role these mechanisms might have in the ecology of disease. Moreover, some reports have given the impression that adhesion alone is the only or at least the most important virulence factor in *Candida* infections, and that simple tests for adhesion (eg, to isolated epithelial cells) can be expected to predict fungal virulence (170, 171). The emphasis on adhesion mechanisms appears, therefore, to have somewhat obscured the recognition and study of other factors which in many instances may be of equal or greater importance in the ecology and pathogenesis of *Candida* infections. Therefore, in the following paragraphs, the role of adhesion in colonization and pathogenesis, as well as factors that affect *Candida* attachment in vivo, will be considered.

Is Adhesion Necessary for *Candida* Colonization and Pathogenesis?

The association of *C. albicans* with any host tissue is a multifactorial process which cannot be shown to be an important virulence or colonization determinant by means of a single test. Thus, although a number of mechanisms of association for *Candida* with animal cell surfaces have been described, a definitive role in colonization or pathogenesis for most has not been demonstrated. To date, the most conclusive evidence for adhesion as a determinant of colonization or pathogenesis by *C. albicans* was presented by Calderone et al. (24) who showed that *C. albicans* cerulenin-resistant mutants unable to attach in vitro to fibrin-platelet clots were also relatively avirulent in the rabbit model of endocarditis. Differences in other factors thought to be involved in *Candida* pathogenesis (eg, germ tube and protease production) between these mutants and the parental strain were not noted. Furthermore, one mutant was as virulent as the wild-type strain in a murine model of systemic candidosis. Moreover, avirulence in the rabbit endocarditis model was not associated with differences in clearance of wild-type and mutant strains from the blood stream, or from differential resistance, for at least one of the mutants, to phagocytosis. The degree of inhibition of protein synthesis for these strains by rabbit peritoneal macrophages was the same. Thus the avirulence of at least one cerulenin-resistant strain of *C. albicans* appeared to be directly correlated with a decrease in adhesion. More recently, this same mutant was also found to adhere less readily to human vaginal mucosal cells in vitro, and was less virulent in a murine model of vaginal candidiasis than the wild-type *C. albicans*. Definitive proof that *Candida* adhesion or association mechanisms are important for colonization or pathogenesis of other body tissues must still come from similar studies showing that inhibition of adhesion prevents colonization or infection, or that adhesion-negative mutants are avirulent or unable to colonize the host.

Nevertheless, although such proof may still be lacking for oral mucosal colonization, it is likely that adhesion is important. Such can be deduced from a number of considerations. For instance, it could be argued that adhesion to the epithelium would be essential because it would allow *C. albicans* to overcome removal from the oral cavity by the continuous flow of saliva. Likewise, competition for adhesion sites by indigenous bacteria was shown to cause a reduction in oral colonization by *C. albicans* in gnotobiotic mice (161). The ultrastructural characterization of thrush, or the observation of plaques on oral and esophageal mucosa infected with *C. albicans*, also suggests that mucosal association is very important. Furthermore, a number of studies have shown a correlation between adhesion, colonization, and infection relative to species of *Candida* (46, 144, 146, 171, 172, 187, 188, 191, 236, 269). Several other arguments could likewise be given to support this association, but all of these arguments may not be conclusive regarding the importance of adhesion in colonization or pathogenesis.

In the cecum, *C. albicans* can associate with intestinal mucosal surfaces by apparently several different mechanisms (140), but whether any or all of these are necessary for colonization has not been proven. Recent studies from our laboratory have demonstrated that in the cecum it is possible to define three different ecological niches for *C. albicans*, namely the intestinal contents, the

TABLE 4-10. Population Levels of *C. albicans* in the Cecal Contents and Cecal Walls of Antimicrobic-Treated and Control Animals at 72 Hours After Challenge*

Animal Treatment	Log_{10} Mean No. cfu (±SD) of *C. albicans* in (per g [wet wt])		% Total *Candida* Population Associated with Cecal Wall
	Wall	Contents	
None	2.1 ± 0.4	3.2 ± 0.3	8.3%
Penicillin G†	5.5 ± 0.2	7.4 ± 0.6	1.2%
Vancomycin†	5.1 ± 0.4	6.9 ± 0.2	1.5%

* From Kennedy et al. (140).
† Antimicrobics were given in the drinking water for 3 days before *Candida* challenge.

mucus gel, and the epithelium proper (140). As is shown in Table 4-10, only about 1% of the total cecal population of *Candida* was associated with the gut wall. Therefore, the latter populations may not have been necessary for colonization, but instead may simply have been associated with the mucosa because of the large numbers of cells proliferating in the lumen contents. Interestingly, the percentage of *Candida* associated with the cecal mucosa was significantly higher in nonantimicrobic-treated control animals. When *C. albicans* enters the large intestine under the latter conditions, it remains in a prolonged lag phase (Kennedy, unpublished data) and is inhibited by normal flora (138), thus suggesting that adhesion would be necessary under normal conditions to avoid removal and colonize the intestine because the doubling time of *C. albicans* is slower than the washout rate.

A comparison of localization between *C. albicans*, *C. parapsilosis*, and inert microspheres in renal tissue was conducted by Lee and King (158). Differences in the numbers of associated *C. albicans* and microspheres of corresponding size led these authors to conclude that *C. albicans* retention in perfused kidneys was not due solely to nonspecific retention. A similar comparison between *C. albicans* (2.8×10^4 cfu/g of kidney) and *C. parapsilosis* (1.5×10^4 cfu/g of kidney) led these authors to further suggest that *C. albicans* "demonstrated a significantly greater propensity for adhering to renal endothelium than did the nonpathogen *C. parapsilosis*," and that "*C. albicans* possess a specific adherence factor(s) which allows it to bind to receptor molecules on renal endothelial cells." Similar comparisons of the adhesion of pathogenic and nonpathogenic *Candida* have led others to similar conclusions (Table 4-11). However, although all of these data support this view, they do not prove it. Differences in surface charge or the production of proteases or germ tubes, for instance, could easily account for the differences of association noted between the two species. Consequently, several factors produced by *C. albicans* (eg, adhesins,

TABLE 4-11. Comparison of Adhesion Between *Candida* Species

Substrate	Order of Adhesion (in Decreasing Order)								References
Acrylic-saliva coated	CT	TG	CA-A	CK					191
Acrylic	CA	CT	CP	CS	CG	CPT	SC		46
	CT	TG	CK	CG	CPT	CP	CA-B	CA-A	191
Buccal epithelial cells	CA	CT	CS	CP	CPT	CG	CK		144
	CA	CT	CS	CP	CG	CPT	SC		46
Vaginal epithelial cells	CA	CT	CS	CP	CG	CK	CPT		144
Hexadecane	CT	TG	CK	CG	CPT	CP	CA-B	CA-A	191
Vascular endothelium	CA	CT	CK	CP	CPT	TG			145
Endothelial cells	CA	CT	CK	CP	SC				236
Endocarditis	CA	CK							269
Fibrin-platelet clots	CA	CS	CT	CP	CPT	SC	CG	CK	172

CA, *C. albicans*; CT, *C. tropicalis*, CP, *C. parapsilosis*; CS, *C. stellatoidea*; CG, *C. guilliermondii*; CPT, *C. pseudotropicalis*; CK, *C. krusei*; SC, *Saccharomyces cerevisiae*; TG, *Torulopsis glabrata*.

enzymes, germ tubes, etc) may act collectively to support adhesion, colonization and pathogenesis (21, 106, 167–169, 223, 254, 288). The importance of a single mechanism, then, should not be overestimated to the point that other factors are overlooked, because the latter may supply that extra increment of resistance which is responsible for colonization and pathogenesis. Several factors that influence adhesion and association are discussed below.

Factors Influencing *C. albicans* Adhesion and Association

Colonization of host tissue is a hazardous event for many pathogens including *C. albicans*. Association with oral and GI mucosal surfaces, for instance, means that *Candida* cells are confronted not only by competition and antagonism by the indigenous microflora (which are adapted specifically for colonization of the niches they occupy [266]), but by the host's normal defense mechanisms (eg, secretory IgA in the gut [66, 184, 270, 304]). In some instances, moreover, several of these defense mechanisms may act synergistically (279) to deter survival of *Candida* at mucosal surfaces (138). Indeed, for significant adhesion, colonization, and dissemination of *C. albicans* from the GI tract to occur the ecology of the indigenous microbiota must first be disrupted (eg, by antimicrobic treatment) before *Candida* cells can proliferate in the gut (137–140, 282), or the *Candida* must be implanted before the mucosal flora has become established (71, 214–217).

Studies from our laboratory clearly demonstrate the importance of the anaerobic intestinal microflora in the suppression of intestinal mucosal association, colonization, and subsequent dissmination by *C. albicans* (138). These data demonstrated that the indigenous microflora inhibited mucosal association of *Candida* by several different mechanisms. In antimicrobic-treated adult animals, *C. albicans* cells were often observed to penetrate deep into intestinal tissue, whereas in untreated animals they were not (138, 140). As the first step in mucosal association must be the penetration of the mucus gel (78, 81), it is likely that the dense layers of bacteria in the mucus gel (62) covering the epithelium provided an important defense mechanism that inhibited mucosal association and dissemination from the GI tract (138). Studies in infant mice, which lack a complete bacterial flora including the dense microbial populations in the mucus gel (52, 268), showed that *C. albicans* can readily associate and pass through the gut wall to initiate systemic infection (71, 215). It appeared that the indigenous wall-associated microflora inhibited mucosal association of *C. albicans* by out-competing yeast cells for adhesion sites and physically blocking the larger yeast cells from penetrating into the mucus gel (138). Furthermore, this inability to penetrate deeply into the mucus gel of untreated animals kept *Candida* cells more localized to the surface of the mucosa, and, apparently, caused the yeast to disassociate from the tissue to a faster and much greater extent than from the mucosa of antimicrobic-treated animals (138).

Moreover, it was also shown that certain chemical factors present in the normal gut environment inhibited mucosal association by *C. albicans* (138). Volatile fatty acids and secondary bile acids, for example, significantly inhibited the association of *Candida* with the mucosa in an in vitro adhesion

TABLE 4-12. Association of *C. albicans* with Cecal Slices*

Assay				
System	Solution†	Source of Intestinal Slices‡	Log_{10} Mean No. of *C. albicans* per Slice	Association Index§
1	IC	Antimicrobic-treated hamsters	2.5	0.08
2	IF	Antimicrobic-treated hamsters	4.0	1.82
3	PBS	Antimicrobic-treated hamsters	4.8	13.04
4	IC	Untreated hamsters	2.4	0.06
5	IF	Untreated hamsters	3.4	0.25
6	PBS	Untreated hamsters	3.7	0.73
7	PBS + BA	Antimicrobic-treated hamsters	4.3	4.19
8	PBS + VFA	Antimicrobic-treated hamsters	4.1	1.86

* From Kennedy and Volz (138).

† PBS + BA, PBS containing bile acids (lithocholic acid, 3.0 mM; deoxycholic acid, 2.6 mM); PBS + VFA, PBS containing VFA (valeric acid, 1.2 mM; isovaleric acid, 2.2 mM; isobutyric acid, 1.4 mM; propionic acid, 20.1 mM; acetic acid, 49.3 mM).

‡ Antimicrobic-treated hamsters given VAG in the drinking water for 3 days.

§ The association index = $(t/t + k) \times 100$, where t is the number of *C. albicans* associating with intestinal slices after rinsing, and k is the number of viable *C. albicans* per ml of assay solution after 2 hours of incubation.

TABLE 4-13. Cecal Characteristics From Antimicrobic-Treated and Control Animals*

Antimicrobic Treatment[†]	Gram Stain	Predominant Bacterial Organisms	Consistency of Cecal Contents	Cecal Size[‖]
None	+[‡]	Gm-rods[§]	Thick and pasty	1–2%
Erythromycin	+	Gm-rods	Thick and pasty	1–2%
Gentamicin	+	Gm-rods	Thick and pasty	1–2%
Vancomycin	–	Large, Gm + rods Small, Gm-rods	Soft	4–8%
Penicillin G	–	Gm + cocci and small Gm-rods	Soft	5–10%
Clindamycin	–	Gm + cocci and small Gm-rods	Soft	5–10%

* From Kennedy and Volz (139).
† Mice received 3 days of antimicrobic given in the drinking water.
‡ Gram stains: – = abnormal; + = normal appearing.
§ Predominant organisms seen on gram stained smears.
‖ Percentage of total body weight.

assay using intestinal tissue slices (Table 4-12). Because environmental parameters are known to influence *Candida* adhesion to vaginal epithelial cell and BECs, it follows that bacterial substances produced in the intestinal tract (probably as a result of the metabolic activity of those organisms which control the indigenous microflora [80]) also reduced the ability of *Candida* cells to attach to certain mucosal receptors. This could be the result of volatile fatty acids or secondary bile acids modifying *Candida* adhesins, mucosal receptors, or both, thus rendering *Candida* cells unable to attach to intestinal tissues. These data are consistent with the findings that intestinal levels of volatile fatty acids (138) and deconjugated bile acids (70a) dropped significantly after treatment with antimicrobics that predispose animals to intestinal colonization by *C. albicans* (138, 139). Tables 4-13 and 4-14 compare cecal characteristics from antimicrobic-treated and normal animals.

A number of similar interactions are likely to occur at other sites (eg, the oral cavity and vagina) where *Candida* can attach and colonize. Liljemark and Gibbons (161), as well as others (134, 174, 250, 253), found that certain oral streptococci can inhibit *C. albicans* adhesion to BECs and acrylic, presumably by similar mechanisms (161). Therefore, a number of factors can influence the association of *C. albicans* with a surface (Table 4-15). Some inhibit attachment, whereas others may enhance attachment. Therefore, to gain a full understanding of the role any particular adhesion or association mechanism may play in colonization and pathogenesis, future studies must assess the impact of environmental factors that are normally present in the ecosystem under study. Otherwise, one may be studying a situation that is far removed from what takes place in vivo.

TABLE 4-14. Concentration of VFA in the Ceca of Antimicrobic-Treated and Control Hamsters*

Animal Treatment[†]	VFA Concentration (mM) of Cecal Content[‡]						
	Acetic	Propionic	Isobutyric	Butyric	Isovaleric	Valeric	Total
None (control)	118.6 ± 19.9	20.4 ± 4.5	4.4 ± 0.8	20.7 ± 6.3	3.6 ± 0.4	1.3 ± 0.1	168.2 ± 31.3
Penicillin	29.1 ± 3.9 (24.5)	6.9 ± 1.0 (33.8)	2.7 ± 1.0 (61.4)	2.7 ± 0.7 (13.0)	3.9 ± 0.7 (108.3)	0.5 ± 0.1 (38.4)	45.6 ± 4.9 (27.1)
VAG	25.8 ± 2.9 (21.8)	3.3 ± 0.4 (16.2)	16.3 ± 2.7 (370.4)	33.3 ± 21 (15.9)	4.0 ± 0.5 (111.1)	0.7 ± 0.6 (53.8)	53.4 ± 5.0 (31.7)

* From Kennedy and Volz (138).

[†] Animals were given nothing, penicillin, or VAG *ad libitum* in the drinking water for 3 days.

[‡] Values are mean ± standard deviation of five animals per group. Values within parentheses are percents of control group.

TABLE 4-15. Factors Influencing *C. albicans* Adhesion In Vivo

Factor	References
Host factors	
Hormonal status	276
Immunologic status	66, 159, 270, 314
Antimicrobic therapy	138–140
Underlying debilitating diseases	197
Environmental factors (eg, pH)	138, 207
Diet	251, 252
Body site	260, 262
Number and type of receptors	
Indigenous microflora	
Colonization of adhesion sites	138, 139, 161
Production of inhibitors	138
Alteration of physiochemical nature of environment	138
Modification of substrate	138, 161
Yeast factors	
Germ tube production	143, 260, 264
Enzyme production (eg, proteinase, phospholipase)	10, 94
Concentration and type of adhesins	182, 264
Surface properties	260, 264

Models for Studying Adhesion and Association Mechanisms and Their Role in Colonization and Pathogenesis

Efforts to study the adhesion of *C. albicans* to mucosal surfaces, certain organs, or prosthetic devices, and the role adhesive mechanisms may play in host colonization and pathogenesis, has led to the development of numerous in vitro and in vivo models. Such models have been used to characterize *C. albicans* adhesion and association mechanisms, and have led several investigators to suggest that these mechanisms may play an important role in colonization and pathogenesis. As noted, however, the relevance to human disease of many of the adhesion mechanisms observed for *C. albicans* in various adhesion assays has not been verified. Thus although any adhesive reaction observed for *C. albicans* in an in vitro adhesion model must be viewed as a real event (87), rigorous proof that adhesion is necessary for colonization or pathogenesis must still come from studies showing that nonadhesive mutants are avirulent (or at least less virulent) or unable to colonize the host. Only then can adhesion be labeled a "virulence factor" or "colonization factor." Likewise, if an adhesion mechanism is observed in an experimental animal model, it cannot be assumed to be important in human disease. Body tissues differ in many ways (eg, host physiology, cell surface receptors, etc) from species to species of animal and, in many instances, from animal to animal within the species. Examples of host specificity in microbial adhesion have been reported in the literature (47, 162, 265, 301, 303, 317). Differences in the composition of the indigenous microbiota of mucosal surfaces, for instance, have been noted for different species of animals (267), from individual to individual and, even, from day to day in the same individual (266). These fluctuations in populations may account, in part, for differences noted in variations of adhesion of microorganisms in different animal models and in humans (87). As Freter and Jones (87) have noted, "this fact ... has been immortalized in the profound statement 'man is not a mouse'"; and the dog, rat, hamster, rabbit or guinea pig might also be added to the list.

Pathogenesis of any fungal infection involves a complex series of separate, interdependent interactions, all of which cannot be reproduced in vitro. Consequently, simple in vitro adhesion tests may be of limited value as they cannot simulate the complex series of interactions that occur in vivo (87). These tests can aid in the identification and characterization of the various adhesion mechanisms of *C. albicans*, but they may contribute little to the more important question of the significance of adhesion in human or animal colonization and pathogenesis (87). As one example, there are a large number of factors that may modify adhesion and association of *C. albicans* with intestinal mucosal surfaces in vivo (138, 140), and there appears to be at least five distinct mechanism by which *C. albicans* can associate with the mucosa (140). The complexity of *Candida*-mucosal association, therefore, makes it difficult to devise a single model system, such as adhesion to isolated epithelial cells, which can be relied on to duplicate in vitro the process of mucosal association as it occurs in vivo. Another example that illustrates this point is the binding of *C, albicans* to mucus material in the gut. As noted by Freter (78), this material is of two types: 1) glycoproteins and glycolipids synthesized by epithelial cells (ie, the glycocalyx [116]), and 2) glycoproteins that differ from that of the glycocalyx that are secreted by specialized (goblet) cells of the mucosa. The latter material, referred to as the "mucus gel," forms a thick layer covering the epithelium (8, 16, 78, 238). Recent studies from our laboratory (140) indicate that *C. albicans* may adhere to both types of mucus material. Thus, the molecular basis of *C. albicans* adhesion to epithelial glycocalyx and the mucus gel may only be understood from studying these interactions in separate adhesion models. Furthermore, if a single model of intestinal mucosal association had been used, it is likely that some of the association mechanisms for *C. albicans* would not have been identified. On the other hand, it is also apparent that very little progress in the understanding of *C. albicans* adhesion mechanisms could be made without the use of simple adhesion assays, because they allow one to make various manipulations to a system that would not be possible to make in vivo or even in more complex in vitro adhesion models. Therefore, whereas in vitro models of adhesion remain valid tools to identify, differentiate and study various adhesion and association mechanisms of *C. albicans* at the molecular level, proper critical interpretation as well as caution must be applied to the data when extrapolating from models to the situation found in vivo. Furthermore, it should be emphasized that the continued use of an in vitro adhesion model after the initial identification of an adhesive process, requires a demonstration of the similarity of the adhesion or association mechanism in vitro to the situation found in vivo (87).

An understanding of the biochemical or molecular basis of an adhesion mechanism, and the role that mechanism plays in host colonization and pathogenesis, may only be gained by initially studying each factor separately in simple in vitro systems. Thereafter, it may be necessary to proceed to more complex in vitro models, followed finally by studies in experimental animals (87). Important supplemental studies, such as determining if a putative adhesin is produced in vivo, have been identified by Freter and Jones (87) and are outlined in Table 4-6. It should be noted that following these procedures has led to the characterization and identification of several adhesion and association mechanisms for a number of microbial pathogens (77, 79). Moreover, analogous studies also have shown that these mechanisms are determinants of colonization, pathogenesis, or both, and, more importantly, that certain other adhesion mechanisms identified in vitro were not important in vivo (82, 88, 89). Different modes of interaction of *Vibrio cholera* with intestinal mucosa, for instance, were identified only after adhesion studies were performed using two different in vitro model systems (86, 120, 121). Additional mechanisms of mucosal association were later identified for this organism when further studies were performed with yet more complex models (88, 89). The latter studies also showed that one of the mechanisms identified orginally was not involved with the association of cholera vibrios with intestinal mucosa in vivo (88, 89).

Finally, important information regarding the regulation and synthesis of *Candida* adhesins in vivo, may only be gained by studying the microecology, physiochemical properties, or both, of the in vivo ecosystem. An examination of factors present in the gut of conventional mice, for instance, has revealed that several substances (some of which are produced by the indigenous microbiota) may inhibit the adhesion of *C. albicans* to intestinal epithelium in vivo (138). Therefore, factors present in a given ecosystem may be as important as the presence of an adhesin itself in controlling adhesion.

In Vitro Models

As noted by Freter and Jones (87), adhesion models are subject to many methodologic pitfalls. Indeed, many factors have been shown to influence the adhesion of *C. albicans* in vitro. These are summarized in Table 4-16 and a few are described in more detail in this section. Although the following general discussion focuses primarily on epithelial cell adhesion assays, it is applicable to other model systems as well. Pertinent examples of important experimental pitfalls will be noted for other systems where relevant. The following examples

TABLE 4-16. Factors Affecting the Adhesion of *Candida albicans* to Mucosal Cells and Nonbiological Surfaces In Vitro

Factors	References
Yeast factors	
Species and strain	46, 144, 145, 180, 191, 236, 269
Viability	142, 157, 248, 249, 289
Morphology	2, 142, 143, 236, 249, 250, 289
Coadhesion	144, 260
"Cell-type" or "phenotype"	Kennedy, unpublished data
Epithelial cell factors	
Body site of origin	144, 260
Cell type	262, 263, 276
Viability	249
Indigenous bacteria	138, 174, 250, 253
Growth factors	
Medium composition	59, 133, 179, 180, 183, 260
Medium viscosity	260
Temperature	157, 260, 274
Growth phase	2, 144, 274
Environmental factors	
Assay medium	142, 143, 157, 179, 248, 250, 251, 253, 289
Assay temperature	142, 144
Incubation time	142–144, 249, 274, 289, 314
Yeast: epithelial cell ratio	44, 142, 144, 249
pH	144, 207, 249, 250, 289
Antibodies	66, 159, 314

are intended, however, only to illustrate the importance of the selection of experimental parameters that might influence *Candida* adhesion. Table 4-17 summarizes in vitro adhesion models that have been described in the literature for *C. albicans*, and the reader is referred to the cited papers for a more detailed description of a particular model.

Of the factors that have been shown to influence *C. albicans* adhesion in vitro, growth conditions are probably the most important (260). Although other factors (eg, composition of the assay medium) can also modify microbial adhesion, growth conditions have been shown to directly influence microbial adhesin production (87). Indeed, Douglas and McCourtie (59, 179, 180) have noted that growth of *C. albicans* in media that enhanced adhesion to BECs and acrylic correlated with changes in yeast cell surface composition. These authors also showed that mannoprotein, possibly the surface component(s) responsible for some of the adhesive activities for *C. albicans*, was more readily produced, and secreted, in media that promoted adhesion. Other media, shown to cause a decrease in *Candida* adhesion to BECs and acrylic, also correlated with cell surface changes (179, 260). Recent studies from our laboratory corroborate this view and suggest further that cell surface hydrophobicity, and other factors, are also affected (260). Likewise, phase of

TABLE 4-17. Models for Studying *C. albicans* Adhesion and Association Mechanisms

Type of Model	Basis of Model	Model Has Been Used with	References
In vitro	Exfoliated epithelial cells	Buccal epithelial cells	10, 25, 44–46, 59, 60, 66, 93, 94, 102, 131, 133, 142–144, 170, 171, 175, 180–182, 258–264, 289, 307, 314
		Corneocytes	41, 228
		Urogenital epithelial cells	33, 175, 262
		Vaginal epithelial cells	2, 25, 144, 157, 159, 160, 170, 171, 207, 234, 262, 274, 276, 289–291
	Tissue culture	HeLa cells	174, 249–251
		Cervical epithelial cells	70
		Vaginal epithelial cells	208, 290
	Tissue slices, disks, or explants	Endothelial tissue	145, 236
		Oral mucosa	111–113
		Gastrointestinal mucosa	138, 275
		Fibrin-platelet matrices	172, 173
		Intestinal mucus gel	140
	Nonbiological surfaces	Acrylic	46, 179–183a, 191, 248, 253
		Glass	230
		Plastic	146, 267
		Denture base resins	188
	Hydrophobicity testing	Phase-partition test	107, 140, 146, 187, 191, 260
		Hydrophobic interaction chromatography (HIC)	230
		Modified HIC	This chapter
		Contact angle measurements	146, 187, 188, 191
		Salting out procedures	NT*
		Replica plate test	NT
In vivo	Gastrointestinal mucosa	Infant mice	71, 108, 214–217
		Adult euthymic mice	5, 109
		Adult germ-free mice	5, 109, 210
		Adult conventional and antibiotic-treated hamsters and mice	137–140, 309–312, 320, 321
		Adult conventional rats	195
		Dogs	294
	Heart	Rabbit	23, 24, 76, 269–271
	Oral mucosa	Mice	5, 109, 292
		Hamsters	75
		Rats	1, 72, 73, 105, 126–128, 203, 239–242, 277
		Monkeys	19, 20
	Renal endothelium	Rabbit	9
	Vaginal mucosa	Mouse	159, 160
		Rats	288

*Not tested

growth, pH, incubation temperature, and whether growth is on solid or liquid medium have been shown to effect adhesin production (157, 207, 260, 264). The adhesiveness of the test cells, therefore, is directly dependent on, and can be manipulated by, conditions under which the cells are propagated, and may depend as much on environmental factors as on the capability to produce an adhesin (87).

Although the importance of culture conditions, particularly growth medium, on *Candida* cell surface composition and adhesion has been noted in the literature (179, 260), it is somewhat surprising to note that more than 15 different culture media have been reported for propagation of *C. albicans* for studies of epithelial cell adhesion (260). Of the investigators that have studied *Candida* adhesion, few investigators have used the same culture medium. Although two or more investigators reported using Sabouraud glucose broth (or other similar peptone based media), it is unlikely that they used exactly the same medium unless they had used the same lot. As noted by Odds, (198, 199), there are major differences in the chemical composition of peptones and "Sabouraud's glucose medium" from laboratory to laboratory, from manufacturer to manufacturer, and from lot to lot from the same manufacturer. In some laboratories, for example, the routine concentration of glucose in Sabouraud glucose agar (SGA) is 20 g/l; in others, the glucose concentration in SGA is 40 g/liter (198). Furthermore, the peptone components of SGA and other peptone based media are highly complex and undefined, and are not standardized from batch to batch of media. Peptone components have been shown to cause "dramatic effects ... on the outcome of tests for acid phosphatase activity in *C. albicans* [which is thought to enhance *Candida* adhesion (198)] ... and considerable variations in colony characteristics and pigment production by dermatophytes" (198). It seems likely, therefore, that differences in the composition of media peptone may account for at least some of the discrepancies reported in the literature regarding *Candida* adhesin(s) and other surface properties thought to be involved in the adhesion process. Furthermore, the use of different lots of the same medium may also account for some of the variation observed for *C. albicans* adhesion to epithelial cells from day to day (260).

The studies of Douglas and McCourtie (59, 179, 180) showed that concentration of carbohydrate (including glucose) directly influenced *C. albicans* adhesion. This was correlated with changes in *Candida* cell surface composition. Similarly, differences in cell surface hydrophobicity, a factor thought to be important in adhesion to plastic (146), and cell surface composition were also noted in our laboratory when *C. albicans* was grown in different peptone-based media (including the same medium from different manufacturers and different lots from the same manufacturer) (260). Dramatic differences in the ability of *Candida* to attach to BECs were also noted when cells of *C. albicans* were grown in these media (260). Apparently, differences in composition of media peptone, as well as amount and type of carbon source, can also influence *Candida* adhesion.

In addition to culture conditions, a number of other experimental factors can have a profound effect on the physiochemical properties of the yeast cell surface, which, in turn, can affect test results. The most obvious of these is composition of the assay medium. Others include pH, molarity, ionic strength, oxygen tension, assay temperature, and buffering capacity of the assay medium. Placing *Candida* cells in media to promote germ tube formation, may also yield cells coated with molecules that might influence adhesion.

Several variations in what might be thought of as miscellaneous test conditions can also have a marked influence on adhesion data. These variables include source of test cells, reaction time, quantitation methods, yeast : epithelial cell ratio, speed of agitation of test mixtures, and the time it takes to process the test cells. The velocity at which *C. albicans* and epithelial cells are mixed, for example, can greatly influence binding kinetics. At high speeds of agitation the greater fluid shear may actually hinder adhesion. For studies using disks of tissues or intestinal slices, *Candida* cells may attach to both the serosal and lumenal sides. Thus, it may be necessary to secure tissue so that the appropriate side is "right side up" to ensure that the surface being studied is where the yeasts are attaching. Klotz et al. (145) used a Lucite template to secure endothelial tissue in such a way to allow the application of *Candida* cells directly to the endothelial surface. Moreover, multiple wells on the apparatus allowed experimental and control observations to be made on the same segment of tissue (145). This Lucite template might easily be adapted for use with other tissues as well. Intestinal slices could be similarly secured for studies on adhesion and penetration of gut mucosa by *C. albicans*.

A number of other factors complicating adhesion studies have been dealt with by Rotrosen et al. (235). Nevetheless, it should be noted that a number of physical and mechanical factors that are used routinely in in vitro assays can greatly influence adhesion data. Every detail in an adhesion assay, therefore, must be carefully considered if meaningful results are to be obtained. No longer can *C. albicans* simply be grown "overnight" in "Sabs" broth, washed and resuspended in "PBS," and mixed with epithelial cells as a means of studying *Candida* adhesion.

Once appropriate measures have been taken to obtain an in vitro model that closely resembles the adhesion found in vivo, some degree of confidence can then be gained in the use of inhibitors to aid in the identification of *Candida* adhesins and mucosal receptors. However, this area too is frought with pitfalls. Agglutination by antibody or potential inhibitors may not necessarily represent identification of an adhesin. It is also important to monitor the influence lectins and potential chemical inhibitors have on the physiochemical properties of a test system, as a number of these may cause changes (eg, pH) that might inhibit adhesion without competing for host cell receptors or binding to adhesins. Likewise, if a chemical substance that is normally present in a given ecosystem (eg, VFA in the gut) inhibits *C. albicans* adhesion when added to the assay mixture, it may be necessary to perform additional tests to determine if the reduction in adhesion was due to modifying *Candida* adhesins, mucosal, receptors, or both. Finally, if two or more specific inhibitors block adhesion, it may indicate that there is more than one adhesin. Alternatively, it may also mean that such inhibitors bind to different sites of the same multifactorial adhesin. Therefore, careful interpretations and appropriate controls are necessary to evaluate test results properly.

It should also be emphasized that in vivo epithelial cell surfaces are bathed by various secretions such as saliva or mucous material, which may cause glycoproteins to bind to receptors of the epithelial glycocalyx. Thus, microbial cells may adhere in vivo not to receptors on the cell surface proper, but to receptors of tissue secretions (eg, the mucus gel) coating the tissue surface or factors adsorbed to the surface (87, 97). Exfoliated epithelial cells that are extensively washed and used in in vitro adhesion assays, then, may reflect adhesion which is different from that occurring in vivo. Likewise, a number of other factors that can also modify adhesion in vivo (87) must be considered in the development of in vitro assays. The fact that most natural foodstuffs contain sugars, polysaccharides, glycoproteins, and glycolipids, suggests a number of possibilities for the promotion as well as inhibition of *Candida* adhesion in vivo. Samaranayake et al. (250–253) have commented on some of these. The above examples do, however, illustrate the importance and the care with which assay parameters must be chosen.

In Vivo Models

A number of animal models for the various manifestations of human candidiasis have been developed and used for studies of antifungal chemotherapy, colonization, and pathogenesis. At least 15 such models have been used to study *C. albicans* adhesion (Table 4-17). Guentzel et al. (103) in their exhaustive review on animal models for candidiasis, described in detail most of the currently available models. Therefore, this subsection makes no attempt to describe in any detail particular in vivo models. Instead, the following discussion focuses on the methods that accompany the use of such models as they relate to studying adhesion mechanisms.

In practice, two general approaches have been used with experimental animals. These have included, with rare exceptions, either visual and/or quantitative methods to determine how *C. albicans* associates with a certain tissue and to estimate *Candida* population sizes associated with the tissue, respectively. Although both types of methods have been used with some success to elucidate particular aspects of adhesion and association, each is limited and can be misleading at times due to a number of accompanying technical difficulties. This suggests that studies combining both types of methods may be required to accurately understand and describe adhesive events.

Visual methods to examine *Candida* adhesion have included visible and ultraviolet light (immunofluorescence), and scanning and transmission electron microscopy. These methods have been used, for example, to demonstrate the mechanisms of association of *C. albicans* with oral and gastrointestinal mucosal surfaces. However, it is important to note that information gained in such a way may only be indicative of the mechanisms by which *C. albicans* adheres or associates with various surfaces. Therefore, these results need to be interpreted cautiously as tissues can, and do, change during specimen processing. Several artifacts, such as shrinkage of tissue, can be induced during specimen preparation, and most drying procedures used can distort the relationship of yeast cells with epithelial surfaces. The outcome can present a picture drastically different from that found in the living animal, because the cells may appear closer to or further away from the tissue. Lee et al. (156), for instance, noted that when intestinal tissues were fixed and viewed by SEM *Campylobacter jejuni* appeared to be attached to the epithelium, whereas when similar unfixed tissues were examined by phase contrast microscopy they were not. Likewise, washing techniques can be misleading. As noted by Savage (267), washing techniques used in tissue preparation may flush microorganisms away from a surface, especially those that colonize overlying mucus (15). Thus, although microscopy remains a valid tool to study microbial adhesion, it must be used with caution, and should be combined with other methods to completely characterize the molecular nature of an adhesive mechanism and its role in tissue colonization.

Numerous studies also have visualized the association of microorganisms with tissues using histologic procedures and viewing stained tissue sections by light microscopy. Methods for preparing tissues in this manner are subject to several of the same pitfalls as those described above, and can, therefore, change the relative position of *Candida* cells to the surfaces being examined. Nevertheless, histologic preparations do have the advantage of noting any accompanying pathologic changes that might take place from the resulting association.

Tissues can be frozen without chemical fixation for histologic sectioning (267) and can be subjected to staining or treatment with antibodies after sectioning so that tissue, yeasts, and antigens can be observed by light or immunofluorescent microscopy (82, 88, 89, 267). Similar frozen sections can also be viewed without staining by phase contrast microscopy (302). Preparation of tissues in this manner has several advantages over more classical techniques that require washing and other manipulations that tend to remove microbial cells from tissue surfaces and cause tissues to shrink. Furthermore, the contents of the gastrointestinal tract, which are usually washed away by conventional paraffin-block histologic procedures, can be frozen along with the mucosa to preserve close relationships between *C. albicans* and tissue cells as they occur in vivo (50, 51). Savage (267) noted that freezing mucosal tissues at $-18^{\circ}C$ or below, with intestinal contents intact, leaves microbial communities intact on the surfaces, which can be used to determine the distribution of microbial populations over the tissue surface. Freter et al. (82, 88, 89) used this technique to examine those factors that influence the passage of bacteria and yeasts through the mucus gel and penetration into the epithelium of the small intestine. Moreover, Davis (50, 51) found that freezing whole intestinal segments at −70°C before sectioning and processing for electron microscopy not only preserved the microbial communities on the epithelial surface, but preserved the overlying mucus gel and associated microorganisms as well. More recently, Rozee et al. (238) showed that treating intestinal mucosa with serum before processing for microscopy also preserved the mucus layers and microorganisms associated with it. Likewise, similar results were obtained by feeding experimental animals phytohemagglutinin lectins (8). However, in the latter studies the mucus layer was often observed only amorphously on intestinal tissues. At present, none of these methods have been applied to studies discussed in this chapter.

Three general types of assays have been used to quantitate the numbers of microbial cells associated with infected tissues (150), and each has its unique advantages and disadvantages (267). The first method includes direct microscopic examination to estimate the number of attached organisms. This can also give information regarding tissue distribution as well as population dynamics. However, this method is incapable of distinguishing between live and dead microorganisms, and cannot be used accurately with certain organ systems. Furthermore, this method is prone to many of the pitfalls mentioned. On the other hand, this method can reveal important information that would be obscured by the mechanical counting methods presented below. The other two methods are estimating the numbers of associated yeasts by culture methods and radioisotope techniques. The greatest asset of culturing is that it determines only those cells that are viable. Both methods have the advantage of being more objective and are able to distinguish between inoculated and indigenous yeasts (which are present in the GI tract of many laboratory rodents [295]). Disadvantages of these techniques are that populations attaching to different receptors would be indistinguishable, and that additional sources of error due to pipetting, inefficiency in tissue grinding, etc, can be introduced during tissue processing. Furthermore, the radioisotope method has the disadvantage that isotope may leak from intact microorganisms or be released from lysing cells and be incorporated into tissues (267). More disturbing, however, are the findings of Freter et al. (88) that results differed significantly between isotopes, and that results correlated more closely with the isotope used than with bacterial strain studied. Consequently, only microscopic and culture methods are suggested here.

Another important consideration regarding in vivo models is the selection of a test animal species. It seems reasonable that such a selection be made on the basis of how closely the model simulates the comparable infection in humans. Yet it is interesting to note that many animal models that are currently being used fail to do just that (185). As one example, oropharyngeal candidiasis has been studied in a number of animal models, including the rat, mouse, monkey and hamster (103). However, in only the rat model have gross lesions comparable to those found in humans been reported to develop (103).

In addition, age, immunologic, and microbial status may also be important in the selection of an in vivo model. Infant mice, which lack a complete bacterial flora including the dense microbial populations in the mucus gel (52, 268), have been used successfully for studies of intestinal colonization and association with the gut mucosa (5, 71, 108, 214–217). Studies using infant mice, for instance, showed that *C. albicans* persisted in the intestinal tract for several weeks (215). Thus, this model may provide an excellent means of studying infant infections, passive immunity, and gastrointestinal carriage of *C. albicans*. On the other hand, it may be inappropriate for studies on acute GI candidiasis that can accompany antimicrobic therapy. An adult antimicrobic-treated model (136–140), therefore, may more closely represent such infections.

It is also important to note that all major animal breeders supply mice which are unsuitable for research on *Candida*-indigenous floral interactions, because these animals are derived from germ-free stock which are deliberately contaminated with a cocktail containing a mixture of a few nonindigenous bacteria (83, 84, 90). Mice are then subsequently contaminated randomly by exposure to environmental and handler microorganisms. These "specific pathogen-free" animals, therefore, do not contain a bacterial flora representative of those species that normally colonize the mouse. According to Freter (83, 84, 90), these animals are characterized by their lack of strictly oxygen-sensitive anaerobes which predominate in the intestinal tracts of conventional mice. Such animals also have been shown to lack certain intestinal mucosa-associated populations (211). Likewise, germ-free mice associated with a diflora of *C. albicans* and any single bacterial species (or even a few bacterial species) cannot be expected to reflect interactions as they normally occur in the oral cavity or intestinal tract (138). In summary, several factors must be considered in the selection of an animal model, which may be just as important as the aforementioned methods by which adhesion and association mechanisms are studied.

Comparison of Epithelial Cell Adhesion Data

Numerous studies have been conducted to assess the ability of *C. albicans* to attach to exfoliated epithelial cells in vitro (2, 25, 33, 49, 59, 131, 133, 142–144, 157, 159, 160, 170, 171, 180, 182, 207, 258–264, 274, 276, 289–291). It is difficult to draw many conclusions, however, because of the wide variation in experimental parameters used between laboratories. These differences include *Candida* strain, growth and assay medium, environmental conditions of the test, concentrations of yeast and epithelial cells in the assay, and the presence or absence of germ tubes to name a few, and probably account for the majority of discrepancies in the literature regarding which surface component(s) serves as the *Candida* adhesin(s). It is therefore apparent that a direct comparison of published *Candida* adhesion data is virtually impossible. Consequently, Table 4-18 was constructed to list nearly all published data on the adhesion of *C.*

TABLE 4-18. Adhesion of *C. albicans* to Human Epithelial Cells

Candida Strain	Source of Isolate	Assay Medium	Epithelial Cell Type and Source*	Ratio Yeast/Epithelial Cells in Assay	Yeast Growth Conditions	Assay Parameters	Germ Tubes Present	Mean No. Yeast Attached per Epithelial Cell[†]	References
"Vaginal strain"	Vaginal secretion	PBS (0.01 M, pH 7.2)	VEC	10 : 1	SDB (37°C, O.N.)	37°C, 1 h	–	13.0	290
"	"	"	VEC	10 : 1	"	37°C, 2 h	–	10.1	290
"	"	Williams (soln pH 7.2)	VEC	10 : 1	"	37°C, 1 h	+	14.4	290
"	"	"	VEC	10 : 1	"	37°C, 2 h	+	21.6	290
"	"	"	VEC	25 : 1	"	37°C, 1 h	+	9.1	290
"	"	"	VEC	25 : 1	"	37°C, 2 h	+	20.0, 28.1	290
"	"	PBS	VEC	25 : 1	"	37°C, 2 h	–	12.7	290
"Patient isolate"	Patient with acute vulvovaginitis	PBS (0.85%, pH 7.2)	VEC	1,000 : 1	PPG (BBL) (25°C, 24 h)	37°C, 30 min	NG[‡]	175.0	144
"	"	PBS	BEC	1,000 : 1	"	37°C, 30 min	NG	~115.0	144
"	"	PBS	VEC	1,000 : 1	"	"	"	117.0	144
"	"	M199	VEC	1,000 : 1	"	"	"	113.0	144
"	"	PBS	VEC	10 : 1	"	"	"	7.0	144
"	"	"	VEC	100 : 1	"	"	"	15.2	144
"	"	"	VEC	1,000 : 1	"	"	"	91.4	144
"	"	"	VEC	10,000 : 1	"	"	"	179.0	144
GDH2023	Patient with denture stomatitis	PBS (0.15 M, pH 7.2)	BEC	1,000 : 1	YNB + 500 mM glactose (37°C, 24 h)	37°C, 45 min	NG	8.7	81
GDH2346	"	"	BEC	1,000 : 1	YNB + 50 mM glucose (37°C, 24 h)	37°C, 45 min	NG	1.1, 0.93, 1.1, 1.5	60, 181
"	"	"	"	1,000 : 1	YNB + 500 mM galactose (37°C, 24 h)	37°C, 45 min	NG	6.3, 8.5, 6.9, 10.9	60, 182
"	"	"	"	1,000 : 1	YNB + 500 mM sucrose (37°C, 24 h)	37°C, 1 h	NG	3.3, 3.9	180
MRL3153	NG	"	BEC	50 : 1	Mycological peptone (37°C, 18 h)	37°C, 1 h	NG	1.2	251
GDH1957	Patient with chronic atrophic candidosis	"	"	50 : 1	SDB (37°C, 18–24 h)	37°C, 2 h	NG	1.5	251

TABLE 4-18. *Continued*

Candida Strain	Source of Isolate	Assay Medium	Epithelial Cell Type and Source*	Ratio Yeast/ Epithelial Cells in Assay	Yeast Growth Conditions	Assay Parameters	Germ Tubes Present	Mean No. Yeast Attached per Epithelial Cell†	References
N-1-5	Human carrier oral cavity	TC199 (pH 7.0)	BEC	50 : 1	"	37°C, 2 h	+	4.9	142
N-1-5	"	"	"	250 : 1	SDB (37°C, 18–24 h)	37°C, 45 min	+	10.5	142
N-1-5	"	PBS (0.01 M, pH 7.0)	BEC	500 : 1	"	37°C, 2 h	NG	1.4, 2.1	143
N-1-5	"	"	"	500 : 1	"	"	NG	~1.2	143
N-1-5	"	"	"	500 : 1	"	"	NG	~0.5	143
N-1-5	"	Saliva	"	500 : 1	"	"	NG	~2.5	143
N-1-5	"	Saliva	"	500 : 1	"	"	NG	~0.5	143
N-1-5	"	TC199 (pH 7.0)	"	500 : 1	"	"	+	24.7	143
N-1-5	"	TC199 (pH 7.0)	"	500 : 1	"	"	+	5.1	143
"Clinical isolate"	"Patient"	PBS (pH 7.2)	UEC (healthy female volunteers)	20 : 1	SDB (37°C, 48 h)	37°C, 1 h	NG	1	33
"Clinical isolate"	"Patient"	PBS (pH 7.2)	BEC	20 : 1	SDB (37°C, 48 h)	37°C, 1 h	NG	1.7, 2, 2.6	33
VW32	"Human candidosis"	PBS (pH 7.2)	BEC	50 : 1	SDB (37°C, 24 h)	37°C, 1 h	NG	2.1	307
MSU-1	"Patient"	PBS (pH 7.2)	BEC	5 : 1	24TSB (BBL) + 4% glucose (37°C, h)* TC1991 h	37°C, 1 h	+	0.75, 2.2, 3.1	259, 264
"Clinical isolate"	Patient with acute vulvoganitis	PBS (pH 7.2)	VEC	1,000 : 1	PPG (25°C, 24 h)	37°C, 30 min	NG	150.3	157
"	"	"	"	1,000 : 1	PPG (37°C, 24 h)	37°C, 30 min	NG	21.3	157
"Clinical isolate"	NG	PBS (pH 7.4)	BEC (human infant 7.5 h old)	1,000 : 1	SDB (37°C, 18 h)	37°C, 1 h	NG	3.7	49
"	"	"	BEC (human infant 2.3 d old)	1,000 : 1	SDB (37°C, 18 h)	37°C, 1 h	NG	3.8	49
"	"	"	BEC (human infant 6.7 d old)	1,000 : 1	SDB (37°C, 18 h)	37°C, 1 h	NG	4.9	49

10231 (ATCC)	NG	PBS (0.02 M, pH 7.4)	BEC	7.5 : 1	10% glucose solution (RT, "overnight")	"room temp", 30 min	–	~9.5	44
"	"	"	"	75 : 1	"	"	–	~15.0	44
"	"	"	"	750 : 1	"	"	–	~22.0	44
"	"	"	"	7,500 : 1	"	"	–	~22.5	44
"	"	"	"	75,000 : 1	"	"	–	~23.0	44
19273	"Lab. strain"	PBS	BEC	500 : 1	LBC agar (37°C, 36 h)	37°C, 45 min	–?	3.5, 0.4, 1.2	133
"	"	"	"	"	Malt agar (37°C, 36 h)	"	"	0.3, 0.3, 0.3	133
19321	"	"	"	"	LBC agar (37°C, 36 h)	"	"	3.0, 0.1, 1.6	133
"	"	"	"	"	Malt agar (37°C, 36 h)	"	"	0.3, 0.1, 0.4	133
21462	"	"	"	"	LBC agar (37°C, 36 h)	"	"	3.0, 0.4, 1.5	133
"	"	"	"	"	Malt agar (37°C, 36 h)	"	"	0.7, 0.3, 0.3	133
22114	"	"	"	"	LBC agar (37°C, 36 h)	"	"	2.6, 0.2, 1.1	133
"	"	"	"	"	Malt agar (37°C, 36 h)	"	"	0.4, 0.2, 0.4	133
B1 (T)	"Clinical isolate"	"	"	"	LBC agar (37°C, 36 h)	"	"	8.5, 5.6, 5.6	133
M4 (C)	"Carrier isolate"	"	"	"	"	"	"	6.7, 4.8, 5.0	133
H5 (T)	"Clinical isolate"	"	"	"	"	"	"	5.8, 2.3, 4.6	133
M3 (C)	"Carrier isolate"	"	"	"	"	"	"	5.1, 1.9, 5.1	133
H19 (T)	"Clinical isolate"	"	"	"	"	"	"	3.0, 2.1, 3.0	133
C1 (C)	"Carrier isolate"	"	""	"	"	"	"	4.7, 2.7, 3.5	133
GDH2346	Denture stomatitis	PBS (0.02 M, pH 7.2)	BEC	1,000 : 1	YNB + 500 mM fructose (37°C, 24 h)	37°C, 45 min	NG	1.9	59
"	"	"	"	"	YNB + 500 mM glucose (37°C, 24 h)	"	"	2.5	59
"	"	"	"	"	YNB + 500 mM maltose (37°C, 24 h)	"	"	7.8	59

TABLE 4-18. *Continued*

Candida Strain	Source of Isolate	Assay Medium	Epithelial Cell Type and Source*	Ratio Yeast/ Epithelial Cells in Assay	Yeast Growth Conditions	Assay Parameters	Germ Tubes Present	Mean No. Yeast Attached per Epithelial Cell†	References
MRL3153	"	"	"	"	YNB + 500 mM glucose (37°C, 24 h)	"	"	0.9	59
"	"	"	"	"	YNB + 500 mM sucrose (37°C, 24 h)	"	"	2.2	59
"	"	"	"	"	YNB + 500 mM galactose (37°C, 24 h)	"	"	5.2	59
GR1681	Cervical smear (symptomless carrier)	"	"	"	YNB + 500 mM glucose (37°C, 24 h)	"	"	0.8	59
"	"	"	"	"	YNB + 500 mM sucrose (37°C, 24 h)	"	"	1.7	59
"	"	"	"	"	YNB + 500 mM galactose (37°C, 24 h)	"	"	1.7	59
GR1682	"	"	"	"	YNB + 500 mM glucose (37°C, 24 h)	"	"	0.9	59
"	"	"	"	"	YNB + 500 mM sucrose (37°C, 24 h)	"	"	1.8	59
"	"	"	"	"	YNB + 500 mM galactose (37°C, 24 h)	"	"	1.6	59

* VEC = vaginal epithelial cells; BEC = buccal epithelial cells.
† Where more than one number is given, the values were taken from replicate experiments reported in the same or different publications.
‡ NG, not given.

TABLE 4-19. Adhesion of *C. albicans* to Buccal Epithelial Cells (BEC) After Growth on Different Media and Under Different Environmental Parameters*

Assay No.	Growth Medium†	Mean No. *C. albicans*/BEC	Relative Adhesion‡	% BEC with Attached *Candida*	Coadhesion§
1	TSB + G	0.7	1.0	36	–
2	TSB + G-S	0.9	1.2	28	–
3	TSB + G25	0.5	0.7	32	–
4	SGB-1	0.8	1.1	44	–
5	SGB-2	0.9	1.2	34	–
6	SGB-1-25	3.1	4.3	70	+
7	SMB	0.5	0.7	36	–
8	FSM	0.7	1.0	32	–
9	MB	0.8	1.1	36	–
10	BHI	3.0	4.3	82	+
11	TSB-1	1.3	1.8	56	+
12	TSB-2	3.4	4.7	64	–
13	PPG	2.2	3.1	70	–
14	YE	2.8	3.9	64	–
15	YNB + G	0.8	1.1	36	–
16	YNB + gal	3.8	5.3	76	±
17	LBC-37	2.9	4.1	72	+
18	LBC-25	6.2	8.7	94	+
19	SGA-37	2.7	3.8	70	+
20	SGA-25	3.8	5.3	76	+

*Adapted from Sandin and Kennedy (260).

†Abbreviations: TSB (assays 1–3) = trypticase soy broth (BBL) + 4% glucose; SGB = Sabouraud glucose broth (Difco); SMB = Sabouraud maltose broth (Difco); FSM = fluid Sabouraud medium (Difco); MB = mycological broth (Difco); BHI = brain-heart infusion broth (Difco); TSB (assays 11 & 12) = tryptic soy broth (Difco); PPG = phytone peptone broth (BBL) + glucose; YE = yeast extract broth (Difco); YNB = yeast-nitrogen base (Difco) + glucose (G) or galactose (gal); LBC = the medium of Lee et al. (154); SDA = Sabouraud glucose agar (Difco). All cultures were grown at 37°C unless given (eg, assay 3, cells were grown at 25°C). Also, different lots of the same medium were used as noted (eg, assays 4 and 5 and 11 and 12).

‡Adhesion relative to that of cells grown in TBS + G (assay 1).

§Indirect attachment to BEC.

‖Cultures not shaken.

albicans to epithelial cells as the only means of examining this data, and to serve as a reference for future experimetnal approaches. Table 4-19 is also included to compare the adhesion of *C. albicans* with BECs after growth on various media (260). In that study, Sandin and Kennedy (260) compared the ability of *C. albicans* to attach to exfoliated buccal mucosal cells after growth on different media, but kept all other parameters constant. As can be noted from the table, there were major differences in the adhesion of *Candida* to BECs. Furthermore studies using these media will be necessary to determine if different adhesins were produced after growth on different media.

A Standardized Buccal Epithelial Cell Adhesion Assay?

In view of the findings discussed, and the importance of a standardized assay to study *Candida* adhesion at the molecular level, the need of reproducible, defined conditions for use in adhesion studies is very apparent. As mentioned, more than 15 different culture media have been used for propagation of *C. albicans* for adhesion studies. This, coupled with the fact that several other assay parameters (eg, assay medium, yeast : epithelial cell ratio, etc [see Table 4-18]) have been used by different investigators, indicates that at present there is little agreement on the selection of criteria required for the standardization of an assay. Therefore, outlined below are guidelines for future experimental approaches to study *Candida* adhesion, and a proposed defined basal medium and assay conditions for a standardized BEC adhesion assay.

Several methods have been used to study the adhesion of *C. albicans* to epithelial cells. These include mixing *Candida* suspensions with: 1) monolayers of HeLa cells (208, 249–251, 290); 2) exfoliated BECs (2, 25, 33, 49, 51, 131, 133, 142–144, 157, 159, 160, 170, 171, 180, 182, 207, 258–264, 274, 276, 289–291); and 3) oral explants from laboratory rodents (111–113). The number of attached yeast are then determined after incubation and washing.

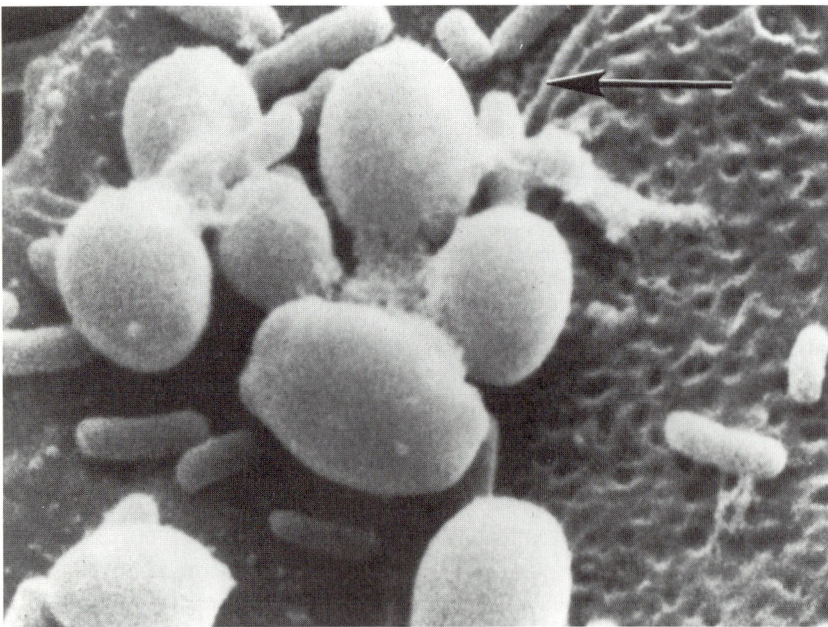

FIG. 4-41. A buccal epithelial cell with adherent *C. albicans* and piliated *Klebsiella pneumoniae*. Note the juxtaposition of yeasts and bacteria. *Arrow* denotes cell border. Bar = 2.5 μm. (From Centeno et al. [33].)

Nonadherent yeasts are usually separated from the epithelial cells by filtration, and the number (or proportion) of attached yeasts are determined by microscopy (eg, 264). The most widely used method is by mixing suspensions of exfoliated BECs with suspensions of *C. albicans*. A modification of this method, the "radiometric adherence test" (144), also has been developed. Although this method has been used previously for studies on *Candida* and bacterial adhesion (102, 144, 150, 157), it allows only for the total number of attached yeasts to be determined, and does not give any information on the number of yeasts that have attached indirectly by coadhesion to adherent organisms (144). In Fig. 4-41, *Candida* cells appear to be indirectly attached to a BEC by coadhesion to adherent bacteria, and it is apparent from Fig. 4-42 that numerous yeasts are attached by coadhesion to adherent yeasts. Adhesion tests using radiolabeling techniques would bypass such information. Therefore, the microscopic method is recommended for its simplicity and relative inexpense. Furthermore, microscopy provides information about factors effecting adhesion and coadhesion, attachment by "tiny" germ tubes, and coadhesion to adherent bacteria and yeasts (33, 175, 260).

A problem that plagues the study of the adhesion of *C. albicans* to exfoliated

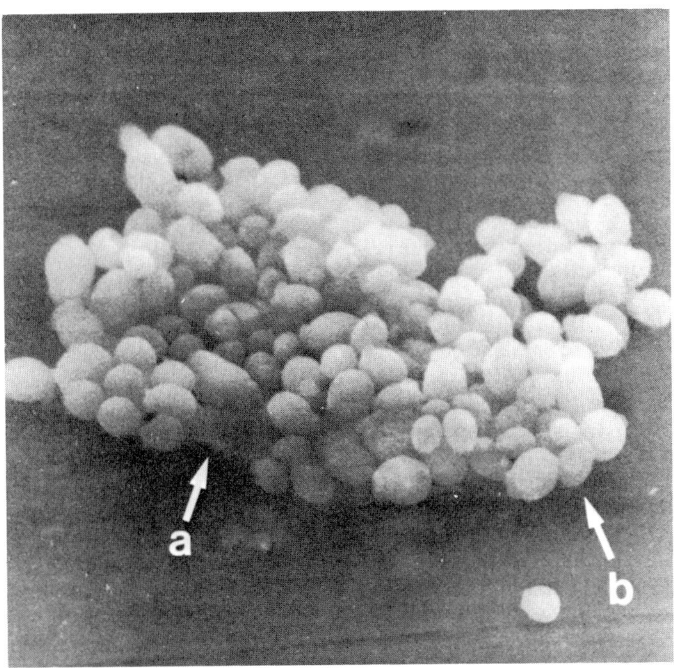

FIG. 4-42. Scanning electron micrograph of a vaginal epithelial cell showing the direct adhesion of yeasts to the epithelial cell (a) and yeast coadhesion (b) (× 1,810). (From King et al. [144].)

epithelial cells in vitro is the observation that *Candida* adhesion varies considerably by changing the mucosal cell donor or even date of collection (44, 49, 133). Sandin et al. (262, 263) studied the influence of collecting mucosal cells from various anatomic sites, and varying the date of collection and cell donor on *C. albicans* adhesion. They found statistically significant differences in the number of attached yeasts between individuals and in the same individual with time. Variations in receptiveness to *C. albicans* of epithelial cells obtained from different sources or at different times, makes it difficult to recommend their routine use in a standardized adhesion assay. To circumvent this problem, it has been proposed that cultured cell monolayers might be used (208, 235, 290). However, before cultured cells can be used routinely in an adhesion assay, they must be shown to retain receptors functionally analogous to those expressed by host cells in vivo. Otherwise the adhesion being studied may be different from that which is important for colonization or pathogenesis in humans. Other important considerations regarding the use of cultured cells have been presented by Rotrosen et al. (235). Until all these are considered, it is recommended that BECs be collected from at least 10 healthy adult volunteers, male and female, who are not taking antimicrobics, and suspending the cells in 0.01 M phosphate-buffered saline (PBS) at pH 7.2. This large batch of cells can be stored at 4°C, and aliquots can be taken from it periodically and used for experimentation. Sandin and Kennedy (260) used this method and found that no difference in adhesion of *C. albicans* to these BECs stored for at least 2 weeks. By using a large group of donors, differences between pools of cells between laboratories should be minimal. It should be noted that this method has only been tested for BECs, and, therefore, epithelial cells from other anatomic sites of the body will have to be tested to determine if they can be used in a similar manner.

The next question to be addressed is that of the selection of culture medium and growth conditions. From the comparison of epithelial cell adhesion data described, coupled with the necessity of a chemically defined medium (260), it is suggested that the medium of Lee et al. (154) or yeast nitrogen base (Difco Laboratories) supplemented with 500 mM galactose (179) be used. Both media are chemically defined, and produce cells of *C. albicans* that are highly adhesive to BECs (260). Furthermore, because these media are defined, several manipulations of the media can be performed to study metabolic pathways and the genetics of adhesin production. Early stationary phase cells are also suggested because stationary phase cells have been shown to adhere more readily than logarithmic phase cells (142, 144, 179, 180, 264). Growth should be at 37°C, and it is recommended that cultures be shaken at 100 rpm. Although in most studies cultures were shaken, in at least one study negligible differences were found in adhesion to BECs when *C. albicans* cultures were static or shaken (260). *Candida* cells have been grown both ways, but in nearly all studies cultures were shaken. Continuous-flow cultures, at flow rates similar to that of the ecosystem under study, may yield cells that are more similar to their in vivo counterparts, and the use of such should be considered and added to a standardized assay once appropriate comparative studies have been performed. Viable cells are recommended because most methods of killing modify the cell surface in some way. Exposure to heat, for instance, releases mannan from the cell wall (289), and has been shown to cause a reduction in *C. albicans* adhesion (172, 289). Prolonged exposure to ultraviolet irradiation releases a glycoprotein of low molecular weight that has been implicated in the adhesion of *C. albicans* to phagocytes (55). Moreover, treatment of *Candida* blastoconidia with heat or ultraviolet irradiation was found to release soluble carbohydrate complexes from the cell wall that partially blocked adhesion (157, 236).

The selection of an assay medium and the conditions of the assay are also very important. Generally, any assay should probably reflect as closely as possible those environmental factors present in vivo. Studies by Persi et al. (207) showed that there were significant differences in the adhesion of *C. albicans* to vaginal epithelial cells in vitro when oxygen tensions were lowered to levels similar to that found in the vagina. Similarly, the adhesion of *C. albicans* to vaginal epithelial cells was shown to be affected by the strain of yeast used, morphologic form of the yeast, side of vaginal cell exposed, and the pH of the assay medium (2, 207, 289). Therefore, the assay parameters recommended here were chosen to represent environmental parameters normally found in the oral cavity. The assay temperature should be 37°C, with an atmosphere of air (ambient pressure) possibly purged with 5% Co_2 (207). KC^1 (0.05M) containing 1–2 mM phosphate (pH 6.0), 1 mM calcium, and 0.1 mM magnesium is recommended as an assay medium, as it mimics the ionic composition of saliva (97). A yeast : BEC ratio of 100 : 1 is suggested because saliva from *Candida* carriers often contains *C. albicans* at concentrations of 100 cfu/ml or greater (67). As noted earlier, at high yeast : epithelial ratios coadhesion and clumping may complicate results. A range of ratios, low (10 : 1), medium (100 : 1) and high (500 : 1), might also be used for comparison. Finally, the test mixtures should be incubated for 1 hour, and processed immediately thereafter.

The question of strain differences must also be raised, as several studies have shown that certain strains are more adhesive than others (46, 59, 180, 183, 207). It may be necessary, therefore, to conduct interlaboratory studies to test the procedures recommended here and select strains of *C. albicans* for use in future studies.

Given the fact that there are few similarities between the results of different investigators, it seems reasonable to conclude that a standard test assay is greatly needed. Although the adhesion assay described is probably incorrect in some respects, its use could lead to the formulation of incisive questions to be addressed in the future. It is therefore urged that this assay be adopted for use with *C. albicans*, even if only to determine which experimental parameters are to be kept and which are to be changed.

Acknowledgments

The author wishes to thank Robert J. Yancey, Jr. for critical review of the manuscript, and Barbara Burton for typing the manuscript. The author also wishes to thank those who provided photographs to be used in this chapter.

References

1. Allen CM, Blozis GG, Rosen S, Bright JS: Chronic candidiasis of the rat tongue: A possible model for human median rhomboid glossitis. *J Dent Res* 61:1287–1291, 1982.
2. Anderson ML, Odds FC: Adherence of *Candida albicans* to vaginal epithelia: Significance of morphological form and effect of ketoconazole. *Mykosen* 28: 531–540, 1985.
3. Bacon JSD, Davidson ED, Jones D, Taylor IF: The location of chitin in the yeast cell wall. *Biochem* 101:36C–38C, 1966.
4. Bagg J, Silverwood RW: Coagglutination reactions between *Candida albicans* and oral bacteria. *J Med Microbiol* 22:165–169, 1986.
5. Balish E, Balish MJ, Salkowski CA, Lee KW, Bartzal KF: Colonization of congenitally athymic, gnotobiotic mice by *Candida albicans. Appl Envrion Microbiol* 47:647–652, 1984.
6. Balish E, Phillipis AW: Growth, morphogenesis, and virulence of *Candida albicans* after oral inoculation in the germ free and conventional chick. *J. Bacteriol* 91:1736–1743, 1966.
7. Ballou C: Structure and biosynthesis of the mannan component of yeast cell envelope. *Adv Microbiol Physiol* 14:93–158, 1976.
8. Banwell JG, Howard R. Cooper D, Costerton JW: Intestinal microbial flora after feeding phytohemagglutinin lectins (*Phaseolus vulgaris*) to rats. *Appl Environ Microbiol* 50, 68–80, 1985.
9. Barnes JL, Osgood W, Lee JC, King RD, Stein JH: Host-parasite interactions in the pathogenesis of experimental renal candidiasis. *Lab Invest* 49:460–467, 1983.
10. Barrett-Bee K, Hayes Y, Wilson RG, Ryley JF: A comparison of phospholipase activity, cellular adherence and pathogenicity of yeast. *J Gen Microbiol* 131: 1217–1221, 1985.
11. Bartnicki-Garcia S: Fungal cell wall composition, in Laskin AI, Lechevalier HA (eds.) *Handbook of Microbiology Vol. II: Microbial Composition.* CRC Press, Cleveland, pp 201–214, 1973.
12. Bartnicki-Garcia S: Cell wall chemistry, morphogenesis, and taxonomy of fungi. *Ann Rev Microbiol* 22:87–108, 1968.
13. Bianchi DE: The lipid content of cell walls obtained from juvenile, yeast like and filamentous cells of *Candida albicans. Antonie van Leeuwenhoek J Microbiol Serol* 33:324–332, 1967.
14. Bishop CT, Blank F, Gardner P: The cell wall polysaccharides of *Candida albicans*, glucan, mannan and chitin. *Can J Chem* 38:869–881, 1960.
15. Blumershine RV, Savage DC: Filamentous microbes indigenous to the murine small bowel: A scanning electron microscopic study of their morphology and attachment to the epithelium. *Microbial Ecol* 4:95–103, 1978.
16. Bollard JE, Vanderwee MA, Smith GW, Tasman-Jones C, Gavin JB, Lee SP:

Location of bacteria in the mid-colon of the rat. *Appl Environ Microbiol* 51:604–608, 1986.
17. Braun P, Calderone R: Chitin synthesis in *Candida albicans*: Comparison of yeasts and hyphal forms. *J. Bacteriol* 133:1472–1477, 1978.
18. Brawner DL, Cutler JE: Changes in surface topography of *Candida albicans* during morphogenesis. *Sabouraudia: J Med Vet Mycol* 23:389–393, 1985.
19. Budtz-Jorgensen E: Denture stomatitis IV. An experimental model in monkeys. *Acta Odont Scand* 29:513–526, 1971.
20. Budtz-Jorgensen E: Effects of triamcinolone acetonide on experimental oral candidiasis in monkeys. *Scand J Dent Res* 83:171–178, 1975.
21. Budtz-Jörgensen E: Proteolytic activity of *Candida* spp as related to the pathogenesis of denture stomatitis. *Sabouraudia* 12:266–271, 1971.
22. Cabib E. Roberts R, Bowers B: Synthesis of yeast cell wall and its regulation. *Ann Rev Biochem* 51:763–793, 1982.
23. Calderone RA, Rotondo MF, Sande MA: *Candida albicans* endocarditis: Ultrastructural studies of vegetation formation. *Infect Immun* 20:279–289, 1978.
24. Calderone RA, Cihlar RL, Lee DDS, Hoberg K, Scheld WM: Yeast adhesion in the pathogenesis of endocarditis due to *Candida albicans*: Studies with adherence negative mutants. *J Infect Dis* 152:710–715, 1985.
25. Calderone RA, Lehrer N, Segal E: Adherence of *Candida albicans* to buccal and vaginal epithelial cells: Ultrastructural observations. *Can J Microbiol* 30: 1001–1007, 1984.
26. Cassone A: Improved visualization of wall structure in *Saccharomyces cerevisiae*. *Experientia* 29:1302–1309, 1973.
27. Cassone A: Cell wall of pathogenic yeasts and implications for antimycotic therapy. *Drugs Exp Clin Res* 12:635–643, 1986.
28. Cassone A, Kerridge D, Gale EF: Ultrastructural changes in the wall of *Candida albicans* following cessation of growth and their possible relationship to the development of polyene resistance. *J Gen Microbiol* 110:339–349, 1979.
29. Cassone A, Mattia E, Boldrini L: Agglutination of blastospores of *Candida albicans* by Concanavalin A and its relationship with the distribution of mannan polymers and ultrastructure of the cell wall. *J Gen Microbiol* 105:263–273, 1978.
30. Cassone A, Simonette N, Strippoli V: Ultrastructural changes in the wall during germ-tube formation from blastospores of *C. albicans*. *J Gen Microbiol* 77: 417–426, 1973.
31. Cassone A, Sullivan PA, Shepherd MG: N-acetyl-D-glucosamine-induced morphogenesis of *Candida albicans*. *Microbiologica* 18:17, 1984.
32. Cawson RA, Rajasingham KC: Ultrastructural features of the invasive phase of *C. albicans*. *Br J Dermatol* 87:435–443, 1972.
33. Centeno A, Davis CP, Cohen MS, Warren MM: Modulation of *Candida albicans* attachment to human epithelial cells by bacteria and carbohydrates. *Infect Immun* 39:1354–1360, 1983.
34. Chaffin LW, Stocco DM: Cell wall proteins of *Candida albicans*. *Can J Microbiol* 29:1438–1444, 1983.
35. Chattaway FW, Bishop R, Holmes MR, Odds FC, Barlow AJE: Enzyme activities associated with carbohydrate synthesis and mycelial forms of *Candida albicans*. *J Gen Microbiol* 75:97–109, 1973.
36. Chattaway FW, Holmes MR, Barlow AJE: Cell wall composition of the mycelial and blastospore forms of *Candida albicans*. *J Gen Microbiol* 51:367–376, 1968.
37. Chattaway FW, Shenolikar S, O'Reilly J: Changes in the cell surface of the dimorphic forms of *Candida albicans* by treatment with hydrolytic enzymes. *J Gen Microbiol* 95:335–347, 1976.

38. Cheng KJ, Irvin RT, Costerton JW: Autochthonous and pathogenic colonization of animal tissues by bacteria. *Can J Microbiol* 27:461–490, 1981.
39. Chiew YY, Shephered MG, Sullivan PA: Regulation of chitin synthesis during germ-tube formation in *Candida albicans. Arch Microbiol* 125:97–104, 1980.
40. Christensen GD, Simpson WA, Beachey EH: Adhesion of bacteria to animal tissues: complex mechanisms, in Savage DC, Fletcher M (eds): *Bacterial Adhesion: Mechanisms and Physiological Significance.* New York, Plenum Press, pp 279–305, 1985.
41. Collins-Lech C, Kalbfleisch JH, Franson TR, Sohnle PG: Inhibition by sugars of *Candida albicans* adherence to human buccal mucosal cells and corneocytes in vitro. *Infect Immun* 46:831–834, 1984.
42. Costerton JW, Irvin RT, Cheng K-J: The role of bacterial surface structures in pathogenesis. *CRC Crit Rev in Microbiol* 8:303–338, 1981.
43. Costerton JW, Marrie TJ, Cheng K-J: Phenomena of bacterial adhesion, in Savage DC, Fletcher M (eds): *Bacterial Adhesion: Mechanisms and Physiological Significance.* New York, Plenum Press, pp 3–43, 1985.
44. Cox F: Adherence of *Candida albicans* to buccal epithelial cells in children and adults. *J Lab Clin Med* 102:960–972, 1983.
45. Cox F: *Candida albicans* adherence in newborn infants. *J Med Vet Mycol* 24:121–125, 1986.
46. Critchley IA, Douglas LJ: Differential adhesion of pathogenic *Candida* species to epithelial and inert surfaces. *FEMS Microbiol Lett* 28:199–203, 1985.
47. Croucher SC, Houston AP, Bayliss CE, Turner RJ: Bacterial populations associated with different regions of the human colon wall. *Appl Environ Microbiol* 45:1025–1033, 1983.
48. Davenport JC: The oral distribution of *Candida* in denture stomatitis. *Br Dent* 129:151–156, 1970.
49. Davidson S, Brish M, Rubinstein E: Adherence of *Candida albicans* to buccal epithelial cells of neonates. *Mycopathologia* 85:171–173, 1984.
50. Davis CP: Postmortem alterations of bacterial localization. *Scan Electron Microsc* 3:523–526, 1980.
51. Davis CP: Preservation of gastronintestinal bacteria and their microenvironmental associations in rats by freezing. *Appl Environ Microbiol* 31:304–312, 1976.
52. Davis CP, McAllister JS, Savage DC: Microbial colonization of the intestinal epithelium in suckling mice. *Infect Immun* 7:666–672, 1973.
53. DeMaria A, Buckly H, vonLichtenberg F. Gastrointestinal candidiasis in rats treated with antibiotics, cortisone, and azathrioprine. *Infect Immun* 13: 1761–1770, 1976.
54. Derjagiun BV, Landau L: Theory of the stability of strongly charged lyophobic sols and of the adhesion of strongly charged particles in solutions of electrolytes. *Acta Physiochim USSR* 14:633–662, 1941.
55. Diamond RD, Krzesicki R: Mechanisms of attachment of neutrophils to *Candida albicans* pseudohyphae in the absence of serum, and of subsequent damage to pseudohyphae by microbial processes of neutrophils in vitro. *J Clin Invest* 61:360–369, 1978.
56. Djaczenko W, Cassone A: Visualization of new ultrastructural components in the cell wall of *Candida albicans* with fixatives containing tapo. *J Cell Biol* 52:186–190, 1971.
57. Douglas LJ: Adhesion of pathogenic *Candida* species to host surfaces. *Microbiol Sci* 2:243–247, 1985.
58. Douglas LJ: Surface composition and adhesion of *Candida albicans. Biochem Soc Trans* 13:982–984, 1985.
59. Douglas LJ, Houston JG, McCourtie J: Adherence of *Candida albicans* to

human buccal epithelial cells after growth on different carbon sources. *FEMS Microbiol Letters* 12:241–243, 1981.

60. Douglas LJ, McCourtie J: Effect of tunicamycin treatment on the adherence of *Candida albicans* to human buccal epithelial cells. *FEMS Microbiol Letters* 16:199–202, 1983.
61. Doyle RJ, Nesbitt WE, Taylor KG: On the mechanism of adherence of *Streptococcus sanguis* to hydroxylapatite. *FEMS Microbiol Letters* 15:1–5, 1982.
62. Dubos R, Schaedler RW, Costello R, Hoet P: Indigenous, normal, and autochothonous flora of the gastrointestinal tract. *J Exp Med* 122:67–76, 1965.
63. Elorza MV, Mugui A. Sentandraeu R: Dimorphism in *Candida albicans*: Contribution of mannoproteins to the architecture of yeast and mycelial cell walls. *J Gen Microbiol* 131:2209–2216, 1985.
64. Elorza MV, Ricco H, Gozalbo D, Sentandreu R: Cell wall composition and protoplast regeneration in *Candida albicans*. *Antonie van Leeuwenhoek* 49: 457–469, 1983.
65. English MP: The saprophytic growth of keratinophilic fungi on keratin. *Sabouraudia* 2:115–130, 1963.
66. Epstein JB, Kimura LH, Menard TW, Truelove EL, Pearsall NN: Effects of specific antibodies on the interaction between the fungus *Candida albicans* and human oral mucosa. *Arch Oral Biol* 27:469–474, 1982.
67. Epstein JB, Pearsall NN, Truelove EL: Quantitative relationships between *Candida albicans* in saliva and the clinical status of human subjects. *J Clin Microbiol* 12:475–476, 1980.
68. Eras P, Goldstein MJ, Sherlock P: *Candida* infection of the gastrointestinal tract. *Medicine* (Baltimore) 51:367–379, 1972.
69. Evron R, Drewe JA: Demonstration of the polysaccharides in the cell wall of *Candida albicans* blastospores, using silver methenamine staining and a sequence of extraction procedures. *Mycopathologia* 84:141–149, 1984.
70. Farell SM, Hawkins DF, Ryder TA: Scanning electron microscope study of *Candida albicans* invasion of cultured human cervical epithelial cells. *Sabouraudia* 21:251–254, 1983.

70a. Fekety R, Brown R, Silva J, Hofmann AF: Fecal bile acids and cholestyramine in hamsters with clindamycin-associated coitis. ICCAC *Abstracts* No. 129, 1978.

71. Field LH, Pope LM, Cole GT, Guentzel MN, Berry LJ: Persistence and spread of *Candida albicans* after intragastric inoculation of infant mice. *Infect Immun* 31:783–791, 1981.
72. Fisker AV, Schiott CR, Philipsen HP: Short-term oral candidiasis in rats, with special reference to the site of infection. *Acta Pathol Microbiol Immunol Scand* 90:49–57, 1982.
73. Fisher AV, Rindon C, Schiott CR, Philipsen HP: Long-term oral candidiasis in rats. *Acta Pathol Microbiol Immunol Scand Sect B* 90:221–227, 1982.
74. Fletcher M: The question of passive versus active attachment mechanisms in non-specific bacterial adhesion, in Berkley RCW, Lynch JM, Rutter PR, Vincent B (eds): *Microbial Adhesion to Surfaces*. London, Ellis Horwood Limited, 1980, pp 197–210,
75. Franklin CD, Martin MW: The effects of *Candida albicans* on turpentine-induced hyperplasia of hamster cheek pouch epithelium. *J Med Vet Mycol* 24:281–287, 1986.
76. Freedman LR, Johnson ML: Experimental endocarditis. *Ann NY Acad Sci* 236:456–465, 1974.
77. Freter R: Association of enterotoxigenic bacteria with the mucosa of the small intestine: Mechanisms and pathogenic implications, in Ouchterlony Õ, Holmgren J (eds): *Cholera and Related Diarrheas*. S Karger, Basel pp 155–170, 1980.

78. Freter R: Bacterial association with the mucus gel system of the gut, in Schlessinger D (ed): *Microbiology—1982.* Washington, DC, American Society for Microbiology, pp 278–281, 1983.
79. Freter R: Mechanisms of association of bacteria with mucosal surfaces, in Elliott K, O'Connor M, Whelan J (eds): *Adhesion and Microorganism Pathogenicity.* Pitman Medical Ltd, London pp 36–55, 1981.
80. Freter R: Mechanisms that control the microflora in the large intestine, in Hentge DJ (ed): *Human Intestinal Microflora in Health and Disease.* Academic Press, New York, pp 33–54, 1983.
81. Freter R: Prospects for preventing the association of harmful bacteria with host mucosal surfaces, in Beachey EH (ed): *Bacterial Adherence.* Chapman & Hall, Ltd, London, pp 439–458, 1980.
82. Freter R, Allweiss B, O'Brien PCM, Halstead SA, Macsai MS: Role of chemotaxis in the association of motile bacteria with intestinal mucosa: In vitro studies. *Infect Immun* 34:241–249, 1981.
83. Freter R, Brickner H, Botney M, Cleven D, Aranki A: Mechanisms that control bacterial populations in continuous-flow culture models of mouse large intestinal flora. *Infect Immun* 39:676–685, 1983.
84. Freter R, Brickner H, Fekete J, O'Brien PCM, Vickerman MM: Testing of host-vector systems in mice. *Recomb DNA Tech Bull* 2:68–76, 1979.
85. Freter R, Brickner H, Fekete J, Vickerman MM, Carey KE: Survival and implantation of *Escherichia coli* in the intestinal tract. *Infect Immun* 39:686–703, 1983.
86. Freter R, Jones GW: Adhesive properties of *Vibrio cholera*: Nature of the interaction with intact mucosal surfaces. *Infect Immun* 6:918–927, 1976.
87. Freter R, Jones GW: Models for studying the role of bacterial attachment in virulence and pathogenesis. *Rev Infect Dis* 5:S647–S658, 1983.
88. Freter R, O'Brien PCM: Role of chemotaxis in the association of motile bacteria with *Vibrio cholerae* mutants in infant mice. *Infect Immun* 34:222–233, 1981.
89. Freter R, O'Brien PCM, Macsai MS: Role of chemotaxis in the association of motile bacteria with intestinal mucosa: In vivo studies. *Infect Immun* 34:234–240, 1981.
90. Freter R, Stauffer E, Cleven D, Holdeman LV, Moore WEC: Continuous-flow cultures as in vitro models of the ecology of large intestinal flora. *Infect Immun* 39:666–675, 1983.
91. Gardiner R, Podgorski C, Day AW: Serological studies on the fimbriae of yeasts and yeast-like species. *Bot Gaz* 143:534–541, 1982.
92. Garrison RG: Vegetative ultrastructure, in Arnold WN (ed): *Yeast Cell Envelopes Ultrastructure, Vol 1.* Boca Raton, Florida, CRC Press, pp 139–160, 1981.
93. Ghannoum MA, Burns GR, Elteen K, Radwin SS: Experimental evidence for the role of lipids in adherence of *Candida* spp to human buccal epithelial cells. *Infect Immun* 54:189–193, 1986.
94. Ghannoum MA, Elteen KA: Correlative relationship between proteinase production, adherence and pathogenicity of various strains of *Candida albicans. J Med Vet Mycol* 24:407–413, 1986.
95. Ghannoum MA, Janini G, Khamis L, Radwan SS: Dimorphism-associated variations in the lipid composition of *Candida albicans. J Gen Microbiol* 32:2367–2375, 1986.
96. Gibbons RJ: Adhesion of bacteria to the surfaces of the mouth, in Berkley RCW, Lynch JM, Rutter PR, Vincent B (eds): *Microbial Adhesion to Surfaces.* London, Ellis Horwood Limited, pp 351–388, 1980.
97. Gibbons RJ, Etherden I, Peros W: Aspects of the attachment of oral streptococci to experimental pellicles, in Mergenhagen SE, Rosan B (eds): *Molecular Basis of Oral Microbial Adhesion.* Washington, American Society for Microbiology, pp 77–84, 1985.

98. Gibbons RJ, Spinell DM, Skobe Z: Selective adherence as a determinant of host tropisms of certain indigenous and pathogenic bacteria. *Infect Immun* 13:238–246, 1976.
99. Gibbons RJ, vanHoute J: Selective bacterial adherence to oral epithelial surfaces and its role as an ecological determinant. *Infect Immun* 3:567–573, 1971.
100. Gooday GW: Biosynthesis of fungal wall: Mechanisms and implications. *J Gen Microbiol* 99:1–18, 1977.
101. Gopal P, Sullivan PA, Sheperd MG: Isolation and structure of glucan from regenerating spheroplasts of *Candida albicans*. *J Gen Microbiol* 130:1217–1225, 1984.
102. Gorman SP, McCafferty DF, Anderson L: Application of an electronic particle counter to the quantification of bacterial and *Candida* adherence to mucosal epithelial cells. *Lett Appl Microbiol* 2:97–100, 1986.
103. Guentzel MN, Cole GT, Pope LM: Animal models for candidiasis, in McGinnis MR (ed): *Current Topics in Medical Mycology, Vol 1*. New York, Springer-Verlag, pp 57–116, 1985.
104. Haley LD: Yeast infections of the lower urinary tract 1. In vitro studies of the tissue phase of *Candida albicans*. *Sabouraudia* 4:98–105, 1964.
105. Hassan OE, Jones JH, Russell C: Experimental oral candidal infection and carriage of oral bacteria in rats subjected to a carbohydrate-rich diet and tetracycline treatment. *J Med Microbiol* 20:291–298, 1985.
106. Hattori M, Yoshiura K, Negi M, Ogawalt: Keratinolytic proteinase produced by *Candida albicans*. *Sabouraudia: J Med Vet Mycol* 22:175–183, 1984.
107. Hazen KC, Plotkin BJ, Klimas DM: Influence of growth conditions on cell surface hydrophobicity of *Candida albicans* and *Candida glabrata*. *Infect Immun* 54:269–271, 1986.
108. Hector RF, Domer JE: Mammary gland contamination as a means of establishing long-term gastrointestinal colonization of infant mice with *Candida albicans*. *Infect Immun* 38:788–790, 1982.
109. Helstrom PB, Balish E: Effect of oral tetracycline, the microbial flora, and the athymic state on gastrointestinal colonization and infection to BALB/c mice with *Candida albicans*. *Infect Immun* 23:764–774, 1979.
110. Horisberger M, Vonlanthen M: Location of mannan and chitin on thin sections of budding yeasts with gold markers. *Arch Microbiol* 115:1–7, 1977.
111. Howlett JA: Candidial infection of the oral mucosa: An in vitro model. *Proc Roy Soc Med* 69:766–770, 1976.
112. Howlett JA: The infection of rat tongue mucosa in vitro with five species of *Candida*. *J Med Microbiol* 9:309–316, 1976.
113. Howlett JA, Squier CA: *Candida albicans* ultrastructure: Colonization and invasion of oral epithelium. *Infect Immun* 29:252–260, 1980.
114. Isaacson RE: Pilus adhesins, in Savage DC, Fletcher M (eds): *Bacterial Adhesion: Mechanisms and Physiological Significance*. New York, Plenum Press, pp 307–336, 1985.
115. Isenberg H, Allerhand J, Berkman JJ, Goldberg D: Immunological and toxic differences between mouse virulent and mouse avirulent *Candida albicans*. *J Bacteriol* 86:1010–1016, 1963.
116. Ito S: Structure and function of the glycocalyx. *Fed Proc* 28:12–25, 1969.
117. Jones GW: The attachment of bacteria to the surfaces of animal cells, in Reissig JL (ed): *Microbial Interactions. Receptors and Recognition*, series B vol 3. New York, Chapman and Hall, pp 139–176, 1977.
118. Jones GW: Adhesion to animal surfaces, in Marshall KC (ed): *Microbial Adhesion and Aggregation*. New York, Springer-Verlag, pp 71–84, 1984.
119. Jones GW: Mechanisms of the attachment of bacteria to animal cells, in Klug

MJ, Reddy CA (eds): *Current Perspectives in Microbial Ecology*. Washington, DC, pp 136–143, 1984.
120. Jones GW, Abrams GD, Freter R: Adhesive properties of *Vibrio cholera*: Adherence to isolated rabbit brush border membranes and hemagglutinating activity. *Infect Immun* 14:232–239, 1976.
121. Jones GW, Freter R: Adhesive properties of *Vibrio cholera*: Nature of the interaction with isolated rabbit brush border membranes and human erythrocytes. *Infect Immun* 14:240–245, 1976.
122. Jones GW, Isaacson RE: Proteinaceous bacterial adhesins and their receptors. *CRC Crit Rev Microbiol* 10:229–260, 1983.
123. Jones GW, Richardson LA: The attachment to, and invasion of HeLa cells by *Salmonella typhimurium*: The contribution of mannose-sensitive and mannose-resistant haemagglutinating activities. *J Gen Microbiol* 127:361–370, 1981.
124. Jones GW, Richardson LA, Uhlman D: The invasion of HeLa cells by *Salmonella typhimurium*: Reversible and irreversible bacterial attachment and the role of bacterial motility. *J Gen Microbiol* 127:351–360, 1981.
125. Jones GW, Rutter JM: Role of the K88 antigen in the pathogenesis of neonatal diarrhea caused by *Escherichia coli* in piglets. *Infect Immun* 6:918–927, 1972.
126. Jones JH, Adams D: Experimentally induced acute oral candidiasis in the rat. *Br J Dermatol* 83:670–673, 1970.
127. Jones JH, Russell C: The histology of chronic candidal infection of the rat's tongue. *J Pathol* 113:97–100, 1974.
128. Jones JH, Russell C, Young C, Owen D: Tetracycline and the colonization and infection of the mouths of germ-free and conventionalized rats with *Candida albicans*. *J Antimicrob Chemother* 2:247–253, 1976.
129. Joshi SN, Garvin PJ, Sunwoo YC: Candidiasis of the duodenum and jejunum. *Gastroenterology* 80:829–833, 1981.
130. Käppeli O, Walther P, Mueller M, Fiechter A: Structure of the cell surface of the yeast *Candida tropicalis* and its relation to hydrocarbon transport. *Arch Microbiol* 138:279–282, 1984.
131. Karaev ZO, Velichko EV, Bykov VL: Main characteristics of the process of adhesion of *Candida* to human epithelial cells. *Zhurnal Mikrobiol Epidemiol Immunol* 7:59–61, 1986.
132. Kaye D: Infecting microorganisms, in Kaye D (ed): *Infective Endocarditis*. Baltimore, University Park Press, pp 45–54, 1976.
133. Kearns MJ, Davies P, Smith H: Variability of the adherence of *Candida albicans* strains to human buccal epithelial cells: Inconsistency of differences between strains related to virulence. *Sabouraudia* 21:93–98, 1983.
134. Kennedy MJ: Inhibition of *Candida albicans* by the anaerobic oral flora of mice in vitro. *Sabouraudia* 19:205–208, 1981.
135. Kennedy MJ: Role of motility, chemotaxis, and adhesion in microbial ecology. *Annal New York Acad Sci* (in press), 1987.
136. Kennedy MJ, Bajwa PS, Volz PA: Gastrointestinal inoculation of *Sporothrix schenckii* in mice. *Mycopathologia* 78:141–143, 1982.
137. Kennedy MJ, Volz PA: Dissemination of yeasts after gastrointestinal inoculation in antibiotic-treated mice. *Sabouraudia* 21:27–33, 1983.
138. Kennedy MJ, Volz PA: Ecology of *Candida albicans* gut colonization: Inhibition of *Candida* adhesion, colonization, and a dissemination from the gastrointestinal tract by bacterial antagonism. *Infect Immun* 49:654–663, 1985.
139. Kennedy MJ, Volz PA: Effect of various antibiotics on gastrointestinal colonization and dissemination by *Candida albicans*. *Sabouraudia: J Med Vet Mycol* 23:265–274, 1985.
140. Kennedy MJ, Volz PA, Edwards CA, Yancey RJ: Mechanisms of association of *Candida albicans* with intestinal mucosa. *J Med Microbiol* (in press), 1987.

141. Kessler G, Nickerson WJ: Glucomannan-protein complexes from cell walls of yeast. *J Biol Chem* 234:2281–2285, 1959.
142. Kimura LH, Pearsall NN: Adherence of *Candida albicans* to human buccal epithelial cells. *Infect Immun* 21:64–68, 1978.
143. Kimura LH, Pearsall NN: Relationship between germination of *Candida albicans* and increased adherence to human buccal epithelial cells. *Infect Immun* 28:464–468, 1980.
144. King RD, Lee JC, Morris AL: Adherence of *Candida albicans* and other *Candida* species to mucosal epithelial cells. *Infect Immun* 27:667–674, 1980.
145. Klotz SA, Drutz DJ, Harrison JL, Huppert M: Adherence and penetration of vascular endothelium by *Candida* yeasts. *Infect Immun* 42:374–384, 1983.
146. Klotz SA, Drutz DJ, Zajic JE: Factors governing adherence of *Candida* species to plastic surfaces. *Infect Immun* 50:97–101, 1985.
147. Kobayashi K, Suginaka H: Comparison of cell wall and membrane proteins from eight *Candida* species. *Sabouraudia: J Med Vet Mycol* 22:341, 334, 1984.
148. Koch Y, Rodemacher KH: Chemical and enzymatic changes in the cell walls of *Candida albicans* and *Saccharomyces cerevisiae* by scanning electron microscopy. *Can J Microbiol* 26:965–970, 1980.
149. Kolarova N, Masler L, Sikl D: Cell wall glycopeptides of *Candida albicans* serotypes A and B. *Biochim Biophys Acta* 328:221–227, 1973.
150. Kotarski SF, Savage DC: Models for study of the specificity by which indigenous lactobacilli adhere to murine gastric epithelia. *Infect Immun* 26:966–975, 1979.
151. Krause W, Matheis H, Wulf K: Fungaemia and funguria after oral administration of *Candida albicans*. *Lancet* 1:498–599, 1969.
152. Kulkarni RK, Hollingsworth PJ, Volz PA: Variation in cell surface features of *Candida albicans* with respect to carbon sources. *Sabouraudia* 18:255–260, 1980.
153. Kuo-SC, Lampen JO: Tunicamycin—an inhibitor of yeast glycoprotein synthesis. *Biochem Biophys Res Comm* 58:287–295, 1974.
154. Lee KL, Buckley HR, Campbell CC: An amino acid liquid synthetic medium for development of mycelial and yeast forms of *Candida albicans*. *Sabouraudia* 13:148–153, 1975.
155. Lee A, Gemmelle E: Changes in the mouse intestinal microflora during weaning: Role of volatile fatty acids. *Infect Immun* 5:1–7, 1972.
156. Lee A, O'Rourke JL, Barrington PJ, Trust TJ: Mucus colonization as a determinant of pathogenicity in intestinal infection by *Campylobacter jejuni*: A mouse cecal model. *Infect Immun* 51:536–546, 1986.
157. Lee JC, King RD: Characterization of *Candida albicans* adherence to human vaginal epithelial cells in vitro. *Infect Immun* 41:1024–1030, 1983.
158. Lee JC, King RD: Adherence mechanisms of *Candida albicans*, in Schlessinger D (ed): *Microbiology—1983*. Washington, DC, American Society for Microbiology pp 269–272, 1983.
159. Lehrer N, Segal E, Barr-Nea L: In vitro and in vivo adherence of *Candida albicans* to mucosal surfaces. *Ann Microbiol* 134:293–306, 1983.
160. Lehrer N, Segal E, Cihlar RL, Calderone RA: Pathogenesis of vaginal candidiasis: Studies with a mutant which has reduced ability to adhere in vitro. *J Med Vet Mycol* 24:1270132, 1986.
161. Liljemark WF, Gibbons RJ: Suppression of *Candida albicans* by human oral streptococci in gnotobiotic mice. *Infect Immun* 8:846–849, 1973.
162. Lin JHC, Savage DC: Host specificity of the colonization of murine gastric epithelium by lactobacilli. *FEMS Microbiol Lett* 24:67–71, 1984.
163. Locci R, Peters G, Pulverer G: Microbial colonization of prosthetic devices. IV.

Scanning electron microscopy of intravenous catheters invaded by yeasts. *Zentralbl Bakteriol Hyg (B)* 173:419–424, 1981.
164. Loeb GI: The properties of nonbiological surfaces and their characterization, in Savage DC, Fletcher M (eds): *Bacterial Adhesion: Mechanisms and Physiological Significance*. New York, Plenum Press, pp 111–129, 1985.
165. Luft JH: Ruthenium red and ruthenium violet. II. Fine structural purification, methods for use for electron microscopy and localization in animal tissues. *Anat Rec* 171:369–416, 1971.
166. Lyon FL, Domer JE: Chemical and enzymatic variation in the cell walls of pathogenic *Candida* species. *Can J Microbiol* 31:590–597, 1985.
167. MacDonald F: Secretion of inducible proteinase by pathogenic *Candida* species. *Sabouraudia: J Med Vet Mycol* 22:79–82, 1984.
168. MacDonald F, Odds FC: Inducible proteinase of *Candida albicans* in diagnostic serology and in the pathogenesis of systemic candidiasis. *J Med Microbiol* 13:423–435, 1980.
169. MacDonald F, Odds FC: Virulence for mice of a proteinase-secreting strain of *Candida albicans* and a proteinase-deficient mutant. *J Gen Microbiol* 129: 431–438, 1983.
170. Macura AB: Adherence of *Candida* to mucosal epithelial cells. *Acta Microbiolog Polon* 34:55–58, 1985.
171. Macura AB, Pawlik B, Wita B: *Candida* adherence to mucosal epithelial cells with regard to its pathogenicity. *Zbl Bakt Hyg I Abt Orig* 254:561–565, 1983.
172. Maisch PA, Calderone RA: Adherence of *Candida albicans* to a fibrin-platelet matrix formed in vitro. *Infect Immun* 27:650–656, 1980.
173. Maisch PA, Calderone RA: Role of surface mannan in the adherence of *Candida albicans* to fibrin-platelet clots formed in vitro. *Infect Immun* 32:92–97, 1981.
174. Makrides HC, MacFarlane TW: Effect of commensal bacteria on the adherence of *Candida albicans* to epithelial cells in vitro. *Microbios Lett* 21:55–61, 1982.
175. Marrie TJ, Costerton JW: The ultrastructure of *Candida albicans* infections. *Can J Microbiol* 27:1156–1164, 1981.
176. Marshall KC: *Interfaces in Microbial Ecology*. Cambridge, MA, Harvard University Press, 1976.
177. Marshall KC (ed): *Microbial Adhesion and Aggregation*. Berlin, Springer-Verlag 1984.
178. Marshall KC, Bitton G: Microbial adhesion in perspective, in Bitton G, Marshall KC (eds): *Adsorption of Microorganisms to Surfaces*. New York, John Wiley & Sons, pp 1–5, 1980.
179. McCourtie J, Douglas LJ: Relationship between cell surface composition of *Candida albicans* and adherence to acrylic after growth on different carbon sources. *Infect Immun* 32:1234–1241, 1981.
180. McCourtie J, Douglas LJ: Relationship between cell surface composition, adherence and virulence of *Candida albicans*. *Infect Immun* 45:6–12, 1984.
181. McCourtie J, Douglas LJ: Extracellular polymer of *Candida albicans*: Isolation, analysis and role in adhesion. *J Gen Microbiol* 131:495–503, 1985.
182. McCourtie J, Douglas LJ: Unequal distribution of adhesins within populations of *Candida albicans*. *FEMS Microbiol Lett* 27:111–115, 1985.
183. McCourtie J, MacFarlane TW, Samaranayake LP: Effect of chlorhexidine gluconate on the adherence of *Candida* species to denture acrylic. *J Med Microbiol* 20:97–104, 1985.
183a. McCourtie J, MacFarlane TW, Samaranayake LP: Effect of saliva and serumon the adherence of *Candida* species to chlorhexidine-treated denture acrylic. *J Med Microbiol* 21:209–213, 1986.

184. McNabb PC, Tomasi TB: Host defense mechanisms at mucosal surfaces. *Ann Rev Microbiol* 35:477–496, 1981.
185. McRipley RJ: Animal models of candidiasis: Experimental chemotherapy, in Schlessinger D (ed): *Microbiology—1981*. Washington, DC, American Society for Microbiology, 1981, pp 218–221.
186. Miles MR, Olsen L, Rogers A: Recurrent vaginal candidiasis. Importance of an intestinal reservoir. *JAMA* 238:1836–1837, 1977.
187. Minagi S, Miyaka Y, Fugioka Y, Tsuru H, Suginaka H: Cell-surface hydrophobicity of *Candida* species as determined by the contact-angle and hydrocarbon-adherence methods. *J Gen Microbiol* 132:1111–1115, 1986.
188. Minagi S, Miyake Y, Inagaki K, Tsuru H, Suginaka H: Hydrophobic interaction in *Candida albicans* and *Candida tropicalis* adherence to various denture base resin materials. *Infect Immun* 47:11–14, 1985.
189. Mirelman D (ed): *Microbial Lectins and Agglutinins: Properties and Biological activity*. New York, John-Wiley & Sons, 1986.
190. Mirelman D, Altmann G, Eshdat Y: Screening of bacterial isolates for mannose-specific lectin activity by aggulation of yeasts. *J Clin Microbiol* 11:328–331, 1980.
191. Miyake Y, Fujita Y, Minagi S, Suginaka H: Surface hydrophobicity and adherence of *Candida* to acrylic surfaces. *Microbios* 46:7–14, 1986.
192. Montes LF, Wilborn WH: Ultrastructure features of host-parasite relationship in oral candidiasis. *J Bacteriol* 96:1349–1356, 1968.
193. Montes LF, Wilborn WH: Fungus-host relationship in candidiasis. *Arch Dermatol* 121:119–124, 1985.
194. Montplaisir S, Nabarra B, Drouhet E: Susceptibility and resistance of *Candida* to 5-Fluorocytosine in relation to the cell wall ultrastructure. *Antimicrob Agents Chemother* 9:1028–1032, 1976.
195. Myerowitz RL: Gastrointestinal and disseminated candidiasis: An experimental model in the immunosuppressed rat. *Arch Pathol Lab Med* 105:138–143, 1981.
196. Myerowitz RL, Pazin GJ, Allen CM: Disseminated candidiasis: Changes in incidence, underlying diseases, and pathology. *Am J Clin Pathol* 68:29–38, 1977.
197. Odds FC: *Candida and Candiosis*. Baltimore, University Park Press, 1979.
198. Odds FC: Biotyping of medically important fungi, in McGinnis MR (ed): *Current Topics in Medical Mycology, Vol 1*. New York, Springer-Verlag, pp 155–171, 1985.
199. Odds FC, Hall CA, Abbott AB: Peptones and mycological reproducibility. *Sabouraudia* 16:237–246, 1978.
200. Ofek I, Beachey EH: Mannose binding and epithelial adherence of *Escherichia coli*. *Infect Immun* 22:247–254, 1978.
201. Ofek I, Lis H, Sharon N: Animal cell surface membranes, in Savage DC, Fletcher M (eds): *Bacterial adhesion: Mechanisms and Physiological Significance*. New York, Plenum Press, pp 71–88, 1985.
202. Okubo Y, Honma Y, Suzuki S: Relationship between phosphate content and serological activities of the mannans of *Candida albicans* strains NIH A-207, NIHB-792, and J-1012. *J Bacteriol* 137:677–680, 1979.
203. Olsen I, Bondevik O: Experimental *Candida*-induced denture stomatiti in the wister rat. *Scand J Dent Res* 86:392–398, 1978.
204. Olsen I, Haanaes HR: Experimental palatal candidiasis and saliva flow in monkeys. *Scand J Dent Res* 85:135–141, 1977.
205. Paerl HW: Influence of attachment on microbial metabolism and growth in aquatic ecosystems, in Savage DC, Fletcher M (eds): *Bacterial Adhesion: Mecha-*

nisms and Physiological Significance. New York, Plenum Press, pp 363–400, 1985.

206. Persi M, Burnham J: Use of tannic acid as a fixative-mordant to improve the ultrastructural appearance of *Candida albicans* blastospores. *Sabouraudia* 19: 1–8, 1981.
207. Persi MA, Burnham JC, Duhring JL: Effects of carbon dioxide and pH on adhesion of *Candida albicans* to vaginal epithelial cells. *Infect Immun* 50:82–90, 1985.
208. Persi MA, Whalen SA, Burnham JC: Use of a controlled environment chamber to study interactions between *Candida albicans* (ATCC 18804) and cultured vaginal cells. *Micron* 12:217–218, 1981.
209. Pethica BA: Microbial and cell adhesion, in Berkley RCW, Lynch JM, Rutter PR, Vincent B (eds): *Microbial Adhesion to Surfaces*. London, Elis Horwood Limited, pp 19–45, 1980.
210. Phillips AW, Balish E: Growth and invasiveness of *Candida albicans* in the germ-free and conventional mouse after oral challenge. *Appl Microbiol* 14:737–741, 1966.
211. Phillips MW, Lee A: Microbial colonization of rat colonic mucosa following intesting pertubation. *Microb Ecol* 10:79–88, 1984.
212. Ponton J, Jones JM: Analysis of cell wall extracts of *Candida albicans* by sodium dodecyl sulfate-polyacrylamide gel elecrophoresis and western blot techniques. *Infect Immun* 53:565–572, 1986.
213. Ponton J, Jones JM: Identification of two germ-tube-specific cell wall antigens of *Candida albicans*. *Infect Immun* 54:864–868, 1986.
214. Pope LM, Cole GT, Guentzel MN, Berry LJ: An experimental model of candidiasis in infant mice: Systemic infection following gastrointestinal colonization, in Kuttin ES, Baum GL (eds): *Human and Animal Mycology*. Amsterdam, Escerpta Medica, 1979, pp 71–74.
215. Pope LM, Cole GT, Guentzel MN, Berry LJ: Systemic and gastrointestinal candidiasis of infant mice after intragastric challenge. *Infect Immun* 25: 702–707, 1979.
216. Pope LM, Cole GT: SEM studies of adherence of *Candida albicans* to the gastrointestinal tract of infant mice. *Scan Electron Microsc* 3:73–80, 1981.
217. Pope LM, Cole GT: Comparative studies of gastrointestinal colonization and systemic spread by *Candida albicans* and nonlethal yeast in the infant mouse. *Scan Electron Microsc* 4:1667–1676, 1982.
218. Poulain D, Hopwood V, Vernes A: Antigen variability of *Candida albicans*. *Crit Rev Microbiol* 12:223–271, 1985.
219. Poulain D, Trouchin G, Dubremetz JF, Bigvet J: Ultrastructure of the cell wall of *Candida albicans* blastospores. *Ann Microbiol* 125:141–153, 1978.
220. Poulain D, Tronchin G, Dubrementz JF, Bigvet J: Ultrastructure of the cell wall of *Candida albicans* blastospores: Study of its constitutive layers by the use of a cytochemical technique revealing polysaccharides. *Ann Microbiol* (*Inst Past*) 129:141–153, 1978.
221. Poulain D, Tronchin G, Jouvert S, Herbant J, Biguet J: Architecture pariétale des blastospores de *Candida albicans* localization de composants chimiques et antigéniques. *Ann Microbiol* 132A:219–223, 1981.
222. Price MF, Cawson RA: Phospholipase activity in *Candida albicans*. *Sabouraudia* 15:179–185, 1977.
223. Price MF, Wilkinson ID, Gentry LO: Plate method for detection of phospholipase activity in *Candida albicans*. *Sabouraudia* 20:7–14, 1982.
224. Pugh D, Cawson RA: The cytochemical localization of phospholipase and lysophoslipase in *Candida albicans*. *Sabouraudia* 13:110–115, 1975.

225. Pugh D, Cawson RA: The cytochemical localization of acid hydrolases in four common fungi. *Cell Mol Biol* 22:125–132, 1977.
226. Pugh D, Cawson RA: The cytochemical localization of phospholipase in *Candida albicans* infecting the chick chorio-allantoic membrane. *Sabouraudia* 15: 29–35, 1977.
227. Pugh D, Cawson RA: The surface layer of *Candida albicans*. *Microbios* 23: 19–23, 1978.
228. Ray TL, Digre KB, Payne CD: Adherence of *Candida* species to human epidermal corneocytes and buccal mucosal cells: Correlation with cutaneous pathogenicity. *J Invest Dermatol* 83:37–41, 1984.
229. Ray TL, Hanson AN, Ray LF, Wuepper KD: Purification of a mannan from *Candida albicans* which activates serum complement. *J Invest Dermatol* 73: 269–274, 1979.
230. Reinhart H, Muller G, Sobel JD: Specificity and mechanism of in vitro adherence of *Candida albicans*. *Ann Clin Lab Sci* 15:406–413, 1985.
231. Reiss E: *Molecular Immunology of Mycotic and Actinomycotic Infections*. New York, Elsevier, 1986.
232. Rippon JW: *Medical Mycology: The Pathogenic Fungi and the Pathogenic Actinomycetes*. WB Saunders Company, Philadelphia, p 842, 1982.
233. Rosenberg M, Gutnick D, Rosenberg E: Adherence of bacteria to hydrocarbons: A simple method for measuring cell-surface hydrophobicity. *FEMS Microbiol Lett* 9:29–33, 1980.
234. Rossano F, Tufano MA: Effect of concanavalin A on the adhesiveness of *Candida albicans* to vaginal cells. *Rass Med Sper* 22:313–317, 1975.
235. Rotrosen D, Calderone RA, Edwards JE: Adherence of *Candida* species to host tissues and plastic surfaces. *Rev Infect Dis* 8:73–85, 1986.
236. Rotrosen D, Edwards JE, Gibson TR, Moore JC, Cohen AH, Green I: Adherence of *Candida* to cultured vascular endothelial cells: Mechanisms of attachment and endothelial cell penetration. *J Infect Dis* 152:1264–1274, 1985.
237. Rotrosen D, Gibson TR, Edwards JE: Adherence of *Candida* species to intravenous catheters. *J Infect Dis* 147:594, 1983.
238. Rozee KR, Cooper D, Lam K, Costerton JW: Microbial flora of the mouse ilieum mucous layer and epithelial surfaces. *Appl Environ Microbiol* 43: 1451–1463, 1982.
239. Russell C, Jones JH: Effects of oral inoculation of *Candida albicans* in tetracycline-treated rats. *J Med Microbiol* 6:275–279, 1973.
240. Russell C, Jones JH: The effects of oral inoculation of the yeast and mycelial phases of *Candida albicans* in rats fed on normal and carbohydrate rich diets. *Arch Oral Biol* 18:409–412, 1973.
241. Russell C, Jones JH: The histology of prolonged candidal infection of the rat's tongue. *J Oral Pathol* 4:330–339, 1975.
242. Russell C, Jones JH, Gibbs ACC: The carriage of *Candida albicans* in the mouths of rats treated with tetracycline briefly or for a prolonged period. *Mycopathologia* 58:125–129, 1976.
243. Rutter PR: Mechanisms of adhesion, in Marshall KC (ed): *Microbial Adhesion and Aggregation*. Berlin, Springer-Verlag, pp 5–19, 1984.
244. Rutter PR, Vincent B: Physiochemical interactions of the substratum, microorganisms, and the fluid phase, in Marshall KC (ed): *Microbial Adhesion and Aggregation*. New York, Springer-Verlag, pp 21–38, 1984.
245. Rutter PR, Vincent B: The adhesion of microorganisms to surfaces: Physiochemical aspects, in Berkley RCW, Lynch JM, Rutter PR, Vincent B (eds): *Microbial Adhesion to Surfaces*. London, Ellis Horwood Limited, pp 79–92, 1980.

246. Ryley JF: Pathogenicity of *Candida albicans* with particular reference to the vagina. *J Med Vet Mycol* 24:5–22, 1986.
247. Samaranayake LP, Huges A, MacFarlane TW: The proteolytic potential of *Candida albicans* in human saliva supplemented with glucose. *J Med Microbiol* 17:13–22, 1984.
248. Samaranayake LP, MacFarlane TW: An in vitro study of the adherence of *Candida albicans* to acrylic surfaces. *Arch Oral Biol* 25:603–609, 1980.
249. Samaranayake LP, MacFarlane TW: The adhesion of the yeast *Candida albicans* to epithelial cells of human origin in vitro. *Arch Oral Biol* 26:815–820, 1981.
250. Samaranayake LP, MacFarlane TW: Factors affecting the in vitro adherence of the fungal oral pathogen *Candida albicans* to epithelial cells of human origin. *Arch Oral Biol* 27:869–873, 1982.
251. Samaranayake LP, MacFarlane TW: The effect of dietary carbohydrates on the in vitro adhesion of *Candida albicans* to epithelial cells. *J Med Microbiol* 15: 511–517, 1982.
252. Samaranayake LP, MacFarlane TW: On the role of dietary carbohydrates in the pathogenesis of oral candidosis. *FEMS Microbiol Lett* 27:1–5, 1985.
253. Samaranayake LP, McCourtie J, MacFarlane TW: Factors affecting the in vitro adherence of *Candida albicans* to acrylic surfaces. *Arch Oral Biol* 25:611–615, 1980.
254. Samaranayake LP, Raeside JM, MacFarlane TW: Factors affecting the phospholipase activity of *Candida* species in vitro. *Sabouraudia: J Med Vet Mycol* 22:201–207, 1984.
255. San-Blas G: The cell wall of fungal human pathogens: Its possible role in host-parasite relationships. *Mycopathologia* 79:159–184, 1982.
256. San-Blas G, San-Blas F: *Paracoccidioides brasiliensis*: Cell wall structure and virulence. A Review. *Mycopathologia* 62:249–258, 1979.
257. Sande MA, Bowman CR, Calderone RA: Experimental *Candida albicans* endocarditis: Characterization of the disease and response to therapy. *Infect Immun* 17:140–147, 1977.
258. Sandin RL: Studies on cell adhesion and concanavalin A induced agglutination of *Candida albicans* after mannan extraction. *J Med Microbiol* (in press), 1987.
259. Sandin RL: The attachment to human buccal epithelial cells by *Candida albicans*: An in vitro kinetic study using concanavalin A. *Mycopathologia* 98: 179–184, 1987.
260. Sandin RL, Kennedy MJ: Influence of growth parameters on *Candida albicans* adhesion, hydrophobicity, and cell wall ultrastructure. *Infect Immun* (submitted for publication), 1987.
261. Sandin RL, Rogers AL: Inhibition of adherence of *Candida albicans* to human epithelial cells. *Mycopathologia* 77:23–26, 1982.
262. Sandin RL, Rogers AL, Beneke ES, Fernandez MI: Influence of mucosal cell origin on the in vitro adherence of *Candida albicans*: Are mucosal cells from different sources equivalent? *Mycopathologia* 98:111–119, 1987.
263. Sandin RL, Rogers AL, Fernandez MI, Beneke ES: Variations in affinity to *Candida albicans* in vitro among human buccal epithelial cells. *J Med Microbiol* (in press), 1987.
264. Sandin RL, Rogers AL, Patterson RJ, Beneke ES: Evidence for mannose-mediated adherence of *Candida albicans* to human buccal cells in vitro. *Infect Immun* 35:79–85, 1982.
265. Savage DC: Localization of certain indigenous microorganisms on the ileal villi of rats. *J Bacteriol* 97:1505–1506, 1969.
266. Savage DC: Microbial ecology of the gastrointestinal tract. *Ann Rev Microbiol* 31:107–133, 1977.

267. Savage DC: Associations of indigenous microorganisms with gastrointestinal epithelial surfaces, in Hentges DJ (ed): *Human Intestinal Microflora in Health and Disease*. New York, Academic Press, pp 55–78, 1983.
268. Schaedler RW, Dubos R, Costello R: The development of the bacterial flora in the gastrointestinal tract of mice. *J Exp Med* 122:59–66, 1965.
269. Scheld WM, Calderone RA, Alliegro GM, Sande MA: Yeast adherence in the pathogenesis of *Candida* endocarditis. *Proc Soc Exp Biol Med* 168:208–213, 1981.
270. Scheld WM, Calderone RA, Brodeur JP, Sande MA: Influence of preformed antibody on the pathogenesis of experimental *Candida albicans* endocarditis. *Infect Immun* 40:950–955, 1983.
271. Scheld WM, Strunk RW, Balian G, Calderone RA: Microbial adhesion to fibronectin in vitro correlates with production of endocarditis in rabbits. *Proc Soc Exp Biol Med* 180:474–482, 1985.
272. Schwartz DS, Larsh HW: An effective medium for the selective growth of yeast or mycelial forms of *Candida albicans*: Biochemical aspects of the two forms. *Mycopathologia* 70:67–75, 1980.
273. Schwartz DS, Larsh HW: Comparative activities of glycolytic enzymes in yeast and mycelial forms of *Candida albicans*. *Mycopathologia* 78:93–98, 1982.
274. Segal E, Lehrer N, Ofek I: Adherence of *Candida albicans* to human vaginal epithelial cells: Inhibition by amino sugars. *Exp Cell Biol* 50:13–17, 1982.
275. Segal E, Savage DC: Adhesion of *Candida albicans* to mouse intestinal mucosa in vitro: Development of the assay and test of inhibitors. *J Med Vet Mycol* 24: 477–479, 1986.
276. Segal E, Soroka A, Schechter A: Correlative relationship between adherence of *Candida albicans* to human vaginal epithelial cells in vitro and candidal vaginitis. *Sabouraudia* 22:191–200, 1984.
277. Shakir BS, Martin MV, Smith CJ: Induced palatal candidiasis in the Wistar rat. *Arch Oral Biol* 26:787–793, 1981.
278. Sharon N, Eshdat Y, Silverbatt FJ, Ofek I: Bacterial adherence to cell surface sugars, in Ciba Foundation Symposium 80: *Adhesion and Microorganism Pathogenicity*. Tunbridge Wells, Pittman Medical, pp 119–141, 1981.
279. Shedlofsky S, Freter R: Synergism between ecological and immunological control mechanisms of intestinal flora. *J Infect Dis* 129:296–303, 1974.
280. Shepherd MG, Poulter RTM, Sullivan PA: *Candida albicans*: Biology, genetics, and pathogenicity. *Ann Rev Microbiol* 39:579–614, 1985.
281. Shepherd MG, Surarit R, Gopal PK, Sullivan PA: Cell wall metabolism of *C. albicans*: B(1→3) and B(1→6) glucan synthesis, in Nombela C (ed). *Microbial Cell Wall Synthesis and Autolysis*. Elsevier Science Publishers, New York, pp 73–83, 1984.
282. Shibl AM: Effect of antibiotics on adherence of microorganisms to epithelial cell surfaces. *Rev Infect Dis* 7:51–65, 1985.
283. Shimokawa O, Nakayama H: A *Candida albicans* rough-type mutant with increased cell surface hydrophobicity and a structural defect in the cell wall mannan. *J Med Vet Mycol* 24:165–168, 1986.
284. Skerl KG, Calderone RA, Sreevalsan T: Platelet interactions with *Candida albicans*. *Infect Immun* 34:939–943, 1981.
285. Skerl KG, Calderone RA, Segal E, Sreevalsan T, Scheld WM: In vitro binding of *Candida albicans* yeast cells to human fibronectin. *Can J Microbiol* 30:221–227, 1984.
286. Smail EH, Jones JM: Demonstration and solubilization of antigens expressed primarily on the surfaces of *Candida albicans* germ tubes. *Infect Immun* 45: 74–81, 1984.
287. Smyth CJ, Jonsson P, Olsson E, Söderlind O, Rosengren J, Hjerten S, Wads-

trom T: Differences in hydrophobic surface characteristics of porcine enteropathogenic *Escherichia coli* with or without K88 antigen as revealed by hydrophobic interaction chromatography. *Infect Immun* 22:462–472, 1978.
288. Sobel JD, Muller G, Buckley HR: Critical role of germ tube formation in the pathogenesis of candidal vaginitis. *Infect Immun* 44:576–580, 1984.
289. Sobel JD, Myers PG, Kaye D, Levison ME: Adherence of *Candida albicans* to human vaginal and buccal epithelial cells. *J Infect Dis* 143:76–82, 1981.
290. Sobel JD, Myers P, Levison ME, Kaye D: Comparison of bacterial and fungal adherence to vaginal exfoliated epithelial cells and human vaginal epithelial tissue culture cells. *Infect Immun* 35:697–701, 1982.
291. Sobel JD, Obedeanu N: Effects of subinhibitory concentrations of ketoconazole in vitro adherence of *Candida albicans* to vaginal epithelial cells. *Eur J Clin Microbiol* 2:445–452, 1983.
292. Sofaer JA, Holbrook WP, Southam JC: Experimental oral infections with the yeast *Candida albicans* in mice with or without inherited iron-deficiency anemia (s la). *Arch Oral Biol* 27:497–503, 1982.
293. Stewart TS, Ballou CE: A comparison of yeast mannans and phosphomannans by acetolysis. *Biochemistry* 7:1855–1863, 1968.
294. Stone HH, Geheber CE, Kolb LD, Litchens WR: Alimentary tract colonization by *Candida albicans*. *J Surg Res* 14:273–276, 1973.
295. Suegara N, Siegel JE, Savage DC: Ecological determinants in microbial colonization of the murine gastrointestinal tract: Adherence of *Torulopsis pintolopesii* to epithelial surfaces. *Infect Immun* 25:139–145, 1979.
296. Sullivan PA, Yin CY, Molloy C, Templeton MD, Shepherd M: An analysis of the metabolism and cell wall composition of *Candida albicans* during germ tube formation. *Can J Microbiol* 29:1514–1525, 1983.
297. Summers DF, Grollman AP, Hasenclever HF: Polysaccharide antigens of *Candida* cell walls. *J Immunol* 92:491–499, 1964.
298. Sunderstrom PM, Kenny GE: Characterization of antigens specific to the surface of germ tubes of *Candida albicans* by immunofluorescence. *Infect Immun* 43:850–855, 1984.
299. Suzuki M, Fukazawa Y: Immunochemical characterization of *Candida albicans* cell wall antigens: Specific determinant of *Candida albicans* serotype A mannan. *Microbiol Immunol* 26:387–402, 1982.
300. Tadros TF: Particle-surface adhesion, in Berkley RCW, Lynch JM, Rutter PR, Vincent B (eds): *Microbial Adhesion to Surfaces*. London, Ellis Horwood Limited, pp 79–92, 1980.
301. Tannock GW, Miller JR, Savage DC: Host specificity of filamentous, segmented microorganisms adherent to the small bowel epithelium in mice and rats. *Appl Environ Microbiol* 47:441–442, 1984.
302. Tannock GW, Savage DC: Indigenous microorganisms prevent reduction in cecal size induced by *Salmonella typhimurium* in vaccinated gnotobiotic mice. *Infect Immun* 13:172–179, 1976.
303. Tannock GW, Szylit O, Duval Y, Raibaud P: Colonization of tissue surfaces in the gastrointestinal tract of gnotobiotic animals by lactobacillus strains. *Can J Microbiol* 28:1196–1198, 1982.
304. Tomasi TB: Mechanisms of immune regulation at mucosal surfaces. *Rev Infect Dis 5: Suppl 4*:S784–S792, 1983.
305. Tronchin G, Poulain D, Herbaut J, Biguet J: Cytochemical and ultrastructural studies of *Candida albicans*. II. Evidence for a cell wall coat using concanavalin A. *J Ultruct Res* 75:50–59, 1981.
306. Tronchin G, Poulain D, Herbaut J, Biguet J: Localization of chitin in the cell wall of *Candida albicans* by means of wheat germ agglutinin. Fluorescence and Ultrastructural Studies. *Eur J Cell Biol* 26:21–128, 1981.

307. Tronchin G, Poulain D, Vernes A: Cytochemical and ultrastructural studies of *Candida albicans*. III. Evidence for modifications of the cell wall coat during adherence to human buccal epithelial cells. *Arch Microbiol* 139:221–224, 1984.
308. Tronchin G, Senet J-M: Binding of human fibrinogen to *Candida albicans* in vitro: A preliminary study. *J Med Vet Mycol* 24:345–348, 1986.
309. Turner JR, Butler TF, Johnson ME, Gordee RS: Colonization of the intestinal tract of conventional mice with *Candida albicans* and treatment with antifungal agents. *Antimicrob Agents Chemother* 9:787–792, 1976.
310. Umenai T: Systemic candidiasis produced by oral *Candida* administration in mice. *Tohoku J Exp Med* 126:173–175, 1978.
311. Umenai T, Konno S, Ishida N: Systemic candidiasis from *Candida albicans* colonizing the gastrointestinal tract of mice. *Experientia* 35:1331–1332, 1979.
312. Umenai T, Konno S, Yamauchi A, limura Y, Fugimoto H: Growth of *Candida* in the upper intestinal tract as a possible source of systemic candidiasis in mice. *Tohoku J Exp Med* 130:101–102, 1980.
313. Verwey EJW, Overbeek JTG: *Theory of the Stability of Lyophobic Colloids*. Elsevier, Amsterdam, 1948.
314. Vudhichamnog K, Walter DM, Ryley HC: The effect of secretory immunoglobulin A on the in vitro adherence of the yeast *Candida albicans* to human oral epithelial cells. *Arch Oral Biol* 27:617–621, 1982.
315. Waid JS: Physiological and biochemical adjustment of fungi to their environment, an advanced treatise, in Ainsworth GC, Sussman AS (eds): *The Fungi, Vol 3*. Academic Press, New York, pp 298–301, 1978.
316. Wain WH, Price MF, Cawson RA: Factors affecting plaque formation by *Candida albicans* infecting the chick chorio-allantoic membrane. *Sabouraudia* 14:149–154, 1976.
317. Wesney E, Tannock GW: Association of rat, pig, and fowl biotypes of lactobacilli with the stomach of gnotobiotic mice. *Microbial Ecol* 5:35–42, 1979.
318. Wilborn WH, Montes LF: Scanning electron microscopy of oral lesions in chronic mucocutaneous candidiasis. *JAMA* 244:2294–2297, 1980.
319. Winblad B: Experimental renal candidiasis in mice and guinea pigs. *Acta Pathol Microbiol Immunol Scand Sect* A83:406–414, 1975.
320. Wingard JR, Dick JD, Merz WG, Sandford GR, Saral R, Burns WH: Pathogenicity of *Candida tropicalis* and *Candida albicans* after gastrointestinal inoculation in mice. *Infect Immun* 29:808–813, 1980.
321. Wingard JR, Dick JD, Merz WG, Sanford GR, Saral R, Burns WH: Differences in virulence of clinical isolates of *Candida tropicalis* and *Candida albicans* in mice. *Infect Immun* 37:833–836, 1982.
322. Yu R, Bishop C, Cooper F, Hasenclever H: Glucans from *Candida albicans* (serotype B) and from *Candida parapsilosis*. *Can J Chem* 45:2264–2267, 1967.
323. Yu R, Bishop C, Cooper F, Hasenclever H, Blank F: Structural studies of mannan from *Candida albicans* (serotype A and B), *Candida parapsilosis*, *Candida stellatoidea*, and *Candida tropicalis*. *Can J Chem* 45:2205–2211, 1967.

5—Peptide Transport in *Candida albicans*: Implications for the Development of Antifungal Agents

FRED NAIDER AND JEFFREY M. BECKER

The yeast *Candida albicans* typically exists in a symbiotic relationship with humans (68). In the event, however, that the host is immunologically weakened upon challenge by disease or medical therapy, *C. albicans* can develop into a virulent pathogen. For many years this microorganism has gained increasing prominence as an opportunistic pathogen in hospital-associated infections and in compromised patients. Recently, this yeast has been documented as an agent in the morbidity and mortality of patients suffering from acquired immune deficiency syndrome (AIDS)(18).

A variety of clinical regimens exist for systemic candidiasis (58). Prominent among these are treatment with amphotericin B, 5-fluorocytosine, and the imidazole antimicrobics. Unfortunately, none of these antifungal agents are completely effective or without serious side effects. Given the medical importance of *Candida*, new approaches to drug design are clearly justified.

Several years ago Ames and co-workers (2) and Fickel and Gilvarg (27) observed that peptides could be used to carry normally impermeant molecules into *Salmonella typhimurium* and *Escherichia coli*. This phenomenon, termed illicit transport, smuggling, or portage (29) by various investigators, was put forth as a route to design antibacterial agents and was brought to fruition in the form of alafosfin (1). The approach has the desirable characteristics of target specificity and the possibility of using lowered blood concentrations of the active (toxic) moiety.

Studies from our laboratory have shown that *Saccharomyces cerevisiae* contains a peptide permease with specific structural requirements different from those found for bacterial cells and intestinal mucosa (9, 54, 55). An obvious extension of these investigations was to determine whether *C. albicans* had a peptide transport system and to attempt to use this system in the design of anticandidal drugs. In this review we discuss the peptide transport phenomenon as found in this pathogenic fungus and critically assess the shortcomings and advantages of using a peptide transport system in antimicrobial chemotherapy.

Techniques of Studying Peptide Transport in Microorganisms

Peptide uptake into cells can be assayed by either direct or indirect measures of transport. Early studies on microorganisms showed that the growth response of amino acid auxotrophs to peptides can be used as an indirect measurement of peptide uptake (6, 69). Despite certain limitations, properly designed growth experiments can and have yielded a great deal of information. Indeed, the structural specificity for peptide transport in *E. coli* was defined using the response of various amino acid auxotrophs to peptides. In the absence of extracellular peptide hydrolysis the growth of auxotrophs was related to peptide transport and consequent intracellular breakdown to component amino acids. The rate-limiting step in this process was peptide transport. However, growth, an indirect measure of transport, is limited to peptides containing a nutritionally required amino acid and does not readily yield information about the kinetics or energetics of the transport process. Consequently, investigators have sought more direct approaches.

Clearly, the most direct assay of peptide transport should use a radioactively labeled peptide that is not metabolized inside the target cell. Because microbial peptidases are ubiquitous and have broad and overlapping specifities, few peptides remain intact upon reaching the cytoplasm. It is rare, therefore, for investigators to have reported recovery of intact peptides from inside the cell. Nevertheless, during the past few years more and more studies have been based on the use of labeled peptides.

In addition to growth assays and the use of radioactive peptides, a variety of other indirect techniques have been reported in studies of peptide uptake. These include measurement of protein synthesis as stimulated by peptides (72), use of physiologic auxotrophs (17), and induction of β-galactosidase (11). Other direct methods used are the determination of disappearance of peptides from culture media or their appearance in the cell by peptide derivatization using the dansyl (70) or the fluorescamine methods (73). The release of thiophenol from a transported "detector peptide" has recently been exploited as a more direct assay of peptide transport (47, 48). This method uses α-substituted glycine-containing peptides and has been applied to both *E. coli* and *C. albicans*. Finally, inhibition by toxic peptides has proved useful in studies of peptide transport systems (71). Most investigations on *C. albicans* have examined uptake of radioactively labeled peptides or inhibition by peptides containing a toxic amino acid.

Mechanisms of Peptide Utilization

Many authors have described routes by which an amino acid in an exogeneous peptide can enter the metabolic pathways of a cell (6, 9, 69, 71). In Fig. 5-1, we

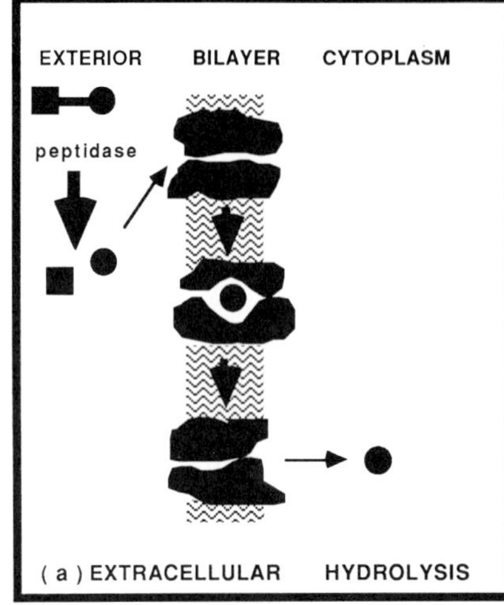

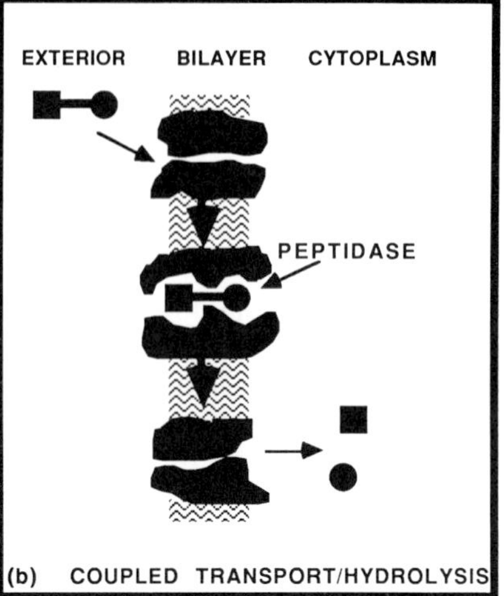

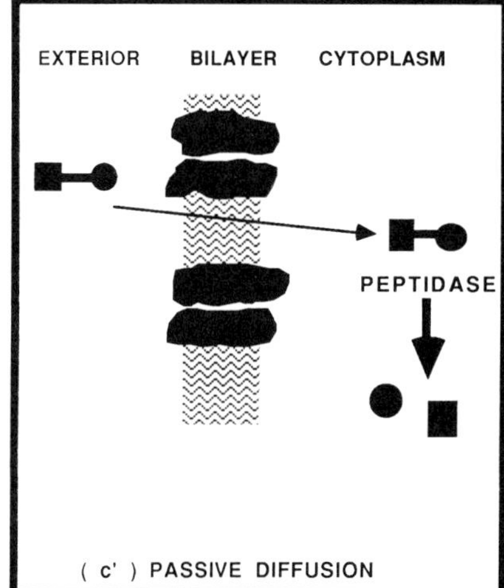

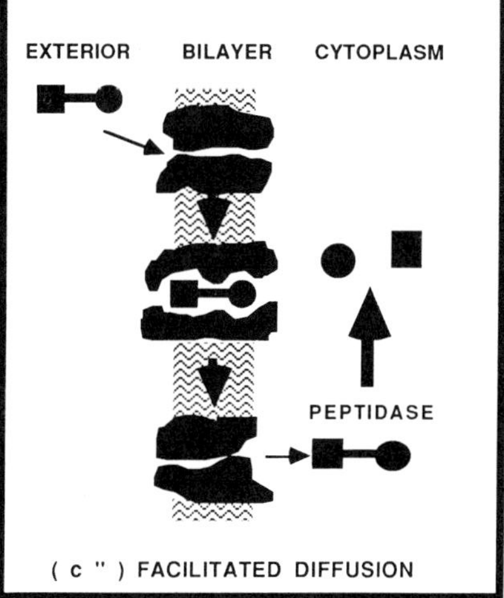

FIG. 5-1. Mechanisms of peptide utilization. The filled square connected to the filled circle represents a dipeptide. The filled circle and filled square represent amino acids. In panel (a) *extracellular hydrolysis*, the dipeptide is hydrolyzed extracellularly by an extracellular peptidase, and the component amino acids are transported into the cell via amino acid transport systems. Panel (b) *coupled transport/hydrolysis* represents the transfer of peptide across the membrane with concomitant peptidase activity possibly inherent in the carrier protein. *Passive diffusion* (c′) is illustrated as the peptide entering the cell unmediated by a specific membrane component. In panel (c″) *facilitated diffusion*, the transfer of peptide across the membrane is mediated by a membrane component, but a concentration gradient across the membrane is not established. For *active transport* (c‴), the peptide is accumulated inside the cell against a concentration gradient, and energy is required in some step of the process to establish this gradient. *Group translocation* (d) represents a covalent modification of the peptide during transport represented by the addition of X to the peptide. Panel (e) *receptor-mediated endocytosis* is illustrated as an internalization of the peptide mediated by a membrane-receptor complex.

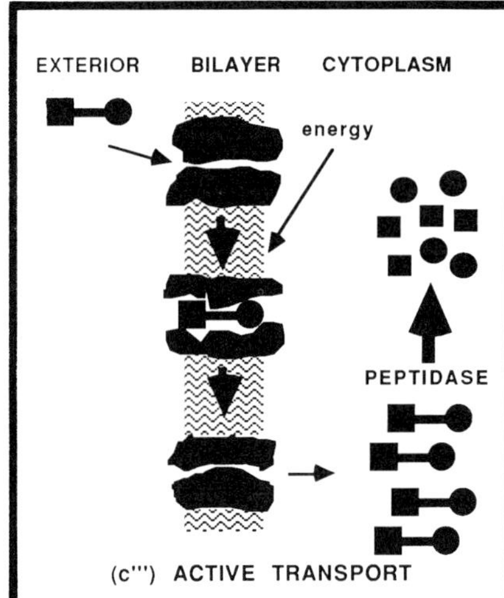

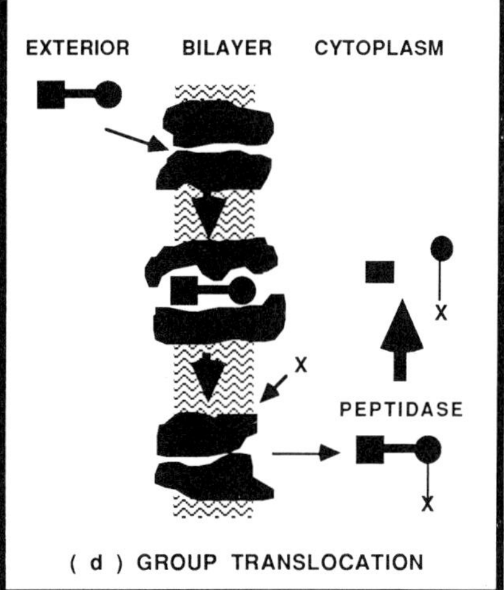

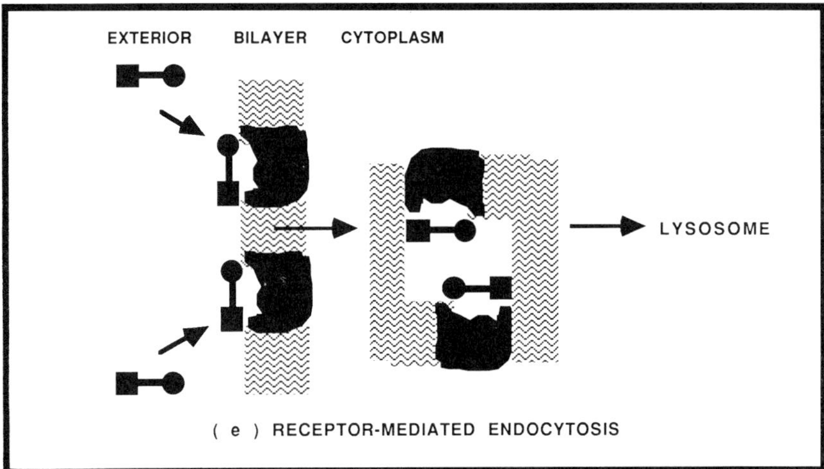

FIG. 5-1 (*Continued*)

represent diagrammatically extracellular hydrolysis followed by amino acid transport (a), vectorial transport coupled to hydrolysis (b), "true peptide transport" (c), group translocation (d), and endocytosis (e). "True peptide transport," which implies passage of the intact peptide across the cell membrane, can be subdivided into passive diffusion (c′), facillitated diffusion (c″), and active transport (c‴). For mechanisms c, d, and e the peptide must be further processed by peptidases contained in either the cytoplasm or in intracellular compartments such as lysosomes or vacuoles. In eukaryotic cells, compartmentalization of peptidase can have a major effect on the kinetics of the transport process. Despite this observation almost no experimental attempts to address the question of intracellular compartmentalization of transported peptides or peptidase have been reported, and most investigators ignore this consideration. Yet the ultimate fate of the peptide within the cell has major implications for both the transport process itself and the design of peptide carriers for drugs.

Many microorganisms contain a well-defined cell wall and do not appear to manifest an endocytic activity. *Candida albicans* is not known to be endocytotic, and it is unlikely that small peptides enter this yeast by mechanism e. Although recent work with *S. cerevisiae* indicates that the tridecapeptide α-factor and its receptor may be internalized by endocytosis (22, 75), we consider this a very specific process. No evidence for a similar mechanism in *C. albicans* exists at this time.

In all studies to date, which include investigations on a broad spectrum of cell types and peptides, there is not to our knowledge one example of a peptide which has been shown to enter a cell via group translocation. Therefore, we exclude mechanism d as a possible method of peptide transport in *C. albicans*. At high concentrations hydrophobic peptides may enter *C. albicans* by passive diffusion (c′). This mechanism, however, probably does not contribute significantly to the uptake of most peptides at physiologic concentrations. In the sections that follow, we will distinguish between the remaining pathways for peptide utilization by this fungus.

Are Intact Peptides Transported into *Candida albicans*?

Extensive investigations in *E. coli* and *S. typhimurium* conclusively show that peptide utilization in these prokaryotes occurs via mechanism c‴ (Fig. 5-1). These bacteria do not secrete extracellular peptidases, but they do contain genetically defined peptide permeases (3, 23, 32, 41). Several studies have recovered intact peptides from the cytoplasm, and calculations show that both di- and tripeptides are concentrated by 100 to 1,000-fold inside the microorganism (1 ,4, 45). Less rigorous studies on *S. cerevisiae* also have shown that mechanism c‴ is operative in this eukaryote (8, 9), although it is difficult to completely rule out pathway b (Fig. 5-1). Based on the above results, one is tempted to conclude that intact peptides also enter *C. albicans*. However, the fact that many fungi secrete a broad spectrum of extracellular proteases indicates that acceptance of the bacterial mechanism for fungal peptide transport requires further study.

Despite the possibility of extracellular peptidase activity, studies have not supported mechanism a (Fig. 5-1) as a mode of peptide use in *C. albicans*. Lichtliter et al (51) observed that spent medium from *C. albicans* WD 18-4 was devoid of peptidase activity. We also reported that several nonutilized peptide substrates were rapidly cleaved by cell extracts of this yeast. These findings suggest that the peptidase activities against the peptides examined are primarily intracellular. Later studies showed that methionine (Met) did not compete with the uptake of *L*-Met-*L*-Met-*L*-[^{14}C]Met into *C. albicans* WD 18-4 (52), and that in *C. albicans* 6406 alanine (Ala) did not inhibit uptake of either Ala-[^{14}C]Ala or Ala-Ala-[^{14}C]Ala (24), and neither glycine (Gly) nor phenylalanine (Phe) prevented entry of Gly-[^{14}C]Phe (24). If these peptides are first cleaved to their constituent amino acids, one would predict that competition at the level of the amino acid permease should occur. Davies (24) reported that in addition to glycine and phenylalanine, intact Gly-Phe was recovered from *C. albicans* 6406 cells incubated with this dipeptide. Alafosfin (*L*-alanyl-*L*-1-aminoethyl phosphonic acid) was recovered intact from the same microorganism. These results suggest that extracellular hydrolysis is not required for peptide transport in strain 6406. However, Logan et al (52) showed that only free methionine could be recovered from *C. albicans* WD 18-4 incubated with labeled trimethionine. Based on this study we concluded that one could not rule out a combination of membrane hydrolysis and vectorial transport in this strain (52, 83).

Yadan and co-workers (87) have shown that mutants of *C. albicans* ATCC 26278 simultaneously lost sensitivity to the antimicrobic nikkomycin Z and the ability to efficiently transport dimethionine. Similarly, mutants of *C. albicans* B-311 simultaneously became cross-resistant to polyoxin B, bacilysin, and m-F-Phe-Ala (59). The peptidyl nucleosides, nikkomycin Z and polyoxin B, are only active in the intact form, whereas both bacilysin and m-F-Phe-Ala must be hydrolized to manifest their toxicity. Therefore, the most reasonable explanation of the above results is that the mutants are peptide transport deficient and that intact peptides normally enter *C. albicans*. Virtually identical results were reported for *C. albicans* B2630 (74). On the basis of all these studies, we favor mode c‴ of Fig. 5-1 for peptide transport in this fungus, although we cannot eliminate the possibility of membrane hydrolysis followed by vectorial transport in some strains of *C. albicans*.

Structural Specificity for Peptide Transport in *Candida albicans*

A Qualification

Much of the investigation on peptide transport systems in microorganisms has been built on the pioneering work by Gilvarg and Payne using *E. coli* (6, 27, 29, 69, 71). These studies revealed a number of general characteristics which applied to virtually all strains of *E. coli*, and which indeed were even applicable to the closely related *S. typhimurium*. Attempts to formulate similar generalizations in eukaryotes have been less successful. In particular, variations in structural specificities for peptide transport have been reported in different strains of *S. cerevisiae* (9), and it will be obvious that this also holds true for *C. albicans*. In discussing features of peptide transport in this yeast, we believe it necessary to mention continually the strain which was examined to avoid incorrect generalizations. In most instances, we present results from our own studies first and then discuss other results that provide supporting or alternative data and conclusions.

Are Distinct Peptide Transport Systems Present?

Most studies on peptide transport in procaryotes concluded that separate amino acid and peptide transport systems exist in these microorganisms. Recent genetic analyses prove distinct amino acid, dipeptide, and oligopeptide permeases are present (3, 32). The situation in *C. albicans* is not conclusive. Competition studies show that a 20-fold excess of methionine did not affect $(Met)_3$ uptake into strain WD 18-4 (52), and identical results were found in *C. albicans* H 317 (Becker and Naider, unpublished results). Similarly, amino acids did not compete with the entry of Gly-Phe, Ala-Ala, or Ala-Ala-Ala into *C. albicans* 6406 (24), and alanine could not reverse the toxicity of the dipeptide antimicrobic tetaine in *C. albicans* AMB-25 (61). Twenty-seven different amino acids present in 20-fold excess did not antagonize the inhibitory activity of *L*-m-F-Phe-*L*-Ala-*L*-Ala against *C. albicans* B311 (46). In addition, peptides containing a toxic amino acid are often significantly more toxic than the amino acid itself. For example, the minimal inhibitory concentration (MIC) of *L*-m-F-Phe against *C. albicans* B311 and *C. albicans* 759 was 250 μg/ml, whereas di- and tripeptides containing the toxic amino acid are 100 to 500-fold more effective (46). Finally, the uptake of trimethionine into *C. albicans* was irreversibly inhibited by photolysis in the presence of 4-azidobenzoyltrimethionine (76). Under identical conditions no effect on methionine transport was observed. Taken independently each of the above experiments is not conclusive. Together, however, the weight of the data strongly argues for separate amino acid and peptide transport systems in *C. albicans*. The question will not be resolved conclusively until genetic analysis of peptide transport is undertaken. However, genetics of *C. albicans* is not well developed because the organism is a diploid with no known haploid stage and transformation techniques have not been very successful.

The evidence pertaining to independent dipeptide and oligopeptide permeases in *C. albicans* is less clear. As stated previously genetically distinct dipeptide and oligopeptide permeases have been characterized in bacteria (3, 32). In contrast several research groups concluded that both di- and tripeptides use one peptide transport system in *S. cerevisiae* (53, 64, 66, 67). Recent studies suggest that this latter conclusion is probably an oversimplification, and that peptide uptake in *S. cerevisae* is actually regulated in a complex manner by a variety of amino acids and nitrogen sources (Island, Becker, and Naider, unpublished results). This regulation hampers genetic analysis and complicates attempts to separate the various genotypes, which control peptide transport in this yeast.

Given the above situation with *E. coli* and *S. cerevisiae*, and the fact that *N. crassa* was reported to lack a dipeptide transport system (86), it is perhaps not surprising that various laboratories have reached different conclusions concerning the multiplicity of peptide permeases in *C. albicans*. Based on the poor competition by $(Met)_2$ for $(Met)_3$ uptake, we suggested that separate di- and oligopeptide transport systems were present in *C. albicans* WD 18-4 (52). We qualified this conclusion by raising the possibility that the system transporting $(Met)_3$ has low affinity for $(Met)_2$. In contrast Davies (24) stated that a common transport system mediated entry of both di- and tripeptides into *C. albicans* 6406 because both di- and tripeptides competed with each other at the level of uptake. Several additional reports support this type of reciprocal competition. Both di- and tripeptides reversed the inhibition of the dipeptidyl antimicrobic tetaine in *C. albicans* AMB-25 (61), and both $(Ala)_2$ and $(Ala)_3$ could relieve the toxicity of either *L*-m-F-Phe-*L*-Ala or *L*-m-F-Phe-*L*-Ala-*L*-Ala in *C. albicans* B311 (46). Recently, both di- and tripeptides were shown to compete with the uptake of *L*-alanyl-*L*-2-thiophenylglycine (Ala-α-TPG) and the analagous tripeptide (Ala-α-TPG-Ala)(56).

None of the above experiments are totally conclusive. However, a mutant of *C. albicans* ATCC 26278 was isolated recently that is resistant to the dipeptidyl antimicrobic nikkomycin Z (87). This mutant simultaneously gained resistance to the toxic dipeptide bacilycin (tetaine) and lost most of its ability to transport radioactive nikkomycin Z and dimethionine. However, the mutant was still able to efficiently transport $(Met)_3$. Although the kinetic analyses described by Yadan et al (87) are somewhat complex and will be described in more detail below, the authors concluded that at least two distinct transport systems mediate peptide transport into *C. albicans*. One of these can accept both di- and tripeptides, whereas the second was more specific for trimethionine. The presence of multiple peptide transport systems in *C. albicans* is supported by data of other authors. Two mutants of *C. albicans* B311 resistant to polyoxin B were cross-resistant to toxic dipeptides but not to a toxic tripeptide (59). In addition, a mutant of *C. albicans* 124 (NIK5) isolated using nikkomycin X and Z was unable to transport dipeptides such as $(Ala)_2$, Ala-α-TPG, and Leu-Gly and was resistant to the dipeptidyl antimicrobics polyoxin and bacilysin (56, 57). This mutant, however, still transported $(Ala)_3$, Ala-α-TPG-Ala, and $(Ala)_4$ and was partially sensitive to m-F-Phe-Ala-Ala. Finally, several mutants of *C. albicans* B2360 showed cross-resistance patterns compatible with separate di- and tripeptide permeases (74). However, we note that certain mutants, for example, *C. albicans* PA8001, which were resistant to the toxic dipeptides polyoxin, nikkomycin, and bacilysin and which did not transport radioactive dialanine, were still sensitive to the toxic dipeptide m-F-Phe-Ala. This latter observation suggests that more than one dipeptide transport system may be present in this strain or that m-F-Phe-Ala has a high affinity for the oligopeptide transport system.

It is certainly true that different *C. albicans* strains may contain different peptide transport systems. We believe, however, that the current evidence supports the conclusion that more than one transport system exists in *C. albicans*. One of these systems appears to be a general system that recognizes di-, tri-, and, perhaps, tetrapeptides. The other system(s) does not take up most dipeptides with an appreciable affinity.

Effect of pH and Nitrogen Source on Peptide Transport

Few investigations of the effect of growth medium on peptide uptake have been reported. A great body of literature suggests, however, that the uptake of nitrogenous substrates is regulated in a complex manner by the nitrogen balance in the cell. As anticipated, the uptake of trimethionine into *C. albicans* WD 18-4 was pH dependent. Optimal uptake occurred between pH 3.5 and 4.5 (52). Similar acidic pH optima were reported for $(Ala)_2$ and Gly-Phe transport into *C. albicans* 6406 (24) and for the uptake of a variety of peptides into *C. albicans* 124 and *C. albicans* 124 (NIK 5) (46). No other reports on the determination of pH optima for peptide uptake in *C. albicans* appear in the literature. However, other studies of peptide transport in *C. albicans* have assessed peptide uptake in the optimal pH range of 3.5 and 4.5. It is important to note that under certain conditions, shifts in medium composition or pH can cause transitions from the yeast to the mycelial form of *C. albicans*. This is a complicating factor in interpreting media and pH effects.

C. albicans WD 18-4 grown on isoleucine as the nitrogen source had six to eight times the peptide transport activity of cells grown on ammonium sulfate (52). Although transport rates were not measured, polyoxin toxicity is highly dependent on the nitrogen source; cells grown on glutamate are 25 to 50-fold more sensitive than cells grown on ammonium sulfate (59). In comparison to results in a nitrogen-poor medium, the Km of trimethionine uptake was much higher in cells harvested from a rich, but undefined, medium. However, nikkomycin uptake was similar in both rich and minimal media (87). Recently, we observed that certain amino acids have a major effect on the uptake rates of dileucine and trimethionine (Becker and Naider, unpublished results). Interestingly, trimethionine uptake is stimulated to a much higher degree than dileucine. These results suggest that peptide transport in *C. albicans*, and probably in *S. cerevisiae* (63), are under nitrogen repression. Detailed studies on this phenomenom are currently in progress by several investigators

Kinetics of Peptide Uptake

Analysis of the kinetics of transport processes can provide detailed insights into factors affecting substrate recognition at the molecular level. Peptide transport in *C. albicans* appears to be energy dependant because metabolic inhibitors such as sodium azide, carbonyl cyanide m-chlorophenylhydrazone (CCCP), dinitrophenol, and sodium arsenate totally inhibit di- and tripeptide uptake (24, 52, 56). Much more work needs to be done on this aspect of peptide uptake into the pathogenic eukaryote.

TABLE 5-1. Kinetic Parameters for Peptide Transport in *Candida albicans*

Strain	Peptide	pH	Nitrogen Source	Km
WD 18-4[51]*	$(Met)_3$	4.0	Isoleucine	3.3×10^{-5}
H 317[78]	$(Met)_3$	4.0	Isoleucine	3.0×10^{-5}
6406[24]	Gly-Phe	5.0	Ammonium sulfate	3.5×10^{-4}
6406[24]	$(Ala)_2$	5.0	Ammonium sulfate	2.5×10^{-4}
6406[24]	$(Ala)_3$	5.6	Ammonium sulfate	1.2×10^{-4}
ATCC 26278	$(Met)_2$	4.5[87]	Yeast extract, peptone	6×10^{-6}
ATCC 26278	$(Met)_3$	4.5[87]	Yeast extract, peptone	4×10^{-6}
ATCC 26278	$(Met)_3$	4.5[76]	Isoleucine	5.5×10^{-5}
ATCC 26278 (Nik)	$(Met)_2$	4.5[87]	Yeast extract, peptone	8×10^{-6}
ATCC 26278 (Nik)	$(Met)_3$	4.5[87]	Yeast extract, peptone	6×10^{-5}
124[56]	Ala-α-TPG	5.0	Peptone	2.8×10^{-5}
124[56]	Ala-α-TPG-Ala	5.0	Peptone	4.9×10^{-5}

* Note reference.

Studies using different strains indicate that peptide uptake is saturable, allowing the determination of both Km and Vm values. As seen in Table 5-1 there is significant variation in the Km values reported by different authors. However, the Km for $(Met)_3$ uptake determined in three different strains are comparable. In most cases the Km values are in the 10^{-5} to 10^{-6} range. These values are close to apparent Km values reported for *S. cerevisiae* (8, 67) and *Neurospora crassa* (86). The values reported by Davies (24) are significantly greater (one order of magnitude) than those reported in other studies using *C. albicans*.

Interestingly, although the growth conditions do not affect the Km for dipeptide uptake, they do have a significant influence on the kinetics of trimethionine uptake (87). Specifically, the Km for $(Met)_3$ uptake changed from 55 μM in cells grown in a rich medium to 4 μM for cells grown in minimal medium. These findings are consistent with different regulation of di- and tripeptide uptake. Moreover, whereas $(Met)_2$ uptake into a wild type and nikkomycin-resistant strain of *C. albicans* was reported to have similar kinetic parameters, the Km for $(Met)_3$ uptake in the mutant was increased by one order of magnitude and the Vm value was 20-fold higher. Finally, competition studies between trimethionine and a toxic dipeptide suggest that more than one transport system is present in *C. albicans* ATCC 26278. In particular, trimethionine is a competitive inhibitor of nikkomycin Z uptake, whereas nikkomycin competition with $(Met)_3$ uptake is not totally linear at high concentrations (87). Despite this observation we have observed that many peptides composed of naturally occurring amino acids are competitive inhibitors of $(Met)_3$ uptake in *C. albicans* (52). Thus, competition studies can provide much information about the structural requirements for peptide uptake into the pathogenic yeast.

Because none of the above studies established that the intact peptide is concentrated inside the yeast, it is possible that peptidase hydrolysis contributes to the measured Km value. This possibility has been discussed and for the most part discounted by many authors. Peptidase activity in most microorganisms is quite high. The fact that no intact trimethionine was found inside *C. albicans* WD 18-4 (52) indicates that this peptide is rapidly cleaved either inside the cell or during the process of peptide transport. Cleavage of detector peptides also was shown to be more rapid than their rate of entry into *C. albicans* 124 and *C. albicans* 124 (NIK5) (56). We believe that peptide hydrolysis is not rate limiting in the kinetics of peptide uptake into *C. albicans*. Given the fact that concentration against a gradient was not demonstrated for peptide uptake in *C. albicans*, and the possibility that peptide uptake may reflect a multistep process, we prefer to consider the measured kinetic parameters as apparent Km values.

The Km values for peptide transport in *C. albicans* and other fungi are one to two orders of magnitude greater than Kms measured for peptide transport in *E. coli* (69). Interestingly, similar differences also have been noted for the "binding affinities" of amino acid permeases in bacteria as compared with *C. albicans* (42). It is not clear to us what ecologic or environmental conditions are faced by the bacteria that would cause them to evolve more efficient peptide and amino acid transport systems than the fungi. However, the Vm values for peptide uptake in *C. albicans* are quite comparable to those in bacteria. Thus, at high concentrations the yeast can rapidly transfer nitrogenous peptides into its interior.

In our discussion of the kinetics of peptide uptake we have not treated the Vm parameter. Most authors have used different units for reporting actual rates of uptake, and the velocity is very sensitive to the metabolic state of the cell (87). Velocity values in the literature are generally in the range of 1–100 nmol peptide per milligram dry weight cell per minute. It is interesting to note that in two studies in which uptake in wild type and nikkomycin-resistant mutants has been compared, the rate of uptake of oligopeptides into the dipeptide transport deficient mutant has actually increased (57, 87). This increased transport activity might reflect an adaptation that is necessary to maintain the nitrogen balance inside the yeast cell.

Side Chain Specificity of Peptide Transport

The oligopeptide permease in bacteria can recognize peptides containing all of the naturally occurring amino acids (6). This broad side chain specificity was extended to unnatural amino acids and has been exploited in the design of antimicrobial agents. In contrast to the extensive studies in bacteria, a smaller number of peptides has been examined in *C. albicans*. In addition, certain peptides have been analyzed by examining their inhibitory effect on the yeast. In such studies the proper controls have not always been reported, and it is not clear whether or not the intact peptide enters the yeast. Finally, no reports have been published that have characterized the side chain specificity of peptide uptake in mutants lacking one or more of the peptide transport systems in *C. albicans*. Thus, in discussing side chain specificity one can only comment on the ability of peptides composed of different amino acids to enter *C. albicans*, and we cannot discuss the specificity of any individual transport system.

Growth studies in a methionine, lysine double auxotroph showed that peptides containing hydrophobic amino acids such as Met, Ala, Val, and Phe, readily entered *C. albicans* WD 18-4 (51). Many peptides containing one Gly residue were also growth substrates. However, except for Lys-Gly no other di-, tri-, tetrapeptide or higher peptide containing lysine was transported into *C. albicans*. Similar conclusions were reached in studies examining the ability of peptides to reverse the toxicity of tetaine (61). Hydrophobic peptides were found to be excellent inhibitors, whereas peptides containing glycine were often ineffective or only weak inhibitors. Interestingly, this latter study showed a marked difference in the ability of certain peptides to reverse tetaine toxicity in the mycelial as compared with the yeast phase. Unfortunately, because this is the only report of a comparison of peptide transport in the different forms of *C. albicans*, it is not possible to make generalizations.

For the most part, data on side chain specificity using growth response have been verified using labeled peptides. As seen in Table 5-2, hydrophobic peptides are more effective competitors of the uptake of label than are peptides composed completely of glycine or those containing lysine or glutamic acid. These findings agree with results in *S. cerevisiae* where, with the exception of one report (67), most studies conclude that peptides containing hydrophobic amino acids are better substrates for the oligopeptide permease.

TABLE 5-2. Competition by Peptides with Peptide Transport in *Candida albicans*

Strain	Labeled Peptide	Competitor	Percent Inhibition
WD 18–4[52†]	Met-Met-[^{14}C]Met	Leu-Leu-Leu (5)*	72
		Ala-Ala-Ala (10)	38
		Lys-Lys-Lys (10)	15
6406[24]	Gly-[^{14}C]Phe	Gly-Gly (10)	26
		Ala-Ala (10)	85
		Glu-Glu (10)	52
6406[24]	Ala-[^{14}C]Ala	Gly-Gly (10)	6
		Leu-Leu (10)	100
		Glu-Glu (10)	18
6406[24]	Ala-Ala-[^{14}C]Ala	Gly-Gly-Gly (10)	0
		Leu-Leu-Leu (10)	100
124[56]	Ala-α-TPG	Glu-Ala (1)	21
		Ala-Ala (1)	47
		His-Ala (1)	91
		Val-Ala (1)	69
		Phe-Ala (1)	63
		Leu-Ala (1)	63

* Parentheses indicate ratio of competitor to labeled peptide.
† Note references.

Given the somewhat sparse data and the variations which occur from strain to strain it is probably prudent to conclude that *C. albicans* can take in peptides composed of most amino acids and that the yeast has a particularly high affinity for peptides with hydrophobic side chains.

Size Restriction for Peptide Transport

There is no report to date that has examined whether or not there is a chain length restriction for peptide uptake in *C. albicans*. Oligopeptides up to and including pentamethionine supported growth of *C. albicans* WD 18-4 (51). Included in these studies were a variety of tetrapeptides composed of Met and Gly. In addition, using the fluorescamine method for measuring uptake, $(Ala)_4$ was judged to efficiently enter *C. albicans* 124 and a nikkomycin-resistant mutant (57). The above findings with tetra- and pentapeptides are in marked contrast to investigations in *S. cerevisiae*, which concluded that a size limit for transport exists and that peptides longer than a tripeptide are not recognized by this yeast (53, 67).

Importance of Termini for Peptide Uptake

In addition to the side chain functionalities, the amino and carboxyl termini of a peptide are potential points for attachment of toxic agents. Studies in bacteria showed that acylation of the α-amino nitrogen resulted in a non-transportable derivative, whereas the carboxyl terminal of an oligopeptide was not essential for transport (6). In *C. albicans* WD 18-4 exactly the opposite was observed (52). A number of di- and tripeptides containing either an acetyl or a t-butoxycarbonyl (Boc) group on the α-amine were excellent growth substrates. However, methyl esters of trimethionine, tetramethionine, and pentamethionine could not serve the nutritional needs of the yeast. Other studies showed that trimethionine acylated with propionic acid, isobutyric acid, or benzoic acid all gave positive growth responses with strain WD 18-4 (10). Similar findings were reported by Milewski et al. (61), in that Ac-Ala-Ala was able to reverse the toxicity of tetaine on the mycelial phase of *C. albicans* AMB-25. Unfortunately, this peptide was not tested against the yeast phase. Interestingly, the homologous tripeptide Ac-Ala-Ala-Ala did not reverse tetaine inhibition of the yeast phase of strain AMB-25.

The results of the growth studies are consistent with competition for radioactive trimethionine uptake into *C. albicans* WD 18-4. Thus, a 10-fold excess of Ac-$(Met)_3$ caused an 80% inhibition of the initial rate of uptake of $(Met)_3$ (52), and Ac-Ala-Ala competed with the uptake of Ala-Ala into an unspecified strain of *C. albicans* (21). Moreover, 4-azidobenzoyltrimethionine competitively inhibited $(Met)_3$ permeation and was a specific photoaffinity label for the system transporting $(Met)_3$ into *C. albicans* ATCC 26278 (76). This latter experiment gives evidence, at the molecular level, that some component of the system transporting $(Met)_3$ can recognize an alpha-N-acylated peptide. In contrast to the above body of evidence, Davies (24) reported that Ac-Ala-Ala-Ala and Ac-Ala-Gly-Ala could not inhibit the uptake of either $(Ala)_2$ or $(Ala)_3$ into *C. albicans* 6406. Thus, the majority of the evidence published suggests the conclusion that α-N-acylated peptides can enter some strains of *C. albicans*, whereas peptide esters are not transported. These findings must be considered when using peptides as carriers for anticandidal drugs.

Stereospecificity of the Peptide Transport System

Peptides containing *D* residues are appreciably more stable to peptidases than their *L* counterparts. In general this aspect of peptide transport and drug design has not been systematically examined in microorganisms. For *C. albicans*, strong evidence exists that a *D* residue at either the amine or carboxyl residue of a dipeptide leads to a nontransportable substrate. For example, neither *L*-Ala-*D*-Ala nor *D*-Ala-*L*-Ala competed with *L*-Ala-*L*-Ala for uptake into *C. albicans* 6406 (24). Similarly neither of these diastereomers reversed tetaine toxicity, whereas *L*-Ala-*L*-Ala was a moderately effective antagonist (61). Direct transport assays by the fluorescamine method and studies using detector peptides showed that *L*-Leu-Gly and *L*-Ala-*L*-α-TPG were efficiently transported into *C. albicans* 124, whereas *D*-Leu-Gly and *L*-Ala-*D*-α-TPG were not taken up by the cells (56).

In contrast to the absolute requirement of *L* residues for dipeptide uptake, the situation with oligopeptides is less clear. Studies with *C. albicans* WD 18-4 showed that *D*-Met-*L*-Met-*L*-Met supported the growth of this methionine auxotroph, whereas *L*-Met-*L*-Met-*D*-Met and *D*-Met-*D*-Met-*D*-Met were not growth substrates (51). Subsequent competition studies suggested that the difference between the three diastereomers represented transport affinity because *D*-Met-*L*-Met-*L*-Met caused 80% inhibition of $(Met)_3$ uptake when present in fivefold excess, whereas neither of the other *D*-Met containing peptides were competitors (52). Virtually identical results have been found with strain H-317, which does not require methionine for growth (Becker and Naider, unpublished results). Other peptides containing *D* residues appear to enter *C. albicans* via a peptide transport system. Peptides isolated from *Aphanoascus fulvescens* (as "*Keratinophyton terrum*") with the sequence Arg-*D*-allo-Thr-Phe have anticandal activity (50). Similarly, a number of analogs (Arg-*D*-X-Phe where X is an amino acid) also inhibit *C. albicans* (60). Because the *D*-X residue itself is not toxic to the cells, the above peptides must reach the cytoplasm to manifest toxicity by the intact peptide or by the smuggled *D*-X residue. In contrast an *L*-*D*-*L* detector peptide did not enter *C. albicans* 124 (56).

Other studies using peptides containing *D*-m-F-Phe are not easily interpreted (60). Although both di- and tripeptides containing *D*-m-F-Phe are poor inhibitors compared with the *L*-m-F-Phe-containing peptide, no data are given on the toxicity of *D*-m-F-Phe. It is impossible, therefore, to distinguish between transport deficiency, peptidase resistance, or the lack of toxicity of *D*-m-F-Phe in explaining the failure of these peptides to prevent growth of *C. albicans*. In conclusion it appears that certain tripeptides containing *D* residues are recognized by the peptide transport system in a number of *C. albicans* strains. The *D* residue cannot be at the carboxyl terminus and at present there is no peptide known with more than one *D* residue that can enter *C. albicans*. Thus, peptide diastereomers can be exploited in designing drugs against the pathogenic yeast.

Other Characteristics of Peptide Uptake

The effect of peptide bond isomerism and replacement of the α-carboxyl group have been examined in *C. albicans* 6406 (24). Dipeptides containing β- or γ-amino groups were significantly less effective inhibitors of both $(Ala)_2$ and $(Ala)_3$ transport than the parent compound. Similarly, γ-Glu-Gly-Gly was a poor inhibitor when compared with α-Glu-Ala-Ala. Because $(Gly)_3$ has a low affinity for the peptide transport system (Table 5-2), the latter comparison is somewhat questionable. Carboxyl group replacement was well tolerated by the peptide transport system in that both Ala-Ala-phosphonate and Ala-Ala-tetrazole inhibited dipeptide and tripeptide transport. All of the above studies were limited to strain 6406. As indicated previously, certain results with this strain differ from those published with other strains. Therefore, additional studies are warranted before the above conclusions can be generalized.

Comparison of Peptide Uptake in *Escherichia coli*, *Saccharomyces cerevisiae*, and *Candida albicans*

Comparison of peptide transport phenomenon in *E. coli*, *S. cerevisiae*, and *C. albicans* reveals both similarities and some striking differences (Table 5-3). The observation that N-acylated oligopeptides, but not oligopeptide esters, are transported into *C. albicans*, whereas the opposite is true in *E. coli* points out that different molecular interactions must be involved in peptide recognition by the permeases in these cells. The preference for hydrophobic peptides by the transport system in a number of yeast strains has no counterpart in bacteria. Again this suggests either environmental or molecular differences in the peptide transport systems of microorganisms. We should reiterate that growth studies are indirect measures of the transport process. To more fully understand the molecular interactions that result in different transport rates, one must determine both the Vm and Km for closely related series of peptides. Such detailed kinetic information is not available at present for peptide uptake in *C. albicans*. Despite this, the results of transport investiga-

TABLE 5-3. Characteristics of Peptide Transport in Microorganisms

Characteristic	*E. coli*	*S. cerevisiae*	*C. albicans*
Separate amino acid and peptide transport	Yes	Yes	Yes
Distinct dipeptide and oligopeptide systems	Yes	No?	Yes
Broad side chain specificity	Yes	Yes	Yes
Oligolysines transported	Yes	No?	No
N-acylated peptides transported	No	No	Yes
Peptide esters transported	Yes	Yes	No
Peptides with *D* residues transported	Yes	Yes	Yes
Size limit for transport	Yes (5–6)*	Yes (3)*	No

* Residues.

tions show that peptides can be used as carriers for toxic agents into *C. albicans*. The fact that different structural specificities are found for peptide uptake in three microorganisms, suggests that, in principle, a carrier might be designed to target a drug against only a specific population of harmful microflora of the body. Possibly the carrier could also discriminate between host and pathogen. The use of peptides in drug design against *C. albicans* is considered in the remaining sections of this review.

Can Peptides Carry Toxic Moieties into *Candida albicans*?

For use in drug design a peptide carrier must meet the following criteria: 1) it must be able to carry normally impermeable toxic agents into the target cell, 2) the peptide-drug conjugate must be stable or have a reasonable half-life in the host serum, 3) the conjugate should be toxic or metabolized to a toxic form inside the target cell, and 4) the conjugate should not be toxic to the host. Given the above criteria the use of peptides in the design of anticandidal agents required the establishment of illicit transport or smuggling in eukaryotic cells.

Prior to systematic attempts to demonstrate smuggling of toxic agents via the peptide transport system, there was evidence that this phenomenon was operative in *C. albicans*. Thus, the naturally occurring antibiotic tetaine (also called bacilysin) was shown to be considerably more toxic than its component amino acids (21, 44), and tripeptides found in the spent media from isolates of *A. fulvescens* were active against *C. albicans* (50).

The first systematic attempt to demonstrate smuggling, used peptides conjugated to the pyrimidines 5-fluorocytosine and 5-fluoroorotic acid (80, 82). Based on the activity of the peptide-pyrimidine conjugates and competition

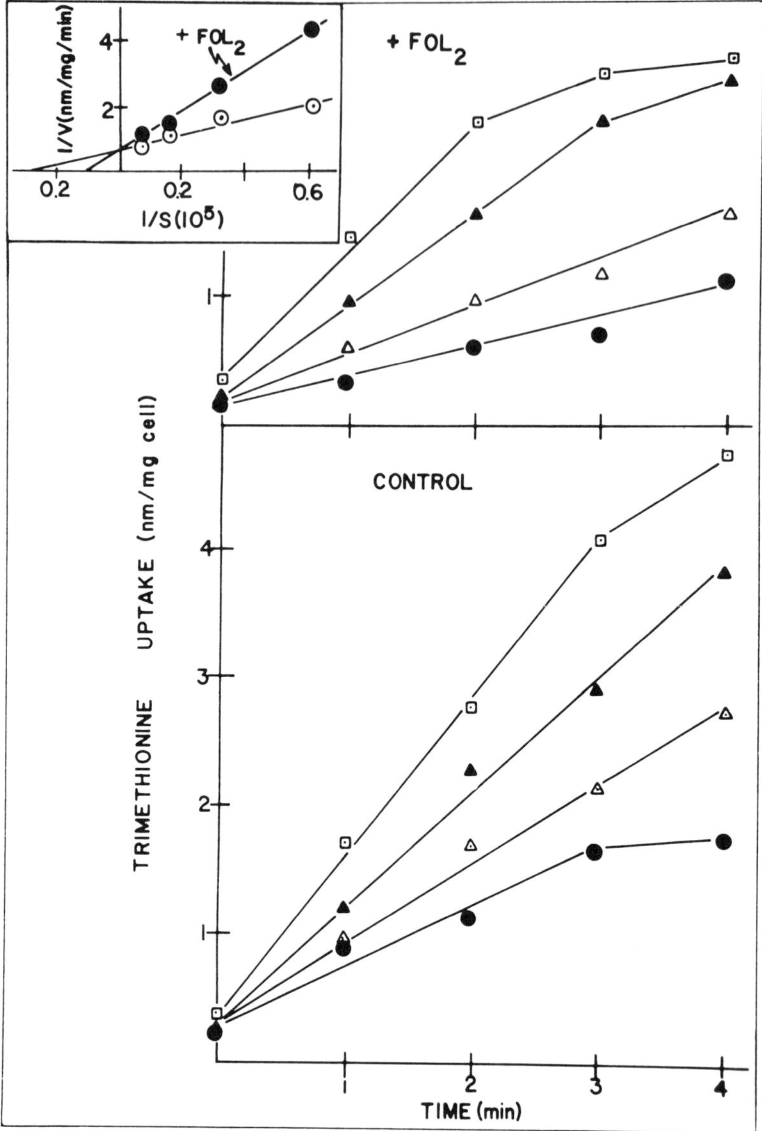

FIG. 5-2. Competition for uptake of radioactive trimethionine by 5-fluoroorotyl-leucyl-leucine (FOL_2). The control panel represents uptake of trimethionine at 12×10^{-5} M (*squares*), 6×10^{-5} M (*closed triangles*), 3×10^{-5} M (*open triangles*), and 1.6×10^{-5} M (*closed circles*). The upper panel labeled FOL_2 represents trimethionine uptake at different trimethionine concentrations (labeled as in the control panel) and in the presence of 3×10^{-4} M FOL_2. The insert panel is a double-reciprocal analysis of the data. Reprinted with permission from *J Med Chem* 23:913–918, 1980.

assays (Fig. 5-2), it was concluded that 5-fluorocytosine and 5-fluoroorotic acid were carried into *C. albicans* using a peptide transport system. Most importantly the conjugate design was based on the structural specificity of the peptide transport system, and the results obtained were consistent with predictions. For example, orotyl-leucyl-leucine, 5-fluoroorotyl-leucyl-leucine, and N^4(succinyl-alanyl-leucyl)-5 fluorocytosine all competed with the uptake of radioactive trimethionine into *C. albicans* WD 18-4, whereas orotyl-methionyl-methionine methyl ester, orotyl-glycyl-glycine, and orotyl-leucine did not compete. As peptide esters, amino acids, and nonpolar peptides have low affinity for the peptide transport system in strain WD 18-4 the above findings were expected. However, the bond conjugating 5-fluorocytosine to the succinyl spacer was quite labile and rapidly hydrolized in the culture medium. The amide linkage between orotic acid and the peptide was not susceptible to enzymatic cleavage by cellular extracts and it was stable in boiled medium. Thus, although we concluded that illicit transport was operative, none of the above conjugates were effective anticandidal agents.

Later studies provided more convincing evidence that peptides could smuggle nonpermeant molecules into *C. albicans*. Di- and tripeptides containing *L*-m-fluorophenylalanine were 100-fold more effective inhibitors of *C. albicans* B311 and *C. albicans* 759 than the amino acid antimetabolite itself (46), and inhibition by these peptides was antagonized by peptides but not amino acids. Peptides containing 5-fluorouracil attached as an α-substituted glycine were shown to enter *C. albicans* via a peptide transport system (47). In addition to the reversal of the toxicity of the fluorouracil-containing peptides by both di- and trialanine, the activity of the conjugates followed the known stereochemical requirements of the peptide permease. Finally, several of the above toxic peptides were not active against peptide transport deficient mutants of *C. albicans* (59). Thus, it appears clear that the peptide transport system can bring certain molecules into *C. albicans* and that the smuggling or portage mechanism is operative in this pathogenic eukaryote.

Are Peptide Carriers Viable Agents in Drug Design?

Despite the body of evidence that demonstrates illicit transport into microorganisms by peptide carriers, there have been few successful applications of this approach in the design of antimicrobial agents. The outstanding achievement in this area was the preparation of alafosfin (*L*-alanyl-*L*-1-aminoethyl phosphonic acid)—a dipeptide mimetic that has excellent antibacterial activity (1). Its mechanism of action clearly establishes entry via dipeptide permease, enzymatic cleavage to the toxic moiety (1-aminoethyl phosphonic acid), and inhibition of cell wall biosynthesis by this antimetabolite. Even given the excellent in vitro activity of alafosfin and its activity against penicillin resistant strains, it has found a very narrow zone of utility.

The reason for limited clinical acceptance of alafosfin is the high rate of serum degradation of the dipeptide, which renders it inactive. This characteristic is of general concern in the application of peptide carriers. The carrier must be stable in the host, yet the carrier or the carrier-toxic agent linkage must be degradable inside the target cell. It has proven difficult to establish this differential host-pathogen stability. At present not enough is known about the structural specificities of host versus pathogen peptidases to allow for a rational design of the "optimum peptide carrier." To circumvent this problem attempts have been made to attach toxic agents via nonpeptide bonds. For example, the use of sulfhydryl linkages (48) and α-substituted glycines (47) results in release by mechanisms independent of specific enzymolysis of the bond between the drug and the peptide carrier. Nevertheless, it is difficult for us to visualize how these approaches can overcome the need to differentiate between host and pathogen. Until this shortcoming is eliminated the application of peptide carriers will likely be limited to fortuitous circumstances where success is obtained for reasons that are not totally obvious.

One should not conclude, however, that the use of peptide transport systems should be discarded completely. Rather, certain restrictions should be considered in the choice of the toxic moiety. In particular, one must define a biochemical target in the pathogen having no counterpart in the host. Inhibitors of this target should have reduced host toxicity, which make them excellent candidates for drug design. If one can then choose such an inhibitor with high in vitro but low in vivo activity because it does not permeate into the target cell, the potential for drug design via peptide carriers becomes more attractive. In the remaining portion of this review we illustrate this approach using the polyoxin antimicrobics.

Chitin Synthetase Inhibitors Use Peptide Transport Systems

Many clinicians have dreamed of having a fungal equivalent of penicillin. Such a dream would be reality if effective inhibitors of fungal cell wall biosynthesis could be developed. Given the fact that mammalian cells do not contain cell walls, it is quite reasonable that the cell wall of *C. albicans* would be an appropriate target for a pathogen-specific drug. *Candida albicans* contains mannan, glucan, and chitin as important structural components of its cell wall (28). Although chitin is only a minor polysaccharide constituent (approximately 1% by weight), it is concentrated in the bud scar formed during reproduction and is more abundant in the hyphal tips of the mycelial phase of *C. albicans* (14, 19, 30, 81). This polymer of N-acetyl glucosamine is formed by the action of the membrane-bound enzyme chitin synthetase, which has been extensively studied in *S. cerevisiae* (16).

Mammalian cells do not contain any enzyme that is analogous to chitin synthetase of *C. albicans*, thus this protein appears to be an ideal target for a cell-specific inhibitor. Indeed, since the late 1960s a number of peptidyl-nucleosides that inhibit chitin synthetase have been isolated from fermentation broths of *Streptomyces* species (38, 39, 40). The antimicrobics originally called polyoxins and more recently nikkomycins (neopolyoxins) are effective against a variety of plant pathogenic fungi (12, 25, 49, 84, 85). However, early investigations reported no toxicity to *C. albicans*. It was puzzling that chitin synthetase inhibitors did not affect these cells, yet recent studies showed that under certain conditions polyoxins do affect *Candida*. Because the polyoxins can be viewed as dipeptides with two very unusual side chains (Fig. 5-3), studies were initiated to determine whether 1) polyoxins inhibited chitin synthetase from *C. albicans*, 2) failure of the polyoxins to kill *S. cerevisiae* and *C. albicans* was the result of low permeation into the cell, and 3) increased permeation could be achieved via the peptide transport system in *C. albicans*.

Investigations in both *S. cerevisiae* (13) and *C. albicans* (14, 15) indicated that polyoxin D and nikkomycin were effective inhibitors against chitin synthetase from these cells. Inhibitory constants derived from kinetic investigations were on the order of 10^{-6} to 10^{-7} M, which was quite similar to values reported for the phytopathogenic fungi. In minimal medium and at high concentrations (mM), polyoxin D was an effective inhibitor of the growth of both *S. cerevisiae* (43) and *C. albicans* (7). Cells treated in this manner became swollen and bulbous and did not form defined septa (7, 13, 14). Studies using staining agents such as calcofluor white, primulin, and wheat germ agglutinin colloidal gold (34) unequivocally proved that the morphologic changes in the cell were due to inhibition of chitin synthesis (Fig. 5-4).

Interestingly, the sensitivity of *C. albicans* to polyoxin-D and nikkomycin varied with both the strain and the medium conditions. For example, although strain H317 showed 50% cell death at 0.5 mM polyoxin-D, three other clinical isolates were 90% inhibited at 0.1 mM (7; and Becker and Naider, unpublished findings). In addition, the sensitivity of *C. albicans* B311 to polyoxin B varied 50-fold when the cells were grown on different nitrogen and carbon sources (59). Significantly, the toxic effects of the polyoxins were reversed by peptides in the growth medium (7, 59, 78). Earlier studies using phytopathogenic fungi also showed that the antifungal action of the polyoxins could be relieved by peptides when included in the growth medium (35, 62).

The above results indicate that if the polyoxins can reach chitin synthetase inside *C. albicans*, they could severely hamper growth of the yeast. Inferences were made that the polyoxins enter the yeast via a peptide transport system because peptides interfered with polyoxin toxicity. Unequivocal evidence that this was the situation came from studies that reported isolation of mutants that were cross-resistant to polyoxins, nikkomycins, and toxic peptides (57, 59). In addition, mutants resistant to nikkomycin Z could not transport radioactive dimethionine (87). Although it is likely that both polyoxins and nikkomycins enter *C. albicans* via a peptide transport system, they do so with

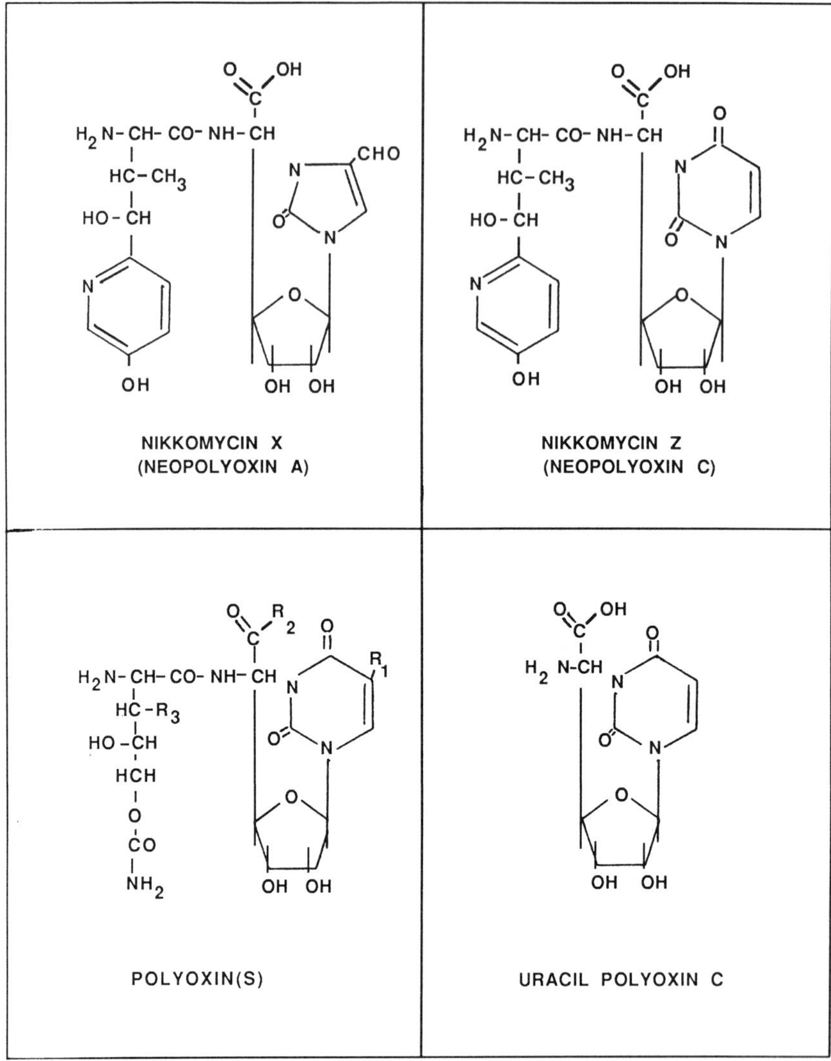

FIG. 5-3. Structural formulae of polyoxins. The panel in the lower left illustrates the general formula for the polyoxins. When R_1 = COOH, R_2 = OH, and R_3 = OH, the compound is polyoxin-D, the form of polyoxin used for many studies of the polyoxins. Uracil polyoxin-C (right lower panel) is the synthetic nucleoside used as the starting compound for synthesis of the synthetic polyoxin analogs. The upper two panels illustrate the complete structural formulae for nikkomycin X (also called neopolyoxin A) and nikkomycin Z (also called neopolyoxin C).

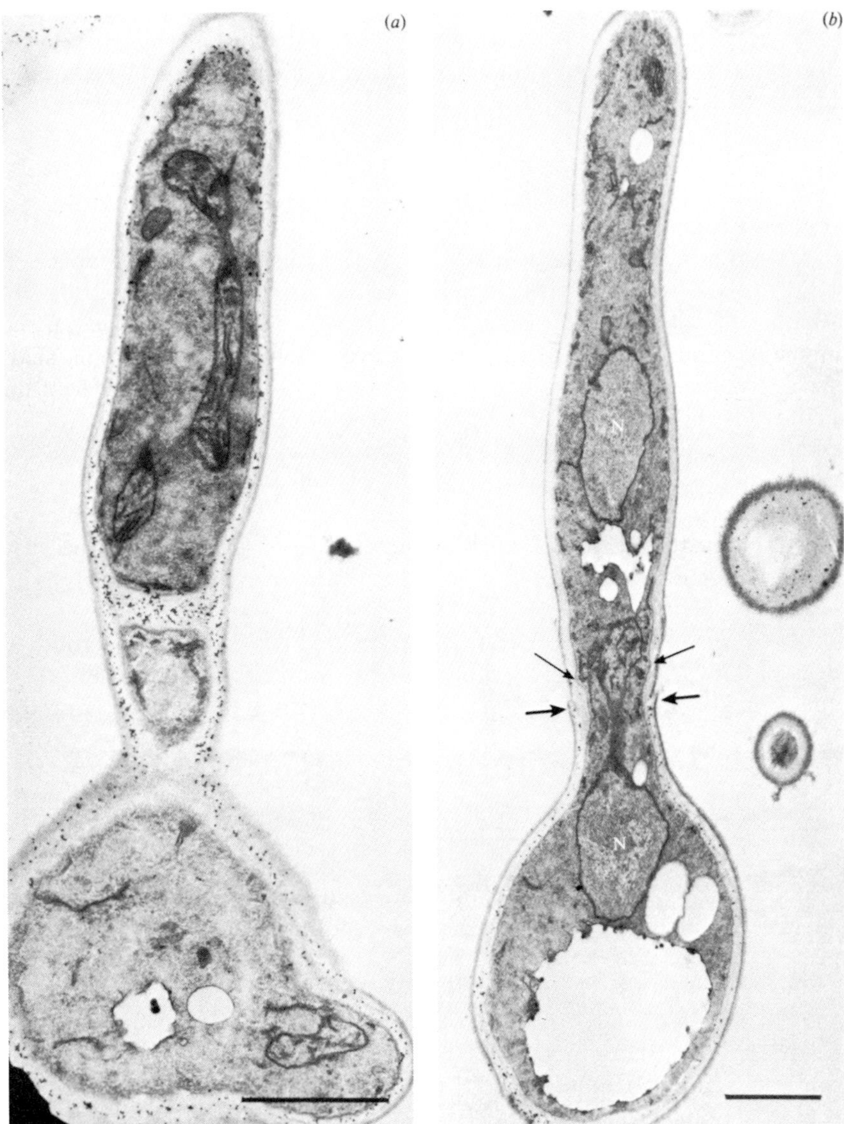

FIG. 5-4. Effect of polyoxin-D on *Candida albicans*. Comparison of germ tubes without (a) and with (b) 4 mM polyoxin-D for 4.5 hours. In the control cell, septum labeled with gold wheat germ agglutinin, a marker for chitin, is denoted by black dots corresponding to the gold label. In the treated cell, no septum is present and labeling is not seen in the germ tube. Bars = 1 μm. Reprinted with permission from *J Gen Microbiol* (34).

very different efficiencies. Thus, the peptide transport system appears to be sensitive to the amino acids contained in the peptide. This is strikingly illustrated by comparing Vm values for nikkomycin Z and dimethionine. Both of these dipeptides have similar Km values (5×10^{-6} M), but the Vm of the antimicrobic is 20 times lower than that of dimethionine (87). Therefore, the possibility was raised that a more effective antimicrobic could be achieved by modifications which would improve recognition and transport by the peptide transport system.

Attempts in this latter direction have been reported and a number of synthetic and semisynthetic polyoxin analogs have been prepared (5, 36). Analogs of polyoxin L in which the naturally occurring amino acid at the amine terminus of the dipeptide was replaced by hydrophobic amino acids such as norleucine, tryptophan, and homophenylalanine were excellent inhibitors of chitin synthetase in *C. albicans* H317 (78). However, none of the synthetic polyoxins inhibited the uptake of radioactive trimethionine or the growth of the yeast. Subsequent metabolic analysis revealed that the synthetic polyoxins were rapidly cleaved by peptidases inside *C. albicans*. This observation explained the lower potency of these synthetic antimicrobics because naturally occurring polyoxin D and nikkomycin were stable to hydrolysis by *C. albicans* peptidases.

A number of methods are available to stabilize peptides against peptidase degradation. These include the insertion of *D*-amino acid residues, N-methyl amino acids, and pseudopeptide linkages (37) into the peptide. For the most part such approaches have not been successful with the polyoxins, because these replacements have resulted in greatly reduced activity against chitin synthetase. Thus, although analogs of polyoxin L-containing *D*-tryptophan, N-methyl norleucine, or aminoxy phenylalanine were not cleaved by candidal peptidases, they were at least 100-fold poorer inhibitors of chitin synthetase than polyoxin D (77). Similar results were reported for polyoxin analogs containing an N-methyl peptide bond or an aminoalkyl linkage in place of the peptide bond (26). Recently, synthetic polyoxins containing amino acids with long hydrophobic side chains were shown to be excellent chitin synthetase inhibitors and at the same time were highly stable inside *C. albicans* (79). It appears that proper choice of the amine terminal residue can lead to a polyoxin analog with properties quite similar to the naturally occurring antimicrobic. Nevertheless, none of the synthetic dipeptidyl polyoxin analogs competed effectively with the uptake of trimethionine or uridine into *C. albicans*. One might conclude that none of the analogs had affinity for the peptide or pyrimidine transport systems. However, a tripeptidyl polyoxin (leucyl-norleucyl-UPOC) prevented trimethionine uptake (65) and it is possible that the dipeptidyl polyoxins use a transport system that does not recognize tripeptides or pyrimidines. It is necessary to examine the competition between the synthetic dipeptidyl polyoxins and a radioactive dipeptide such as dileucine or dimethionine before any final conclusions are reached.

Despite the above reservations, it is clear that very small molecular differences seem to exert a major influence on the ability of chitin synthetase inhibitors to use the peptide transport system. The fact that nikkomycin Z is a much more effective substrate for the peptide transport system than polyoxin D does not result from the different amino terminal residues in these antimicrobics. Comparison of biologic activities of the neopolyoxins shows that three isomeric antimicrobics with an identical amino terminal residue have markedly different anticandidal activities (12, 49), even though they have virtually identical inhibitory constants against chitin synthetase. Two of these with high activity have carboxyl terminal residues with neutral pyrimidine rings. The inactive isomer contains a 5-carboxy uridine moiety. Although no studies of the transport characteristics of these neopolyoxins have been reported, it is interesting to note that polyoxin D also contains a 5-carboxy uridine functionality. Thus, it is possible that small changes in the carboxyl terminal side chain have an influence on the transportability of these chitin synthetase inhibitors.

In summary, a number of synthetic polyoxin analogs with high activity against chitin synthetase and good intracellular stability have been prepared. Except for nikkomycin Z, which enters the pathogen slowly compared with normal di- and tripeptides, no evidence exists that these inhibitors can efficiently use the peptide transport system in *C. albicans*. Given the medical importance of *C. albicans* and the limited number of effective therapeutic regimens for this pathogen, further attempts to prepare chitin synthetase inhibitors with better affinity for the peptide transport system are warranted.

Conclusion

The exciting recent discoveries of Chen et al (20) and Gross et al (31) have intensified interest in the study of peptide transport. These investigators have cloned the genes for multiple drug resistance (MDR) in mammalian cells and have discovered homology of the MDR genes with bacterial transport proteins including OPPD, a protein involved in peptide transport in *Salmonella*. Thus, investigations on peptide transport systems in microorganisms may reveal information relevant to cancer chemotherapy and aid in the development of new and better therapeutic regimens.

Peptide transport systems provide cells with an opportunity to take up a variety of nitrogenous compounds rapidly and efficiently. Such transport systems have been encountered in many cells studied from simple bacteria to germinating barley embryos (33) and the mammalian gut (54). The yeast *C. albicans* appears to be no exception; it possesses a peptide transport phenomenon and exhibits a variety of structural characteristics that could prove beneficial to drug design. Future success in this area will depend on the proper choice of target and the ability of the investigator to overcome strain variations, differential target cell and host peptidase activity, and other problems related to the pharmacodynamics of drugs.

Civilization is currently battling a number of insidious diseases that attack immunologic processes. Until these diseases can be effectively prevented, the opportunistic pathogens will be prominent public health problems. The clinical mycologist requires improved and more sophisticated drugs to control candidal infections. Active transport systems provide an interesting and attractive alternative in the rational design of such agents.

Acknowledgments

Support for our studies came from the The National Institute of Allergy and Infectious Disease grant AI-14387 and contract AI-42651, and the American Cancer Society grant CH-290. We are grateful for the collaboration of the following students and postdoctoral fellows whose assistance was essential for our work: Charlotte Boney, Nancy Covert, Ali Gulumoglu, Lula Hilenski, Bijoy Kundu, Wayne Lichliter, David Logan, Ponniah Shenbagamurthi, Herb Smith, Alvin Steinfeld, and Jen-Shing Ti.

References

1. Allen JG, Atherton FR, Hall MJ, Hassall CH, Holmes W, Lambert RW, Nisbet LJ, Ringrose PS: Phosphonopeptides as antibacterial agents: Alaphosphin and related phosphonopeptides. *Antimicrob Agents Chemother* 15:684–695, 1979.
2. Ames BN, Ames GF, Young JD, Isuchiya D, Lecocq J: Illicit transport: The oligopeptide permease. *Proc Natl Acad Sci USA* 70:456–458, 1973.
3. Andrews JC, Short SA: Genetic analysis of *Escherichia coli* oligopeptide transport mutants. *J Bacteriol* 161:484–492, 1985.
4. Atherton FR, Hall MJ, Hassall CH, Lambert RW, Lloyd WJ, Lord AV, Ringrose PS, Westmacott: Phosphonopeptides as substrates for peptide transport systems and peptidases of *Escherichia coli. Antimicrob Agents Chemother* 24:522–528, 1983.
5. Azuma T, Saita T, Isono K: Polyoxin analogs, III. Synthesis and biological activity of aminoacyl derivatives of polyoxin C and L. *Chem Pharma Bull* 25:1740–1748, 1977.
6. Barak Z, Gilvarg C: Peptide transport, in Eisenberg H, Katchalski-Katzir E, Manson LA (eds): *Biomembranes*, vol. 7. New York, Plenum Press, 1975, pp 167–218.
7. Becker JM, Covert NL, Shenbagamurthi P, Steinfeld AS, Naider F: Polyoxin D inhibits growth of zoopathogenic fungi. *Antimicrob Agents Chemother* 23:926–929, 1983.
8. Becker JM, Naider F: Peptide transport in yeast: Uptake of radioactive trimethionine in *Saccharomyces cerevisiae. Arch Biochem Biophys* 278:245–255, 1977.
9. Becker JM, Naider F: Transport and utilization of peptides by yeast, in Payne JW (ed): *Microorganisms and Nitrogen Sources*. Chichester, United Kingdom, Wiley & Sons, 1980, pp 258–279.
10. Becker JM, Steinfeld A, Naider F: Novel Approach to the Development of Anticandidal Drugs. *Proc Fourth International Conf Mycoses, Pan American Health Organization Scientific Publication* No. 356, 1978, pp 303–308.

11. Bell G, Payne GM, Payne JW: Monitoring enzyme synthesis as a means of studying peptide transport and utilization in *Escherichia coli. J Gen Microbiol* 98:485–491, 1977.
12. Bormann C, Huhn W, Zahner H, Rathman R, Huhn H, Konig WA: Metabolic products of microorganisms: New nikkomycins produced by mutants of *Streptomyces tendae. J Antibiot* 38:9–16, 1985.
13. Bowers B, Levin G, Cabib E: Effect of polyoxin D on chitin synthesis and septum formation in *Saccharomyces cerevisiae. J Bacteriol* 119:564–575, 1974.
14. Braun P, Calderone RA: Chitin synthesis in *Candida albicans*: Comparison of yeast and hyphal forms. *J Bacteriol* 133:1472–1477, 1978.
15. Braun PC, Calderone RA: Regulation and solubilization of *Candida albicans* chitin synthetase. *J Bacteriol* 14:666–670, 1979.
16. Cabib E, Roberts R, Bowers B: Synthesis of the yeast cell wall and its regulation. *Ann Rev Biochem* 51:763–793, 1982.
17. Cascieri T, Mallette MF: New method for study of peptide transport in bacteria. *Appl Microbiol* 27:457–463, 1974.
18. Chandler FW: Pathology of the mycoses in patients with acquired immunodeficiency syndrome (AIDS), in McGinnis MR (ed): *Current Topics in Medical Mycology*, Vol. 1. New York, Springer-Verlag, 1985, pp 1–23.
19. Chattaway FW, Holmes MR, Barlow AJE: Cell wall composition of the mycelial and blastospore forms of *Candida albicans. J Gen Microbiol* 51:367–376, 1968.
20. Chen C, Chin JE, Ueda K, Clark DP, Pastan I, Gottesman MM, Roninson IB: Internal duplication and homology wth bacterial transport proteins in the *mdr* 1 (P. glycoprotein) gene from multidrug-resistant human cells. *Cell* 47:381–389, 1986.
21. Chmara H, Smulkowski M, Borowski E: Growth inhibitory effects of amidotranferase inhibition in *Candida albicans* by epoxy-peptides. *Drugs Under Exp Clin Res* 6:7–14, 1980.
22. Chvatchko Y, Howald I, Riezman H: Two yeast mutants defective in endocytosis are defective in pheromone response. *Cell* 46:355–364, 1986.
23. Cowell JL: Energetics of glycylglycine transport in *Escherichia coli. J Bacteriol* 120:139–146, 1974.
24. Davies MB: Peptide uptake in *Candida albicans. J Gen Microbiol* 114:181–186, 1980.
25. Dahn U, Hagenmaier H, Konig WA, Wolf G, Zahner H: Stoffwechselprodukte von mikroorganismen 154 Mitteilung. Nikkomycin ein neuer Hemmstoff der Chitinsynthase bei Pilzen. *Arch Microbiol* 197:143–160, 1976.
26. Emmer G, Ryder NS, Grassberger MA: Synthesis of new polyoxin analogs and their activity against chitin synthetase from *Candida albicans. J Med Chem* 28:278–281, 1985.
27. Fickel TE, Gilvarg C: Transport of impermeant substances in *Escherichia coli* by way of oligopeptide permease. *Nature (London)* 241:161–163, 1973.
28. Fleet GH: Composition and structure of yeast cell wall in, McGinnis MR (ed): *Current Topics in Medical Mycology*. New York, Springer-Verlag, 1985, pp 24–56.
29. Gilvarg C: Portage transport, in Ninet L, Bost PE, Bouanchaud DH, Florent J (eds): *The Future of Antibiotherapy and Antibiotic Research*. New York, Academic Press, 1981.
30. Gooday GW, Gow NAR: A model of the hyphal septum of *Candida albicans* during germ tube formation. *Exp Mycol* 7:370–373, 1983.
31. Gross P, Croop J, Housman D: Mammalian multidrug resistance gene: Complete cDNA sequence indicates strong homology to bacterial transport proteins. *Cell* 47:371–380, 1986.
32. Higgins CF, Hardie MM, Jamieson D, Powell LM: Genetic map of the *opp* (oligopeptide permease) locus of *Salmonella typhimurium. J Bacteriol* 153:830–836, 1983.

33. Higgins CF, Payne JW: Characterization of active dipeptide transport by germinating barley embryos: Effects of pH and metabolic inhibitors. *Planta* 136:71–76, 1977.
34. Hilenski LL, Naider F, Becker JM: Polyoxin D inhibits colloidal gold-wheat germ agglutinin labelling of chitin in dimorphic forms of *Candida albicans*. *J Gen Microbiol* 132:1441–1451, 1986.
35. Hori M, Kakiki K, Misato T: Antagonistic effect of dipeptides on the uptake of polyoxin A by *Alternaria kikuchiana*. *J Pest Sci* 2:139–149, 1977.
36. Hori M, Kakiki K, Suzuki S, Misato T: Studies on the mode of action of polyoxins. III. Relation of polyoxin structure to chitin synthetase inhibition. *Agric Biol Chem* 35:1280–1291, 1971.
37. Hruby VJ, Rich DH (eds): *Peptides Structure and Function: Proceedings of the Eighth American Peptide Symposium*. Rockford, IL, Pierce Chemical Company, 1983.
38. Isono K, Azuma T, Suzuki S: Polyoxin analogs. I. Synthesis of aminoacyl derivatives of 5′-amino-5′deoxyuridine. *Chem Pharmacol Bull* 19:505–512, 1971.
39. Isono K, Nagatsu J, Kawashima Y, Suzuki S: Studies on polyoxins, antifungal antibiotics. I. Isolation and characterization of polyoxins A and B. *Agric Biol Chem* 29:848–854, 1965.
40. Isono K, Nagatsu J, Kobinata K, Sasaki K, Suzuki S: Studies on polyoxins, antifungal antibiotics, V. Isolation and characterization of polyoxins C, D, E, F, G, H, and I. *Agric Biol Chem* 31:190–199, 1967.
41. Jackson MB, Becker JM, Steinfeld A, Naider F: Oligopeptide transport in proline peptidase mutants of *Salmonella typhimurium*. *J Biol Chem* 251:5300–5309, 1976.
42. Jayakumar A, Singh M, Prasad R: Characteristics of proline transport in normal and starved cells of *Candida albicans*. *Biochim Biophys Acta* 514:348–355, 1978.
43. Keller FA, Cabib E: Chitin and yeast budding. Properties of chitin synthetase from *Saccharomyces carlsbergensis*. *J Biol Chem* 246:160–166, 1971.
44. Kenig M, Abraham EP: Antimicrobial activities and antagonists of bacilysin and anticapsin. *J Gen Microbiol* 94:37–45, 1976.
45. Kessel D, Lubin M: On the distinction between peptidase activity and peptide transport. *Biochim Biophys Acta* 71:656–663, 1963.
46. Kingsbury WD, Boehm JC, Mehta RJ, Grappel SF: Transport of antimicrobial agents using peptide carrier systems: Anticandidal activity of m-fluorophenylalanine-peptide conjugates. *J Med Chem* 26:1725–1729, 1983.
47. Kingsbury WD, Boehm JC, Mehta RJ, Grappel SF, Gilvarg C: A novel peptide delivery system involving peptidase activated prodrugs as antimicrobial agents. Synthesis and biological activity of peptidyl derivatives of 5-fluorouracil. *J Med Chem* 27:1447–1451, 1984.
48. Kingsbury WD, Boehm JC, Perry D, Gilvarg C: Portage of various compounds into bacteria by attachment to glycine residues in peptides. *Proc Natl Acad Sci USA* 81:4573–4576, 1984.
49. Kobinata K, Uramoto M, Nishii M, Kusakabe H, Nakamura G, Isono K: Neopolyoxins A, B, and C, new chitin synthetase inhibitors. *Agric Biol Chem* 44:1709–1711, 1980.
50. Koenig WA, Loffler W, Meyer-Glauner WH, Uhman R: *L*-arginyl-*D*-allo threonyl-*L*-phenylalanin ein aminosaureantagonist aus dem pilz *Keratinophyton terrreum*. *Chem Berichete* 106:816–823, 1973.
51. Lichliter WD, Naider F, Becker JM: Basis for the design of anticandidal agents from studies of peptide utilization in *Candida albicans*. *Antimicrob Agents Chemother* 10:483–490, 1976.
52. Logan DA, Becker JM, Naider F: Peptide transport in *Candida albicans*. *J Gen Microbiol* 114:179–186, 1979.
53. Marder R, Rose R, Becker JM, Naider F: Isolation of a peptide transport-deficient mutant of yeast. *J Bacteriol* 136:1174–1177, 1978.

54. Matthews DM: Intestinal absorption of peptides. *Physiol Rev* 55:537–608, 1975.
55. Matthews DM, Payne JW: Transmembrane transport of small peptides. *Curr Top Membr Transp* 14:331–425, 1980.
56. McCarthy PJ, Nisbet LJ, Boehm JC, Kingsbury WD: Multiplicity of peptide permeases in *Candida albicans*: Evidence from novel chromophoric peptides. *J Bacteriol* 162:1024–1029, 1985.
57. McCarthy PJ, Troke PF, Gull K: Mechanism of action of nikkomycin and the peptide transport system of *Candida albicans*. *J Gen Microbiol* 131:775–780, 1985.
58. Medoff G, Brajtburg J, Kobayshi GS: Antifungal agents useful in the therapy of systemic fungal infection. *Annu Rev Pharmacol Toxicol* 23:3030–330, 1983.
59. Mehta RJ, Kingsbury WD, Valenta J, Actor P: Anti-*Candida* activity of polyoxin: Example of peptide transport in yeasts. *Antimicrob Agents Chemother* 25:373–374, 1984.
60. Meyer-Glauner W, Bernard E, Armstrong D, Merrifield B: The antifungal activity of carrier peptides, *L*-arginyl-X-*L*-phenylalanine, containing amino acid antagonists or atypical non-biogenic *D*-amino acids in the central position. *Zbl Bakt Hyg Orig A* 252:274–278, 1982.
61. Milewski S, Chmara H, Borowski E: Growth inhibitory effect of antibiotic tetaine on yeast and mycelial forms of *Candida albicans*. *Arch Microbiol* 135:130–136, 1983.
62. Mitani M, Inoue Y: Antagonists of antifungal substance polyoxin. *J Antibiot* 21:492–496, 1968.
63. Moneton P, Sarthou P, LeGoffic F: Role of the nitrogen source in peptide transport in *Saccharomyces cerevisiae*. *FEMS Microbiol Lett* 36:95–98, 1986.
64. Moneton P, Sarthou P, LeGoffic F: Transport and hydrolysis of peptides in *Saccharomyces cerevisiae*. *J Gen Microbiol* 132:2147–2153, 1986.
65. Naider F, Shenbagamurthi P, Steinfeld AS, Smith HA, Boney C, Becker JM: Synthesis and biological activity of tripeptidyl polyoxins as antifungal agents. *Antimicrob Agents Chemother* 24:787–796, 1983.
66. Nisbet TM, Payne JW: Specificity of peptide uptake in *Saccharomyces cerevisiae* and isolation of a bacilysin-resistant, peptide transport deficient mutant. *FEMS Microbiol Lett* 7:193–196, 1979.
67. Nisbet TM, Payne JW: Peptide uptake in *Saccharomyces cerevisiae*. Characteristics of a transport system shared by dipeptides and oligopeptides. *J Gen Microbiol* 115:127–133, 1979.
68. Odds FC: *Candida and Candidosis*. Baltimore, University Park, Press, 1979.
69. Payne JW: Transport and utilization of peptides by bacteria, in Payne JW (ed): *Microorganisms and Nitrogen Sources*. Chichester, United Kingdom, Wiley & Sons, 1980, pp 211–256.
70. Payne JW, Bell G: Direct determination of the properties of peptide transport systems in *Escherichia coli* using a fluorescent labelling procedure. *J Bacteriol* 137:447–455, 1979.
71. Payne JW, Gilvarg C: Transport of peptides in bacteria, in Rosen BP (ed): *Bacterial Transport*. New York, Marcel Dekker, 1978, pp 325–383.
72. Payne JW, Nisbet TM: Limitations to the use of radioactively labeled substrates for studying peptide transport in microorganisms. *FEBS Lett* 119:73–76, 1980.
73. Payne JW, Nisbet TM: Continuous monitoring of substrate uptake by microorganisms using fluorescamine: Application to peptide transport by *Saccharomyces cerevisiae* and *Streptococcus faecalis*. *J Appl Biochem* 3:447–458, 1981.
74. Payne J, Shallow DA: Studies on drug targeting in the pathogenic fungus *Candida albicans*: Peptide transport mutants resistant to polyoxins, nikkomycins, and bacilysin. *FEMS Microbiol Lett* 28:55–60, 1985.
75. Riezman H, Chvatchko Y, Dulic V: Endocytosis in yeast. *Trends Biochem Sci* 11:325–328, 1986.

76. Sarthou P, Gonneau M, Le Goffic F: Photaffinity inhibition of peptide transport in yeast. *Biochem Biophys Res Commun* 110:884–889, 1983.
77. Shenbagamurth P, Smith HA, Becker JM, Naider F: Synthesis and biological properties of chitin synthetase inhibitors resistant to cellular peptidases. *J Med Chem* 29:802–808, 1986.
78. Shenbagamurthi P, Smith HA, Becker JM, Steinfeld A, Naider F: Design of anticandidal agents: Synthesis and biological properties of analogues of polyoxin L. *J Med Chem* 26:1518–1522, 1983.
79. Smith HA, Shenbagamurthi P, Naider F, Kundu B, Becker JM: Hydrophobic polyoxins are resistant to intracellular degradation in *Candida albicans*. *Antimicrob Agents Chemother* 29:33–39, 1986.
80. Steinfeld AS, Naider F, Becker JM: Synthesis and biological studies of 5-fluorocytosine conjugates as antifungal agents. *J Med Chem* 22:1104–1109, 1979.
81. Sullivan PA, Yin CY, Molley C, Templeton MD, Shepherd M: An analysis of the metabolism and cell wall composition of *Candida albicans* during germ-tube formation. *Can J Microbiol* 29:1514–1525, 1983.
82. Ti JS, Steinfeld As, Naider F, Gulumoglu A, Lewis SV, Becker JM: Anticandidal activity of pyrimidine-peptide conjugates. *J Med Chem* 23:913–918, 1980.
83. Ugolev AM, DeLaey P: Membrane digestion, a concept of enzymic hydrolysis on cell membranes. *Biochim Biophys Acta* 300:105–128, 1973.
84. Uramoto M, Kobinata K, Isono K, Higashijima T, Miyazawa T, Jenkins EE, McCloskey JA: Structure of neopolyoxins A, B, and C. *Tetrahedron Lett* 21: 3395–3399, 1980.
85. Uramoto M, Kobinata K, Isono K, Higashijima T, Miyazawa T, Jenkins EE, McCloskey JA: Structure of neopolyoxins A, B, and C. *Tetrahedron Lett* 38: 1599–1603, 1982.
86. Wolfinbarger L, Marzluf GA: Specificity and regulation of peptide transport in *Neurospora crassa*. *Arch Biochem Biophys* 171:637–644, 1979.
87. Yadan JC, Gonneau M, Sarthou P, LeGoffic F: Sensitivity to Nikkomycin Z in *Candida albicans*: Role of peptide permeases. *J Bacteriol* 160:884–888, 1984.

6—Epidemiology of Coccidioidomycosis

DEMOSTHENES PAPPAGIANIS

Coccidioidomycosis (San Joaquin Fever or Valley Fever) is an infection caused by the soil-inhabiting fungus *Coccidioides immitis*. The infection is usually acquired by inhalation of the arthroconidia, rarely by their introduction percutaneously. Although many infections are asymptomatic, symptomatic primary acute infection usually appears to be confined to the lungs and regional (thoracic) lymph nodes. Recovery is often complete although occasionally (5–10% of symptomatic cases and an unknown portion of asymptomatic cases) the patient is left with a pulmonary residuum: cavity, solid coccidioidoma, bronchiectasis, or fibrosis. In a few cases, *C. immitis* is borne beyond the thoracic (including supraclavicular) lymphatic system leading to a serious, disseminated form of the disease.

The perception of coccidioidomycosis varies with one's experience with the disease: broad field studies have indicated that there is extensive *infection*, less *disease*, and relatively few serious cases (162). On the other hand, in certain clinical settings, coccidioidomycosis appears predominantly as an infection that takes advantage of immunologically or physiologically impaired hosts (142). In the major referral military medical center, severe coccidioidomycosis may be the usual form, whereas the station hospital personnel in the endemic area see the gamut of mild to severe disease. The individual pediatrician only occasionally takes note of the disease, and rarely sees a serious case, though collectively such serious cases can be seen in a substantial portion of children ill with coccidioidomycosis. In veterinary small animal practice in endemic areas, serious cases are recognized with some frequency in the dog, whereas larger (livestock) species are noted only infrequently to have clinically significant disease despite the frequent occurrence of infection.

The epidemiology (and epizootiology) is affected by properties of *C. immitis*, conditions of the environment in which the organism is found, and characteristics of the populations at risk; the varied—acute and chronic—forms of the infection provide many faces of this mycosis approaching the "great imitator" status of syphilis.

Characteristics of the Organism

Coccidioides immitis is a dimorphic fungus of uncertain taxonomic placement (192). (Currah (23a) has suggested that *C. immitis* fits in the Ascomycotina, order Onygenales, family Onygenaceae.) In infected tissue and under special laboratory conditions, it grows as a sporangium-like structure, the spherule (20–150 μm) with endospores (3–4 μm). The latter are liberated into the surrounding tissue, lymph, or blood, and under the influence of several factors, for example, polymorphonuclear neutrophile leukocytes (49) and CO_2 (85), in turn enlarge to form new mature, endosporulating spherules. These then may liberate more endospores unless development is arrested by the host response.

In nature and in the usual laboratory culture (infrequently in the infected host) *C. immitis* produces septate hyphae 1–2 μm in diameter some of which differentiate into cells that evolve into cylindrical or barrel-shaped 2 × 5-μm arthroconidia in about 5 days (in vitro). The arthroconidia (enteroarthric), usually alternate with empty, degenerate cells and readily can be released by disruption of the latter cells; in a dry environment, the arthroconidia become dispersed, airborne, and are inhaled. The infective dose for humans is unknown, but 10 arthroconidia suffice to infect and cause disease in the dog, monkey (21), or mouse. Variation in arthroconidial size and shape has been noted (47), but the significance of such variation in infectivity is unknown. The settling rate in air of the 2 × 5-μm arthroconidia appears to be that of particles 0.1–0.2 μm in size (R Dimmick, personal communication). This slow settling is indicated also by Lacey (93), who states that *C. immitis* (conidia) have a terminal velocity of 0.003 cm/second, contrasted with 2.0–2.8 cm/second for *Bipolaris sorokiniana* (as "*Helminthosporium sativum*"). Whether this influences their retention or expulsion after inhalation is apparently unknown. When arthroconidia were labeled with $^{32}PO_4^{-3}$ and aerosolized for inhalation by mice, a substantial portion (mean 44%) of the label was detected in the stomach, the remainder in the upper respiratory tract (mean 40%), and (mean 16%, range 1–47%) in the lower respiratory system (trachea, bronchi, lungs) (D Pappagianis, unpublished). Thus, arthroconidia deposited in the upper respiratory tract may be swallowed directly or swept up and out of the tracheobronchial system.

The arthroconidia may remain suspended in air for considerable periods of time as was evident when a dust storm in Kern County, California, led to dispersion of conidia some 400 miles distant where they settled 24 hours later causing may infections in humans outside the usual endemic area (125). Another factor that may be pertinent to the infectivity of the arthroconidia is their apparent hydrophobicity—in the laboratory dry arthroconidia often float on water or saline, but are readily wetted and become suspended in the aqueous milieu if subjected to negative pressure. Perhaps entrapped gas (air?) and relative dehydration provide buoyancy and this is reduced by evacuating air from the container. On the other hand, based on ultrastructure, the hydrophobicity has been related to the presence of certain "rodlets" apparently associated with the outer hyphal wall (20). It is not known if the hydrophobicity in any way affects interaction of *C. immitis* with pulmonary surfactant. However, in limited studies in humans (8) it appears that *C. immitis* becomes deposited and establishes infection initially in small bronchi rather than in the alveoli (although the pneumonitis that ensues must extend to the latter structures too).

The influence of electric charge on the dispersion, settling, inhalation, and infectivity of arthroconidia may be significant. Under experimental conditions, mice infected intranasally with *C. immitis* arthroconidia and maintained in an atmosphere of positively charged air ions developed illness earlier and had a higher cumulative mortality than mice maintained in the usual laboratory air (88).

In contrast to the infectivity of arthroconidia, the spherule-endospore phase found in infected hosts is not transmitted from human to human (or between mammalian hosts in general). The only and unusual instance of transmission directly from person to person is that of the embalmer infected through an abrasion of a finger while handling the body of an individual who died with disseminated coccidioidomycosis (188). Castleberry et al (18) reported that an infant monkey developed a pulmonary lesion containing an immature spherule after exposure to a draining purulent lesion on the forearm of its mother. *Coccidioides immitis* has been demonstrated in the prostate gland and even semen, but there appears to have been no evidence of conjugal transmission as with *Histoplasma capsulatum* and *Blastomyces dermatitidis*. Although the hyphal form including apparent arthroconidial structures can be found in vivo in pulmonary cavities, there has been no documentation of transmission from an individual with cavitary coccidioidomycosis to another. An unusual mode of transmission of *C. immitis* was demonstrated by Borelli and Marcano (9). The bodies of mice infected with *C. immitis* were fed to rats which developed infected cervical lymph nodes. Possibly, *C. immitis* was introduced through the oropharyngeal mucosa traumatized by ingested mouse bones.

Pleural fluid or pus containing *C. immitis* should pose no risk to others, including medical personnel if these transudates and exudates are disposed of promptly, that is, in less than the approximately 5 days required for arthroconidiation. Wound dressings should be changed daily and decontaminated by autoclaving, incineration, or exposure to 5% hypochlorite solution for 15 minutes. If the dressings have dried, they should be wetted before removal from the patient to preclude release of dry arthroconidia. The arthroconidia as well as spherule phase are readily rendered sterile by hypochlorite, iodophor, phenolic compounds, and formaldehyde (90, 91). The hazard of formation of arthroconidia from exudate was evident from the infection of several hospital personnel from a contaminated plaster of Paris cast (36).

Although apparently not adapted or in the proper milieu for transmission between patient and others, spherules discharged from a host can survive and

TABLE 6-1. Mean Relative Humidity (RH)—30 Years' Observation, Phoenix, Arizona

Month	RH%	Month	RH%
January	50.1	July	33.4
February	43.5	August	40.4
March	39.8	September	42.0
April	30.3	October	36.1
May	22.4	November	47.2
June	20.1	December	54.2

Courtesy B. Chaiken, Arizona Lung Association, and Sky Harbor Airport, Phoenix.

germinate to produce hyphae and arthroconidia. Burke (12) reported survival of *C. immitis* for 7 months in pus sealed in a microcope slide. Sorensen (166) showed that spherules suspended in blood, presumably a protective colloid, survived in sterile sand for at least 4 days, sufficient time for germination into the mycelial phase. On the other hand arthroconidia are hardy. They survived 6 months at 4°C and 25°C in saturated (approximately 36 g/dl) NaCl (48). (Stewart and Meyer (168) had demonstrated that mycelial phase *C. immitis* survived in 30–35% NaCl solution for 3–4 hours.) Dry arthroconidia kept at 50°C died in 2 weeks, but survived well for at least 6 months at temperatures of −15°C–37°C provided the relative humidity (RH) was greater than 10% (up to 95%). Interestingly, at RH 10% and 37°C, there was significant loss of viability. This may seem paradoxical as these conditions resemble those observed in endemic areas; however, such a low (10%) RH does not appear to be sustained for long in a given day (95). The mean monthly relative humidity determined over the past 30 years in Phoenix, Arizona is shown in Table 6-1. Mycelial fragments inoculated into soil in the laboratory survived at least 4 months at 42°C (103). However, 4-day-old cultures directly exposed to 42°C were dead within 8 days. It is possible that the 4-day-old cultures had not yet developed arthroconidia and were therefore vulnerable to this temperature.

Maddy (106) pointed out that development of *C. immitis* in nature took place in environments (such as the Lower Sonoran Life Zone) that had mean temperatures of 26–32°C in July and 4–12°C in January, that, hot summers and relatively few freezes in winter.

The first isolation of *C. immitis* from the soil was accomplished in 1932 (168) next to a bunkhouse at Delano, California. This sampling was carried out because Filipino farm workers housed in the bunkhouse developed coccidioidal granuloma. *Coccidioides immitis* was recovered from the soil in 1942 by Emmons (41) in Arizona and by Davis et al (25) in California. In 1954 Plunkett and Swatek (130) recovered *C. immitis* from California soil directly on culture medium without using animals as "selective media."

Mycelial growth of *C. immitis* in soil was observed by Maddy (109) in nature and by Sorensen (166) in the laboratory. In the soil *C. immitis* can survive for considerable though incompletely determined periods. The organism could be recovered from the soil near Phoenix, Arizona 7 years after burying infected canine, murine, or bovine tissues (110). Soil obtained about 64 m away remained negative except for one specimen, during these 7 years (109). Swatek et al (172) showed survival for 12 years.

Lacy and Swatek (94) concluded that the production of "blooms" (growth) required 56–90% RH for several weeks (see reference above to RH requirements for survival of arthroconidia).

The persistence of *C. immitis* in the soil assures a new cycle of infections yearly. That persistence may be quantitatively affected at different times of year by rainfall, sunlight, temperature, and salt concentration of the soil. For example, Egeberg and Ely (38) studied the recovery of *C. immitis* from the soil in Kern County, California (southern San Joaquin Valley), finding that 4.2% of the samples yielded the fungus in January at the end of the dry season, whereas 16% of the samples were positive at the end of the wet season in April. All of the latter were surface samples, whereas only one of six positive cultures obtaned at the end of the dry season was from the surface, the other five being recovered from depths of 10–30 cm. Exposure to ultraviolet rays and elevated temperature at the surface would be lethal as would the temperature at 1 cm below the surface, which may reach 60–67°C for 5 hours in a given day (108). It had previously been shown that *C. immitis* can survive in the laboratory for only 4 minutes at 60°C, and even 2 hours at 52°C reduced the viability by 95% (140).

Egeberg et al (39) and Elconin et al (40) proposed that increasing salinity (eg, $CaCl_2$ and NaCl) of surface soil along with elevated temperature, for example, 40°C, would progressively enhance growth and survival of *C. immitis* while inhibiting or killing microbial adversaries of *C. immitis* in the soil such as *Bacillus subtilis* and *Penicillium janthinellum*. The increasing salt concentration was recognized as the result of the leaching (solubilization) effect of heavy rains and subsequent movement of water and salts by capillarity toward the surface where evaporation would lead to deposition of the salts. *Coccidioides immitis* grows in media containing sea water (3.4% salts, 2.9% NaCl) in place of plain water, again illustrative of its salt tolerance (35, 174). This has an interesting relationship to the occurrence of coccidioidal infections at sites where marine fossils can be found, for example, Coalinga and Shark Tooth Mountain (Bakersfield), California. Sorensen (166) also showed that *C. immitis* grew in Sabouraud glucose agar containing as high as 8% $CaCl_2$ or KNO_3 and 4% NaCl, although survival was diminished in 6 and 8% NaCl. There also appeared to be a selective effect of borate. At a concentration of 0.25% $Na_2B_4O_7$ in Sabouraud glucose agar, *C. immitis* flourished, and it grew to some extent at 0.5 and 1% concentrations. Neither *Histoplasma capsulatum* nor *Candida albicans* grew at any of these concentrations of borate. The presence of a high concentration of boron salts in soil yielding *C. immitis* than in those not yielding *C. immitis* had also been noted by Egeberg et al (39).

In the laboratory *C. immitis* can grow in the pH range of 3.5–9.0. Long before the advent of the selective media using cycloheximide and chloramphenicol, CE Smith (153) devised a selective medium that took advantage of the tolerance by *C. immitis* of high pH and of 0.04% $CuSO_4$. Although *C. immitis* did not grow profusely, contaminant organisms were repressed even more. Maddy (106) pointed out that the endemic areas are characterized by alkaline soil; Lacy and Swatek (95) related the recovery of *C. immitis* from the soil of old American Indian middens to sandy soil and alkalinity. *Coccidioides immitis* can grow also in soil likely to contain substantial organic material, for example, rodent burrows (38), or in deserted mine tunnels containing bat guano (78, 92), but there appears to be no great predilection for such sites.

The variation in rainfall in the areas endemic for *C. immitis* make it difficult to generalize about its influence. This variation, 12.5–50 cm, applies both within North America (southern Kern County, California to northern Tehama County, California) and South America (Argentina to Venezuela). In California, rainfall usually occurs between November and April, leaving a long dry season. Primary infection is usually acquired in the dry summer and fall. The number of cases during the dry season is greater after a heavy winter rainfall (Fig. 6-1) (161). Such a heavy rainfall would be expected to provide a wet environment for a longer period for hyphal growth and formation of

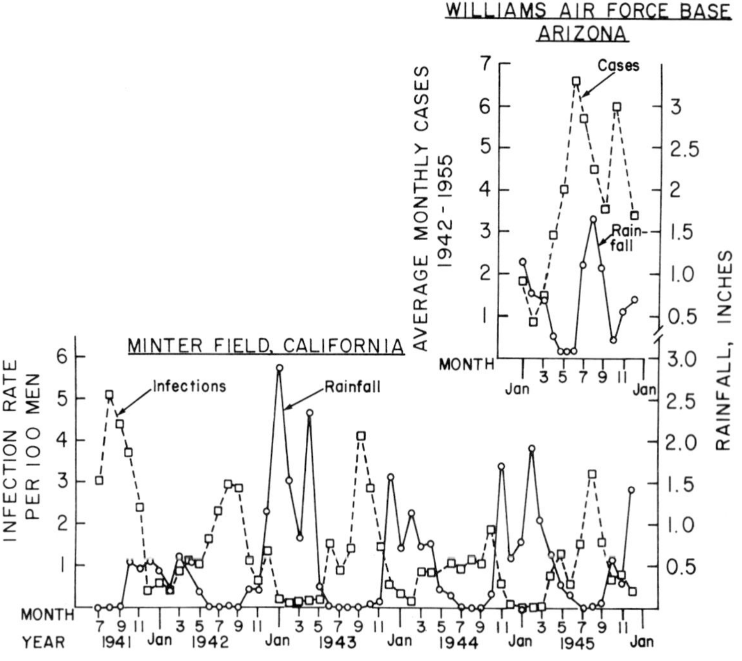

FIG. 6-1. Relationship between occurrence of coccidioidomycosis and rainfall.

arthroconidia. A prolonged, moist environment would be expected along stream beds and their banks. *Coccidioides immitis* was isolated from the air near a stream bed at Camp Roberts, California (62) and from soil near a dry stream bed and along dry washes (172). Duran et al (34) reported isolation of *C. immitis* from an arroyo and from fertile river bottom soil adjacent to a drainage ditch (as well as from other sites). Heavy rain may lead to an increased deposition of salts near the surface of the soil providing a selective advantage to *C. immitis* as indicated (40). Clearly, rainfall also influences the number of cases of coccidioidomycosis by wetting the soil, reducing airborne dust and arthroconidia. This is evident in the reduction in cases during the winter wet season in California and the reduction of cases in the winter and after the usual summer rain in Arizona (Fig. 6-1) (162, 165).

There has been limited success in recovering *C. immitis* from the air. Hoggan et al (62) recovered *C. immitis* from 169,883 L of air sampled at Camp Roberts, California, at a time of little disturbance of the soil. Ajello et al (2) recovered *C. immitis* from the air in Phoenix, Arizona, 3–4 days after a windstorm in July 1959.

Coccidioides immitis and cases of coccidioidomycosis appear broadly encountered, but within the endemic zones the fungus appears spottily distributed. It is apparently present at sea level, for example, in Venezuela (16) (also see sea otter below under Epizootiology), but the better known endemic sites are at various elevations: in Red Bluff, California at 304 ft, Bakersfield at 421 ft, Inyokern at 3200 ft; in Phoenix, Arizona at 1083 ft, Tucson at 2300 ft; in Venezuela at 2600 ft; and in El Paso, Texas at 3710 ft. Despite the various influences cited, there is no clear explanation of the confinement of *C. immitis* to such enclaves. Several outbreaks of coccidioidomycosis have occurred after excavation of "virgin" or at least long undisturbed, uncultivated soils (77, 106, 172, 184). Although sporadic cases occur among agricultural workers, perhaps *C. immitis* must cope with more microbial competitors in cultivated and fertilized soil. The increase in primary coccidioidomycosis that occurs (in California) in late summer and fall rather than during the earlier springtime cultivation of soil may be a result of the restriction of microbial competitors by heat, dehydration, and increased salinity; the more ready disarticulation and launching into the air of arthroconidia occurs in the relative dehydration of late summer and fall.

Geographic Distribution

Coccidioides immitis and coccidioidomycosis are in limited areas of the New World (Figs. 6-2, 6-3, and 6-4). These lie between 40° North 120° West in Northern California and 40° South 65° West in Argentina. Rarely, arthroconidia are transported out of the endemic areas on some agricultural product, soil, or other artifact to cause primary infection in someone who has not

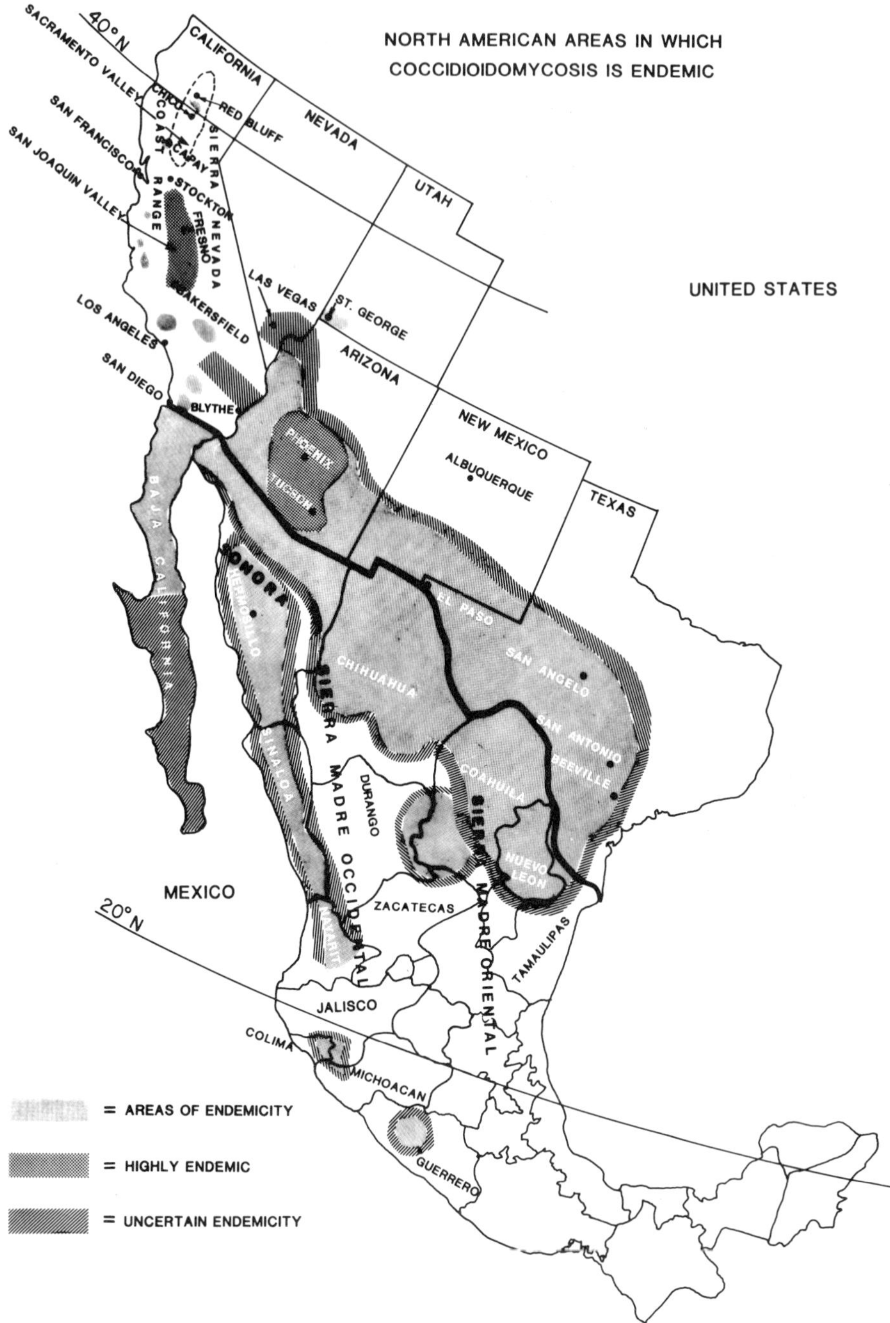

FIG. 6-2. Distribution of *C. immitis* and endemic coccidioidomycosis in North America.

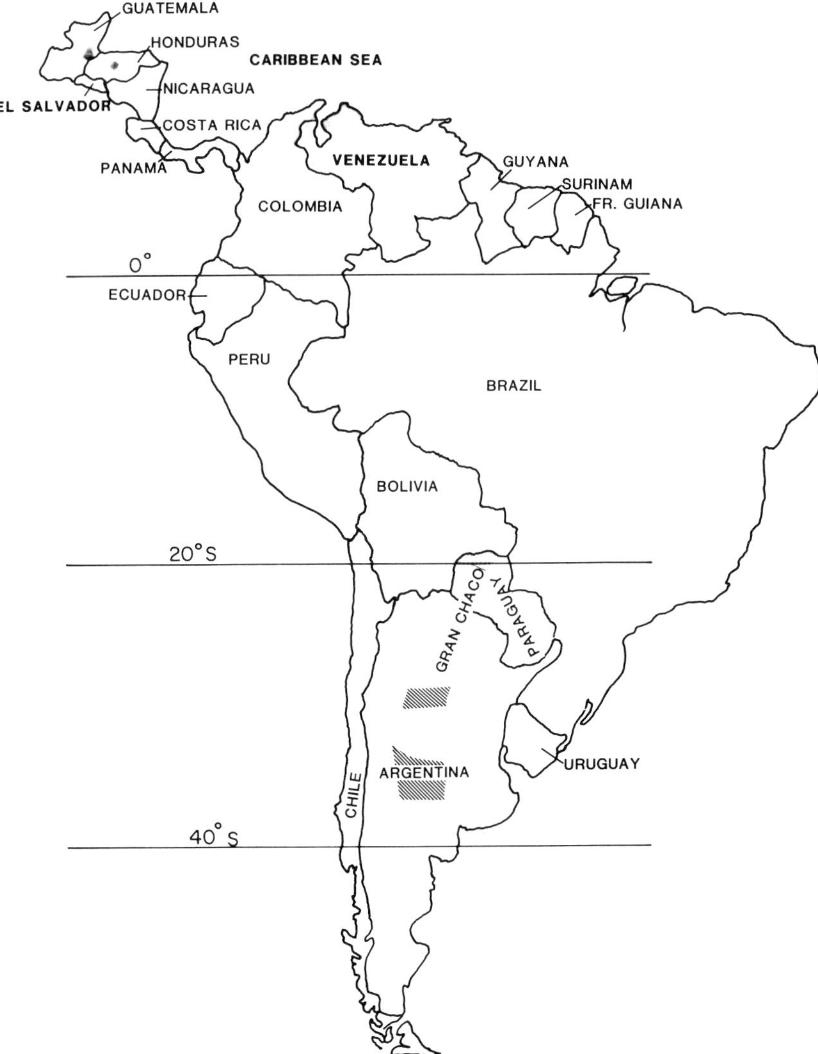

FIG. 6-3. Distribution of *C. immitis* and endemic coccidioidomycosis in Central and South America.

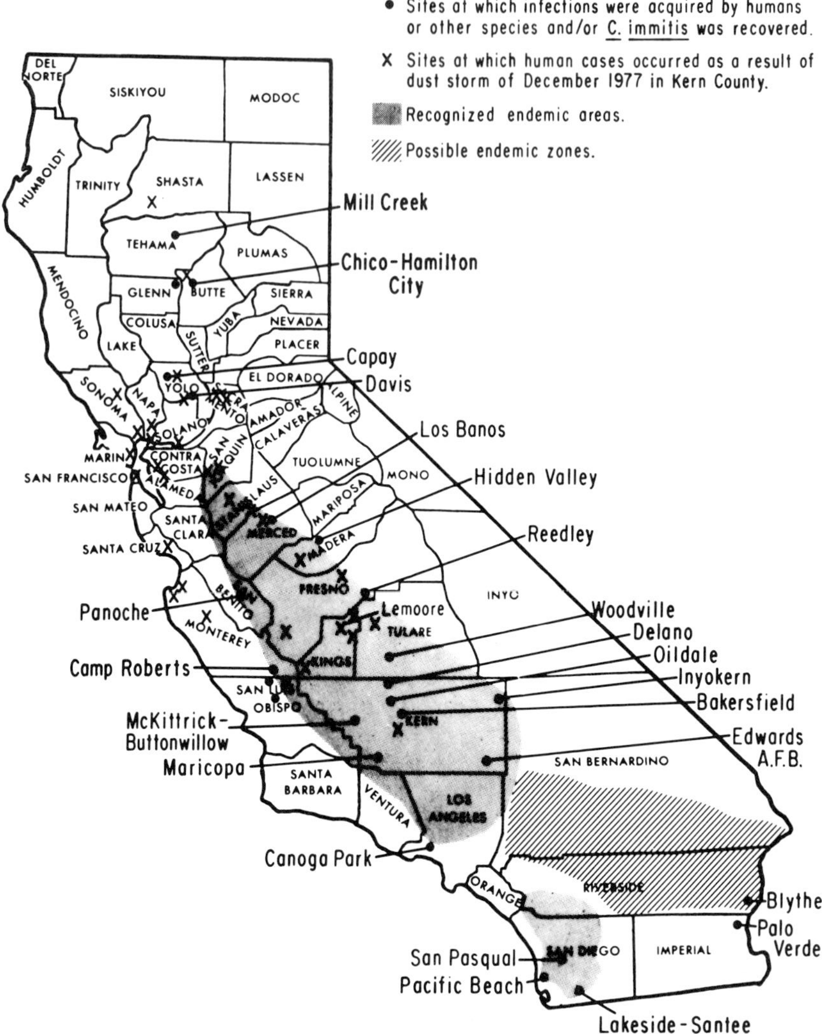

FIG. 6-4. Sites in California at which *C. immitis* was recovered in nature or where cases of coccidioidomycosis occurred.

been in the endemic area (see Fomites). With increasing travel, however, coccidioidomycosis is encountered far from the endemic areas in those returning home after a visit, for example, to the "sun belt" of the southwest United States.

Arizona, California, Nevada, New Mexico, Texas, and Utah, which include greater than 20% of the national population, contain the endemic areas of the United States (Fig. 6-2). In California, parts of the following counties represent endemic zones: Tehama, the northernmost, Butte, Glenn, Yolo, San

Joaquin, Alameda, Stanislaus, Merced, Madera, Fresno, San Benito, Tulare, King, Monterey, Kern, San Luis Obispo, Los Angeles (87, 133), Ventura, Riverside, a limited area of Imperial County, and probably part of San Bernardino, and San Diego, the southernmost (Fig. 6-4). Most of the affected areas lie inland, for example, along the San Joaquin River Valley, and to a limited extent the Sacramento River Valley, bordered on the east by the Sierra Nevada mountains, and on the west by the Coast Range, although *C. immitis* resides in some foci west of the Coast Range, for example, Camp Roberts and other sites in San Luis Obispo County; and loci in San Diego County lie within 5–10 miles of the sea without a significant mountain range interposed.

The distribution of *C. immitis* in Northern California is spotty, and despite deposition of *C. immitis* in nonendemic areas in Northern and Coastal California by a dust storm in December, 1977, (125) there is no clear evidence that new endemic foci were established.

Arizona is an important coccidioidal region. Infections are recognized among the immigrants who continue to seek the warmth and among the Native American population many of whom reside on reservations that lie within endemic counties. These are Gila County, Pima County (which includes the Tucson area), Maricopa County (containing Phoenix), and Pinal County (containing Florence). Florence had been recognized as a highly endemic area, with 50% of susceptible individuals becoming infected within 6 months after arrival (159). The northwestern Mohave County also includes an endemic area.

The endemic zone(s) of Nevada is not clearly defined, although some physicians believe that coccidioidal infections are acquired somewhere in the vicinity of Las Vegas. The area of St. George, Utah, in the southwest corner of that state harbors *C. immitis*. An ill-defined southern portion of New Mexico yields cases.

Southwest Texas is endemic from El Paso, which lies south of New Mexico, east to Beeville (176), roughly between San Antonio and Corpus Christi in the south.

In Mexico, three zones of endemicity were recognized based largely on coccidioidin skin testing (54): 1) the Northern zone lying adjacent to the endemic southwestern United States, including the northern half of Baja California, the states of Sonora, Chihuahua, Coahuila, Nuevo Leon, and Tamaulipas. Rates of skin test reactivity decreased from west to east; 2) the Pacific Littoral zone, south to Guerrero, parts of Sonora, Nayarit, Jalisco, and Michoacan; and 3) The Central zone, Coahuila, into Nuevo Leon, and southward into Durango and San Luis Potosi. Most of these areas resemble the arid southwestern United States, including the presence of the creosote bush, *Larrea tridentata*. However, two tropical regions are included: the Tecoman Valley of Colima and Apatzingan Valley of Michoacan, both in the Pacific Littoral zone, with skin test reactivity rates of 10–30%, and Arcelia's Valley further south in Guerrero, with skin test reactivity of 5–10%. Gonzalez-Ochoa (54) pointed also to the diagnosis of disseminated coccidioidomycosis in children who had never been out of Apatzingan and Arcelia in support of coccidioidal endemicity in these tropical areas.

In Central America coccidioidomycosis appears to have been recognized infrequently. These cases were summarized as follows: Guatemala, 8 in humans, 2 in cattle, 7 in dogs; Honduras, 2 in humans; and Nicaragua, 1 in a dog. In Northeastern Guatemala, 42% of the residents of the endemic part of Motagua Valley were reactive to coccidioidin skin tests. Another part of the Motagua Valley showed 3.8% reactors. Skin test reactivity in Honduras ranged from 16% in the Comayagua Valley to 4% or less in other areas. Costa Rica and Panama had fewer than 1% reactors (112).

South America is recognized to be endemic in Argentina, Paraguay, Venezuela, and Colombia (16). The number of cases reported in the literature has been limited so that the prevalence and incidence of coccidioidomycosis are hard to discern. In his summary of Venezuelan cases, Campins (16) recorded a total of 35 pulmonary and disseminated cases mostly from the northwestern states of Lara, Falcon, and Zulia. Although Argentina was the site of the first described case of coccidioidomycosis in 1892, no other case was reported until 1927. By 1967 Negroni (117) had compiled but 25 confirmed cases naturally acquired in Argentina; two additional cases included one laboratory infection and one from Paraguay. Organisms resembling *C. immitis* were recovered from the soil in Argentina, but there was no confirmation of identity by demonstration of mature endosporulating spherules (10). Paraguay appeared to have an endemic zone in its drier south- and northwestern Chaco regions where coccidioidin reaction rates of 16–44% were recorded. Two clinically apparent cases with erythema nodosum and pneumonia were deduced from positive skin tests (53).

Colombia may be endemic as indicated by reports of two cases of coccidioidomycosis, one poorly documented, and by coccidioidin skin testing (139). Skin test reactivity ranged from 3.3–6.3% (up to 18% in adults) in the northeastern area of Guajira y Magdalena. No case of coccidioidomycosis was found in a clinicopathologic study of 162 cases of deep mycoses in Colombia (127).

With the exception of the areas of tropical character in Mexico, most of the endemic areas are characterized as arid, with rainfall in the range of 5–20 inches (12.5–50 cm), with hot summers, few winter freezes, and alkaline soil. These factors (alluded to above as influences on growth and survival of *C. immitis*) fit the characteristics of the bioclimatic zone called the Lower Sonoran Life zone (LSLZ). Maddy (106) made the striking observation that the distribution of *C. immitis* generally conforms to the LSLZ. The creosote bush, *L. tridentata*, represents a regular part of the flora of much of the LSLZ. The map of the LSLZ can be strikingly superimposed on much of the area endemic for *C. immitis* and coccidioidomycosis; however, although there is general conformity between these zones it is not precise. Lacy and Swatek (94) indicated that the soil of American Indian middens from which *C. immitis* was recovered was alkaline and sandy in texture, and *L. tridentata* is not present in some of these sites. Indeed, some of these were characterized as "mediterranean woodland with its rolling grasslands, scattered oak trees and California laurel" (94, 171) (Fig. 6-5). Such endemic areas are found in the San Joaquin and Sacramento Valleys, Monterey County, San Luis Obispo County, and San Diego County of California. Conversely, Imperial County of California is virtually all in the creosote bush LSLZ, and yet indigenous coccidioidomycosis appears to have been confirmed only in the northeastern corner of the county.

Although "point source" epidemics can be tied to certain specific sites, for example, archeologic digs at Indian middens (see below) and digging activities of children (52, 190, 132, 176), cases usually occur singly, perhaps reflecting the existence of microendemic foci. Soil of the Indian middens may contain more organic substances (as in rodent burrows) and inorganic ash (from camp-fires), and the former may support but does not determine the distribution of *C. immitis*. There is no satisfactory explanation of the existence of such apparently scattered microfoci in the LSLZ or Mediterranean woodland.

Outside the endemic areas, cases have been recognized in visitors from numerous states in the United States (57, 116, 83) and in foreign countries: the Netherlands (60), France (32), Belgium (187), Germany (169), and Canada (79). The resemblance of coccidioidomycosis to other diseases had delayed its recognition and diagnosis. However, there is now an awareness of the disease among some physicians abroad (149).

Populations Affected

Because coccidioidomycosis is a notifiable (reportable) disease only in California and Arizona, it is difficult to obtain precise figures on its incidence. In Table 6-2 are shown the numbers of reported cases for the past 5 years in California and total in the United States. The recently recorded deaths due to coccidioidomycosis in the United States average some 58 per year.

The degree of underreporting can only be guessed; we have compiled the cases reported to the California State Department of Health Services from the endemic Tulare County and those detected through our diagnostic serologic studies for the period 1981 through 1984 (Table 6-2). This provides some indication of the underreporting. In the state of Arizona coccidioidomycosis was a reportable disease for many years until 1972. At that time, when its population was in the neighborhood of 1,000,000 persons, less than 10% of the population of California, it reported more than 500 cases per year, usually exceeding those reported in California. Since resumption of reporting in Arizona in 1979, the cases have not achieved their erstwhile numbers despite continuing expansion of the population, with about 200 cases being reported per year.

Attack rates and incidence rates are difficult to calculate for the states in which coccidioidomycosis is endemic because the limited parts of the total

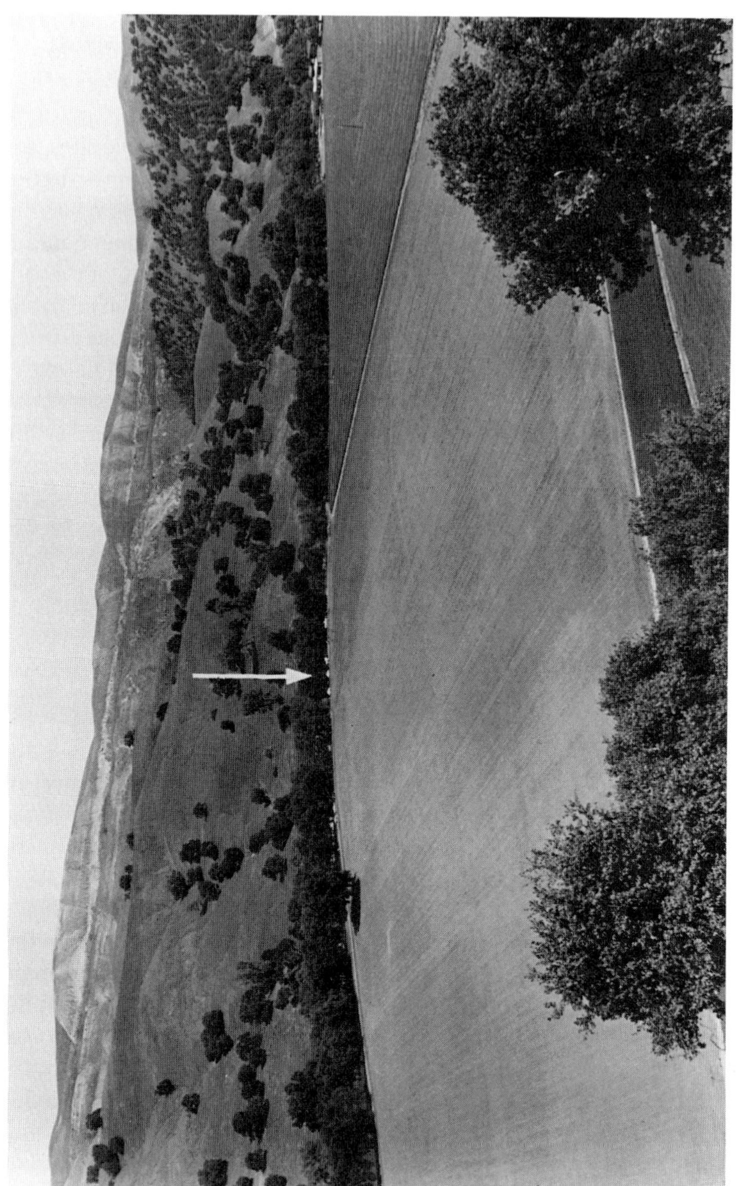

FIG. 6-5. Capay Valley, California (*arrow*), where archaeology students acquired coccidioidomycosis. This area resembles Mediterranean Woodland (Swatek) rather than the usual Lower Sonoran Life zone associated with coccidioidomycosis (Photograph courtesy J. Loofbourow).

TABLE 6-2. Reported Cases of Coccidioidomycosis by Year

	1980	1981	1982	1983	1984
United States*	825[†]	833	695	559	NA
California					
CSDHS[‡]	607	464	414	309	414
UCD[§]	739	515	508	533	498
Tulare County, CA					
CSDHS[‡]	14	18	20	18	8
UCD[§]		94	84	56	93

Mean member of deaths per year in United States for 1972–1981 = 58.
* From Annual Summary, Morbidity & Mortality Weekly Report, US Dept. Health and Human Services, Centers for Disease Control, Atlanta, GA.
[†] California cases are included that were originally omitted from US Annual Summary.
[‡] California State Department of Health Services, California Morbidity.
[§] Department of Medical Microbiology, School of Medicine, University of California, Davis.
NA = not available at this writing.

population are exposed. Thus, the 500 or so cases per year reported for California's 20,000,000 persons would give an incidence rate of 2.5 per 100,000, but the endemic Tulare County has an incidence of 33 per 100,000.

In localized outbreaks, attack rates with clinically evident disease of 60–93% have been recorded (183, 95). However, in the general exposed population, approximately 40% of persons infected with *C. immitis* develop symptomatic illness (157), the asymptomatic exposures being detected by skin test reactivity with coccidioidin. Because more reactors are detected with spherulin, there may actually be a greater than 60% rate of asymptomatic infections.

Occupation

Occupational aspects of coccidioidomycosis have been reviewed by Johnson (75) and Pappagianis (121). One can readily infer from the terricolous nature of *C. immitis* the often occupationally related nature of coccidioidomycosis. The second reported case was that of an Azorean-Portuguese agricultural worker in the San Joaquin Valley (136), starting a long line of patients in this category.

Beck (5) compiled 254 cases of coccidioidal granuloma, the severe form of coccidioidomycosis, that had been recognized between 1893 and 1931 in the United States. This and subsequent tabulation (Table 6-3) showed an agricultural association not only with the serious forms of the infection, but also nonfatal "Valley Fever" (157). Work in fruit orchards, vineyards, cotton fields, and digging potatoes exposes workers to *C. immitis*.

TABLE 6-3. Coccidioidomycosis in California Among Various Occupations (Percent of Total)

	Coccidioidal Granuloma 1893–1931* $N = 254$	All Coccidioidomycosis 1960–1972† $N = 233$	Nonfatal Coccidioidomycosis 1973–1976† $N = 49$
Agriculture	22.5	17.10	32.65
Construction, laborer	20.1	21.00	8.16
Mining (mineral, oil)	2.7	2.15	2.04
Transportation, utilities	5.9	11.16	12.24
State and local government		34.33	32.65
Services		7.30	2.04
Manufacturing		3.86	4.08
Office (finance, insurance, real estate)	16.1	0.43	2.04
Others (children, unknown)	32.7	0.86	

* Adopted from Beck (1931).
† State of California, Department of Industrial Relations.

TABLE 6-4. Coccidioidomycosis Among Anthropologists, Archaeologists, Paleontologists, and Zoologists Conducting Field Studies—California

Location	County	Year	Number Exposed	Number Ill	Confirmed Skin Test and/ or Serology
Panoche[1]	San Benito	1942	14	7	7
Inyokern[2]	Inyo	1954	Not given	4 (+ 1 in lab)	
Los Banos[3]	Merced	1962	16	16	16
Marciopa[4]	Kern	1966	Not given	3	3
Capay[5]	Yolo	1968	23	11	8
Chico[6]	Butte	1970	103	61	27
Madera County[7]		1970	30	28	
Buchanan Reservoir	Madera	1970	20	17	
Dye Creek[8]	Tehama	1972	34	17	10
Hamilton City	Glenn	1974	24		8
Hidden Valley Reservoir	Madera	1975	49		12
Buchanan Reservoir	Madera	1975	8		4
Maricopa[9]	Kern	1983	2	2	2

[1] Davis et al. (1942); [2] Plunkett and Swatek (1957); [3] Huberty (1963); [4] Schmidt and Howard (1968); [5] Loofbourow et al. (1969); [6] Werner et al. (1972); [7] Lacy and Swatek (1977); [8] Werner and Pappagianis (1973); [9] Larsen et al. (1985).

Other occupations involved in moving soil are also highly represented among patients: construction, laborers, and persons involved in transportation.

Other high-risk individuals are archaeologists, anthropologists, paleontologists, and zoologists. Their exposure is often in a confined area, exposure to excavated and sifted dust intense, and high attack rates as described above (Table 6-4). Three epidemics of coccidioidomycosis occurring among archaeology students provided confirmation of the existence of endemic foci not previously recognized in Northern California (101, 183, 184). Perhaps the most striking of such epidemics was that among 103 archaeology students, most of whom were from nonendemic New York State (183). The attack rate was estimated to be 65% of the entire group, 77% of those with a positive coccidioidin skin test (the latter contrasts with prior reports of 30–40% symptomatic cases among skin test reactors (162).

Other such field exposures resulted in small epidemics of acute coccidioidomycosis; seven of 14 participants on a zoology field trip who attempted to dig a rattlesnake from its refuge in a squirrel hole (25); four students excavating an old Indian campsite 10 miles south of Inyokern (173); all of 16 (including two children) participants in an anthropologic dig of an Indian site at Los Banos at the northern end of the San Joaquin Valley (64, 135); three volunteer participants in a paleontologic dig in 1960 (146) and two in 1983 (96) at Maricopa, California. Such exposure can provide severe infection, for example, acute respiratory failure (96), but of at least 95 or so infections shown in Table 6-4 only one had confirmed dissemination (ultimately fatal case of coccidioidomycosis meningitis).

The first recognized case of coccidioidomycosis was in an Argentinian soldier stationed on the Pampa (Chaco) (131). His was also the first of many cases among military personnel stationed in the endemic region [we have already pointed out that cases have been recognized in Europe and these include Belgian (187) and German military personnel who had undergone military training in Texas or Arizona (169)]. During the year 1941 and into the 1950s large numbers of individuals were assigned to duty, training or were prisoners of war in California, Arizona, and Texas where they encountered *C. immitis*. Smith et al (161, 162, 159) demonstrated that 25–50 per 100 susceptible individuals became infected per year at three Army Air Fields in the San Joaquin Valley. From these studies, Smith demonstrated that serious and even fatal cases of coccidioidomycosis occur among military troops; it was through these studies and those of Willett and Weiss (186) that the heightened susceptibility to disseminated disease among blacks was recognized. The skin test conversion rate per year at the Lemoore Naval Air Station in the 1963–1964 period was 1.58% (Drips and Smith, 1964) similar to the 1.4% recorded for the adjacent Lemoore Army Air Field in 1944–1945 (162).

Hugenholtz (65) and Scogins (148) described coccidioidomycosis as the first and second causes of human-days lost due to illness at Williams and Luke Air Force Bases (AFB) southeast and west of Phoenix, Arizona, respectively. These air bases and Davis-Monthan AFB near Tucson, Lemoore Naval Air Station in the San Joaquin Valley, and military installations in Texas continue to yield cases of coccidioidomycosis. Additional infections as indicated by coccidioidin or spherulin skin test conversions have resulted from desert warfare training in Fort Irwin and possibly Twenty-Nine Palms, California (63, 113). During the 6-year period of 1969 through 1974 when we maintained serologic surveillance of coccidioidomycosis at some military installations, we detected 400 new cases from these installations, 8% of the total cases (4,799) reported in the United States.

Hugenholtz (65) and Scogins (148) estimated that there was an average of 35 days lost per case of coccidioidomycosis per year, the same figure as that previously reported (World War II) for military personnel in Southern California (98).

The infectivity of *C. immitis* cultures poses a threat to laboratory and other hospital personnel (Table 6-5). A high index of suspicion is essential so that suspect cultures are handled very carefully.

The marked infectivity of arthroconidia was manifested when several nurses, residents, and interns were infected during removal of a plaster of Paris cast that had been contaminated with exudate from a lesion of the leg (36). The risk of infection with *C. immitis* in the laboratory deserves to be stressed. Some of these have been severe infections with dissemination. One involved a laboratory technician in Milwaukee virtually incapacitated by coccidioidal meningitis that allegedly resulted from exposure to a slide culture (114).

In 1927, what was apparently the first recognized laboratory infection

TABLE 6-5. Laboratory-Acquired Coccidioidomycosis

Location	No. Infected	Symptomatic	Laboratory and/or Skin Test Conversion
Respiratory			
Frederick, MD*	207*	3	207
Various*	96	30	59
Oakland, CA†	2	2	2
West Germany‡	6	6	6
Milwaukee, WI§	2	2	2
Cutaneous			
New Orleans, etc. (reviewed by Carroll et al. 1977)	7‖	7	7

* Johnson et al. (1964)—reviewed cases to 1964.
‡ Smith et al. (1957), plus one unpublished case.
† Wegmann and Plempel (1974).
§ Milwaukee Journal (1979), November 8, 1979, pp 1, 11.
‖ Three of these cutaneous infections also included in the cases reported by Johnson et al. (1964).

occurred in a medical student in Nebraska who had a typical primary infection that then disseminated to the leg and foot (177, 178, 179). A second medical student, at Stanford (San Francisco), was infected by opening a petri dish for the purpose of a closer examination of *C. immitis*. He developed a severe primary coccidioidomycosis with erthema nodosum (a rash long recognized as part of the Valley Fever syndrome), but had no apparent dissemination (29, 30). Retrospectively, this case provided a clue that ultimately helped to identify *C. immitis* as the etiology of Valley Fever.

Medical laboratory workers have been infected in Alabama (13), London, England (115, 175), Mexico City (55), and West Germany (182). A laboratory researcher with a prior positive coccidioidin skin test developed an acute but self-limited coccidioidal infection after respiratory exposure to dry arthroconidia (163). A fatal case developed in a 74-year-old black male glassware washer who collected glassware in the mycology laboratory at Duke University in 1946 (156) (Imagine the legal proceedings and expenses if such a mishap occurred today!) Several summaries have emphasized the hazard associated with *C. immitis* in the laboratory (89, 72, 129, 147). The "first recorded case" cited by Pike (129) was not laboratory acquired in Chicago, and was likely naturally acquired in Texas.

Influence of Race

By the early 1930's, the disproportionate representation of certain ethnic groups among the cases of disseminated coccidioidomycosis (coccidioidal granuloma) was recognized (6, 51). From those findings it was apparent that adult Filipino and black males were much more likely to develop disseminated and lethal coccidioidal disease than whites. The data also indicated that others, such as Mexicans, Native Americans, and Asians other than Filipinos, were at risk of more severe disease. However, the rate of dissemination among Mexicans, although higher than that in whites, was markedly lower than that in Filipinos and blacks. Filipinos were said to be 175 times as likely as whites to develop disseminated coccidioidomycosis. This was based on the fact that although Filipinos represented only 0.25% of the population, they contributed 22% of the cases. This has been demonstrated more recently also in connection with coccidioidal meningitis: 4.2% of the cases involved Filipino males, who made up only 0.4% of the population of California and Arizona; and 16% of the coccidioidal meningitis was in black males who constituted 3.4% of the population. White males who constituted 44% of the population, contributed essentially the same (43%) proportion of cases of meningitis (124).

Some have questioned whether these differences are truly racial or are based on environment, for example, occupational exposure of agricultural workers (68, 152). Direct evidence bearing on this is derived from both military (162, 186, 126) and civilian populations (126).

Dissemination occurred in 12% of black male soldiers with clinically apparent coccidioidomycosis compared with 1% of white male soldiers living and training under the same conditions (162). It was significant that inapparent and symptomatic infections, the latter detected by conversion of the coccidioidin skin test to positive, were similar for both groups: blacks 63.1% inapparent, 36.9% symptomatic; and whites 60% inapparent, 40% symptomatic. The recent study of marine infantry and tank battalions near Twenty-Nine Palms, California, indicated that a higher proportion of blacks had an asymptomatic conversion of skin test reactivity to spherulin than did white or "other" marines (63). Various factors including absence of clinically apparent coccidioidomycosis make it difficult to assess the significance of these findings. In military personnel and their dependents (virtually all adults 21 years of age or older) for whom living conditions and duties were similar, dissemination occurred in 23.5% of clinically apparent coccidioidomycosis in blacks, and 21% in Filipinos compared with 2.3% among whites (Table 6-6). An "experiment of nature" was provided by a dust storm in Kern County in December 1977 that led to infections far from the agricultural and other soil moving occupations of the endemic area (125). The dust storm was followed by rain within 24–48 hours thus limiting exposure to arthroconidia to a short, well-defined time, and unrelated to occupation involving movement of soil. Symptomatic infections in whites yielded a higher than usual rate of dissemination (11.2%), but in blacks the rate of dissemination was 53.8%, and in Asians (other than Filipinos) it was 38.4%, statistically significantly different from the rate in whites. [The three Filipino patients, two of whom underwent dissemination of their infection, were too few for proper evaluation (126).]

Several additional studies provide evidence of such racial differences.

TABLE 6-6. Racial Distribution of Coccidioidomycosis at Lemoore US Naval Air Station, 1961–1977

Ethnic Derivation	Number of Patients*	%	Disseminated Number	Disseminated %
White	173	77.0	4	2.3
Black	17	7.5	4	23.5
Filipino	19	8.4	4	21.0
Mexican	6	2.7		
Asian	4	1.8		
Guamanian	2	0.9		
"Caucasian"/Indian	1	0.4		
Filipino/Italian	1	0.4	1	
Hawaiian	1	0.4		
Spanish	1	0.4		
Total	225	100.0	13	5.7

*A total of 231 cases were detected, but the ethnic background of 6 was not known. The calculations are based on the 225 cases. After Pappagianis (1980), with permission of Plenum Medical Book Co., NY.

TABLE 6-7. Racial Distribution of Fatal Cases of Coccidioidomycosis in Arizona

	% of Population	% of Total Coccidioidomycosis
Black	3	15
Mexican-American	19	9
Native American Indian	5	10
White	72	66

From Johnson, 1977.

Johnson (74) examined data on morbidity and mortality due to coccidioidomycosis in Arizona. Of 122 deaths ascribed to coccidioidomycosis for the period 1968–1975, he offered the racial breakdown shown in Table 6-7. The mortality of blacks disproportionate to their representation in the population once again is shown by these data. Johnson pointed out the difficulty in assessing the significance of the racial factor in the face of underlying diseases and use of immunosuppressant drugs in some of the population; however, he also pointed out that whites had the highest proportion of deaths known to be associated with underlying disease, a factor not assessed for blacks and Native American Indians. The report of Kelly et al (81) showed no significant difference in deaths due to coccidioidomycosis among black and nonblack patients in the Maricopa Medical Center of Phoenix.

In his studies of coccidioidomycosis in Indians, Sievers (151) had reported that the rate of dissemination of some tribes in Arizona was the same (3.5 times that in whites) as that which had been reported earlier by Gifford et al (51) for Indians and Mexicans, not surprising in view of the American Indian antecedence of most Mexicans. Later Sievers (152) estimated that dissemination occurred in 0.2% of southwestern Indians who had been infected based on 44 disseminated cases and skin test results in 20,600 individuals. The mortality rate for Indians in Arizona was 3.75 per 100,000, similar to that for blacks in Arizona, 3.99 per 100,000, both of which were significantly higher than for whites (0.54 per 100,000). However, there was a significant disparity in the morbidity and mortality rates for disseminated coccidioidomycosis among different tribes, the highest being among the Athapascan (apparently mainly San Carlos Apache in this study) and Piman (Pima and Papago tribes). Sievers suggested that a dominant environmental influence may be involved in this difference based on the higher annual incidence rate of disseminated disease among the Athapascans (14 per 100,000) than the Pimans (4.5 per 100,000) or whites (2.2 per 100,000). But he also suggested a possible genetic effect in that the Pimans may be protected by virtue of their greater carriage (87%) of the blood group 0 trait and lower carriage of blood group A (13%), whereas 58% of Athapascans have the 0 blood group, and 42% have blood group A. However, these factors become difficult to assess in view of the seeming paradox that the case fatality rate for the Pimans with disseminated coccidioidomycosis (83%) was much higher than that of the Athapascans (32%).

Additional indications of racial or ethnic differences in response to primary coccidioidomycosis are provided by other studies. Iger (69) studied 112 cases of coccidioidal osteomyelitis in Kern County, California, for the years 1949–1976. The distribution of these cases is shown in Table 6-8. Huntington (67) reported on 45 cases of fatal coccidioidal pneumonia drawn from five hospitals in four counties. Sixty-two percent (28) were blacks, (18 males, 10 females). Neither of these latter two studies provided a baseline of total coccidioidal

TABLE 6-8. Racial Makeup of 112 Cases of Coccidioidal Osteomyelitis in California,* 1949–1976

	% of Patients	% of Population in Kern County
Blacks	51.0 (34.0 male) (17.0 female)	5.7
Filipino	9.8 (all males)	0.6
Mexican	9.8 (5.0 males) (4.8 females)	14.0

* Most of these were from Kern County.

infections and their racial distributions for comparison. The high attack rates previously described among archaeology, anthropology, etc., "digs" indicate heavy exposure to arthroconidia. Yet these groups, largely consisting of whites, have had rare disseminations.

In his review of the literature on racial factors, Johnson (76) indicates that the available information does "support an increased susceptibility among blacks and Filipinos although in selected instances high dose occupational exposures may be the most important risk factor." Nevertheless, the aggregate of the evidence indicates that, whatever the underlying basis, racial differences exist in the risk of metapulmonary dissemination for symptomatic primary coccidioidomycosis. As a result, particular care is justified in the management of black, Filipino, and other Asian patients in anticipation of possible dissemination.

Influence of Intercurrent Conditions

Although *C. immitis* is usually a primary pathogen affecting apparently normal hosts, it also has found an appropriate setting for pathogenesis in hosts altered physiologically or immunologically (138, 27, 120, 143). The course of primary acute infection may be adversely affected, and old, seemingly arrested disease may be reactivated. For example, in one hospital in Phoenix, Arizona, of all (25) inpatients with fatal coccidioidomycosis who were studied in the 5-year period from January 1971–January 1976, most (84%) were recognized to have an underlying compromising condition and/or therapy, for example, malignant neoplasm, collagen vascular disease, diabetes mellitus, renal failure with or without renal transplant, and pregnancy (142). As noted the nature of the malignant neoplasms has a bearing. Thus, neoplasms not of the hematopoietic-lymphoreticular system(s) appear to exert no adverse effect on the coccidioidal infection unless accompanied by cytotoxic or other therapy (120). Corticosteroid therapy appeared to represent a risk factor, although this appears related to dose (143). In one study, lymphocytopenia appeared related to occurrence of disseminated coccidioidomycosis (28), but in another study lymphocytopenia alone did not add a significant risk of dissemination to the patient already receiving immunosuppressive therapy (143).

Renal transplantation has proved to be a significant risk factor in at least some parts of the endemic areas (14, 19, 164). Thus, of 152 renal transplants performed at the University of Arizona, Tucson, between 1970 and 1976, seven (4.6%) developed disseminated coccidioidomycosis (164); in an expansion of the same study over a 10-year period and inclusion of patients from the Phoenix area, there was a similar incidence (5%) of disseminated coccidioidomycosis (19).

During the period 1971–1984, there was a progressive diminution in deaths from coccidioidomycosis in patients with renal transplants: 1971–1973, 67% deaths; 1974–1976, 71% deaths; and 1977–1979, 44% deaths (14). This decrease may indicate more awareness of coccidioidomycosis as a risk and prompt diagnosis, as well more experience in the management of the immunosuppressive factors. Indeed, in patients with a known prior coccidioidomycosis, subject to relapse with immunosuppression, antifungal therapy afforded a means of precluding serious reactivation of coccidioidomycosis. Coccidioidomycosis also has been recognized in at least five patients undergoing cardiac transplants, both as a relapse of prior coccidioidomycosis, and, apparently, occurrence of acute primary coccidioidomycosis after the transplantation (11, 14). Two of these died, and three survived, although the time of follow up was not given.

It is not surprising that patients with acquired immune deficiency syndrome (AIDS) should be subject to coccidioidomycosis. At least four cases have been reported all of whom died (1, 61, 86, 137); additional unpublished cases have been recognized. One of these four cases appeared to represent recent acute coccidioidomycosis that disseminated; two represented reactivation of prior, apparently arrested coccidioidomycosis. In the fourth, it could not be determined whether the coccidioidomycosis represented a recently acquired or reactivated infection.

The overall influence of diabetes mellitus (DM) is not well defined. Whereas some patients with DM appear at risk, dissemination has not been clearly shown to occur at an unusually high rate. One study directed at this showed no difference in skin test reactivity to coccidioidin between nondiabetics and diabetics, although fewer of the latter reacted to spherulin (15). There does appear to be an increased rate of pulmonary cavitation (120), but from such cavities no apparent increased likelihood of metapulmonary dissemination.

Pregnancy has long been recognized as imposing an additional risk (4, 58, 59, 119, 154, 155, 180, 181). Dissemination occurs at a very high rate (Table 6-9) when primary coccidioidomycosis develops during the third trimester of pregnancy. Thus, although the numbers are small, the contrast between outcome when infection is acquired in the first trimester and third trimester, respectively, was evident as follows: 12% dissemination and 6% fatality

TABLE 6-9. Influence of Stage of Pregnancy on Outcome of Coccidioidomycosis

	Number		
Infection Acquired	Cases	Disseminated	Fatal
First trimester	16	2	1 (or 2)
Second trimester	12	6	5
Third trimester	22	20	19
Total	50	28	25

From various sources, cited in Pappagianis (1980), with permission of Plenum Medical Book Co., NY.

versus 91% dissemination and 86% fatality. This vulnerability applies to white women who ordinarily exhibit relative resistance to dissemination. These findings apply to clinically evident and diagnosed coccidioidomycosis. The baseline of benign subclinical coccidioidomycosis as evidenced by skin test and/or serologic conversion during pregnancy has not been established. In a study involving 95 pregnant women skin tested at parturition, the mean skin test reactivity to coccidioidin and spherulin was 44%. In a control group of 174 nonpregnant women, the mean skin test reactivity was 32% (80). There was no indication that such skin test reactivity was a result of infection during pregnancy. The evidence to date indicates that coccidioidomycosis incurred and arrested previously is not likely to be reactivated during pregnancy.

Coexistent tuberculosis and coccidioidomycosis have been recognized in many patients, and the course of these diseases appears independent of each other (23), although antituberculous therapy with rifampin and isoniazid concomitantly with the antifungal ketoconazole lead to mutually adverse interaction between these compounds (42).

Coexistent coccidioidomycosis and histoplasmosis (128, 144) and disseminated coccidioidomycosis and blastomycosis (24) have been reported.

Influence of Blood Group and Histocompatibility Complex

Sievers (152) called attention to the the higher rate of disseminated coccidioidomycosis in Athapascan Indians than in Piman Indians and suggested a relationship between resistance in the Piman and the higher prevalence of blood group 0 (87%) and lower blood group A (13%) than in the Athapascans (58% group 0, 42% group A). However, in the reports of Deresinski et al (28) and Cohen et al (19), there appeared to be a greater risk of dissemination among those of blood group B.

Scheer et al (145) had reported on a possible association between histocompatibility type HLA-9 and disseminated coccidioidomycosis. In their study of coccidioidomycosis in patients undergoing dialysis or renal transplantation, Cohen et al (19) could discern no relationship between HLA-A9 or HLA-B5 and coccidioidomycosis. The differences in results both in regard to blood group and HLA influences on coccidioidomycosis and the limited studies invite expansion of studies to determine whether these genetic factors have an influence on the response to *C. immitis*.

Age

Coccidioidomycosis has been observed in newborns and in those older than 80 years of age. The rate of infection in various age groups in the Phoenix, Arizona area as indicated by coccidioidin skin test reactivity was recently studied by DuQuette et al (33). In 1983, the 5–18-year age group showed a 16.4% reactivity. This represented a steady decline when compared with rates of 42% in 1951, and 32% in 1961. Larwood (97) had previously shown a decrease in the prevalence of skin test reactors between 1939 and 1964 among elementary (55–8%) and high school students (68–24%) in Kern County, California. Although environmental changes, for example, greater urbanization and fewer students employed in agricultural pursuits, could lead to fewer individuals being sensitized by *C. immitis*, some of the decrease could be by reversion from positive to negative (26, 88, 111). The change in reactivity with age shown by Sievers (151) among Indians from endemic areas also suggests such a reversion from positive to negative.

Of the reports concerned with coccidioidomycosis in neonates, none appears to establish that infection was transplacental (7, 150, 167, 185). Some of the cases were acquired from a mother with coccidioidomycosis (perhaps intrapartum), but some appeared to have been acquired independently of the mother. The fatality rate was very high (> 80%), but this is difficult to assess without additional background information of infections in neonates in the endemic areas.

Faber (43) regarded children under 4 years of age to be more susceptible to dissemination than older individuals. Sievers (151, 152) reported that the likelihood of dissemination (in Indians in Arizona) was greater in children under 5 years of age (case fatality rate 69%) and in adults over 50 years of age. Birsner (8) described 124 cases of coccidioidomycosis in the age group 3 weeks to 13 years. Twenty-six (20%) of these underwent dissemination, and seven (5.6%) died. As 21 of the 26 disseminated cases involved bone, possibly without other sites involved, this could account for the good survival rate in that preamphotericin B era. Interestingly, our own compilation of cases in children in 1970 (119) showed that 21% of the cases underwent dissemination. Those cases were clearly weighted toward more severe infections that had come to our attention for serodiagnosis. A subsequent survey of 240 infections (skin test and/or seropositive) between 1974 and 1978 showed a dissemination rate of 2.9%. The tissue sites involved in dissemination in children were comparable to those in adults, also reflected in the study of Kafka and Catanzaro (77) of 14 patients 2.5–15 years of age. Whereas the disseminations were disproportionately greater among black children in Birsner's (8) series, no appropriate baseline of symptomatic infections was available from the other studies to provide adequate analysis of the racial distribution.

Birsner (8) described the characteristics of coccidioidal infection in 352 cases in the age group 14–60 years. Sixty-seven (19%) disseminated, and 12.5% died. In his "geriatric" group of 24 patients over 60 years of age, Birsner (8) noted a lack of "benignity," as 10 (42%) of these underwent dissemination and six (25%) died. Sievers (152) gave case fatality rates of 83% for the 50 and older group, markedly greater than the 13% for the 6–49-year age group. However, Sievers pointed out that 45.5% of the patients with disseminated disease had some underlying immunocompromising condition.

Sex

It has long been held that the adult white female is the least likely to undergo dissemination of a primary infection, 1 per 500 clinically apparent cases versus 1 per 100 in the adult white male, and more likely to have the erythema nodosum of Valley Fever (157, 162). In the recent study of university students with coccidioidomycosis in Tucson (104), the greater frequency of erythema nodosum in women than in men was again noted; the primary infection was said to be more severe in men than in women. It has been pointed out, however, that pregnancy significantly increases the risk of dissemination when primary coccidioidomycosis occurs in the later stages of pregnancy (see above). In some studies of coccidioidal meningitis, males have exceeded females by 3 to 5 : 1 (66, 73, 124, 189).

Among patients in California, males with fatal coccidioidal pneumonia exceeded females by 2 : 1 (67), and the ratios in osseous and articular coccidioidomycosis were 2 : 1 and 5 : 1, respectively (70). These comprised mainly but not solely adult patients.

In his earlier analysis of Kern County cases, Birsner (8) found the sex-related dissemination and death rates shown in Table 6-10. These data indicate possible higher rates of dissemination and mortality among older males than females. Johnson (74) also indicated that deaths associated with coccidioidomycosis in Arizona were greater in males than females (1.54 : 1). Recent observations by Kelly et al (81) in Maricopa County, Arizona, however, show mortality greater in females (86% versus 33%) in the older than 50 year old group, and in the younger than 50 year olds (46% to 17%). The numbers were small in this study (20 females and 32 males), but they do call attention to a possibility that differences based on sex may be changing at least in some settings.

TABLE 6-10. Male-Female Distribution of Disseminated (D) and Fatal (F) Coccidioidomycosis

Age (years)	*N**	Male		(%)	*N**	Female		(%)
0–13	64	15	D	(23.4)	60	9	D	(15.0)
		5	F	(7.8)		2	F	(33.3)
14–60	216	41	D	(19.0)	136	26	D	(19.0)
		28	F	(12.9)		16	F	(11.7)
>60	12	7	D	(58.0)	12	3	D	(25.0)
		4	F	(33.3)		2	F	(16.6)
Total	292	63	D	(21.6)	208	38	D	(18.3)
		37	F	(12.7)		20	F	(9.6)
			F/D =	(58.7)			F/D =	(52.6)

* Includes all diagnosed cases of coccidioidomycosis. After Birsner (1954).

Percutaneous Infection

Primary inoculation coccidioidomycosis acquired through the skin is relatively rare. Some 20 cases have been reported [reviewed by Carroll et al (17)] most of which involved introduction of the hyphal form of the organism. Wilson et al (188) established criteria for distinguishing primary cutaneous coccidioidomycosis from cutaneous lesions resulting from metapulmonary dissemination from a primary pulmonary focus. Trauma to the skin may set the stage for development of a lesion resulting from *C. immitis* already present in a host without visible cutaneous manifestations (122).

Fomites as Vehicles for *Coccidioides immitis*

Transportation of *C. immitis* on inanimate objects has led to infections near to and thousands of miles from the endemic area [reviewed by Rothman et al (141)]. Soil brought from an area near Los Angeles was used by a movie director to create an artificial dust storm which led to a stiff coccidioidomycosis infection in the movie director (1979, Director, Los Angeles County Health Department, personal communication). Some "western" movies filmed in endemic areas likely represent a dusty exposure that is followed by coccidioidomycosis.

Exportation of San Joaquin Valley cotton to San Francisco (160), to Georgia (3), and to North Carolina (50) has led to coccidioidal infections. Indian pottery and its packing material from Arizona led to infection in Great Britain (175). Archeologic artifacts carried to urban Los Angeles have led to infection (130). Clothing sent to the South Pacific (31) and agricultural products to Italy (165) led to exotic infections.

The first systematic coccidioidin skin test studies by CE Smith in the 1930s and 1940s were made in populations that to a large extent were newly arrived in the San Joaquin Valley. Thus, 87.5% of the civilian patients with Valley Fever had arrived since the preceding census (1930), more than half from Arkansas, Oklahoma, and Texas (157). Their susceptibility was apparent as nearly half of the patients had been in the Valley less than 1 year, two thirds less than 2 years, and only about one tenth had lived there for 10 or more years. Within 5 years' residence in Tulare and Kern County, 80% of the population was found to have been infected (157).

Recent skin test studies in the known endemic areas of Bakersfield, Lemoore, and Visalia in California, and Tucson, Arizona, showed that 42% of 5,263 adults tested were positive (118). The average annual incidence of infection in university students in Tucson, Arizona, as indicated by positive culture or serologic or skin test conversion was 0.43% (82). The prevalence rate of coccidioidin sensitivity in Scottsdale, Arizona, was found to be 20–25% in adults 19–74 years of age (33). Such skin test reactivity in the endemic areas is usually sufficient to provide confidence in the results, whereas the weak reactions (< 10 mm) recorded outside the endemic area (191) are enigmatic although possibly suggestive of cross-sensitization by some other organism. The introduction of spherulin as a skin test reagent appeared to provide a more sensitive tool for epidemiologic studies (100). It is recognized, however, that some subjects will give a stronger response to coccidioidin than to spherulin. Additional studies indicate and reaffirm the need, earlier stated by CE Smith, to make readings at both 24 and 48 hours (63).

Epizootiology

Although this chapter is titled "Epidemiology," properly it should include reference to the nonhuman species that also have acquired coccidioidal infection. The list is extensive as it includes wild rodents (41), lagormorphs as well as domestic food animals (5) and pets (107), and exotic species housed in zoologic parks (Table 6.11) (123, 134).

Reed et al (134) provided an extensive review of coccidioidomycosis in zoo animals in Arizona. Most of these were recognized to have disseminated and were usually fatal. But there is a range of responses varying from relative resistance to dissemination in cattle, sheep, and swine, to a broad range of disease types in domestic dogs, similar to patterns found in humans, and marked susceptibility to dissemination in primates (123). Two calves in Guatemala were reported to have coccidioidomycosis with bronchopneu-

TABLE 6-11. Mammals with Naturally Acquired Coccidioidomycosis

Aardvark*	Horse, Przewalski*
Baboon,* mandrill*	Impala*
Badger*	Jackrabbit
Binturong,* civet	Kangaroo,* wallaby,* wallaroo*
Burro	Kit fox
Cat, domestic	Llama*
Cattle, domestic	Monkey*: tropical American, sooty mangabey, rhesus, bonnet macaque, Celebes macaque, lion tail macaque, spider, squirrel, wooly
Cheetah*	Otter: river,* sea
Chimpanzee*	Rodents: pocket mouse, grasshopper mouse, kangaroo rat, ground squirrel
Chinchilla*	Sea lion* (also free living)
Coyote	Sheep
Dog, cape hunting*	Skunk,* hognose
Dog, domestic	Swine
Ferret*	Tapir*
Genet*	Tiger,* Bengal
Gorilla*: mountain, lowland	
Guenon*	
Horse, domestic	

*Zoo or captive animals.

monic involvement perhaps causing more severe illness than usually encountered in cattle (44). Several horses have been infected and appear to incur severe infections, but the possible existence of benign equine coccidioidomycosis has not been excluded. A sea otter with coccidioidomycosis was discovered in the wild on a California beach (22), raising the possibility of infection in other free-living marine mammals.

Swatek and Plunkett (173) observed mature endosporulating spherules in lizards inoculated intraperitoneally, and these were found in the lungs and liver. Indeed some of these lizards died after inoculation. Goldfish and crayfish yielded only hyphal phase *C. immitis* after intracoelomic injection. On the other hand, heroic (or foolhardy) attempts to infect rattlesnakes and lizards by intrapharyngeal route, or lizards by intraperitoneal route, yielded no apparent illness (37).

Impact of Coccidioidomycosis

It is difficult to arrive at a clear figure on the impact of coccidioidomycosis because of the variability of its clinical manifestations. Estimates of the number of cases have varied: Birsner (8) estimated 25,000–35,000 new cases per year, and Fiese (45) 35,000 new infections per year in California. The inclusion of the other endemic states could double these figures. However, we are restricted by the lack of precise figures. We do have the reported cases, and some figures for average hospitalization time, on which to base estimates.

Fraser et al (46) estimated the total number of days of hospitalization for coccidioidomycosis per year at 32,000. Projected costs for hospitalization for coccidioidomycosis were \$12.56 $\times$ 10^6 for those hospitalized with coccidioidomycosis as the primary diagnosis and \$5.3 $\times$ 10^6 for those with coccidioidomycosis as the secondary diagnosis. Those costs were based on \$175.00 per day and an average of 11 days' hospitalization per case. Based on the case rate calculated by Fraser et al, 82 per 10^6 in California and 20 $\times$ 10^6 for the total population, 18,040 days would represent the total hospitalization time for California. At \$250.00 per day this would yield \$4,510,000. We estimate through our serologic testing that some 32 cases of disseminated coccidioidomycosis occur per year in the population whose sera we test. We estimate conservatively that those 32 cases represent one fourth of the new disseminations per year, that is, California alone would have 120 new disseminated cases. Johnson (74) reported an average of 17 deaths per year from coccidioidomycosis in Arizona, which probably indicates at least 34 new disseminations per year, giving a total of 154 new disseminated cases for California and Arizona. Assuming that these disseminated cases require 20 days' initial hospitalization and the equivalent of 20 additional days for hospital visits and treatments, using \$250 per day for hospitalization costs would be 154 patients $\times$ 40 days $\times$ \$250 per day = \$1,500,000 for room costs alone.

Kerrick et al (82) provided an estimate of the costs of nondisseminated coccidioidomycosis for 170 patients in a university student health service. Diagnosis and management of these patients (average of 42 patients per year) costs $34,000 per year. These workers correctly point out, however, a greater expense is generated by having to test for and rule out coccidioidomycosis in other patients. No estimate was made of the cost for care of the two patients (1.1% of total) with disseminated coccidioidomycosis for whose care costs could have exceeded those of all the patients with nondisseminated coccidioidomycosis.

None of the foregoing have included considerations of the costs due to coccidioidomycosis in Texas, New Mexico, or elsewhere; nor have the costs involved veterinary diagnosis and therapy. All of these indicate that costs related to coccidioidomycosis in the United States alone exceed $5,000,000 per year.

Medicolegal Aspects

At least three particular areas of medicolegal responsibility can be related to coccidioidomycosis (56, 99, 121):

1. Medical responsibility in making a timely and correct diagnosis, and providing appropriate therapy.
2. Determination of employment-related coccidioidomycosis for compensation purposes.
3. Appropriately informing individuals of the potential risk of acquiring coccidioidomycosis. The latter is particularly applicable to those who might be exposed through employment or academic work. In fact the University of California and the California State Department of Health Services established guidelines that indicated that no student or faculty should be required to participate in field work that would likely expose them in endemic areas; that skin testing should be done and those who are coccidioidin positive can generally be considered resistant to infection, and nonreactors are susceptible; dust control should be attempted to reduce exposure.

Recognition of various aspects of the epidemiology of coccidioidomycosis are of great importance in such matters.

Summary

Coccidioides immitis naturally occurs in the soil and air of certain areas of the New World. These are generally arid to semiarid areas that have relatively modest rainfall, mild winters, and prolonged hot seasons. Coccidioidomycosis is usually a disease of human and nonhuman residents of these areas; but visitors may develop the disease after entering these areas and returning home long distances from the endemic areas. Inhalation (rarely percutaneous introduction) of arthroconidia of *C. immitis* leads to usually benign but occasionally severe and even fatal infection. Recovery from or asymptomatic infection leads to resistance to reinfection. Exposure to soil (dust) means that certain occupations are more likely to be exposed to *C. immitis*. Persistence of the organism in the soil means that infections will be encountered in the future, particularly as long as susceptible newcomers continue to enter endemic areas. Those who have been infected and recovered generally will be resistant to later infection, although exacerbation may occur as a result of superimposed immunosuppression.

References

1. Abrams DI, Robia M, Blumenfeld W, Simonsen J, Cohen MB, Hadley WK: Disseminated coccidioidomycosis in AIDS. *N Engl J Med* 310:986–987, 1984.
2. Ajello L, Maddy K, Crecelius G, Hugenholtz PG, and Hall LB: Recovery of *Coccidioides immitis* from the air. *Sabouraudia* 4:92–95, 1965.
3. Albert BL, Sellers TF: Coccidioidomycosis from fomites. *Arch Intern Med* 112:253–261, 1963.
4. Baker RL: Pregnancy complicated by coccidioidomycosis: Report of 2 cases. *Am J Obstet Gynecol* 70:1033–1038, 1955.
5. Beck MD: Epidemiology, in *Coccidioidal Granuloma*. Special Bulletin No. 57, California Department of Public Health, p 19–37, 1931.
6. Beck MD, Traum J, Harrington ES: Coccidioidal granuloma. *J Am Vet Med Assoc* 78:490–499, 1931.
7. Bernstein DI, Tipton JR, Schott SF, Cherry JD: Coccidioidomycosis in a neonate: Maternal-infant transmission. *J Pediatr* 99:752–754, 1981.
8. Birsner JW: The roentgen aspects of five hundred cases of pulmonary coccidioidomycosis. *Am J Roentgen* 72:556–573, 1954.
9. Borelli D, Marcano C: Transmission experimental de micoses profunda por "predacion." *Med Cut* VI:193–198, 1972.
10. Borghi AL, deBenetti MSR, de Bracalanti: *Coccidioides immitis*: Su aislamiento de muestras de suelos de las provincias de de San Luis y Mendoza. *Sabouraudia* 15:51–57, 1977.
11. Brewer JH, Parrott CL, Rimland D: Disseminated coccidioidomycosis in a heart transplant recipient. *Sabouraudia* 20:261–265, 1982.
12. Burke RC: Viability of *Coccidioides immitis*. 1. Isolation from a seven-month-old sealed microscope slide. *J Invest Dermatol* 23:1–2, 1954.
13. Bush JD: Coccidioidomycosis. *J Med Assoc Alabama* 13:159–166, 1943.
14. Calhoun DL, Galgiani JN, Zukoski C, Copeland JG: Coccidioidomycosis in recent renal or cardiac transplant recipients, in Einstein HE, Catanzaro A (eds): *Coccidioidomycosis*. Washington, DC, National Foundation for Infectious Disease, pp 312–318.
15. Campbell SC, Smith JP: An evaluation of reactivity to *Cooccidioides immitis* skin tests in subjects with diabetes mellitus. *Mycopathologia* 80:133–136, 1982.
16. Campins H: Coccidioidomycosis in South America. A review of its epidemiology and geographic distribution. *Mycopathol Mycol Appl* 40:25–34, 1970.
17. Carroll GF, Haley LD, Brown JM: Primary cutaneous coccidioidomycosis. *Arch Dermatol* 113:933–936, 1977.

18. Castleberry MW, Converse JL, DelFavero JE: Coccidioidomycosis transmission to infant monkey from its mother. *Arch Pathol* 75:459–461, 1963.
19. Cohen IM, Galgiani JN, Potter D, Ogden DA: Coccidioidomycosis in renal replacement therapy. *Arch Intern Med* 142:489–494, 1982.
20. Cole GT, Sun SH: Arthroconidium-spherule-endospore transformation in *Coccidioides immitis*, in Szaniszlo PJ (ed): *Fungal Dimorphism*. New York, Plenum Publishing, 1985, pp 281–333.
21. Converse JL, Reed RE: Experimental epidemiology of coccidioidomycosis. *Bacteriol Rev* 30:678–695, 1966.
22. Cornell L, Osborn KG, Antrim JE: Coccidioidomycosis in a California sea otter (*Enhydra lutris*). *J Wild Dis* 15:373–378, 1979.
23. Cotton BH, Penido JRF, Birsner JW, Babcock CE: Coexisting pulmonary coccidioidomycosis and tuberculosis. *Am Rev Tuberc* 70:109–120, 1954.
23a. Currah, RS: Taxonomy of the Onygenales: Arthrodermataceae, Gymnoascaceae, Myxotrichaceae, and Onygenaceae. *Mycotaxon* 24:1–216, 1985.
24. Davidson W, Sarosi GA: Disseminated blastomycosis and coccidioidomycosis in the same patient. *Am Rev Respir Dis* 124:179, 1981.
25. Davis BL, Smith RT, Smith CE: An epidemic of coccidioidal infection (coccidioidomycosis). *JAMA* 118:1182–1186, 1942.
26. Denenholz EJ, Cheney G: Diagnosis and treatment of chronic coccidioidomycosis. *Arch Intern Med* 74:311–330, 1944.
27. Deresinski S, Stevens D: Coccidioidomycosis in compromised hosts. *Medicine* 54:377–395, 1974.
28. Deresinski SC, Pappagianis D, Stevens DA: Association of ABO blood group and outcome of coccidioidal infection. *Sabouraudia* 17:261–264, 1979.
29. Dickson EC: *Coccidioides* infection. *Arch Intern Med* 59:1029–1044, 1937.
30. Dickson EC: "Valley Fever" of the San Joaquin Valley and fungus *Coccidioides*. *Calif West Med* 47:151–155, 1937.
31. Donohugh DL: Paragonimiasis in the Samoan Islands. *Trans Roy Soc Trop Med Hyg* 58:94–95, 1964.
32. Drouhet E: Coccidioidomycose d'importation en France. *Bull Soc Pathol Exot* 54:1002–1007, 1961.
33. DuQuette RC, Jogerst GJ, Wurster SR: Prevalence of coccidioidin skin test sensitivity in an ambulatory population, in Einstein HE, Catanzaro A (eds): *Coccidioidomycosis*. Washington, DC, National Foundation for Infectious Diseases, 1985, pp 67–74.
34. Duran F Jr, Robertstad GW, Donowbo E: The distribution of *Coccidioides immitis* in the soil in El Paso, Texas. *Sabouraudia* 11:143–148, 1973.
35. Dzawachiszwili N, Landau JW, Newcome VD, Plunkett OA: The effect of sea water and sodium chloride on the growth of fungi pathogenic to man. *J Invest Dermatol* 43:103–109, 1964.
36. Eckmann BN, Schaefer GL, Huppert M: Bedside interhuman transmission of coccidioidomycosis via growth on fomites. *Am Rev Respir Dis* 89:175–185, 1964.
37. Egeberg RO: Socioeconomic impact of coccidioidomycosis, in Einstein HB, Catanzaro A (eds): *Coccidioidomycosis*. Washington, D.C., National Foundation for Infectious Diseases, 1985, pp 27–33.
38. Egeberg RO, Ely AF: *Coccidioides immitis* in the soil of the southern San Joaquin Valley. *Am J Med Sci* 23:151–154, 1956.
39. Egeberg RO, Elconin AE, Egeberg MC: Effect of salinity and temperature on *Coccidioides immitis* and three antagonistic soil saprophytes. *J Bacteriol* 88:473–476, 1964.
40. Elconin AE, Egeberg RO, Egeberg MC: Significance of soil salinity on the ecology of *Coccidioides immitis*. *J Bacteriol* 87:500–503, 1964.

41. Emmons CW: Isolation of *Coccidioides* from soil and rodents. *Pub Health Rep* 57:109–111, 1942.
42. Engelhard D, Stutman HR, Marks MI: Interaction of ketoconazole with rifampin and isoniazid. *N Engl J Med* 311:1681–1683, 1984.
43. Faber HK: Coccidioidomycosis, in McQuarrie (ed): *Brenneman's Practice of Pediatrics*, Vol. 2. Hagerstown, Prior, 1951, pp 17–26.
44. Ferri AG, Correa WM, Villagran E: Coccidioidomicosis en bovinos de Guatemala. *Rev Univ San Carlos Guatemala* 54:137–142, 1961.
45. Fiese MJ: *Coccidioidomycosis*. Springfield, IL, Charles C Thomas, 1958.
46. Fraser DW, Ward JI, Ajello L, Plikaytis BD: Aspergillosis and other systemic mycoses: The growing problem. *JAMA* 242:1631–1635, 1979.
47. Friedman L, Pappagianis D, Berman RJ, Smith CE: Studies on *Coccidioides immitis*: Morphology and sporulation capacity of forty-seven strains. *J Lab Clin Med* 42:438–444, 1953.
48. Friedman L, Smith CE, Pappagianis D, Berman RJ: Survival of *Coccidioides immitis* under controlled conditions of temperature and humidity. *Am J Pub Health* 46:1317–1324, 1956.
49. Galgiani JN, Hayden R, Payne CM: Leukocyte effects on the dimorphism of *Coocidioides immitis*. *J Infect Dis* 146:56–63, 1982.
50. Gehlbach SH, Hamilton JD, Conant NF: Coccidioidomycosis—an occupational disease in cotton mill workers. *Arch Intern med* 131:254–255, 1973.
51. Gifford M, Buss WC, Douds RJ: Data on *Coccidioides* fungus infection, Kern County, 1900–1936. Kern County Health Department Annual Report 1936–1937, pp 39–54.
52. Gilman DW, Wehrle PF, Cowper H: Coccidioidomycosis—Canoga Park, California. *Morbid Mortal Weekly Rep* US Public Health Service, Atlanta, 1965, pp 302–303.
53. Gomez RF: Endemism of coccidioidomycosis in the Paraguayan Chaco. *Calif Med* 73:35–38, 1950.
54. Gonzalez-Ochoa A: Coccidioidomycosis in Mexico, in Ajello L (ed): *Coccidioidomycosis*. Tucson, University of Arizona Press, 1967, pp 293–299.
55. Gonzalez-Ochoa A: Coccidioidomicosis: Algunos conceptos actuales del padecimento con especial mencion del problema Mexicano. *Prensa Med Mex* 14:246–252, 1949.
56. Gorman WF: Legal terms for physicians: Cause, injury, disability, in Einstein H, Catanzaro A (eds): *Coccidioidomycosis*. Washington, DC, National Foundation for Infectious Diseases, 1985, pp 34–42.
57. Harrell ER, Honeycutt WM: Coccidioidomycosis: A traveling fungus disease. *Arch Dermatol* 87:188–196, 1963.
58. Harris RE: Coccidioidomycosis complicating pregnancy. Report of 3 cases and review of the literature. *Obstet Gynecol* 28:401–405, 1966.
59. Harrison HN: Fatal maternal coccidioidomycosis. *Am J Obstet Gynecol* 75:813–820, 1958.
60. Hartmann M: Demonstration eines neuen menschenpathogenen Protisten. *Zentralblatt f Bakt* (Abteilung 1-referate) LIV:253–255, 1912.
61. Hendel E, Hui AN, Diaz J, Boylen CT: *Pneumocystis carinii* pneumonia and malignant lymphoma in a homosexual male with disseminated coccidioidomycosis, in Einstein H, Catanzaro A (eds): *Coccidioidomycosis*. Washington, DC, National Foundation for Infectious Diseases, 1985, pp 305–311.
62. Hoggan MD, Ransom JP, Pappagianis D, Danald GE, Bell AD: Isolation of *Coccidioides immitis* from the air. *Stanford Med Bull* 14:190, 1956.
63. Hooper R, Poppell G, Curley R, Husted S, Schillaci R: Coccidioidomycosis among military personnel in Southern California. *Mil Med* 145:620–623, 1980.

64. Huberty G: An epidemic of coccidioidomycosis. *J Am Coll Health Assoc* 12:131, 1963.
65. Hugenholtz P: Climate and coccidioidomycosis, in *Proc Symp Coccidioidomycosis*. Public Health Service, Publ. #575, 1957, pp 136–143.
66. Huntington RW Jr: Pathologic and clinical observations on 142 cases of coccidioidomycosis with necropsy, in Ajello L (ed): *Coccidioidomycosis*. Tucson, University of Arizona Press, Tuscon, 1967, pp 143–167.
67. Huntington RW: Acute fata coccidioidal pneumonia, in Ajello L (ed): *Coccidioidomycosis: Current Clinical and Diagnostic Status*. Miami, Florida, Symposia Specialists, 1977, pp 127–137.
68. Huppert M: Racism in coccidioidomycosis? *Am Rev Respir Dis* 118:797–798, 1978.
69. Iger M: Coccidioidal osteomyelitis, in Ajello L (ed): *Coccidioidomycosis: Current Clinical and Diagnostic Status*. Miami, Florida, Symposia Specialists, 1977, pp 177–190.
70. Iger M, Coppola AJ: Review of 135 cases of bone and joint coccidioidomycosis, in Einstein H, Catanzaro A (eds): *Coccidioidomycosis*. Washington, DC, National Foundation for Infectious Diseases, 1985, pp 379–389.
71. Joffe B: An epidemic of coccidioidomycosis probably related to soil. *N Engl J Med* 262:720–722, 1960.
72. Johnson JE, Perry JE, Fekety FR, Kadull PJ, Cluff LE: Laboratory—acquired coccidioidomycosis: A report of 210 cases. *Ann Intern Med* 60:941–956, 1964.
73. Johnson RH, Brown JF Jr, Holeman CW, Helvie SJ, Einstein HE: Coccidioidal meningitis: A 25-year experience with 194 patients, in Einstein HE, Catanzaro A (eds): *Coccidioidomycosis*. Washington, DC, National Foundation for Infectious Diseases, 1985, pp 411–421.
74. Johnson WM: Coccidioidomycosis mortality in Arizona, in Ajello L (ed): *Coccidioidomycosis: Current Clinical and Diagnostic Status*. Miami, Florida, Symposia Specialists, 1977, pp 33–44.
75. Johnson WM: Occupational factors in coccidioidomycosis. *J Occup Med* 23: 367–374, 1981.
76. Johnson WM: Racial factors in coccidioidomycosis: Mortality experience in Arizona. *Arizona Med* 39:18–24, 1982.
77. Kafka JA, Catanzaro A: Disseminated coccidioidomycosis in children. *J Pediatr* 98:355–361, 1981.
78. Kajihiro ES: Occurrence of dermatophytes in fresh bat guano. *Appl Microbiol* 13:720–724, 1965.
79. Kapicka L, Matouk E, D'Halewyn MA: Diagnosing coccidioidomycosis outside an endemic area. *Mycopathologia* 82:95–99, 1983.
80. Kelly PD, Rowland V, Doto I: Coccidioidin and spherulin skin tests in pregnant women. *Proc Annual Coccidioidomycosis Study Group*, 1983, p 3.
81. Kelly PC, Thomas AR, Sazie ESM: The outcome of disseminated coccidioidomycosis, in Einstein H, Catanzaro A (eds): *Coccidioidomycosis*. Washington, DC, National Foundation for Infectious Diseases, 1985, pp 360–368.
82. Kerrick SS, Lundergan LL, Galgiani JN: Coccidioidomycosis at a university health service. *Am Rev Respir Dis* 131:100–102, 1985.
83. Key GF, Smith IM: Coccidioidomycosis in Iowa: 12 cases in a nonendemic area. *J Iowa Med Soc* October:531–535, 1972.
84. Klotz AL, Biddle M: Coccidioidin skin test survey of San Fernando Valley State College students over a five year period, in Ajello L (ed): *Coccidioidomycosis*. Tucson, University of Arizona Press, 1967, pp 251–253.
85. Klotz SA, Drutz DJ, Huppert M, Sun SH, DeMarsh P: Critical role of CO_2 in the morphogenesis of *Coccidioides immitis* in cell-free subcutaneous chambers. *J Infect Dis* 150:127–134, 1984.

86. Kovacks A, Forthal DN, Kovacs JA, Overturf GD: Disseminated coccidioidomycosis in a patient with acquired immune deficiency syndrome. *West J Med* 140:447–449, 1984.
87. Kritzer MD, Biddle M, Kessel JF: An outbreak of primary pulmonary coccidioidomycosis in Los Angeles County, California. *Ann Intern Med* 33:960–990, 1950.
88. Krueger AP, Levine HB: The effect of unipolar positively ionized air on the course of coccidioidomycosis in mice. *Int J Biometerorol* 11:279–288, 1967.
89. Kruse RH: Potential aerogenic laboratory hazards of *Coccidioides immitis*. *Am J Clin Pathol* 37:150–158, 1962.
90. Kruse RH, Green TH, Chambers RC, Jones MW: Disinfection of aerosolized pathogenic fungi on laboratory surfaces I. Tissue phase. *Appl Microbiol* 11:436–445, 1963.
91. Kruse RH, Green TH, Chambers RC, Jones MW: Disinfection of aerosolized pathogenic fungi on laboratory surfaces. II. Culture phase. *Appl Microbiol* 12:155–160, 1964.
92. Krutzsch PH, Watson RH: Isolation of *Coccidioides immitis* from bat guano and preliminary findings on laboratory infectivity of bats with *Coccidioides immitis*. *Life Sci* 22:679–684, 1978.
93. Lacey J: The aerobiology of conidial fungi, in Cole GT, Kendrick B (eds): *Biology of Conidial Fungi*, Vol. 1. New York, San Francisco, Academic Press, 1981, p 400.
94. Lacy GH, Swatek FE: Soil ecology of *Coccidioides immitis* at Amerindian middens in California. *Appl Microbiol* 27:379–388, 1974.
95. Lacy GH, Swatek FE: *Coccidioides* in California, in Ajello L (ed): *Coccidioidomycosis: Current Clinical and Diagnostic Status*. Miami, Florida, Symposia Specialists, 1977, p 79–90.
96. Larsen RA, Jacobson JA, Morris AH, Benowitz BA: Acute respiratory failure caused by primary pulmonary coccidioidomycosis. *Am Rev Respir Dis* 131:797–799, 1985.
97. Larwood T: Further drop in Kern County coccidioidin reactivity. *Trans Ninth Annual Coccidioidomycosis Conference*. Los Angeles, California, 1964, p 8–9.
98. Lee RV, Nixon N: Syllabus on coccidioidomycosis. Headquarters Army Air Forces Western Flying Training Command. Office of the Surgeon, Santa Ana, California, 1944.
99. Levan N: Workmen's compensation legislation and coccidioidomycosis: Legal and sociocultural considerations, in Ajello L (ed): *Coccidioidomycosis: Current Clinical and Diagnostic Status*. Miami, Florida, Symposia Specialists, 1977, pp 11–17.
100. Levine HB, Gonzalez-Ochoa A, Ten Eyck DR: Dermal sensitivity to *Coccidioides immitis*. A comparison of responses elicited in man by spherulin and coccidioidin. *Am Rev Respir Dis* 107:379–386, 1973.
101. Loofbourow J, Pappagianis D, Cooper T: Endemic coccidioidomycosis in Northern California: An outbreak in the Capay Valley of Yolo County. *Calif Med* 111:5–9, 1969.
102. Looney JM, Stein T: Coccidioidomycosis: The hazard involved in diagnostic procedures, with report of a case. *N Engl J Med* 242:77–82, 1950.
103. Lubarsky R, Plunkett OA: Some ecological studies of *Coccidioides immitis* in soil, in Sternberg TH, Newcomer VD (eds): *Therapy of Fungus Diseases*. Boston, Mass, Little, Brown, & Co., 1955, pp 308–310.
104. Lundergan LL, Kerrick SS, Galgiani JN: Coccidioidomycosis at a university outpatient clinic: A clinical description, in Einstein H, Catanzaro A (eds): *Coccidioidomycosis*. Washington, DC, National Foundation for Infectious Diseases, 1985, pp 47–54.

105. Maddy KT: Coccidioidomycosis of cattle in the southwestern United States. *J Am Vet Med Assoc* 124:456–464, 1954.
106. Maddy KT: Ecological factors of the geographic distribution *Coccidioides immitis*. *J Am Vet Med Assoc* 130:475–476, 1957.
107. Maddy KT: Disseminated coccidioidomycosis of the dog. *J Am Vet Med Assoc* 132:483–489, 1958.
108. Maddy KT: A study of a site where a dog apparently acquired a *Coccidioides immitis* infection. *Am J Vet Res* 20:642–646, 1959.
109. Maddy KT: Observations on *Coccidioides immitis* found growing naturally in soil. *Arizona Med* 22:281–288, 1965.
110. Maddy KT, Crecelius GT: Establishment of *Coccidioides immitis* in negative soil following burial of infected animals and animal tissues, in Ajello L (ed): *Coccidioidomycosis*. Tucson, University of Arizona Press, 1967, pp 309–312.
111. Masters JB, Harader FR, Gaines RS: Coccidioidin skin sensitivity among high school students in Los Angeles County. *Trans Ninth Annual Coccidioidomycosis Conference, Los Angeles, Calif*, 1964, p 9.
112. Mayorga RP, Espinoza H: Coccidioidomycosis in Mexico and Central America. *Mycopathol Mycol Appl* 40:13–23, 1970.
113. Miller RN, Takafuji ET, McKenna MK, Gertz C, Sampson G: Coccidioidomycosis surveillance of US Army personnel training at Fort Irwin, California. *Proc Twenty-Sixth Annual Coccidioidomycosis Study Group Meeting*, abstract 5, 1981.
114. Milwaukee Journal: $1 million Awarded in Malpractice Case. November 8, 1979, pp 1, 11.
115. Nabarro JDN: Primary pulmonary coccidioidomycosis: Case of laboratory infection in England. Lancet 1:982–984, 1948.
116. Nedwicki EG: Coccidioidomycosis in Michigan. *Postgrad Med* 45:106–110, 1969.
117. Negroni P: Coccidioidomycosis in Argentina, in Ajello L (ed): *Coccidioidomycosis*. Tucson, University of Arizona Press, 1967, pp 273–278.
118. Nichols JW, the Vaccine Study Group: Progress report on the coccidioidomycosis vaccine trial, in Einstein HE, Catanzaro A (eds): *Coccidioidomycosis*. Washington, DC, National Foundation for Infectious Diseases, 1985, p 347.
119. Pappagianis D: Epidemiology of coccidioidomycosis. Proceedings of the International Symposium on Mycoses. *Pan Am Hlth Org Sci Publ* no. 205, 1970, pp 195–201.
120. Pappagianis D: Opportunism in coccidioidomycosis, in Chick EW, Balows A, Furcolow ML (eds): *The Proceedings of the Second International Conference on Opportunistic Fungal Infections*. Springfield, IL, Charles C. Thomas, 1975, pp 221–234.
121. Pappagianis D: Coccidioidomycosis (San Joaquin or Valley Fever), in DiSalvo A (ed): *Occupational Mycoses*. Philadelphia, Lea & Febiger, 1983, pp 13–28.
122. Pappagianis, D: The phenomenon of locus minoris resistentiae in coccidioidomycosis, in Einstein HE, Catanaro A (eds): *Coccidioidomycosis*. Washington, DC, National Foundation for Infectious diseases, 1985, pp 319–329.
123. Pappagianis D: Coccidioidomycosis, in Maibach HI, Lowe NJ (eds): *Models in Dermatology*, Vol. 1. Dermatology. New York, S. Karger, 1985, pp 98–104.
124. Pappagianis D, Crane R: Survival in coccidioidal meningitis since introduction of amphotericin B, in Ajello L (ed): *Coccidioidomycosis: Current Clinical and Diagnostic Status*. Miami, Florida, Symposia Specialists, 1977, pp 223–237.
125. Pappagianis D, Einstein H: Tempest from Tehachapi takes toll. *West J Med* 129:527–530, 1978.
126. Pappagianis D, Lindsay S, Beall S, Williams P: Ethnic background and the clinical course of coccidioidomycosis. *Am Rev Respir Dis* 120:959–961, 1979.

127. Pena CE: Deep mycotic infections in Colombia. A clinicopathologic study of 162 cases. *Am J Clin Pathol* 47:505–520, 1967.
128. Perry LV, Jenkins DE, Whitcomb FC: Simultaneously occurring pulmonary coccidioidomycosis and tuberculosis. *Am Rev Respir Dis* 92:952–957, 1965.
129. Pike RM: Laboratory-associated infections: Incidence, fatalities, causes, prevention. *Ann Rev Microbiol* 33:41–66, 1979.
130. Plunkett OA, Swatek FE: Ecological studies of *Coccidioides immitis*, in *Proc Symposium on Coccidioidomycosis*. Public Health Service Publication no. 575, 1957, pp 158–160.
131. Posadas A Un nuevo caso de micosis fungoides con psorospermias. *An Circ Med Argent* 15:587–597, 1892.
132. Ramras DG, Walch HAA, Murray JP, Davidson BH: An epidemic of coccidioidomycosis in the Pacific Beach area of San Diego. *Am Rev Respir Dis* 101:975–978, 1970.
133. Rao S, Biddle M, Balchum OJ, Robinson JL: Focal endemic coccidioidomycosis in Los Angeles County. *Am Rev Respir Dis* 105:410–416, 1972.
134. Reed RE, Bicknell EJ, Hood HB: A thirty-year record of coccidioidomycosis in exotic pets and zoo animals in Arizona, in Einstein HE, Catanzaro A (eds): *Coccidioidomycosis*. Washington, DC, National Foundation for Infectious Diseases, 1985, pp 275–281.
135. Riley WC, Huberty GT: Coccidioidomycosis in a university archeological group. *Trans 8th Annual Mtg. VA-Armed Forces Coccidioidomycosis Study Group*, 1963, p 8.
136. Rixford E: A case of protozoic skin disease. *Occ Med Times* 8:703–704, 1894.
137. Roberts CJ: Coccidioidomycosis in acquired immune deficiency syndrome. Depressed humoral as well as cellular immunity. *Am J Med* 76:734–736, 1984.
138. Roberts PL, Knepshield JH, Wells RF: *Coccidioides* as an opportunist. *Arch Intern Med* 121:568–570, 1968.
139. Robledo VM, Restrepo MA, Restrepo LM, Ospina OS, Gutierrez AF: Encuesta epidemiologica sobre coccidioidomycosis en algunas zonas aridas de Colombia. *Antioq Med* 18:505–522, 1968.
140. Roessler WG, Herbst CJ, McCullogh WG, Mills RC, Brewer CR: Studies with *Coccidioides immitis*. I. Submerged growth in liquid media. *J Infect Dis* 79:12–22, 1946.
141. Rothman PE, Graw RG Jr, Harris JC Jr, Anslow JM: Coccidioidomycosis—possible fomite transmission. *Am J Dis Child* 118:792–801, 1969.
142. Rowland VS, Westfall RE, Hinchcliffe WA: Fatal coccidioidomycosis: Analysis of host factors, in Ajello L (ed): *Coccidioidomycosis*, Miami, Flordia, Symposia Specialists, 1977, pp 91–106.
143. Rutala PJ, Smith JW: Coccidioidomycosis in potentially compromised hosts: The effect of immunosuppressive therapy in dissemination. *Am J Med Sci* 275:283–295, 1978.
144. Salfelder K, Mendelovici M, Schwarz J: Multiple deep fungus infections: Personal observations and a critical review of the world literature. *Curr Top Pathol* 57:123–177, 1973.
145. Scheer M, Opelz G, Terasaki P, Hewitt W: The association of disseminated coccidioidomycosis and histocompatibility type. *13th Interscience Conference on Antimicrobial Agents and Chemotherapy*. Washington, DC, Am Soc Microbiol, abstract 157, 1973.
146. Schmidt RI, Howard DH: Possibility of *C. immitis* infection of museum personnel. *Pub Health Rep* 83:882–888, 1968.
147. Schwarz J: Laboratory infections with fungi, in DiSalvo A (ed): *Occupational Mycoses*. Philadelphia, PA, Lea & Febiger, 1983, pp 215–227.
148. Scogins JT: Comparative study of time loss in coccidioidomycosis and other

respiratory diseases, in *Proc Symp Coccidioidomycosis*. Public Health Service Publ. no. 515, 1957, pp 132–135.

149. Seeliger HPR, Sturde HC: *Coccidioides*-Mykose (coccidioidomycosis). *Intern Welt* 7:29–65, 1984.
150. Shafai T: Neonatal coccidioidomycosis in premature twins. *Am J Dis Child* 132:634, 1978.
151. Sievers M: Disseminated coccidioidomycosis among southwestern Indians. *Am Rev Respir Dis* 109:602–612, 1974.
152. Sievers ML: Prognostic factors in disseminated coccidioidomycosis among southwestern Indians, in Ajello L (ed): *Coccidioidomycosis: Current Clinical and Diagnostic Status*. Miami, Florida, Sumposia Specialists, 1977, pp 63–78.
153. Sievers ML: Coccidioidomycosis and race. *Am Rev Respir Dis* 119:839, 1979.
154. Smale LE, Birsner JW: Maternal deaths from coccidioidomycosis. *JAMA* 140:1152–1154, 1949.
155. Smale LE, Waechter KG: Dissemination of coccidioidomycosis in pregnancy. *Am J Obstet Gynecol* 107:356–361, 1970.
156. Smith DT, Harrell ER Jr: Fatal coccidioidomycosis: A case of laboratory infection. *Am Rev Tuberc* 57:368–374, 1948.
157. Smith CE: Epidemiology of acute coccidioidomycosis with erythema nodosum. *Am J Pub Health* 30:600–611, 1940.
158. Smith CE: Coccidioidomycosis. *Med Clin North Am* 27:790–807, 1943.
159. Smith CE: Coccidioidomycosis, in *Communicable Diseases, Preventive Medicine in World War II*, Vol. IV. Washington, DC, Office of the Surgeon General, Medical Department. U.S. Army, 1958, pp 285–316.
160. Smith CE: Reminiscences of the flying chlamydospore and its allies, in Ajello L (ed): *Coccidioidomycosis*. Tucson, Arizona, University of Arizona Press, 1967, pp xiii–xxii.
161. Smith CE, Beard RR, Rosenberger HG, Whiting EG: Effect of season and dust control on coccidioidomycosis. *JAMA* 132:833–838, 1946.
162. Smith CE, Beard RR, Whiting EG, Rosenberger HG: Varieties of coccidioidal infection in relation to the epidemiology and control of the disease. *Am J Pub Health* 36:1394–1402, 1946.
163. Smith CE, Pappagianis D, Saito MT: The public health significance of coccidioidomycosis, in *US Public Health Service* Publication no. 575, Atlanta, Ga, 1957, pp 3–9.
164. Smithline N, Ogden DA, Cohn AL, Johnson K: Disseminated coccidioidomycosis, in Ajello L (ed): *Coccidioidomycosis: Current Clinical and Diagnostic Status*. Miami, Florida, Symposia Specialists, 1977, pp 201–106.
165. Sotgiu G, Corbelli G: Micosi rare: Osservazione dei primi casi di isoteoplasmosi in Italia e di un caso di coccidioidomicosi. *Bull Sci Med (Bologna)* 127:85–92, 1955.
166. Sorensen RH: Survival characteristics of diphasic *Coccidioides immitis* exposed to the rigors of a simulated natural environment, in Ajello L (ed): *Coccidioidomycosis*. Tucson, Univ. of Arizona Press, 1967, pp 313–317.
167. Spark RP: Does transplacental spread of coccidioidomycosis occur? *Arch Pathol Lab Med* 105:347–350, 1981.
168. Stewart RA, Meyer KF: Isolation of *Coccidioides immitis* (Stiles) from the soil. *Proc Soc Exp Biol Med* 29:937–938, 1932.
169. Sturde HC: Skin test reactivity and residue of coccidioidal pulmonary infections in German airmen, in Einstein H, Catanzaro H (eds): *Coccidioidomycosis*. Washington, DC, National Foundation for Infectious Diseases, 1985, pp 43–46.
170. Swatek FE: Ecology of *Coccidioides immitis*. *Mycopathol Mycol Appl* 40:3–12, 1970.

171. Swatek FE: The epidemiology of coccidioidomycosis, in Al-Doory Y (ed): *The Epidemiology of Huamn Mycotic Diseases*. Springfield, IL, Charles C Thomas, 1975, pp 74–102.
172. Swatek FE, Omieczynski DT, Plunkett OA: *Coccidioides immitis* in California, in Ajello L (ed): *Coccidioidomycosis*. Tucson, University of Arizona Press, 1967, pp 255–264.
173. Swatek FE, Plunkett OA: Ecological studies on *Coccidioides immitis*: Experimental infections of wild rodents and animals other than mammals. *Pub Health Ser Publ* no. 575, 1957, pp 161–167.
174. Swatek LB, Swatek FE: Growth of *Coccidioides immitis* under marine conditions. Abstract F32. *Annual Meeting, Am Soc Microbiol*, 1978, p 318.
175. Symmers W St C: Cases of coccidioidomycosis seen in Britain, in Ajello L (ed): *Coccidioidomycosis*. Tucson, University of Arizona Press, 1967, pp 301–305.
176. Teel KW, Yow MD, Williams TW Jr: A localized outbreak of coccidioidomycosis in southern Texas. *J Pediatr* 17:65–73, 1970.
177. Tomlinson CC: Granuloma *Coccidioides*. *Med Clin North Am* 12:457–462, 1928.
178. Tomlinson CC, Bancroft P: Granuloma *Coccidioides*: Report of a case responding favorably to antimony and potassium tartrate. *JAMA* 91:947–951, 1928.
179. Tomlinson CC, Bancroft P: Granuloma *Coccidioides*; further observations on the use of antimony and potassium tartrate and the Roentgen rays in treatment: Report of an additional case. *JAMA* 102:36–38, 1934.
180. VanBergen W, Fleury FJ, Cheatle EL: Fatal maternal disseminated coccidioidomycosis in a nonendemic area. *Am J Obstet Gynecol* 124:661–663, 1976.
181. Vaughn JE, Ramirez H: Coccidioidomycosis as a complication of pregnancy. *Calif Med* 74:121–125, 1951.
182. Wegmann T, Plempel M: Das Krankheitsbild der Coccidioidomycose. *Deutsch Med Wochenscr* 99:1653–1656, 1974.
183. Werner SB, Pappagianis D, Heindl I, Mickel A: An epidemic of coccidioidomycosis among archeology students in northern California. *N Engl J Med* 286:507–512, 1972.
184. Werner SB, Pappagianis D: Coccidioidomycosis in northern California—an outbreak among archeology students near Red Bluff. *Calif Med* 119:16–20, 1973.
185. Westley CR, Haak W: Neonatal coccidioidomycosis in a southwestern Pima Indian. *South Med J* 67:855–857, 1974.
186. Willett FM, Weiss A: Coccidioidomycosis in southern California: Report of a new endemic area with review of 100 cases. *Ann Intern Med* 23:349–375, 1945.
187. Williot J: Apropros de deux observations de coccidioidomycose. *J Franc Med Chir Thorac* 20:545–555, 1966.
188. Wilson JW, Smith CE, Plunkett OA: Primary cutaneous coccidioidomycosis. *Calif Med* 79:233–239, 1953.
189. Winn WA: The treatment of coccidioidal meningitis. *Calif Med* 101:78–79, 1964.
190. Winn WA, Levine HB, Broderick JE, Crane RW: A localized epidemic of coccidioidal infection. *N Engl J Med* 268:867–870, 1963.
191. Woodruff WW III, Buckley CE III, Gallis HA, Cohn JR, Wheat RW: Reactivity to spherule-derived coccidioidin in the southeastern United States. *Infect Immun* 43:860–869, 1984.
192. Zimmer BL, Pappagianis D: Taxonomic and physiologic characteristics of *Coccidioides immitis*, in Schlessinger D, Leive L (eds): *Microbiology—1986*. Washington, DC, American Scoiety for Microbiology, 1986.

7—Immune Response to *Paracoccidioides brasiliensis* in Human and Animal Hosts

ANGELA RESTREPO M.

During the past decade, host-parasite interactions in paracoccidioidomycosis have received special attention (23). A number of studies conducted in both the natural host, humans, and in experimental animals have indicated the existence of an active interplay between host defenses and the microorganism's capacity to evade such defenses. From the standpoint of immunology, we have passed from the mere description of the tissue reactions to the study of the sequential steps in granuloma formation and the possible contribution of humoral and cellular factors to such a phenomenon. From the practical applications of serology and skin testing, we now find researchers engaged in studying the timing and significance of immune responses (42, 72, 88). Yet, we are still only beginning to understand the immunologic events that follow infection with *Paracoccidioides brasiliensis*. For progress to ensue, there is need of compiling and analyzing the available information so as to render it useful to those interested in infectious diseases in general, and in the mycoses in particular.

Definitions and Classifications

Paracoccidioidomycosis, a disease geographically limited to several Latin American countries, may be defined as a chronic disease of the adult male. It is manifested by involvement of the lungs, the reticuloendothelial system, the teguments, and the adrenal glands (3, 33). It is now accepted that the primary lesion occurs in the lungs after inhalation of the infective fungal propagule (63). A sizeable proportion of those infected remain asymptomatic and only a few show signs of overt disease (105). Many years may elapse between the initial contact and the manifestations of the disease process as revealed by those cases reported outside of the known endemic areas (60, 105, 110, 115).

Other important epidemiologic aspects are the following: Age distribution is peculiar as children (1.5%) and youngsters (8.8%) are rarely afflicted (3, 33). The disease, on the other hand, predominates in adults, especially those who are 30–50 years-old. Also notorious is the predominance of overt disease in male patients (1 : 15) (3, 33). Concerning the latter, it is interesting that the rate of infection as demonstrated by skin tests, is equal for both sexes (1, 60, 105, 110, 115).

Paracoccidioidomycosis afflicts an important proportion of the working populations of Brazil, Colombia, Venezuela, Ecuador, and Argentina; in the former country it constitutes an important public health problem. In endemic regions the estimated annual incidence of overt clinical cases is 1–3 per 100,000 inhabitants. This means 3,000–10,000 new cases per year for a population estimated to be 350 million. Although the disease can be diagnosed with relative facility, the clinical manifestations are compatible with those of tuberculosis, and, consequently, treatment is often delayed (2, 60, 105, 110, 115).

The host interactions with the fungus forms the basis for the present classification of this mycosis (80) as follows: when there is a balance between the two forces, the process is asymptomatic (paracoccidioidomycosis infection); however, the microorganism does remain latent and may, later on, give rise to endogenous reactivation and overt disease. If the balance is upset either during the earlier or the later stages of the host-parasite interactions, the disease becomes manifested. Depending on the host and on the quantity and/or virulence of the etiologic agent, the disease progresses and bcomes either acute (subacute) or chronic. The former is usually seen in children and young adults and has a poor prognosis. The chronic adult progressive form may remain localized in the lungs, with gradual involvement of the parenchyma, or it may disseminate to other organ systems (skin, mucosa, adrenals, liver, spleen, etc). With few exceptions, once overt disease has become manifested, therapeutic intervention is required to save the patient's life (2, 43).

Paracoccidioides brasiliensis is a dimorphic fungus, which grows as a mould in cultures maintained at room temperature and presumably also in nature. It grows as a yeast in the tissues of humans, experimental animals, and in cultures incubated at 37°C. In the latter phase, the fungus reproduces by multiple budding and acquires the characteristic "pilot's wheel" appearance. Although the fungus' natural habitat is exogenous to humans, it has not been determined with certainty; this fact has hindered the study of the early events of the host-parasite interaction, as well as the precise determination of the portal of entry. The tendency of the fungus to remain latent in tissue partly explains why epidemic outbreaks have not been reported. There is only limited information concerning the existence of hosts other than humans (60, 105).

Fungal Factors that Play a Role in the Expression of Virulence

It has been repeatedly demonstrated that isolates of *P. brasiliensis* vary in their capacity to produce infection in experimental animals (14, 54, 62, 67, 69, 111, 116). Few researchers, however, have investigated the reasons for such a variation; noteworthy among these are the studies by San Blas and coworkers (116, 117, 118). These authors have shown that when *P. brasiliensis* undergoes dimorphic transformation, a parallel modification in the constitution of the cell wall glucans takes place. The yeast cell wall contains α-1,3-glucan while in the cell wall of the mycelium, this polysaccharide is replaced by β-1,3-glucan. Because the yeast form is the one present in tissue, these authors have explored the possible role of the α-glucan in virulence; to this effect, they produced a series of mutants in which the particular glucan was either present or absent. They found that virulence, as determined by the ability to produce disseminated infection in experimental animals, was exhibited only by those isolates producing α-glucan (116, 117, 118). It is thought that the mural α-1,3-glucan present in the yeast cell wall cannot be degraded by phagocytic cells because they lack the necessary enzymes; consequently, the fungus is undamaged and escapes the host's first line of defense. It has been shown that avirulent isolates, those with limited α-glucan content, are digested faster by polymorphonuclear phagocytes than cells from virulent strains which have lots of α-glucan (117). The above results clearly indicate that α-glucan plays an antiphagocytic role.

Another study by the same group (118) revealed an important difference in the soluble fraction obtained from cell walls of mycelial and yeast forms. No major variation was noticed between the mycelial form of a virulent and an avirulent isolate; however, there was a change when the former isolate was reverted to the yeast form. The mycelium of this particular isolate had galactose, glucose, and mannose, whereas the yeast exhibited only mannose. It is possible that this immunogenic polysaccharide may also influence the host's response. To this effect, a recent publication indicated that a polysaccharide fraction isolated form *P. brasiliensis* cell wall induced granuloma formation and stimulated peritoneal macrophages. This fraction influenced the weight and health of the infected animals (120).

The lipid content and composition of four different isolates of *P. brasiliensis* was determined by Manocha (67). No correlation could, however, be established between total lipid or phospholipid and virulence of the various strains. More recently, Silva (119) investigated the role of lipids in granuloma formation; charcoal particles coated with lipid extracts and given intravenously evoked an intense pulmonary inflammation shortly after inoculation. Fractionation of lipids allowed separation of various fractions; those containing free fatty acids and triglycerides were shown to be most active. It was postulated that tissue reaction may depend on the chemical composition of the agent and that polysaccharides as well as lipids (120), might be able to evoke granuloma formation.

The yeast form of six different *P. brasiliensis* isolates was characterized recently by means of growth rate and pathogenicity for sensitive inbred mice (54). There was no correlation between mean generation time and ability to produce infection, as two strains that were similar in growth rate were the most and the least virulent of the isolates tested, respectively. Nor was there a correlation between age of the strain and pathogenicity. The authors concluded that genetic background of the mice and of the fungus influenced the outcome of the experimental infection (54).

Immune Responses in Humans

Considerable progress has been made in recent years in defining both the cellular and the molecular bases of host resistance to infection. The host defense system is complex and entails the coordinated activity of highly specialized cells and of their soluble mediators. However, it is still useful to classify host defenses into three major systems: humoral response, defense by the polymorphonuclear phagocyte (PMN), and cell-mediated immunity (97).

The Humoral Response

Humoral defenses include antibody responses and the activities of complement components, lymphokines and monokines, and immune complexes. These factors may function independently or in concert with each other or with cellular defense mechanisms (97, 114).

Antibody Production

Specific antibodies are regularly produced by patients with paracoccidioidomycosis, and serologic tests have been extensively used with the purpose of establishing reliable diagnostic methods. Because current knowledge has been recently reviewed (99), this topic will be treated only briefly here.

Most (80–95%) patients with active paracoccidioidomycosis have circulating antibodies detectable by complement fixation, agar gel immunodiffusion, counterimmunoelectrophoresis, indirect immunofluorescence, ELISA, erythroimmune absorption, and other tests (12, 26, 27, 31, 32, 37, 41, 68, 71, 76, 78, 90, 99, 100, 121, 124, 126). Furthermore, there is a good correlation between the severity of the disease process and the antibody titers, the latter being higher in patients with disseminated disease. Patients with limited organic involvement, as well as those responding to antimycotic therapy, present with lower titers. Relapses are often accompanied by increased antibody concentrations (22, 78, 91, 99, 100).

The fact that therapy results in decreased antibody formation, whereas relapses produce the opposite effect, illustrates the benefits of serologic testing for the evaluation and follow-up of patients with paracoccidioidomycosis (22, 68, 90, 99, 104). Antibodies may not disappear completely after therapy but may persist for years at low, stationary titers, even in patients whose lesions have healed and who appear in good health. This may well indicate the presence of a persistent antigenic stimulus (99, 100, 101).

Within normal limits, most of the currently available tests are considered specific and sensitive. The agar gel immunodiffusion test and its congeners are among the most specific procedures. Complement fixation, ELISA, immunofluorescence, and others appear more sensitive but less specific (26, 55, 99, 100, 101). Histoplasmosis antigens and sera are the cause of important cross-reactivity (93, 99). It should be remembered that the characteristics of the various tests only reflect the quality of the *P. brasiliensis* antigens used, many of which are crude preparations (12, 71, 91, 99, 125). Consequently, standardization of such antigens and of procedures is highly desirable.

Immunoglobulin Classes

Total immunoglobulin G (IgG) is elevated in most patients at the time of diagnosis and of the first year during therapy; a certain correlation was shown to exist between severity of the disease and IgG concentration (4, 9, 11, 28, 104, 112, 128). On the other hand, in most patients studied, total IgM was found to be within normal limits (9, 28, 84, 104, 112, 121). These findings indicate that paracoccidioidomycosis is not being diagnosed at the time of the primary infection but later when the IgM antibodies are leveling off and being replaced by those of the IgG class. Regarding IgA levels, some authors have indicated normal figures (28, 104), whereas others have reported either increased (11) or diminished levels (112). This interesting difference could be explained by the preferential mucosal involvement seen in certain patients; however, no studies have been done to corroborate this possibility. Some studies have revealed hypergammaglobulinemia E, especially in patients with severe disseminated disease (4, 127).

The indirect immunofluorescent techniques have allowed determination of the specific anti-*P. brasiliensis* antibodies in sera of patients. In these studies, antibodies of the IgG class have been detected in nearly all patients, of the IgA class in 61%, and of the IgM class in 33–68.0% of the patients (9, 11, 84). The three classes of specific antibodies were simultaneously detected in 17% of the cases, IgG plus IgM in 20%, and IgG and IgA in 18.0%. Immunoglobulin G alone was present in 40% of all patients studied. Anti-*P. brasiliensis* IgG antibodies were detectable in 95% of the patients (11). The latter study also indicated that IgG antibody levels correlated with the clinical forms of the disease; anti-*P. brasiliensis* IgG antibody titers were highest in patients with the acute, progressive form (83.4%). In contrast, patients with more limited organic involvement and better physiologic condition, had lower frequencies of IgG antibodies (58–68.0%). Immunoglobulin M antibodies were lower in patients already treated for the mycosis (11).

Attempts have been made to correlate total immunoglobulin concentration with the specific antibodies detected by the various diagnostic tests. Total IgG correlated well with the level of complement-fixing antibodies (28, 37, 59, 90, 112) and also with precipitating antibodies as detected by both tube precipitation and immunodiffusion tests (11, 28). Immunoglobulin A appeared also as a precipitating antibody (90). Immunoglobulin M antibodies were not found in the tube precipitation test (84), a procedure which is known to detect early cases (37). Yet, by immunofluorescence IgM anti-*P. brasiliensis* antibodies were detected in more than 50% of the cases; this finding did not, however, correlate with the duration of disease (84). The IgE class of immunoglobulins was shown to be elevated in severe cases, but specific anti-*P. brasiliensis* antibodies accounted for only 0.6% of the total IgE concentration (4, 127).

Fiorillo and Martinez (40) purified human anti-*P. brasiliensis* antibodies by sephadex columns and used counterimmunoelectrophoresis to determine the activity of the purified immunoglobulins. They found that only IgG-rich fractions were able to reproduce the results previously obtained with the corresponding whole serum, that is, production of one or more precipitin arcs. Sera with normal or elevated concentrations of IgM, IgA, or those with low IgG levels, were unreactive.

It is clear that in active paracoccidioidomycosis there is no deficiency of antibody production, on the contrary, there is a polyclonal activation of the humoral immune system, with a close relationship existing between increased antibody production and severity of the disease (11, 104). When specific therapy is instituted and the disease is brought under control, immunoglobulin levels, especially those of the IgG class, return to normal levels (104, 112).

Role of Antibodies

Antibodies have been shown to be protective against a variety of infections caused by extracellular microorganisms. Among other functions, antibodies promote opsonization and activate the complement system (97, 114). In paracoccidioidomycosis, however, the evidence argues against effective protection. Thus, and as discussed previously, the highest antibody titers are found in those patients with severe disease. The obvious ineffectiveness of those antibodies detectable by the usual serologic tests, does not rule out the possibility that other antibodies with a protective function do exist and could, perhaps, have been formed in response to antigens not permanently expressed by the fungus and which may be undetectable by the usual diagnostic antigens.

As an example, in vitro studies (18) have shown that incubation of yeast cells in the presence of hyperimmune mouse serum or patient serum plus complement, resulted in lysis of an important proportion (30–50%) of fungal cells. It has been recently shown (95) that anti-*P. brasiliensis* lytic antibodies can be detected in various clinical forms of paracoccidioidomycosis. Although these antibodies attempt to destroy the fungus, their protective role in defense has not been confirmed.

It is also interesting that in patients, elevated antibody titers and polyclonal immunoglobulin activation coincided with diminished cell-mediated immune responses (4, 72, 73, 79, 90, 104, 112, 121). This pattern changed when the pathologic alterations were brought under control by appropriate therapy (104).

Antibodies have various possible roles in the overall immune response. They may act as opsonins in the phagocytic process, kill the offending microorganism, activate the complement cascade, participate in the formation of immune complexes, or exert inhibitory functions on cell-mediated immunity (97, 114).

Recent studies by Carvalhaes (23) demonstrate that antibodies may, indeed, constitute an important element of defense. Mouse strains known to be high and low antibody producers, were infected with *P. brasiliensis*. The highest mortality and the most extensive dissemination occurred in low-antibody producers. Furthermore, transfer of ascitic fluid from high-producer animals brought about increased resistance. Attractive as they are, these results may also indicate high and low genetic susceptibility of the mouse strains to the fungus.

It has been demonstrated that in patients, the presence of high serum antibody titers (1:512–1:1024), correlates with increased in vitro phagocytic activity of the patients PMNs, at least in the initial stages (attachment and ingestion) of the disease process (102). Further stages, such as intracellular digestion, appeared not to be mediated by antibodies (44). In experimental animal infection antibodies were shown to promote phagocytosis by peritoneal macrophages (16).

Paracoccidioides brasiliensis activates the alternative complement pathway, but a direct relation between antifungal antibodies and complement activation has not been demonstrated (17). Soluble immune complexes have been detected in the sera from patients with the disease (5, 121); however, it has not been determined which of the immunoglobulin classes participates in this process. Nor has it been shown that the soluble serum factor involved in the blocking of T-lymphocyte function corresponds to an antibody.

In summary, circulating antibodies have only one apparent protective role, that of opsonins for the phagocytic process. From the practical point of view, however, their presence and detection in serologic tests facilitates the establishment of the diagnosis.

Complement System

Complement amplifies the humoral response and as such, various investigators have shown interest in its role in paracoccidioidomycosis. Riberio and Fava-Netto (109), titrated total contents and fractions C7 and C3 in the sera of patients with active disease. They found normal values for both total complement and C7. The C3 component was elevated. On the other hand, Silva et al (121) found decreased values of C3.

As previously mentioned, complement was shown to participate in the phagocytic process (18). Experiments revealed that although *P. brasiliensis* yeast cells were poorly phagocytosed in vitro by mouse peritoneal macrophages, addition of either homologous or heterologous fresh sera greatly enhanced the phagocytic ability of macrophages. The opsonic activity of such sera was eliminated by heating the sera at 56°C, addition of ethylenediaminetetraacetic acid (EDTA), cobra venom factor, and depletion of properdin or B factor. Conversely, ethylene-bis (oxyethylenenitirile) tetraacetic acid (EGTA)-treatment had no effect. These data indicate that the alternative pathway was involved in the increased phagocytosis noted, and that complement and specific antibodies cooperated in the process (17). It must be remembered that *P. brasiliensis* can activate the alternative pathway directly, without the intervention of antibody (17).

It has been suggested that the alternative and possible, also the classic, pathway could mediate some of the tissue alterations (cell migration, edema formation and phagocytosis) seen in patients with paracoccidioidomycosis (17). However, this hypothesis was not confirmed experimentally as normal, C5 defficient, and cobra venom-treated mice mounted the same tissue reaction once inoculated with the fungus. The latter two groups, however, exhibited less edema than controls (17, 19). Thus, in vivo activation of complement does not completely explain the histologic aspect of the lesions.

In vitro the fungus appears not to produce chemotactic substances that may attract phagocytes to the site of fungal deposition and multiplication. Apparently, the sequence of tissue reactions begins with the fungus activating the complement cascade; this results in cell migration and edema formation. Finally, phagocytosis by either PMNs or resident tissue macrophages occurs (17, 19, 42).

Immune Complexes

The prolonged antigenic stimulus occuring in chronic diseases may result in the formation of immune complexes (5, 6, 11). Circulating *P. brasiliensis* antigens have indeed been demonstrated in the sera of patients with the disease (113). Consequently, it was not surprising to find that circulating immune complexes exist in paracoccidioidomycosis, because both antibodies and antigen are present in the circulation (5, 113, 121). The Clq-binding technique detected complexes in patients with the mycosis, whether active or inactive. The Raji cell radioimmunoassay, on the other hand, was more specific as it detected complexes mostly in patients with active and severe disease. Furthermore, a relationship was established between impaired cell-mediated immunity and circulating immune complexes (5, 121). It has been postulated that such complexes represent one of the factors responsible for deficient T-cell-mediated immunity; as such, the complexes would act directly on the effector system or indirectly by inducing suppressor cells (5). In one study (121), circulating immune complexes were associated with decreased levels of the C3 factor of complement, suggesting that such a factor was involved in complex formation.

If circulating immune complexes form regularly, one would expect that their deposition in target tissues would cause damage. However, there are no alterations that could be attributed to such a process, unless one considers the pulmonary damage commonly observed in paracoccidioidomycosis. Alternatively, complexes need not necessarely lead to immune damage, but may be involved in antigen elimination and immune regulation (5).

According to Silva et al (121), in paracoccidioidomycosis the antigen-antibody complexes would be of high molecular weight and formed in the presence of antibody excess. Such complexes do not induce vasculitis but appear to promote granuloma formation. To account for both continued antibody production and immune complex formation, it would be necessary to have a persistent antigenic stimulus, which would be provided by the fungus or its products. Also, antiidiotype antibodies could result in similar prolonged stimulation. More work is needed to prove this hypothesis (121).

Plasma Inhibitory Factors

Various authors have found that certain plasma factors interfere with the expression of cellular immunity (4, 29, 30, 88, 89). Observations have been made concerning the effect of the patient's serum on lymphocyte blastogenic transformation; when autologous serum was used in this test, the transformation index was lower than the one obtained using normal AB serum. Incubation of lymphocytes from normal persons in the serum of patients showing the above suppressor effect, resulted in diminished blast transformation. The inhibitory factor disappeared with treatment, at a time when lymphocyte function had been restored (88, 89). The responsible factors have not been characterized, but there is some evidence indicating that antibodies (8, 19), immune complexes (5), or other factors (87) can be responsible for the suppression. It should be stated that studies by other authors have not confirmed the existence of inhibitory factors (104). A recent ultrastructural study (30) revealed that lymphocytes from patients with diffuse paracoccidioidomycosis exhibited morphologic abnormalities when incubated in autologous plasma which appeared to alter their biologic function. Furthermore, such abnormalities could be reproduced in normal lymphocytes by incubating them in plasma from patients with the mycosis.

As shown previously, immune complexes can also interfere with the expression of cellular immunity. Arango et al (5) showed that the serum of a patient with generalized infection and depressed lymphocyte responsiveness contained a factor capable of arresting transformation of normal lymphocytes. Preincubation of the patient's lymphocytes before stimulation restored their proliferative capacity; furthermore, immune complexes were demonstrated in the culture supernatant. This finding, as well as that of Musatti et al (89), clearly indicates a complex relation among the various cells and factors in charge of the humoral and cellular immune responses in paracoccidioidomycosis.

Phagocytosis by Polymorphonuclear Leukocytes and Macrophages: Natural Killer Cells

For PMNs to perform their role in host defense, they must be capable of carrying out highly coordinated activities, including margination along vascular endothelium, emigration through the capillary wall, chemotaxis, and phagocytosis. Polymorphonuclear phagocytes exert their final microbicidal role by means of both oxygen-dependent and independent mechanisms (97).

Phagocytosis of *P. brasiliensis* yeast cells by PMNs, macrophages, and giant cells is regularly observed in fresh preparations of pathologic specimens, such as sputum and pus, as well as in tissue sections (42). Some of the ingested yeasts appear deformed, whereas others continue to multiply inside the phagocytes. Consequently, the microorganisms are not always killed as a result of the encounter.

In vitro studies using circulating PMNs obtained from patients and control persons, revealed no difference in the rate of phagocytosis (adherence and ingestion) (102). When the phagocytic cells were incubated in the patient's serum, containing antibodies, instead of normal human serum, there was an increase in the phagocytic index, as well as in killing of the fungus (102). The sera used in these experiments were fresh, and consequently the complement system also may have intervened.

Studies by Goihman-Yahr et al (44, 45) revealed that although phagocytosis was normal, there were important alterations in the ability of the patient's PMN to lyse the engulfed yeast cells. Such alterations were not modified by the use of either normal or immune sera. It also was demonstrated that those phagocytes with impaired digestive capacity came from patients with severe organic involvement, whereas those cells from patients in better clinical condition resulted in death of the fungus. Their work also showed that a high phagocyte/fungus ratio resulted in adequate killing. This type of ratio may well be encountered in vivo. Arechavala et al (6) found that PMNs from patients had increased phagocytic activity for *Candida albicans* after appropriate treatment. The increase was more pronounced at the time of diagnosis in patients who were severely ill.

It has recently been shown that in mice previously vaccinated with *P. brasiliensis*, peritoneal PMNs were able to lyse a significant proportion of the yeast cells, especially when such PMNs had been elicited by intraperitoneal injection of the corresponding fungal antigen (70). Furthermore, it was shown that the killing accomplished by such cells correlated with their ability to produce an enhanced oxidative burst. The authors postulated that in *P. brasiliensis*-sensitized hosts, the inflammatory reaction so frequently observed in tissue is the result of PMNs activation for significant killing of the pathogen (70).

Recent in vitro studies by McEwen et al (69) indicated that the yeast phase of the fungus was susceptible to hydrogen peroxide (H_2O_2) but at a concentrations higher than those obtained in the body; however, addition of halides augmented the lethality of the H_2O_2 system and made it compatible with the in vivo activity. It is therefore possible that the impaired digestive capacity could be related to suppression of the phagocyte respiratory burst or to inhibition of the phagosome-lysosome fusion. The latter aspect has been explored by electron microscope studies, using mouse peritoneal macrophages (16). It was found that although the macrophages readily ingested the fungus, growth was not halted but continued and resulted in death of the phagocyte. No fusion of the phagosome with the lysosome occurred.

The roles played by antibodies and complement on the phagocytic process have already been mentioned and shown to be important in the initial (adherence, ingestion) and later (digestive) stages (17, 18).

Mouse peritoneal cells that have been induced by inoculation of yeast cells in the peritoneal cavity, were capable of producing a soluble factor. Such a factor induced an in vivo chemotactic stimulus for PMNs (19). Complement was shown not to play a role in the PMN influx induced by intraperitoneal inoculation, as C5-deficient mice or cobra venom factor-treated animals could still evoke PMN accumulation. Characterization of the factor has revealed that it is produced by adherent cells and has a molecular weight of approximately 15,000 daltons, corresponding to a peptide. Addition of puromycin to the adherent cell population inhibited production of the factor. Previous depletion or inhibition of the activities of histamine, serotonin, prostaglandins, leukotrienes, and coagulation system did not result in altered PMN accumulation, indicating that the factor described does not correspond to any of the above substances (19).

Taking into consideration that the primary lesion occurs in the lungs, various authors have analyzed bronchoalveolar fluids from patients with paracoccidioidomycosis (13, 46). One study (13) revealed that irrespective of the chronicity of the pulmonary process, there was an accumulation of PMNs, an event that occurs seldom in other granulomatous conditions. It was observed that although these cells outnumbered lymphocytes, their efficacy in protecting the host was not apparent. The fungicidal capacity of bronchoalveolar exudate cells was reduced in patients, both in vitro in the presence of yeasts taken from cultures and in vivo with the patient's own fungus (46).

Natural killer cells may still be another cellular mechanism of defense. Jimenez and Murphy (53) have shown that naturally occurring, nonphagocytic cells, classified as NK cells, are capable of arresting the growth of *P. brasiliensis* yeast cells. NK activity is present in the lungs of mice. If this activity could also be demonstrated in the human lung, NK cells would certainly play a role in the infectious process by controlling fungal multiplication at the site of the primary infection.

The Cellular Response

The clinical and immunologic study of numerous patients with paracoccidioidomycosis clearly indicates that there is a spectrum of immunopathologic responses (6, 42, 43, 72, 74, 89, 112). Patients appear distributed in three categories: the hyperergic pole, the anergic pole, and the intermediate zone. Patients in the former category are able to mount a granulomatous response, posses functional T-lymphocytes, and have low titers or no circulating anti-*P. brasiliensis* antibodies; usually, fungal cells are scarce in the affected tissues. In the anergic pole, granulomas are not formed, T-lymphocytes have impaired functions, and fungal antibodies are detected at high titers. At the site of lesions, *P. brasiliensis* yeast cells are numerous and in active multiplication. In the intermediate zone, patients have either impaired or preserved T-cell-mediated immune functions and antibodies are absent or detectable at low titers (80).

The hyperergic pole is represented by patients who spontaneously resolve their primary infection (65), or by those who, aided by prompt therapy, can control the disease process. The anergic pole is regularly observed in severely compromised patients, most of whom exibit the juvenile type of progressive disease, but also by others who have the chronic, progressive adult disease with multiple organ lesions. In between these two extremes, one finds cases exhibiting characteristics of the two polar forms (42, 43, 80, 112). Lacaz et al (59) summarized the characteristics of these types in relation to various features Table 7-1).

Measurement of cell-mediated immune responses has been conducted in patients by skin testing for delayed hypersensitivity (DTH), dinitrochlorobenzene sensitization (DNCB), lymphocyte transformation test (LTT), and migration inhibitory factor (MIF), using both homologous and heterologous

TABLE 7-1. Characteristics of the Polar Types of Human Paracoccidioidomycosis*

Feature	Hyperergic Type	Anergic Type
Predominant clinical manifestations	Chronic, subclinical to mild, localized, adult form	Acute to subacute, severe, disseminated, juvenile form
Sites of extrapulmonary involvement	Mucocutaneous lesions	Mononuclear macrophage system
Histopathology	Compact granulomata	Necrotizing lesions, loose granulomata ± suppuration
Yeast cells in lesions	Scarce	Numerous
Cell-mediated immunity	Normal, intact	Impaired, depressed
Antibody titers	Low to intermediate	Elevated
Immune complexes	Rare	Present
Prognosis	Good	Poor

* Adapted from Lacaz et al. (59).

fungal antigens (paracoccidioidin, candidin), as well as nonspecific mitogens like phytohemagglutinin M (PHA). Studies also have assessed numbers of circulating T-lymphocytes and, more recently, characterization of T-cell subpopulations (8, 86, 87).

Skin Testing

This is the oldest of the tests and it has been used both diagnostically and with the purpose of determining previous contact with the fungus in normal populations of the endemic areas. As a diagnostic tool, paracoccidioidin skin testing soon demonstrated that not all patients reacted positively. Epidemiologic surveys revealed that a certain proportion of healthy persons recognized *P. brasiliensis* antigens indicating that a subclinical infection had taken place (1, 39, 63).

Cutaneous hyporeactivity is a common characteristic of patients with active, progressive disease (88). Skin test studies carried out in patients have all revealed that patients with severe disease such as the progressive juvenile and the adult progressive form fail to react to paracoccidioidin, candidin, and PHA intradermal tests. In contrast, patients with restricted, unifocal dissemination or localized disease, tend to give positive intradermal tests (4, 72, 74, 79, 86, 89, 104). There is a clear trend of conversion from nonreactive to reactive after successful therapy (2, 4, 6, 92, 104, 106, 107).

The histopathologic study of the skin at site of the intradermal test with paracoccidioidin, has revealed an Arthus-type reaction, instead of the typical delayed hypersensitivity (121). It has been shown that intradermal paracoccidioidin tests peak at 24 hours, not at 48 hours (79). Although there is variation in the proportion of patients who failed to react with skin test antigens (from 30–70%), this could, in part, be attributed to the type of antigen used (39, 63, 106). To some extent, the differences observed may be related to the varying severity of the disease.

Dinitrochlorobenzene Sensitization

This procedure has been used by several workers (4, 5, 9, 73, 74, 86, 89). Their results are in close agreement, and show that 70% of the patients with active disease failed to become sensitized. In one study, patients with inactive disease were also tested, and it was found that the proportion of cases not becoming sensitized was lower (40%) (4).

Lymphocyte Transformation Test

This is one of the in vitro tests more frequently used to assess the immune competence of patients. Initially used by Mendes et al (74), the LTT was shown to be depressed (both to PHA and paracoccidioidin) in active patients (4, 79, 86, 89, 104, 112, 121). Costa et al (29) found that lymphocyte PHA-mediated blastogenesis was more frequently reduced in active patients with disseminated disease than in those with lesions restricted to the lungs. The former group consisted of patients with serious impairment of their general condition. Mota et al (86, 87) also found that there was marked impairment of the LTT to both PHA and paracoccidioidin; these authors subdivided their patients according to the degree of organic involvement (chronic, chronic mixed forms, and acute progressive form), but they found that all three groups were equally immune depressed.

Some studies have attributed the degree of LTT hyporeactivity to inhibitory factors present in the patient's plasma. Musatti et al (89), Arango and Yarzabal (4), and Costa et al (29, 30) found that if lymphocytes were cultured in the patient's autologous plasma, one encountered LTT percentages below the lower limit of confidence for normal individuals. When the same lymphocytes were cultured in AB plasma, the blast transformation index increased. Lymphocytes from normal persons incubated in patient's plasma, also exhibited reduced LTT in comparison to values obtained in normal AB serum. These studies also revealed that LTT approaches normal values after therapy or are normal to start with in patients with healed, inactive disease (4, 29, 30, 89).

When lymphocytes from patients with disseminated infections were cultured in autologous plasma, microscopic alterations (fewer blast cells which were deeply stained) were detected. Normal morphology and increased blast cells were found when the lymphocytes were cultured in homologous serum (29, 30). This finding tends to support the hypothesis of a plasma factor as the cause of impaired LTT (88). According to Mota (87), the suppressor activity appears to be related to products liberated by the patient's cultured macrophages (lymphokines).

Leukocyte Migration Inhibition

This in vitro test for lymphocyte function has been used by Mok and Greer (79), Musatti et al (89), Silva et al (121), and Mota et al (86). No complete agreement has been found, as one study showed that all patients, symptomatic and asymptomatic, had positive reactions of PHA (79). From the remaining studies none revealed altered reactivity, with 50–70% of the tests being positive (88, 89). When *P. brasiliensis* was the antigen used, the results of the various studies were in accordance. As expected, leukocytes from normal controls were not inhibited in their normal migration. Silva et al (121) demonstrated that active patients were hyporeactive in the MIF test with PHA. They did not react with paracoccidioidin, and, as such, patients behaved as if they have had no previous contact with the fungus.

Total Numbers of T-Lymphocytes and E-Rosette Forming Cells

Regarding absolute T-lymphocyte numbers, significant differences have been reported between healthy controls and patients with paracoccidioidomycosis, the lower figures predominating in adult patients with chronic forms (4, 86, 89, 104, 121) of the disease.

Concerning E-rosetting, percentage values have shown no major changes, albeit a decrease was noted in a group of patients both before and after therapy (104). The same study revealed diminished total number of lymphocytes. Silva et al (121) showed that diminished activity of the T-lymphocytes persisted after therapy. Other investigators have reported normal total lymphocyte counts (4, 6, 8, 89, 121).

Disseminated mycotic infections are able to produce changes in the normal regulatory mechanisms. Attempts also have been made to classify T-lymphocytes according to their helper and suppressor activities. One study found that the latter type of T-cells were within normal limits (121). However, more precise investigations using monoclonal antibodies (85, 86) indicated a decreased helper/suppressor ratio (CD4/CD8) in the peripheral blood of 60% of the patients with chronic and acute progressive paracoccidioidomycosis. Those patients with acute (subacute) forms had larger suppressor cell populations than did patients with the chronic type of disease. It has been suggested that the altered CD4/CD8 ratio might be related to the depressed cellular immune response exhibited by patients with this mycosis. Recently, Mota (87) found a significant increase in the percentage and total numbers of T-lymphocytes, both suppressor and cytotoxic. Thymic and "null" cells were elevated too.

Correlation of Tests Measuring Cell-Mediated Immune Responses

Not all the procedures mentioned coincide in any one patient; actually, there are discrepancies among them. This should not be surprising because some of these tests need cooperation between B- and T-lymphocytes, whereas others may reflect the functional activity of a particular cell population, or be induced by soluble lymphocyte products (86). Consequently, the differences in T-cell function indicated by several in vivo and in vitro tests may well reflect the extent and severity of the fungal process.

Interactions Between Humoral and Cellular Immunity

The results of the various investigations mentioned clearly demonstrate that in paracoccidioidomycosis there is lack of equilibrium between the cellular immune responses mediated by T-lymphocytes (which are depressed) and those mediated by B-lymphocytes (manifested by increased antibody production). This uneven relation is, in turn, expressed by varying degrees of clinopathologic alterations, with the more pronounced disequilibrium occurring in severely compromised patients (80, 86, 88).

The causes for the immune imbalance have not been clearly defined. Data suggest various possibilities : 1) decreased numbers of active T-lymphocytes; 2) presence of certain plasma factors which inhibit expression of cellular immunity; 3) increased populations of suppressor T-cells; 4) immune suppression due to circulating immune complexes; 5) production of suppressor factors by the fungus; 6) predisposing genetic factors; and 7) polyclonal activation of B-lymphocytes, including hyperimmunoglobulinemia E (4, 6, 86, 88) and others. It is clear, however, that paracoccidioidomycosis patients do not all exhibit the same type of immune disequilibrium but present a spectrum of immunoregulatory perturbations, many of which resolve with treatment (4, 6, 74, 86, 87, 88, 104).

During the past decade, efforts have been made to classify paracoccidioidomycosis as an entity with polar and intermediate forms. This classification takes into consideration the immunologic behaviour of the host (42, 80, 88, 89). Significant impairment of cell-mediated immune responses, polyclonal activation of B-lymphocytes, immune complexes, and numerous fungal cells in lesions are found in the severest forms (anergic pole). Varying degrees of effective cell-mediated responses, normal T-lymphocyte functions, granuloma formation, and scarce numbers of fungal cells are found in patients with subclinical infections or in those patients with chronic, nonlethal paracoccidioidomycosis (hyperergic pole). A gamut of clinical manifestations occurs between the two extremes (6, 86, 88). A significant proportion of the patients can be assigned to the anergic, nonimmune pole at the time of diagnosis, but they move toward the immune pole under the influence of specific therapy (104, 112). Consequently, the clinicoimmunologic manifestations exhibited by the patient reflect his or her overall resistance to fungal invasion.

Histopathology

The morphologic alterations found in the tissue of patients with paracoccidioidomycosis do not greatly differ from those observed in other chronic inflammatory and granulomatous conditions. The only finding that distinguishes paracoccidioidomycosis is the presence of the etiologic agent (3, 42).

Paracoccidioidomycosis is predominantly a chronic and progressive infection that tends to exhibit periods of regression and exacerbation which in turn, result in different histologic presentations. Yet, the inflammatory process evoked by *P. brasiliensis* is relatively uniform in all organs affected and consists of either epithelioid granulomata or of exudating, necrotizing lesions, both of which may coexist in certain cases.

Epithelioid granulomata may be either compact or loose; the former presents firm nodules with both Langhans and foreign body giant cells, central suppuration, lymphocytes, macrophages, plasmocytes, and eosinophils. Usually the fungal cells are few, multiply little, and appear degenerated. The loose granuloma, on the other hand, is ill defined and maintains its epithelioid configuration with variable numbers of giant cells. Exudative inflammation, characterized by edema and congestion, is an important component of this particular tissue reaction. Cellular composition is similar to those of compact granulomata with the PMNs tending to be more numerous (3, 42).

In some deep organs, destructive inflammation with exudation and necrosis occurs. The predominanting cell is also the PMN. Its presence confers to the lesion a suppurative aspect, one which exhibits varying degrees of liquefaction. Usually, large numbers of small, actively multiplying fungal cells are observed in the suppurative lesions (3, 42).

Necrotizing reactions can be associated with epithelioid granulomata, the latter being more apparent on the periphery of the necrotic areas. Fibrosis becomes an important and, at times, intense component of the tissue reaction. Fibrosis is usually found around the epithelioid granulomata or the necrotic areas and replaces them progressively (3, 42, 123).

By the time the patient seeks medical attention, the mycotic process is already well established. Consequently, both exudative-purulent and productive-granulomatous lesions are present. The former pattern is seen in patients with the acute (subacute) progressive, juvenile forms, and is characterized by a poor prognosis due to the body's low defenses. The productive granulomatous lesions, on the other hand, are reported to occur mainly in the adult chronic progressive form. Patients in this group usually respond well to specific therapy (3, 42). Experimental evidence indicates that the granuloma evoked by *P. brasiliensis* is intimately connected to the host's cellular immune response (52), with the two polar types (hyperegic and anergic) being observed regularly. Lacaz et al (59) summarized the characteristics of these types in relation to various features (Table 7-1).

In a recent histopathologic study (123) done using biopsy specimens of skin and mucosal lesions obtained from patients with active paracoccidioidomycosis, it was found that granulomatous inflammation and suppuration was a common denominator to these cases. Affected tissues eliminated the fungus by means of pseudoepitheliomatous hyperplasia and transepidermic elimination; the latter function was aided by formation of progressive edema and exocytosis. Although several phagocytic cells were present in the lesions (PMNs, epithelioid, Langhans, and foreign body giant cells), only Langhans giant cells were able to ingest *P. brasiliensis*. There was, however, no evidence for intracellular killing of the fungus. These results indicate that the host's response to fungal invasion is multifactorial but not always effective.

Recently, attempts have been made to determine the constitution of the immunoregulatory T-cells in peripheral blood and in tissue obtained from the lesions of patients with the disease. Using monoclonal antibodies, Mota et al

(85, 86, 87) and Bacchi et al (8) found great variability in cell numbers and subsets with no specific relationship between T-helper and T-suppressor populations in blood and tissue. The ratio of helper-suppressor cells in tissue was high, indicating predominance of the former subset. In blood, this same ratio was lower but by no means constant. It was concluded that the underlying regulatory mechanism in the lesion was independent of that in peripheral blood. Obviously, much remains to be done before we clearly understand the interreactions between the tissue's defensive system and the invading capacity of the microorganism.

Influence of the Genetic Background

Genetic characteristics do not appear, at first glance, to play an important role in susceptibility to paracoccidioidomycosis. Familial cases are rare and appear to be linked to common exposure and not to heredity (33, 60, 115). It has been observed that immigrants to the endemic areas tend to develop severe disseminated disease (3, 60), irrespective of their race. This indicates that lack of exposure, which could have resulted in acquired resistance, rather than genetic susceptibility is important. All races acquire the disease in similar proportions and in relation to occupation and area of residence (60).

However, the possible role played by genetics is presently under study. Blood groups and HLA antigens have been determined in a series of patients. The B blood group was found to predominate in Brazilian but not in Colombian patients (75, 81). Regarding HLA types, the B40 antigen was present in a significant proportion of Brazilian but not in the Colombian or Venezuelan patients (47, 61, 81). In Colombia, HLA-A9 and B13 were the predominating specificities, with the former being detected more often in patients with the progressive pulmonary type of disease (81). In Venezuela (47) antigen B12 had a much higher frequency in patients in comparison to the controls. Thus, the results are not clear-cut.

As will be discussed in the section on experimental animal infection, genetic traits were implicated in susceptibility of certain mice breeds to infection with the fungus (20).

Resistance Conferred by Hormones

Of late, a new factor in resistance to paracoccidioidomycosis has come into focus, namely, sex hormones. This tropical disease is diagnosed much more frequently in males than in females, at a ratio of 13 : 1–78 : 1. When the disease is manifested in prepubertal patients, there are no significant differences based upon sex (60, 63, 105). Furthermore, skin testing with paracoccidioidin in normal populations of the endemic areas, has revealed that paracoccidioidal infection occurs at equal proportions in males and females (11, 63, 105). This means that contact with the fungus occurs equally in males and females. In females, however, they control the infection and hinder its progression into overt disease.

Paracoccidioides brasiliensis has been found to produce a protein that selectively binds 17-β-extradiol and successfully competes with it (64). Binding results in inhibition of the normal, temperature-mediated mycelial-to-yeast transformation. The inhibition occurred at concentrations compatible with physiologic hormonal levels. No other natural estrogen investigated has caused this alteration. A similar effect has been observed by the synthetic compound diethylstilbestrol (DES) (108), which is also active in vivo.

It has been postulated that in menstruating women, circulating estradiol binds to the infective *P. brasiliensis* propagule (mycelial fragments, conidia), and by so doing temporarely blocks the mycelial-to-yeast transformation process. During this time, specific defenses become available, cooperating in the destruction of the fungus or in controlling its tissue multiplication (64, 108). These interesting findings have not been confirmed in animals, where male and female mice appear equally susceptible (20, 111).

Immune Responses in Experimental Animals

Because some aspects of the host-parasite interaction are not amenable to study in patients with paracoccidioidomycosis, for example, early immune responses, importance of inoculum size, virulence of particular isolates, effect of age, etc., animal studies acquire particular importance.

To be useful, an animal model should include a knowledge of the genetic makeup of the animal strain used, feasibility of using routes of inoculation that mimick the natural infection in humans, production of a disease similar to the one observed in humans, and, finally, information concerning the immune responses of the chosen animal. These criteria are only partially fulfilled by some of the animal systems that have been used. The historical aspects as well as a more detailed account of all experiments conducted in animals have been reviewed by Iabuki et al (52).

The animals most frequently used have been the hamster and the mouse. In both, the degree of lesion formation depends on various factors such as the particular fungal isolate used (14, 62, 116); the type and viability of fungal cell used as inoculum (mycelial, yeast) (52, 103); the age, breed, and sex of the animal (14, 20, 34); the size of the inoculum (14, 58); and the route of inoculation (52). As indicated in Tables 7-2 and 7-3, a number of variations have been studied. Most animals were adult males, but not all were genetically characterized. Immunosuppression or vaccination was frequently used to establish or modulate the mycotic process. Several forms of inoculation were used and, with one exception, all animals were infected with yeast cells, probably because of the difficulty in obtaining homogeneous suspensions of the mycelial phase (52, 62, 103).

TABLE 7-2. Paracoccidioidomycosis: Experimental Mouse Studies Emphasizing Pathogenesis and/or Immune Responses

Strain	Sex	Age	Special Characteristics	Route of Infection	*P. brasiliensis* Inoculated as	Reference
CD	M	Adult	Corticosteroid treated	IV	Yeast	Linares and Friedman, 1972[62]
Swiss	M	Adult	Corticosteroid treated	IN	Mycelium	Restrepo, 1976[103]
Swiss	M	Young	Vaccinated, non-vaccinated	IP	Yeast	Moscardi and Franco, 1980, 1981[82,83]
Swiss	M, F	Young	None	ITr	Yeast	De Faveri et al, 1982[34]
RJ	M	Adult	Irradiated, cyclophosphamide	IP	Yeast	Kerr et al, 1982[56]
BALB/c	M, F	Adult	Nu/nu, Nu/+, +/+	IP	Yeast	Robledo et al, 1982[111]
BALB/c	M	Adult	Nu/nu, Nu/+	IV	Yeast	Miyaji et al, 1983[77]
BALB/c B10.A, A/SN, C57B1/10	M, F	Adult	None	IP	Yeast	Calich et al, 1983[18]
BALB/c	M	Young	None	IN	Yeast	Brummer et al, 1984[14]
BALB/c	M	Adult	Untreated, ketoconazole treated	IN	Yeast	Hoyos et al, 1984[50]
BALB/c	M	Adult	None, vaccinated, nonvaccinated	IN	Yeast	Catañeda, 1985[24]
BALB/c	M	Adult	None	IN	Yeast	Bedoya et al, 1986[10]
Swiss	M	Young	Vaccinated, non-vaccinated	IP IV	Yeast	De Faveri et al, 1986[36]

IN, intranasally; IV, intravenously; IP, intraperitoneal; Itr, intratracheal; ID, intradermal; IT, intratesticular.

TABLE 7-3. Paracoccidioidomycosis: Experimental Studies Emphasizing Pathogenesis and/or Immune Response in Animals Other than the Mouse

Animal Studied	Strain	Sex	Age	Special Characteristics	Route of Infection	*P. brasiliensis* Inoculated as	Reference
Hamster		M	Adult	None	IT	Yeast cells (from biopsy)	Guimaraes, 1951[49]
Hamster		M	Adult	None	IP	Yeast	San Blas et al, 1977[116]
Hamster		M	Adult	None	IT	Yeast	Iabuki and Montenegro, 1979[51]
Hamster		M	Adult	None	IT	Yeast	Peracoli et al, 1982[96]
Hamster		M	Adult	Levamizole treated	IT	Yeast	Rezkallah-Iwasso et al, 1984[98]
Rat	Wistar	M	Adult	None	IP	Yeast	Gosis and Negroni, 1981[48]
Rat	Albino	M	Adult	Silica-treated, untreated	IP	Yeast	Kerr et al, 1983[57]
Guinea pig	Albino	M	Adult	None	IC	Yeast	Negroni et al, 1979[94]

IC, intracardiac; IP, intraperitoned; IT, intratesticular.

Studies in Normal Animals

Experiments have been conducted in several animal species to obtain models paralleling the human disease. We will review only those studies focusing on the immune responses.

Hamster

The hamster was used in 1951 by Guimaraes (49) and found to be susceptible. Important studies using the intratesticular route have since been conducted (51, 96). Sequential observations revealed that after 24 hours postinoculation, tissue responses were nonspecific, exudative, and characterized by edema and PMN accumulation. After 36 hours, PMNs diminished in number and began to be replaced by macrophages. The latter cells organized themselves in loose nodules, and at day 5 multinucleated giant cells were present. Epithelioid granulomata soon became established; the center of the nodule showed suppuration, and simultaneously lymphocytes and plasma cells were noticed.

Throughout this process, fungal cells were easily detectable, although some appeared degenerated. In suppurative macrophagic lesions there was a large number of yeast cells, usually small and actively engaged in multiplication. When compact, epithelioid granulomata became apparent, the number of yeast cells decreased, budding was less active, and some of the cells appeared broken. Degenerated fungal cells predominate in fibrotic foci (51, 96). The precise relationship among size, abundance of fungal sporulation, and type of tissue reaction has not been established. There are no reports on the variation in size and number of buds of any particular *P. brasiliensis* isolate. These aspects merit study.

In certain animals the disease process did not heal but exacerbated, instead causing "loosening" of the formerly compact granulomata. Necrotic foci also appeared about this time. Concomitantly, there was an explosion of fungal growth, with predominance of small yeast cells. Dissemination then ensued and the regional lymph node became involved, reacting with the production of large numbers of plasma cells. In fact, antibody titers were at their peak at this stage. Necrotic foci appearanced and persisted until the end of the infectious process. It is not known why the hamster is more prone to develop disseminated disease rather than the mouse (51, 52).

Cell-mediated immunity, as assessed by lymphokine production in the MIF test and using PHA and *P. brasiliensis* antigen, was studied; animals reacted normally to the former mitogen up to the 10th week postinoculation, after which reactivity gradually disappeared and the test became negative. *Paracoccidioides brasiliensis* antigen produced a positive test after week 1, that peaked by weeks 7–10, and faded in a manner similar to that described for PHA (51, 52).

There was adequate correlation between depression of cell-mediated immunity (CMI) and loosening of compact granulomata, both events becoming noticeable at the time of fungal cell explosion. It has been postulated that the compact epithelioid granuloma represents the best defense the host has against fungal invasion. Once this capacity is lost, as shown in the hamster model, the fungus thrives, the granuloma dissolves, and the host loses the battle (51).

With this postulate in mind, immune reconstitution with levamizole was attempted by Rezkallah-Iwasso et al (98). When this treatment was given during the early stage of the experimental infection, treated animals were able to form epithelioid granuloma and developed heightened CMI responses. If levamizole was administered at a later stage, when the animal was already immunosuppressed, treatment had little effect. This clearly shows that in the hamster model the host-parasite interation is dimorphic. During the first stage the host controls the infection by walling off the microorganism inside the epithelioid granulomata. During the second stage and probably due to diminished cellular immune defense, the fungus proliferates and the animal dies with disseminated infection.

Mice

Mice, if immunologically competent, tend to develop a self-limited infection regardless of route of inoculation; the intensity of the infection is, however, dose-dependent (14, 52). One of the pioneer works by Mackinnon (66) revealed that the intranasal route led to progressive lung lesions and to extrapulmonary dissemination. The author postulated, for the first time, that paracoccidioidomycosis is acquired by inhalation, with the lungs being the site of the primary infection and all other lesions secondary to the original process.

Moscardi and Franco (82, 83) studied by histologic and immunologic parameters the course of intraperitoneal infection in Swiss mice. They found that the peritoneal process was chronic and progresed steadily for the first 4 weeks; after this time, the tissue response, formerly characterized by exudation and necrosis, changed and healing began. Simultaneously, there was marked destruction of fungal cells. After 16 weeks, lesions were small and exhibited scarring, fibrosis, and there were few fungal cells. Dissemination to liver and lungs occurred early after inoculation (1–4 weeks), but it was a restricted, nonprogressive event. Immunologic studies showed detectable antibody levels after 2 weeks, with peak titers at week 4, at the time when the peritoneal process was improving. Antibody titers decreased afterwards. Delayed hypersensitivity response as measured by foot pad testing, fluctuated from positive (week 1 to 4) to negative (weeks 8 to 16), and after this time they became reactive once more. Despite the fact that lesions were healing and both DTH and antibody responses were present, there was no granuloma formation.

De Faveri et al (34) studied the host-parasite interaction in Swiss mice infected intratracheally with yeast cells. Here again, the experimental disease proved limited and progressed slowly, with dissemination occurring infrequently and reaching only the nearby lymph nodes. Sequential histopathologic studies, as well as measurements of humoral and CMI responses, were carried out regularly. Lesions were initially exudative, nonspecific, and rich in PMNs, leading to a pneumonitis after 15 days. Contrary to what was found in the intraperitoneal-infected mice, in this study epithelioid granuloma became noticeable at 30 days and persisted for the entire observation period (1 year). Antibodies were detected after 2 weeks, peaked between days 30–60, and became nondetectable by the end of the study. Positive CMI responses (footpad and MIF tests) were recorded after 15 days, peaked between 60–90 days, and persisted for the rest of the observation period. This particular study showed a better correlation between granuloma formation and CMI responses. The major variation between experiments was the route of inoculation, and, consequently, one may conclude that the respiratory route, a more natural way to acquire the infection, reflects the pattern of the pathologic events observed in humans (34).

In 1984, Brummer et al (14) infected young and adult BALB/c mice by the intranasal route using an inoculum mostly composed of single yeast cells of quantitated viability. In this manner, the model avoided the variability represented by the presence of either nonviable cells or groups of cells; dead cells can probably act as imunogens and groups of cells may be too large to reach the alveolar lumen. This study determined that age was critical for the infectious process to take place, as immature animals (3–4 weeks of age) rapidly developed a lethal infection, whereas adult mice (7–8 weeks old) had a chronic, disseminated, nonlethal disease. Despite the fact that the inoculum was high for both groups of animals ($5–10 \times 10^6$), the results of the study parallel the human situation. It is well-known that the most severe cases of paracoccidioidomycosis, those with an acute or subacute course, occur in children. Adults, on the other hand, tend to develop a chronic, progressive disease (80).

Brummer et al (14) also studied the histopathology and the immune responses in these two groups of animals and found that the acute and chronic forms were distinct. The acute form showed consolidated bronchopneumonia with large numbers of PMNs and fungal cells. The chronic form had an acinonodular pattern, granulomata were present during the whole of the infectious process, and fungi were relatively few and appeared degenerated. Preliminary studies concerning CMI responses revealed that during this same period, spleen cells but not lymph node cells had significantly depressed responses to Con A in comparison with those cells obtained from uninfected mice. At 12 weeks, however, such responses were normal in infected animals. The results indicate that immunosuppression had occurred at a time when the disease process was not severe.

In a series of studies conducted by Castañeda (24), who used the model already described (14), modified by the use of an animal-passage isolate for inoculation purposes. Immune responses were assessed during the course of the progressive lung disease. Determinations of the fungal load present in the lungs and the spleen were made at regular periods. At the same time, humoral and cellular responses (LT and DTH) were measured. It was found that antibody response was intact throughout the experiment (26 weeks). In contract, there was a depression of immunity in vivo and in vitro, to homologous as well as to heterologous antigens (sheep red blood cells) and to mitogens (Con A). Immunoregulation studies revealed that the percentages of T- and B-cells in the peripheral blood (PB) of infected mice were similar to those in normal mice. In vitro, however, PB cells from infected mice depressed the response of PB cells from normal mice to Con A. Treatment of PB cells from infected animals with anti-Lyt-2.2 antibody plus complement, abolished the observed depression. Immune serum containing anti-*P. brasiliensis* antibodies given to mice before or after infection, regulated the induction or expression of DTH to the homologous antigen (24).

Using the same model of Brummer (14), Bedoya et al (10) explored the histopathologic responses of the chronic, disseminated experimental disease produced by the intranasal inoculation of yeast cells in BALB/c mice. Sequential autopsies were done from 0 hours–20 weeks postchallenge. Controls included noninfected animals, which exhibited no tissue reaction. In infected mice lung pathology became noticeable 3 hours postinoculation and persisted for the observation period. There was an initial bronchopneumonic process characterized by PMN accumulation. The infiltrate changed in cell composition with time and lymphocytes, macrophages, histiocytes, and plasmocytes appeared later. Granulomata were noticed at around the 5th week postchallenge, with multinucleated giant cells being noticed at 9 weeks. The lung process reactivated at this time, and the pulmonary lesions became permanent for the rest of the observation period.

The studies by De Faveri et al (34) and Bedoya et al (10) do not fully agree. The former concluded that mouse infections were self-limited and nondisseminating, whereas the latter indicated a progressive disease, apparently controlled by host defenses at the beginning with exacerbation occurring later. There were methodologic variations in the two studies that could explain the differences, for instance, mouse strain, age, route of inoculation, and inoculum preparations.

Other Animals

Guinea pigs were used in the past as models for studying paracoccidioidomycosis. In 1961, Fava-Netto et al (38) demonstrated that the intratesticular inoculation produced an array of histologic changes, leading to tissue necrosis. When this happened, circulating antibodies were at their peak. In contrast, when fibrosis began to replace the active lesions, antibody production declined.

More recently, Negroni et al (94) experimented with this animal using the intravenous route. A disseminated infection developed, the severity of which was at its maximum 8 weeks postchallenge. Circulating antibodies were present at an earlier time (2–4 weeks), whereas the DTH became positive later (4–6 weeks). That is, immune reactivity was well established before the peak of dissemination had occurred. No relation between immune defenses and progression of the infection could be established, but the guinea pigs were not isogenic. In this study, 13.5% of the animals failed to develop lesions, although circulating antibodies and DTH reactions were demonstrated.

Other animals, such as rats, wild rodents, and cold-blooded animals have been sporadically used but the results of the corresponding studies have not been revealing (48, 52).

Genetic Susceptibility of Mice to Experimental *Praracoccidioides brasiliensis* Infection

The genetic background may have important consequences on the infectious process; consequently, Calich et al (20) attempted to define this point. Groups of female mice of various lineages (BALB/c, B10.A, C57B1/10, A/SN) were inoculated intraperitoneally with yeast cells of known viability and the animals were observed for 592 days; mortality was the criterion chosen to assess susceptibility. Infected animals had shorter survival times than the noninfected controls. Of importance, BALB/c mice had a shorter survival time than 57B1/10 or A/SN animals, but such time was similar to that of the B10.A mice. Also interesting was the significantly higher survival rate shown by strain A/SN in comparison to the remaining groups of animals. This strain is deficient in C5, and, consequently, it appears that this complement factor is not crucial in resistance (15, 20). Because C57B10 and B10.A, which had different survival times, are congenital and only have a variation in the H2 locus, susceptibility to the fungus appears independent of this locus.

The histopathologic picture of the infection in B10.A and A/SN strains of mice also was studied (16). It was found that both types of animals, whether male or female, experienced disseminated disease with well-defined granulomata at the inoculation site as well as in the epiplon, intestines, mesenteric areas, liver, spleen, kidney, and diaphragm. However, 10 weeks after challenge, the B10.A animals developed further dissemination (lungs, brain, face), something not observed in the A/SN mice. Macrophage activity and prompt influx of inflammatory cells appeared to help in controlling the microorganism. The above differences certainly point toward the need to further explore genetic composition as a determinant factor in resistance. Calich (21) concludes that resistance to pathogenic fungi is related to factors of both the host and the parasite. In humans, it is extremely difficult to explore racial susceptibility, because natives of the endemic countries are usually of mixed origin (60, 63). However, immigrants, specially orientals, tend to develop severe forms of paracoccidioidomycosis (3, 33).

In Vitro Immune Studies Using Animal Cells or Fluids

McEwen et al (69) have shown that in vitro *P. brasiliensis* yeast cells are susceptible to the components of the myeloperoxidase system. Later (70), it was shown that BALB/c mice previously vaccinated with *P. brasilensis* and which had been inoculated with killed *P. brasiliensis* yeast cells, produced PMNs that destroyed the fungus at a higher rate than those from control, nonvaccinated animals. This indicates that the immune system is important in controlling fungal invasion.

Calich (16) has shown that stimulated mouse peritoneal macrophages avidly ingest *P. brasiliensis* yeast cells but that fungal destruction was less efficient and depended upon the time and the yeast-macrophage ratio. Despite being actively phagocytosed, the yeast cells were able to multiply and, at times, destroy the macrophage. By electron microscopy it has been shown that there was no fusion of the lysosomes with the phagocytic vacuole.

An in vitro study (17) explored the reasons for the inefficient phagocytosis of mouse macrophages. Homologous antibodies, as well as fresh normal serum, had phagocytosis-promoting activity in the system. Complement also was implicated, because treatments known to destroy it resulted in loss of the opsonic activity. *Paracoccidioides brasiliensis* was shown to activate the complement system especially, but not exclusively, by the alternative pathway. Consequently, some of the tissue reactions observed in vivo such as cell migration, edema formation, and phagocytosis could be attributed to complement activation. In an attempt to define this, the fungus was inoculated into the subcutaneous tissue of normal mice (15). After 48 hours there was a massive PMN infiltration. However, such a histologic picture remained constant if the mice were pretreated with cobra venom factor or if the fungus was inoculated on C5-deficient mice. Thus, neither complement activation nor a fungus-secreted factor seemed to explain the initial tissue events.

Recently, Jimenez and Murphy (53) explored the possible role of natural killer (NK) cells against *P. brasiliensis* yeast cells. They used murine splenic cells and treated the corresponding effector cells by different mechanisms. Using the chromium assay technique and in vitro growth inhibition, a correlation was shown between levels of NK cells and ability of effector cells to inhibit the in vitro growth of the fungus. The effector cell population responsible for the NK activity was further demonstrated to consist of nylon wool nonadherent cells, having no detectable Thyl-antigen or immunoglobulins but having the asilo-GM1 determinant on their surface. The data support the hypothesis that NK or NK-like cells are responsible for growth inhibition of the fungus. They suggest that these cells could play a role in limiting the growth of *P. brasiliensis* at the portal of entry, that is the lungs.

Studies in Animals Treated to Increase Normal Resistance

A series of experiments have been conducted to determine if antifungal treatment, previous vaccination, and treatment with drugs increasing the immune response exert favorable effects on infected animals.

Hoyos et al (50) used a BALB/c murine model of chronic pulmonary and disseminated paracoccidioidomycosis and treated some animals with the antifungal drug ketoconazole. At certain periods, circulating antibody and intradermal tests were done in control and treated mice. In controls, antibodies were first detected 77 days after infection, at the time when the animals were exhibiting severe disease. On the other hand, ketoconazole-treated mice did not produce detectable antibody levels at any time. There was no difference in dermal reactivity, which in both groups of animals peaked after 25 days following inoculation. Levamizole, a compound known to increase CMI responses, was used in hamsters by Rezkalla-Iwasso et al (98). In this particular model, the intratesticular inoculation of yeast cells produced a chronic, progressive, and lethal disease (51). The immunomodulating capacities of levamizole were assessed by intradermal tests and MIF assays. Antibodies were also determined. When levamizole was given early after the infection, MIF assays usually negative in untreated animals became positive for both antigens and remained so for prolonged periods. This was not the situation when levamizole was administered at a later stage of the experimental infection. However, levamizole did not affect the cutaneous responsiveness to *P. brasiliensis* antigen, as both groups tended to become skin test-negative with time. Concerning antibody titers there were no major differences among the two groups studied (98).

In the same study (98), it was further demonstrated that levamizole influenced the intensity and pattern of the inflammatory response. Early-treated hamsters produced and maintained for a long time compact, epithelioid granulomata lesions, which contained few fungal cells. Such a pattern was observed only sporadically in those animals receiving levamizole when the infectious process was already advanced. The authors concluded that the hamster model parallels the subacute juvenile form of the disease in humans, and that immunotherapy with levamizole may prove helpful in patients with this form of the disease. (98).

Attempts have been made to increase the resistance or to modify the course of the infection in experimental animals by vaccination with killed fungal cells. Moscardi and Franco (82) used Swiss male mice and divided them into four groups. One group was infected intraperitoneally with live yeast cells, another group served as the noninfected control, a third was sensitized intradermally with killed yeasts 4 weeks before intraperitoneal challenge with live cells, and a fourth group was sensitized with killed cells. Histopathologic studies were done and the immune response evaluated 1 week before sacrifice by skin testing and measuring antibody titers. The results indicated that sensitization with killed yeast cells had been successful. The animals developed intense DTH and had moderate antibody titers. In animals infected with live cells, antibodies were present but no DTH could be demonstrated. The animals sensitized before intraperitoneal infection had the highest antibody responses and maximal skin test reactions. The authors concluded that intraperitoneal infection acted as a booster dose for previously sensitized animals. Furthermore, these animals did not exhibit the immune depression described for nonvaccinated hamsters (96).

When attempting to correlate the heightened immune responses with the histologic aspects of the mouse lesions, Moscardi and Franco (82, 83) were unable to observe differences between newly infected and previously sensitized animals. Both groups of mice had a cellular infiltrate composed of neutrophils and macrophages, which surrounded the inoculated yeast, with no formation of epithelioid granulomata. In other words, there was no relation between DTH and acquired resistance to intraperitoneal challenge. However, a more recent study (7) indicated that previous immunization was protective as there was a positive correlation among heightened cell-mediated responses, restricted foci of infection, small numbers of fungal cells in granuloma, and resistance to infection.

De Farevi et al (35) continued the study of sensitized mice in order to characterize the immunologic inflammation evoked by *P. brasiliensis* antigens. Bentonite particles were coated with either a crude soluble yeast homogenate or a polysaccharide antigen and injected (intradermally or intravenously) in normal and previously sensitized animals. Uncoated bentonite was used as a control. In nonimmunized mice, both types of particles caused minimal, nonspecific local inflammation. In sensitized animals, *P. brasiliensis*-coated particles evoked an intense inflammatory reaction. In intradermally injected mice there was a cellular infiltrate composed of PMNs, macrophages, and lymphocytes together with early granulation tissue. In intravenous-sensitized animals, the infiltrate was characterized by PMNs and macrophages, as well as by incipient granuloma formation. None of the animals, however, was able to develop the typical epithelioid granuloma, despite the fact that previously sensitized mice had exhibited DTH to paracoccidioidin. It was suggested that in the absence of intact fungal cells, cellular immunity alone was not conducive to granuloma formation.

In a more recent study (36), De Faveri et al observed that *P. brasiliensis*-sensitized mice, which were skin test-positive, lost this hypersensitivity upon challenge with the homologous particulate antigen. These animals exhibited an intense pneumonitis, which was attributed to the development of lung hypersensitivity. To explore the reasons for this reaction, animals were immunized with the same particulate antigen and challenged intratracheally with live yeast cells. Nonimmunized animals were also challenged. In sensitized mice, pulmonary inflammation was intense and macrophages predominated. Fungal cells were scarce, the tissue reaction occurred promptly and lasted for a month, control animals had only focal lesions with PMNs but here, there were numerous fungal cells. It was suggested that pulmonary resistance is related to development of local (and systemic) DTH.

A different approach to the study of acquired resistance was taken by Castañeda (24). Initially this author determined the immune responses in BALB/c mice following sensitization with killed yeast cells. It was found that the concanavalin (Con A) LTT carried out with spleen and lymph node cells, was normal in all animals. The LTT test to *P. brasiliensis* antigen became apparent after week 1 and persisted for 3–5 weeks. Antibodies were demonstrated only during weeks 2 and 3 postvaccination. On this basis, intranasal challenge with live yeast cells was done postsensitization. Unsensitized animals were also challenged. Resistance was measured by determining the intensity of fungal proliferation in the lungs and spleen by counting colony-forming units (CFU) in a medium supplemented with growth factors (25). Cultures from lung homogenates obtained from vaccinated mice had significantly lower CFU than those from control animals. A similar picture was observed in the spleens. Consequently, previous sensitization allowed the animals to efficiently control fungal multiplication and resist pulmonary challenge. This resistance could, however, be abolished by a large challenge dose. Also, there was no clearance of the fungus from the tissues. The exact relationship among increased resistance and cellular and humoral responses was implied but not established.

Studies in Immunologically Incompetent Animals

The importance of the thymus in the defense against experimental *P. brasiliensis* infection was explored in two studies (77, 111). Robledo et al (111) showed that homozygous athymic nu/nu mice when challenged intraperitoneally with the fungus, developed a progressive disease that proved fatal, whereas thymus-containing (+/+) animals survived the challenge and had disseminated lesions only at the time of sacrifice, when 88% of the nu/nu littermates had already died. Histologic analyses revealed that tissues of the athymic animals were devoid of both epithelioid and giant cells and that true granulomata were absent. Inflammatory changes were observed in the lungs and liver but were unrelated to protection; the infection proved fatal in most animals. In contrast, tissues of the intraperitoneal-challenged, thymus-containing mice exhibited normal granulomatous lesions, which, furthermore, resolved spontaneously by the time of sacrifice.

In a subsequent experiment, the same investigators (111), attempted intraperitoneal challenge in nu/nu, nu/+, and +/+ animals, as wells as in a group of homozygous nu/nu mice that had received thymus transplantation. The animals behaved as described above; all of the nu/+ mice and most (approximately 85%) of the reconstituted mice, survived in comparison to 100% deaths in the nu/nu controls. Thus, thymus function conferred heightened resistance. It remains to be shown whether cell-mediated immunity or thymus-dependent antibody formation, or both, were the critical elements in host defense.

In the study by Miyaji and Nishimura (77), emphasis was placed on formation and killing function of granulomata. Using established lines of BALB/c, nu/nu, and nu/+ mice, these authors infected mice with *P. brasiliensis* yeast cells by the intravenous route. Based upon the microscopic appearance of the budding yeast as well as by the recovery of the fungus in culture from organ homogenates, these authors (77) concluded that the nu/+ mice were able to control the infection process; granulomata were apparent but fungal cells were scarce and appeared nonviable. By contrast, the nu/nu mice, although able to recruit mononuclear cells to form granuloma, were unable to prevent fungal multiplication. Cultures remained positive from homogenates of brain, kidneys, and lungs but became negative from the liver. The assumption was made that two factors played a key role in the defense, namely, the acute reaction mediated by PMNs and the CMI response which became established later. It is not clear, however, if the granuloma the authors describe in the nude mice, correspond to the classical description (and connotation) of the protective granuloma.

Mice immunosuppressed by various treatment schedules have been studied. Corticosteroid treatment in CDI normal mice was used by Linares and Friedman (62) and by Restrepo and Guzman (103). The former workers found that intranasally infected animals, pretreated with corticosteroides had a higher morbidity (61%) than normal controls (34%). In intravenous-infected mice such a difference was not observed. Histopathologically, no differences were observed between animals receiving corticosteroids and those that did not, except that the size of the lesions in the pretreated animals were larger.

Regarding the outbred mice studied by Restrepo and Guzman (103), corticosteroids were used to augment the rate of infection in animals injected intranasally with the mycelial phase. Using this method, 38% of the mice acquired progressive pulmonary disease, which disseminated to other organs in half of the animals.

Judging from the results of the latter two studies, corticosteroids tend to depress the natural resistance of normal mice to either phase of the fungus. However, it does not appear that this type of treatment renders the animals highly susceptible to fungal infection. This is in accordance with what is known in humans, as there is no relationship between steroid treatment and increased incidence of paracoccidioidomycosis (122).

Irradiation and cyclophosphamide treatments have been explored in RJ-1 intraperoneally infected mice (56). Control, uninfected animals were studied simultaneously. All mice, treated and untreated, developed lesions at the inoculation site. Metastatic lesions, however, were observed more frequently in irradiated (100%) and cyclophosphamide-treated (67%) animals than in controls (33%). It was also observed that both groups of treated animals exhibited more intense dissemination. Others (52) have indicated that macrophages appear to lose their capacity to metabolize phagocytized organisms, a fact that could explain the propagation of lesions to the viscera. Also, treatment with cyclophosphamide may disturb the immune system by delaying antibody formation and eliminating suppressor T-cells, thus aggravating the infection (56). These findings do not fully agree with the human situation as few cases have been reported in immunosuppressed hosts (122).

Attempts have been made to evaluate in rats, the role of macrophages in the local reaction evoked by intraperitoneal infection (57). Because silica is known to alter macrophage function, this compound was injected intraperitoneally before fungal inoculation. The results indicate that silica favors intraperitoneal colonization and dissemination to the lungs and other viscera. Furthermore, rats so treated exhibited poorly fibrotic lesions and numerous fungi. In control animals the infection did not disseminate, and in the circumscribed inflammatory areas few microorganisms were present. This study clearly demonstrated that macrophages play an important role as effector cells in the early experimental stages of infection and might also be implicated in natural resistance to infection (57).

In conclusion, animal experimentation allows for in depth interpretation of the host-parasite interactions. Such experimentation is also pointing toward provocative areas of future research, even if clear-cut explanations for all the normal responses are not yet in sight.

Acknowledgments

The author expresses her appreciation to Ms. Consuelo Agudelo for typing the manuscript and to Drs. Alvaro Henao and Juan G McEwen for their cooperation in organizing the text.

References

1. Albornoz MCG: Resultado de las encuestas epidemiológicas realizadas con paracoccidioidina en Venezuela. *Castellania* 3:37–40, 1975.
2. Albornoz MCG: Paracoccidioidomicosis. Estudio clĭnico e inmunológico en 40 pacientes. *Arch Hosp Vargas* 5-6:5–22, 1976.
3. Angulo-Ortega A, Polak L: Paracoccidioidomicosis, in Baker RD (ed): *The Pathological Anatomy of the Mycosis: Human Infections with Fungi, Actinomycetes and Algae*. Berlin, Springer-Verlag, 1970, pp 507–576.
4. Arango M, Yarzabal LA: T-cell dysfunction and hyperimmunoglobulinemia E in paracoccidioidomycosis. *Mycopathologia* 79:115–124, 1982.
5. Arango M, Oropeza F, Anderson O, Contreras C, Bianco N, Yarzabal LA: Circulating immunocomplexes and in vitro cell-reactivity in paracoccidioidomycosis. *Mycopathologia* 79:153–158, 1982.
6. Arechavala A, Robles AM, Finquelievich J, Negroni R: Estudio inmunológico de pacientes portadores de micosis sistémicas y las modificaciones producidas por el tratamiento. *Bol Acad Nac Med* Buenos Aires 59:59–73, 1981.
7. Bacchi M, Franco MF: Experimental paracoccidioidomycosis in the mouse. II. Histopathological and immunological findings after intravenous infection in the presence or absence of previous immunization. *Rev Soc Bras Med Trop* 18:101–108, 1985.
8. Bacchi M, Mota NGS, Lastoria JC, Mendes RP, Franco MF: Identificao de subpopulacoes linfocitaries no granuloma da paracoccidioidomicose com anticorpos monoclonais e tecnicas de imunoperoxidasa, in *Proceedings ISHAM*

International Colloquium on Paracoccidioidomycosis. Colombia, Medellín, 1986, p 105.
9. Barbosa JFC, Takeda HL, Chacha J, Cua LC, Fava-Netto C: Anticuerpos especificos das classes IgG, IgM, IgA para el *P. brasiliensis* dosados a traves de reacao de imunofluorescencia. *Rev Inst Adolfo Lutz* 41:120–126, 1981.
10. Bedoya V, McEwen JG, Tabares A, Uribe Jaramillo F, Restrepo A: Pathogenesis of paracoccidioidomycosis. Histopathological study of experimental murine infection. *Mycopathologia* 94:133–144, 1986.
11. Biagnoni L, Souza MJ, Chamma LG, Mendez RP, Marquez SA, Mota NGS, Franco MF: Serology of paracoccidioidomycosis. II. Correlation between class specific antibodies and clinical forms of the disease. *Trans Roy Soc Med Hyg* 78:617–621, 1984.
12. Blumer SO, Talbert M, Kaufman L: Rapid and reliable method for production of a specific *P. brasiliensis* immunodiffusion test antigen. *J Clin Microbiol* 19:404–407, 1984.
13. Boscardini RN, Brandao H, Bulla A: Bronchoalveolar lavage findings in pulmonary paracoccidioidomycosis. *Sabouraudia* 23:143–146, 1985.
14. Brummer E, Restrepo A, Stevens DA, Azzi R, Gomez AM, Hoyos GA, McEwen JG, Cano LE, de Bedout C: Murine model of paracoccidioidomycosis. Production of fatal acute pulmonary or chronic pulmonary and disseminated disease. Immunological and pathological observations. *J Exp Pathol* 1:241–255, 1984.
15. Burger E, Singer LM, Calich V: Role of C 5 in experimental murine paracoccidioidomycosis. *J Infect Dis* 152:425–425, 1985.
16. Calich VLG: Interaction of mouse peritoneal macrophages with *P. brasiliensis*. Abstract # 14, *Proceedings II Encontro Paracoccidioidomicose*. Brazil, Botucatú, 1983.
17. Calich VLG, Kipnis TL, Mariano M, Fava-Netto C, da Silva WD: The activation of the complement system by *P. brasiliensis* in vitro: Its opsonic effect and possible significance for an in vivo model of infection. *Clin Immunol Immuno Pathol* 12:20–30, 1979.
18. Calich VLG, Teixeira RVC: Antibody and complement-dependent cytotoxicity against *P. brasiliensis*. Abstract no. 15, *Proceedings II Encontro Paracoccidioidomicose*. Brazil, Botucatú, 1983.
19. Calich VLG, Vaz CAC, Burger E: PMN chemotactic factor produced by glass-adherent cells in the acute inflammation caused by *P. brasiliensis*. *Br J Exp Pathol* 66:57–66, 1985.
20. Calich VLG, Singer-Vermes LM, Siqueira AM, Burger E: Susceptibility and resistance of inbred mice to *P. brasiliensis*. *Br J Exp Pathol* 66:585–594, 1985.
21. Calich VLG: Experimental paracoccidioidomycosis: Mechanisms of resistance to fungi, in *Proceedings ISHAM International Colloquium on Paracoccidioidomycosis*. Colombia, Medellín, 1986, p 54.
22. Campos EP, Sartori JC, Hetch ML, Franco MF: Clinical and serologic features of 47 patients with paracoccidioidomycosis treated by amphotericin B. *Rev Inst Med Trop* São Paulo 26:212–217, 1984.
23. Carvalhaes MS, Silva WD, Birman EG, Sant'Anna ON, Abrahamshon P, Kipnis TL: Experimental paracoccidioidomycosis in high and low antibody-producer mice. I. Evolution of the disease; its correlation with the humoral immune response and the pattern of tissue lesions. *Ann Inst Pasteur (Immunologie)* 137C:127–141, 1986.
24. Castañeda E: Immunological studies in murine paracoccidioidomycosis. Doctoral disertation, University of California, San Francisco, 1985.
25. Castañeda E, Brummer E, McEwen JG, Stevens DA: A culture medium for *P. brasiliensis* with high plating efficience. *J Clin Microbiol* (in press).
26. Chamma LG, Fabio WF, Bacchi MM, Franco MF: Indirect fluorescent test for

detection of anti-*P. brasiliensis* antibodies using bentonite-coated particles. *Trans Roy Soc Trop Med Hyg* 77:181–184, 1983.
27. Conti-Diaz LA, Soma Moreira RE, Gezuela E, Gimenez AC, Peña MI, Mackinnon JE: Immunoelectrophoresis immunodiffusion in paracoccidioidomycosis. *Sabouraudia* 11:39–41, 1973.
28. Correa A, Giraldo R: Study of immune mechanisms in paracoccidioidomycosis. Changes in immunoglobulins (IgG, IgM, IgA). *Proceedings 1st Panamerican Symposium*, 1972. PAHO Scientific Publication no. 254, Washington, DC, pp 245–253.
29. Costa JC, Pagnano PMG, Bechelli LM, Fiorillo AM, Lima-Filho EC: Lymphocyte transformation test in patients with paracoccidioidomycosis. *Mycopathologia* 84:55–63, 1983.
30. Costa JC, Concalves RP, Pagnano PMG, Bechelli LM: Ultrastructure of lymphocytes from patients with paracoccidioidomycosis in the lymphocyte transformation test by phytohemaglutinin. *Mycopathologia* 93:155–161, 1986.
31. De Camargo ZP, Guesdon IL, Drouhet E, Improvici L: Sensitive tritation of antibodies to *P. brasiliensis* by erythroimmunoassay *Sabouraudia* 22:73–78, 1984.
32. De Camargo ZP, Guesdon IL, Drouhet E, Improvisi L: Enzyme-linked immunosorbent assay (ELISA) in the paracoccidioidomycosis. *Mycopathologia* 88:31–37, 1984.
33. Del Negro G, Lacaz CS, Fiorillo AM (eds): *Paracoccidioidomicose (Blastomicose Sul-Americana)*. São Paulo, Brazil, Sarvier Editores, 1982.
34. De Faveri J, Rezkallah-Iwasso MT, Franco MF: Experimental pulmonary paracoccidioidomycosis in mice. Morphology and correlation of lesions with humoral and cellular immune responses. *Mycopathologia* 77:3–11, 1982.
35. De Faveri J, Tamanini J, Tonolli L, Franco MF: Skin and pulmonary models using coated bentonite particles for the study of the inflammation evoked by *P. brasiliensis* antigens in previously immunized mice. *Sabouraudia* 22:477–486, 1984.
36. De Faveri J, Rezkallah-Iwasso MT, Franco MF: Pneumonite de Hipersensibilidad a antygeno de *P. brasiliensis*, in *Proceedings ISHAM International Colloquium on Paracoccidioidomycosis*, Medellín, Colombia, 1986, p 55.
37. Fava-Netto C: The immunology of South American Blastomycosis. *Mycopathol Mycol Appl* 26:349–358, 1965.
38. Fava-Netto C, Lacaz CS: Experimental South American blastomycosis of the guinea pig. An immunologic and pathologic study. *Pathol Microbiol* (Basel) 24:192–206, 1961.
39. Fava-Netto C, Guevara MAG, Costa EO: Contribucao a estudo imunologico de paracoccidioidomicose. Reacoes intradermicas en pacientes com dos antigenos homólogos e dos heterólogos. *Rev Inst Med Trop*, São Paulo 18:186–190, 1976.
40. Fiorillo AM, Martinez R: Naturaleza de anticorpos precipitantes especificos da paracoccidioidomicose revelados por contraimunoelectroforese. *Rev Inst Med Trop*, São Paulo 26:25–30, 1984.
41. Franco MF, Fava-Netto C, Chamma LG: Reacao de imunofluorescenĉia indirecta para o diagnóstico de Blastomicose Sul-Americana. *Rev Inst Med Trop*, São Paulo 15:395–398, 1973.
42. Franco MF, Montenegro MR: Anatomia patológica, in Del Negro G, Lacaz CS, Fiorillo AM (eds): *Paracoccidioidomycosis* (Blastomicose Sul-Americana). São Paulo, Brazil Sarvier Editores, 1982, pp 97–117.
43. Giraldo R, Restrepo A, Gutierrez F, Robledo M, Londoño F, Hernandez H, Sierra F, Calle G: Pathogenesis of paracoccidioidomycosis. A Model based in the study of 46 patients. *Mycopathologia* 58:63–70, 1976.
44. Goihman-Yahr M, Essenfeld E, Albornoz MC, Yarzabal L: Defect on in vitro

digestive ability of polymorphonuclear neutrophils in paracoccidioidomycosis. *Infect Immun* 28:557–566, 1980.
45. Goihman-Yahr M, Rothenberg A, Rosquete R, Avila Millan E, Albornoz MC, Gomez MH, San Martin B, Ocanto A, Pereira J, Molina T: A novel method for estimating killing ability and digestion of *P. brasiliensis* by phagocytic cells in vitro. *J Med Vet Mycol* 23:248–251, 1985.
46. Goihman-Yahr M, Rothenberg A, Avila EM, Rosquette R, Albornoz MC, Kanski A, Pereira K, Gomez MH, Román A, San Martin B: Las células fagocitarias. Su funcionamiento en las enfermedades granulomatosas producidas por agentes vivos. El modelo de la paracoccidioidomicosis. *Cien Tecnol Venezol* 2:183–198, 1985.
47. Gonzalez MM, Albornoz MC, Rios R, Prado L: HLA y paracoccidioidomicosis. *Cien Tecnol Venezol* 2:229–234, 1985.
48. Gosis A, Negroni R: Desarrollo de un modelo animal para el estudio de la paracoccidioidomicosis diseminada. *Rev Argent Micol* 4:5–9, 1981.
49. Guimaraes F: Infecao do hamster (*C. auratus*). Waterhouse, pelo agente de micose de Lutz (Blastomicose Sul-Americana). *Hospital* (Rio) 40:515–520, 1951.
50. Hoyos GA, McEwen JG, Brummer E, Castañeda E, Restrepo A, Stevens DA: Chronic murine paracoccidioidomycosis. Effect of ketoconazole on clearance of *P. brasiliensis* and immune response. *Sabouraudia* 22:419–426, 1984.
51. Iabuki KRC, Montenegro MR: Experimental paracoccidioidomycosis in the syriam hamster. Morphology, ultrastructure and correlation of lesions with presence of specific antigen and serum levels of antibodies. *Mycopathologia* 67:131–141, 1979.
52. Iabuki KRC, De Faveri J, Rezkallah-Iwasso MT, Peracoli MT, Mota NGS: Paracoccidioidomicose experimental, in Del Negro G, Lacaz CS, Fiorillo AM (eds): *Paracoccidioidomycose* (South American Blastomycose). Sarvier Editores, São Paulo, Brazil, 1982, pp 69–84.
53. Jimenez B, Murphy JA: In vitro effects of natural killer cells against *P. brasiliensis* yeast phase. *Infect Immun* 46:552–558, 1984.
54. Kaschino SS, Calich VLG, Burger E, Singer-Vermes ML: In vivo and in vitro characteristics of six *P. brasiliensis* strains. *Mycopathologia* 92:173–178, 1985.
55. Kaufman L: Evaluation of serological tests for paracoccidioidomycosis. Proceedings 1st. Panamerican Symposium. PAHO Scientific Publication no. 254, Washington, DC 1972, pp 221–223.
56. Kerr IB, da Costa SCG, Alencar A: Experimental paracoccidioidomycosis in immunosuppressed mice. *Immunol Lett* 5:151–154, 1982.
57. Kerr IB, da Costa SCG, Shaffer GVS, Lagrange H: Paracoccidioidomycosis in silica-treated rats. *Immunol Lett* 7:129–133, 1983.
58. Kerr IB, de Oliveira PC, Shaffer GV: Influence of inoculum size on the development of intraperitoneal paracoccidioidomycosis in rats. *J Infect Dis* 149:821, 1984.
59. Lacaz CS, Zamith VA, Del Negro G, Martins-Siqueira A: Aspects clinicos generales. Formas polares de la paracoccidioidomycosis. Particulari-dades Clĭnicas Infecto-juvenis, in Del Negro G, Lacaz CS, Fiorillo MM (eds): *Paracoccidioidomycosis* (South American Blastomycosis). Sarvier Editores, São Paulo, Brazil, 1982, pp 141–187.
60. Lacaz CS, Porto E, Costa-Martinez JE: (eds): *Paracoccidioidomycose*, in *Micologia Medica* (7th ed. Sarvier Editores, São Paulo, Brazil, 1984, pp 189–216.
61. Lacerda GB, Arce-Gomez B: HLA en paracoccidioidomicose. Proceedings 2nd Meeting Paracoccidioidomycose, Abstract no. 17, Botucatú, Brazil, 1983.
62. Linares LI, Friedman L: Pathogenesis of paracoccidioidomycosis in mice. *Infect Immun* 5:681–687, 1972.
63. Londero AT: Epidemiologia, in Del Negro G, Lacaz CS, Fiorillo AM (eds):

Paracoccidioidomicose (Blastomicose Sul-Americana). Sarvier, Editores, São Paulo, Brazil, 1982, pp 85–90.

64. Loose DS, Stover EP, Restrepo A, Stevens DA, Feldman D: Estradiol binds to a receptor-like cytosol binding protein and initiates a biological response in *P. brasiliensis*. *Proc Nat Acad Sci USA* 80:7659–7663, 1983.
65. Lopez R, Restrepo A: Spontaneous regression of pulmonary paracoccidioidomycosis. *Mycopathologia* 83:187–189, 1983.
66. Mackinnon JE: Blastomicosis Sudamericana evolutiva por via pulmonar. *Anal Fac Med*, Montevideo 44:355–362, 1959.
67. Manocha MS, San Blas G, Centeno S: Lipid composition of *P. brasiliensis*: Possible correlation with virulence of various strains. *J Gen Microbiol* 117: 147–154, 1980.
68. Martins-Siqueira A: Diagnostico imunologico, in Del Negro G, Lacaz CS, Fiorillo AM (eds): *Paracoccidioidomycosis*, (Blastomicosis Sul-Americana). Sarvier Editores, São Paulo, Brasil, 1982, pp 253–264.
69. McEwen JG, Sugar AM, Brummer E, Restrepo A, Stevens DA: Toxic effects of products of oxidative metabolism on the yeast phase of *P. brasiliensis*. *J Med Microbiol* 18:423–428, 1974.
70. McEwen JG, Brummer E, Stevens DA, Restrepo A: Effect of murine polymorphonuclear leukocytes on the yeast form of *P. brasiliensis*. *Am J Trop Med Hyg* 36:603–608, 1987.
71. McGowan KL, Buckley HR: Preparation and use of cytoplasmic antigens for the serodiagnosis of paracoccidioidomycosis. *J Clin Microbiol* 22:39–43, 1985.
72. Mendes G: Paracoccidioidomycosis (South American Blastomycosis) and keloid blastomicosis, in *Immunopathology of Tropical Diseases*, (1st ed). Sarvier Editores, São Paulo, Brazil, 1981, pp 107–118.
73. Mendes E, Raphael A: Impaired delayed hypersensitivity with South American Blastomycosis. *J Allerg* 47:17–22, 1971.
74. Mendes NF, Musatti CC, Leao RG, Mendes E, Napitz CK: Lymphocyte and skin allograft survival in patients with South American blastomycosis. *J Allerg Clin Immunol* 48:40–45, 1971.
75. Mendes RP: Frecuencia de sistemas sanguineos en doentes com paracoccidioidomicose. *Proceedings 2nd Meeting Paracoccidioidomicose*. Abstract no. 16, Botucatú, Brazil, 1983.
76. Mendes-Giannini MJS, Camargo ME, Lacaz CS, Ferreira AW: Immunoenzymatic absorption test for serodiagnosis of paracoccidioidomycosis. *J Clin Microbiol* 20:103–108, 1984.
77. Miyaji M, Nishimura K: Granuloma formation and killing functions of granuloma in congenitally athymic nude mice infected with *B. dermatitidis* and *P. brasiliensis*. *Mycopathologia* 82:129–141, 1983.
78. Mistreta T, Souza MJ, Chamman LG, Pinho SZ, Franco MF: Serology of paracoccidioidomycosis. I. Evaluation of the indirect immunofluorescent test. *Mycopathologia* 89:13–18, 1985.
79. Mok PWY, Greer DL: Cell-mediated immune responses in patients with paracoccidioidomycosis. *Clin Exp Immunol* 28:89–98, 1977.
80. Montenegro MRG: Clinical forms of paracoccidioidomycosis letter to the editor. *Rev Inst Med Trop*, São Paulo 28:203–204, 1986.
81. Montoya F, Restrepo M, Restrepo A: Blood groups and HLA antigens in paracoccidioidomycosis. *Sabouraudia* 21:35–40, 1983.
82. Moscardi M, Franco MF: Paracoccidioidomicose experimental do camundongo. I. Aspectos imunologicos de infeccao intraperitoneal. *Rev Inst Med Trop*, São Paulo 22:286–293, 1980.
83. Moscardi M, Franco MF: Paracoccidioidomicose experimental do camundongo. II. Infeccao intraperitoneal apos sensibilizacao previa. *Rev Inst Med Trop*, São Paulo 23:204–211, 1981.

84. Mota FT, Franco MF: Observacoes sobre a pesquisa de anticorpos IgM anti-*P. brasiliensis* por imunofluorescencia no soro de pacientes com paracoccidioidomicose. *Rev Inst Med Trop*, São Paulo 21:82–89, 1979.
85. Mota NGS: Studies on immune function and mononuclear cell subsets in human paracoccidioidomycosis abstract. ISHAM IX International Congress, Atlanta, 1985.
86. Mota NGS, Rezkallah-Iwasso MT, Peracoli MT, Audi RC, Mendes RP, Marcondes J, Marques SA, Dillon NS, Franco MF: Correlation between cell-mediated immunity and clinical forms of paracoccidioidomycosis. *Trans Roy Soc Trop Med Hyg* 79:765–772, 1985.
87. Mota NGS: Imunoregulacao na paracoccidioidomicose humana, in *Proceedings ISHAM International Colloquium on Paracoccidioidomycosis*. Medellín, Colombia, 1986, p 58.
88. Musatti CC: Imunidade celular, in Del Negro G, Lacaz CS, Fiorillo AM (eds): *Paracoccidioidomicose* (Blastomicose Sul-Americana). Sarvier, São Paulo, Brasil 1982, pp 119–126.
89. Musatti CC, Rezkallah-Iwasso MT, Mendes E, Mendes NF: In vivo and In vitro evaluation of cell-mediated immunity in patients with paracoccidioidomycosis. *Cell Immunol* 24:365–378, 1978.
90. Negroni R: Serologic reactions in paracoccidioidomycosis. *Proceedings 1st Panamerican Symposium*, 1972 PAHO Scientific Publication no. 254, Washington, DC, pp 203–208, 1972.
91. Negroni R, Negroni P: Antĭgenos del *P. brasiliensis* para las reacciones serológicas. *Mycopathologia* 34:285–286, 1968.
92. Negroni R, Robles AM: El valor pronóstico de la prueba cutánea en la paracoccidioidomicosis. *Med Cut Ibero-Latinoam* 6:453–458, 1974.
93. Negroni R, Iovannetti C, Robles AM: Estudio de las reacciones serológicas cruzadas entre antigenos de *P. brasiliensis* en *H capsulatum*. *Rev Asoc Argent Microbiol* 8:68–73, 1976.
94. Negroni R, Iovannetti C, Iglesia de Elias-Costa MR, Lescano J: Paracoccidioidomicosis diseminada del cobayo. *Rev Argent Micol* 2:5–10, 1979.
95. Nogueira MES, Mendes RP, Marques SA, Franco MF: Complement-mediated lysis: Detection of antibodies in paracoccidioidomycosis. *Brazil J Med* 19: 241–247, 1986.
96. Peracoli MRS, Mota NGS, Montenegro MR: Experimental paracoccidioidomycosis in the syriam hamster. Morphology and correlation of lesions with humoral and cell-mediated immunity. *Mycopathologia* 79:7–17, 1982.
97. Peterson PK: Host defense abnormalities predisponsing the patient to infection. *Am J Med* 76:2–10, 1984.
98. Rezkallah-Iwasso MT, Mota NGS, Gomez MCG, Montenegro MR: Effect of levamizole on experimental paracoccidioidomycosis of the syriam hamster. Immunology and histopahtologic correlations. *Mycopathologia* 84:171–180, 1984.
99. Restrepo A: Procedimientos serológicos en la paracoccidioidomicosis. *Adel Microbiol Enfermed Infec* 3:183–211, 1984.
100. Restrepo A, Moncada LH: Serologic procedures in the diagnosis of paracoccidioidomycosis. Proceedings International Symposium on Mycosis 1970. PAHO Scientific Publication no. 205, Washington, DC, pp 101–110, 1970.
101. Restrepo A, Moncada LH: Characterization of the precipitin bands detected in the immunodiffusion test for paracoccidioidomycosis. *Appl Microbiol* 28:138–144, 1974.
102. Restrepo A. Velez H: Efectos de la fagocitosis in vitro sobre el *P. brasiliensis*. *Sabouraudia* 13:10–21, 1975.
103. Restrepo A, Guzman GE: Paracoccidioidomicosis experimental del ratón inducida por via aerógena. *Sabouraudia* 14:299–311, 1976.
104. Restrepo A, Restrepo M, Restrepo F, Aristizabal LH, Moncada LH Velez H:

Immune responses in paracoccidioidomycosis. A controlled study of 16 patients before and after treatment. *Sabouraudia* 16: 151–163, 1978.
105. Restrepo A, Greer DL: Paracoccidioidomycosis, in Di Salvo A (ed): *The Occupational Mycoses*. Philadelphia, Lea & Febiger, 1983, pp 43–64.
106. Restrepo A, Cano LE, Tabares AM: A comparison of mycelial filtrate and yeast lysate paracoccidioidin in patients with paracoccidioidomycosis. *Mycologia* 84:49–54, 1983.
107. Restrepo A, Gomez I, Cano LE, Arango MD, Gutierrez F, Sanin A, Robledo MA: Postherapy status of paracoccidioidomycosis patients treated with ketoconazole. *Am J Med* (suppl. 1b): 53–57, 1983.
108. Restrepo A, Salazar ME, Cano LE, Stover EP, Feldman D, Stevens DA: Estrogens inhibit mycelial-to-yeast transformation in the fungus *P. brasiliensis*. Implications for resistance of females to paracoccidioidomycosis. *Infect Immun* 46:346–353, 1984.
109. Ribeiro MAG, Fava-Netto C: Complemento hemolitico total e os componentes C3 e C7 em pacientes de paracoccidioidomicose. *Rev Inst Med Trop* 23: 106–110, 1981.
110. Rippon JW: Paracoccidioidomycosis, in *Medical Mycology. The Pathogenic Fungi and the Pathogenic Actinomycetes*, 2nd ed. Philadelphia, WB Saunders, 1982, pp 459–483.
111. Robledo MA, Graybill JR, Ahrens J, Restrepo A, Drutz D, Robledo M: Host defenses against experimental paracoccidioidomycosis. *Am Rev Respir Dis* 125: 563–567, 1982.
112. Robles AM, Negroni R: Estudios inmunológicos en pacientes con micosis sistémicas. *Arch Argent Dermatol* 35: 61–86, 1985.
113. Rodriguez MC, Cassaguerra CM, Lacaz CS: Antigenemia in paracoccidioidomycosis. Probable demonstration of circulating antigen by counter immunoelectrophoresis test. *Rev Inst Med Trop*, São Paulo 26:285–287, 1984.
114. Root RK: Humoral immunity and complement, in, Mandell GL, Douglas RG, Bennett JE (eds): *Principles and Practice of Infection Disease (2nd ed)*. New York, Wiley and Sons, 1985, pp 31–57.
115. Rubinstein P, Negroni R (eds): *Micosis Broncopulmonares del Adulto y del Niño* (2nd ed). Editorial Beta, Buenos Aires, Argentina, pp 194–248.
116. San Blas G, San Blas F, Serrano LE: Host parasite relationship in the yeast-like form of *P. brasiliensis*. *Infect Immun* 15: 343–346, 1977.
117. San Blas G: The cell wall of fungal human pathogens: Its possible role in host-parasite relationship. *Mycopathologia* 79: 159–184, 1982.
118. San Blas G, San Blas F: Variability of cell wall composition in *P. brasiliensis*. A study of two strains. *Sabouraudia* 20: 31–40, 1982.
119. Silva CL: Granulomatous reaction induced by lipids isolated from *P. brasiliensis*. *Trans Roy Soc Trop Med Hyg* 79: 70–73, 1985.
120. Silva CL, Fazioli RA: A *P. brasiliensis* polysaccharide having granuloma-inducing, toxic and macrophage stimulating activity. *J Gen Microbiol* 131: 1497–1501, 1985.
121. Silva MR, Marques AJ, Campos DS, Taboada DC, Soares GH, Broscher HM, Vargens N, Cruz MQ, Labordhe NV, Rochas GL, Lima AO: Imunologia de paracoccidioidomicose. *An Brasil Dermatol* 56: 227–234, 1981.
122. Sugar A, Restrepo A, Stevens DA: Paracoccidioidomycosis in the immunosuppressed host. Report of a case and review of the literature. *Am Rev Respir Dis* 129: 340–342, 1984.
123. Uribe Jaramillo F, Zuluaga AI, Leon W, Restrepo A: Histopathology of cutaneous and mucosal lesions in human paracoccidioidomycosis. *Rev Inst Med Trop*, São Pualo 29: 90–96, 1987.
124. Yarzabal LA: Anticuerpos precipitantes especificos de la Blastomicosis Sud-

americana revelados por inmunoelectroforesis. *Rev Inst Med Trop*, São Paulo 13:320–327, 1971.
125. Yarzabal LA: Composición antigénica de *P. brasiliensis*, in Del Negro G, Lacaz CS, Fiorillo AM (eds): *Paracoccidioidomycosis* (South American Blastomycosis). Sarvier, São Paulo, Brazil, 1982, pp 59–67.
126. Yarzabal LA, Cabral NA, Santiago AR: Evaluación de una técnica especîfica de doble difusión en el diagnóstico de la paracoccidioidomicosis. *Acta Cient Venezol* 30:93–97, 1979.
127. Yarzabal LA, Desaint IP, Arango M, Albornoz MD, Campins H: Demonstration and quantification of IgE antibodies against *P. brasiliensis* in paracoccidioidomycosis. *Int Arch Allerg* 62:346–351, 1980.

8—Morphogenetic Transformation of Fungi

MAXWELL G. SHEPHERD

An extraordinary feature of the majority of human pathogenic fungi is that they exhibit dimorphism and in many cases pleomorphism. In addition it is common to find that the morphology of the fungus in the infected tissue is different from that of the propagule that initiated the infection. It is generally assumed, but not well established experimentally, that the morphogenesis accompanying the parasitic infection in some way confers a survival advantage on the fungus. Basic studies on the phenomenon of fungal morphogenesis are important for at least two reasons: firstly, to expand our understanding of the mechanism of mycotic pathogenicity, and, secondly, to use these fungi as relatively simple systems for studying eukaryotic differentiation. For a more detailed treatment of fungal dimorphism the reader is referred to the excellent monograph of Szaniszlo (133). This review summarizes the salient features of the different morphogenic forms of a number of the human pathogenic fungi and where possible relates these to the infection process.

Traditionally medical mycologists have used the term "dimorphism" to describe the ability of pathogenic fungi to grow in distinctly different morphologic forms in the saprobic and parasitic phases (61, 85). In this article morphogenetic transformation and dimorphism will be used to define vegetative phase transitions for those fungi capable of growing in at least two distinct morphologies. Many of the pathogenic fungi exhibit a number of distinct morphologic forms under different environmental conditions; in some cases several morphologies coexist in a particular environment. For example, *Candida albicans* can grow as budding yeast cells (blastoconidia), pseudohyphae (elongated yeast cells which appear as filamentous cell chains), true hyphae, and chlamydospores. Therefore, a more accurate general description for human pathogenic fungi is that they exhibit pleomorphism, although some species, for example, *Histoplasma capsulatum*, are restricted to dimorphic growth. Finally, care has been taken in this review not to use the term germination to describe the emergence by evagination of a hypha from a yeast cell. This process will be called germ-tube formation.

Dimorphism and Pathogenic Fungi

Medical mycologists have long had a special interest in dimorphic fungi and the term dimorphism has historically been used in reference to the fungi that cause systemic infections in humans with a yeast-like parasitic phase and a mycelial saprobic phase (2, 26). *Coccidioides immitis* is an exception because it forms spherules in tissue. Of the approximately 100,000 known species of fungi, only some 200 are pathogenic to humans: about 20 cause systemic infections, 20 are isolated from cutaneous infections, and the remainder are associated with opportunistic infections (104). These pathogenic fungi are classified in four of the six phyla of the kingdom Fungi: the Zygomycota, Ascomycota, Basidiomycota, and Fungi Imperfecti. All of the dimorphic pathogenic fungi discussed in this review belong to the phylum Fungi Imperfecti. Teleomorphs are known for *Blastomyces dermatitidis* and *Histoplasma capsulatum* which are classified in the genus *Ajellomyces*. The basic characteristics of this phylum are:

1. Vegetative growth occurs in either a unicellular or filamentous septate hyphal form.
2. Asexual reproduction is used as the basis for their classification.
3. Sexual reproduction is absent (21).

The taxonomy of many of the pathogenic fungi is refractory to further analysis because of their anamorphic life cycles. There are, however, reports of teleomorphic states for some of the emerging pathogenic fungi (73), which will lead to a better phylogenetic understanding of these species.

Generally the pathogenic fungi occur in nature as saprobes in soil, composts, and plants (74). However, the pathogenic *Candida* species are associated with warm-blooded animals, and indeed these fungi are unique among opportunistic pathogens because they are part of the normal flora of mucosal tissue.

The majority of animal mycoses are initiated by conidia (including yeast cells) making contact with, adhering to, and invading the host tissue. In the dimorphic fungi, conidia are asexual, nonmotile, usually deciduous propagules produced often either by fragmentation of hyphae or by developing at the tips and along the sides of conidiophores which may be distinct or hyphalike. The morphogenetic changes occur in the fungus after contact with the tissue, but the mechanisms of adherence, invasion, host response, and biochemical events stimulating morphogenesis are not well defined. It is tempting to speculate that the potentially infectious agent that originates outside the host (exopropagule) (27) and survives the defense system undergoes morphogenetic transformation to a cellular form, which is adapted to survive and propagate within or on the host.

General Features of Cell Wall Morphogenesis

In cellular terms, fungal dimorphism can be defined as the ability of a species to grow either as hyphae (linear or apical growth) or yeast (spherical growth). The shape of the cell is determined by the cell wall because protoplasts always assume a sphere, and thus we can refer to fungal dimorphism as cell wall morphogenesis. Consequently, it is the temporal and spatial arrangement of the wall components that dictate the final shape of the cell. *Coccidioides immitis* forms an exception to this general description of dimorphism. This mold forms arthroconidia, which act as infectious propagules for humans. Infection is associated with transformation of the conidia to spherules that release endospores. This parasitic cycle is unique among pathogenic fungi.

A summary of the general features of morphogenesis associated with some of the pathogenic fungi is given below.

Histoplasma capsulatum

Histoplasma capsulatum, the etiologic agent in histoplasmosis, is a dimorphic pathogenic fungus, in which the hyphae represent the saprobic form, and yeast cells are the parasitic form. The hyphae of *H. capsulatum* produces macro- and microconidia which, after inhalation by the host, develop as budding yeasts. Owing to their small size, it is believed that the microconidia initate the infectious process.

The mycelial phase of *H. capsulatum* is characterized by a classic hyphal structure with a Spitzenkorp, coated vesicles, mitochondria, rough endoplasmic reticulum, and a Golgi-like membranous apparatus. The septa possess a narrow central pore that may be occluded with a Woronin body. The yeast phase is composed of oval budding yeast cells of an average diameter of 2–4 μm (43), which give rise to blastoconidia. The mycelium has simple growth requirements and can be grown by incubating cultures at 25°C with glucose as a carbon source and ammonia as an inorganic source of nitrogen. The yeast phase requires cysteine, biotin, and thiamine as growth factors (reviewed in 49). The requirement for sulfhydryl-containing compounds to maintain yeast phase growth led Scherr (111) to speculate that *H. capsulatum* cells lacked the ability to reduce sulfur-containing compounds at 37°C and that, further to Nickerson's hypothesis (88), the sulfhydryl compounds regulated the oxidation-reduction potential of the growing cells. The role of respiration and sulfhydryls has been well studied in *H. capsulatum* dimorphism and is detailed under Metabolic Alterations Associated with Dimorphism.

Blastomyces dermatitidis

Blastomyces dermatitidis is the causative agent of blastomycosis, and this fungus exists in both a yeast and mycelial form depending upon the growth conditions. Conidia are the asexual propagules in nature, and after invasion of the tissue the parasitic yeast cells are formed; hyphae represent the saprobic form. The yeast form has an optimal growth temperature of 35–37°C whereas the mycelial phase has a growth temperature of 31–33°C. There is some controversy over the mechanism of mycelial-to-yeast transition. In one school of thought (29, 62) it is believed that yeast cells are formed within the mycelial elements that eventually break apart, releasing single yeast cells that reproduce by budding. On the other hand, Garrison and Boyd (44) have presented evidence that only conidia are capable of becoming yeast mother cells. The latter concept is considered to be correct.

The most obvious difference between the yeast and hyphal cells lies in the composition of the cell wall material: in yeast cell walls, 95% of the glucan is α-1, 3-linked, whereas only 60% of the mycelial wall has this α-1, 3-linkage (30, 67). The remaining glucan linkages of mycelial cells are β-1, 3-linked. Mannose and galactose are found in higher concentrations in the mycelial cell wall than in the yeast cell wall. There are also different proteins present in the yeast and mycelial cell walls; in one study the yeast extract had four clearly defined proteins, only one of which could be detected in the mycelial extract (107).

Candida albicans

Candida albicans is frequently encountered as a normal commensal of the digestive tract. It is an important human opportunistic pathogen, and the disease it causes generally takes two forms: superficial (mucosal) and invasive (disseminated). *Candida albicans* may infect any tissue in the human body, but by far the most common manifestations of candidiasis are lesions of the mucous membranes. In most instances the more serious invasive form follows dissemination of the yeast from a mucosal focus.

Candida albicans is a polymorphic fungus, as several different morphologic forms can be found in a single environment. At temperatures below 33°C yeast cell growth is favored. The ovoid cells reproduce by budding and produce blastoconidia that are approximately 3 × 5 μm in size. Initiation of new bud formation occurs preferentially at the polar region of the cell distal to the birth scar (20, 63). As with *Saccharomyces cerevisiae* (10), the formation of the septum in *C. albicans* is preceded by the appearance of a filament ring (86), containing a large amount of chitin, and the nucleus migrates into the neck region between the mother and developing daughter cell before dividing. At elevated temperatures and neutral pH mycelial growth is favored. The hyphal cell develops via the intermediate formation of a germ-tube from a yeast cell (112). The first stage of germ-tube formation is the emergence of up to five protuberances from the surface of the mother cell (Fig. 8-1A) (63). An inspection of many cells (see Fig. 8-1) shows that these protuberances and germ-tubes emanate from all aspects of the cell surface (63, 79). In a suitable environment germ-tubes are visible in the light microscope after 60–90 minutes. Hubbard et al (63) showed that the protuberances were extensions of

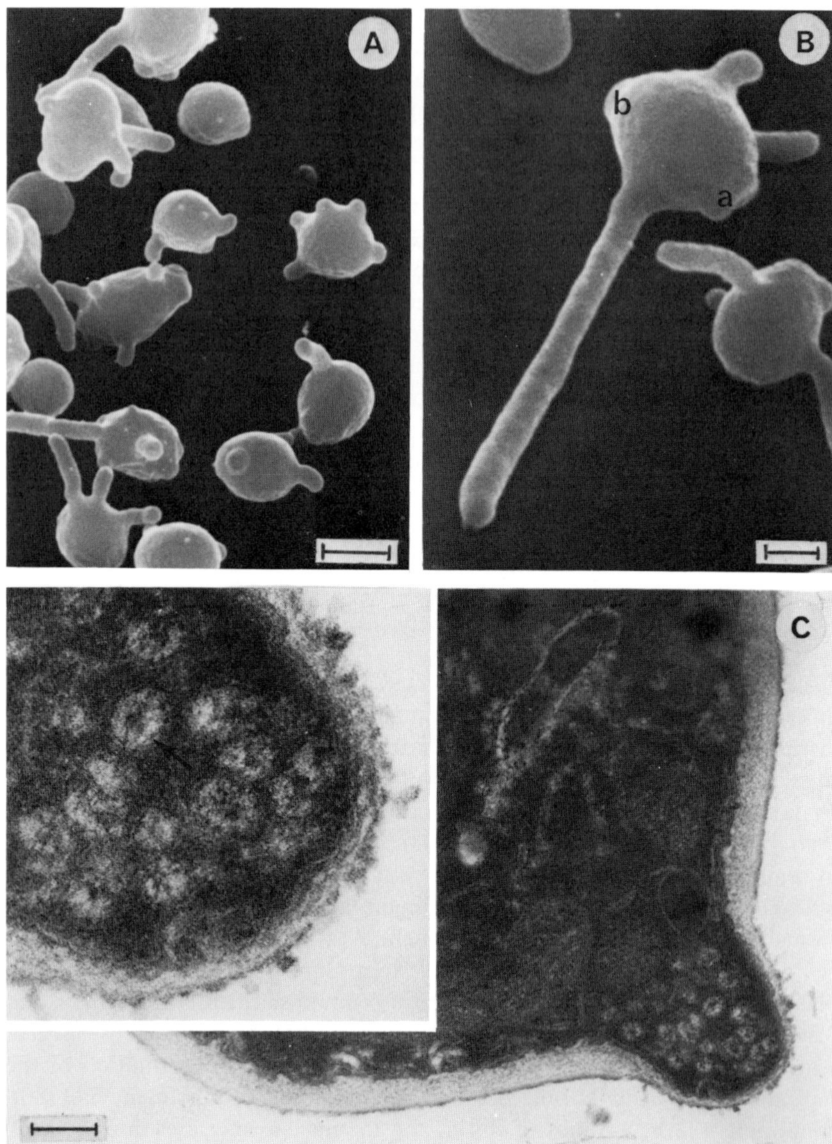

FIG. 8-1. (A) Scanning electron micrograph of early germ-tube forming *C. albicans* cells 90 minutes after induction with N-acetylglucosamine. A cell with five rounded protrusions is visible to the right of center field. Marker bar = 2 μm. (B) Scanning electron micrograph of a germ-tube forming cell which exhibits one elongated and two short germ-tubes. The germ-tubes are nonpolar and emanate from surfaces other than those in the long axis of the cell (a and b). The profile of the elongated germ-tube is smooth (not segmented) and adjoins the cell without any constriction. Marker bar = 1 μm. a and b show the budding pole and birth scar, respectively. (C) Transmission electron micrograph of an early germ-tube forming cell 90 minutes after induction,

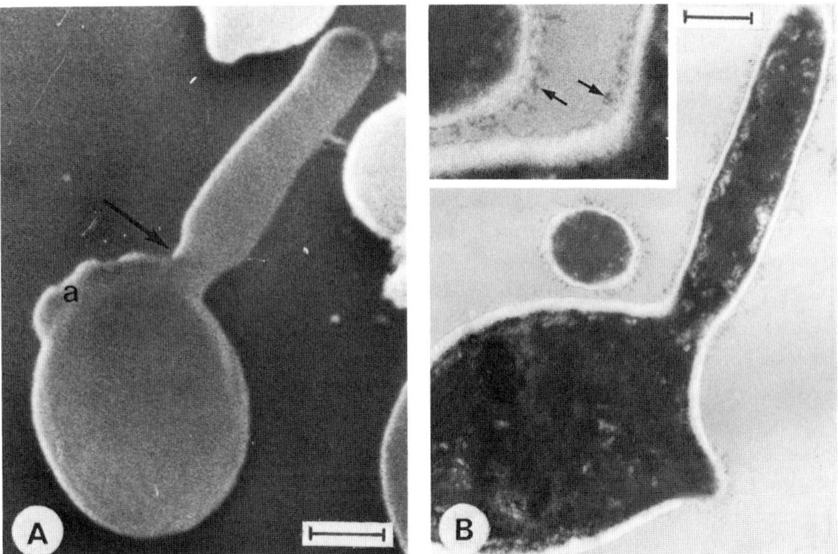

FIG. 8-2. (A) Scanning electron micrograph of *C. albicans* pseudohyphal cell. The pseudohypha originates from the budding pole (a) of the cell with the site of emergence characterized by a constriction (*arrow*). Marker bar = 1.2 μm. (B) Transmission electron micrograph of cell walls. Ultrathin section through a germ-tube forming cell which was fixed in paraformaldehyde plus glutaraldehyde and postfixed with osmium. The cell wall is predominantly electron-lucent with a thin electron-dense outer layer. An electron-dense fibrillar border is visible external to the electron-dense outer layer of the germ-tube wall (*arrows* in inset). In the cross-sectioned germ-tube, the fibrils are seen to be arranged radially and perpendicular to the cell wall. Stained with lead citrate for 45 minutes. Marker bar = 0.6 μm. (Reproduced with permission from *Can J Microbiol* [63].)

the cytoplasm and contained round electron-luscent vesicles (Fig. 8-1C). Unlike budding yeast cells and pseudohyphae (Fig. 8-2), germ-tubes do not have constrictions at the junction with the mother cell because they grow by linear elongation rather than budding. Although multiple protuberances are observed in the early stage of germ-tube formation, most of these subside and usually only one germ-tube, but occasionally two, develops. As the germ-tube continues to grow, a septum is formed 1–2 μm across the germ-tube (86). Once the septum is formed, the germ-tube is considered to be a hypha. Gow and

---

◁ illustrating a protuberance which contains electron-lucent vesicles. The cell wall of the protuberance is of reduced thickness compared with the rest of the cell and is covered by a fibrillar layer. Marker bar = 0.3 μm. The inset shows the protuberance at higher magnification. The apical vesicles appear to be membrane-limited (*arrow*) and to have granular electron-dense contents. Stained with lead citrate for 60 minutes. (Reproduced with permission from *Can J Microbiol* [63].)

Gooday (54) have examined germ-tube formation and mycelial growth of *C. albicans* and found that most of the cytoplasm within the parent yeast cell migrates into and with the extending germ-tube, leaving behind an extensively vacuolated yeast cell. Growing hyphae similarly are subtended by migrating "slugs" of protoplasm and leave behind vacuolated intercalary compartments. For a hyphal cell to develop a branch it must first regenerate protoplasmic contents within the vacuolated cell compartment. Pseudohyphae are essentially long branching filaments composed of elongated yeast cells formed by polar budding that are constricted at the septa. In contrast to germ-tubes, elongate blastoconidia and pseudohyphae have a marked constriction at the site of emergence (Fig. 8-2A). Recent reviews of *C. albicans* dimorphism include Shepherd et al (121) and Odds (92).

There is a large body of literature that claims a causal relationship between mycelial formation and infection. This is based on the premise that hyphae penetrate tissues more readily than do yeast cells and are more difficult to phagocytose. Experimentally it has been observed that 1) mycelium is the predominant form found in scrapings of lesions, and 2) yeast cells inoculated into animals rapidly form mycelium. However, other workers (32, 80, 125) have presented evidence for increased virulence of the yeast form of *C. albicans* over the mycelial form, although both forms were shown to be pathogenic. The ability of tissue fluids to interconvert the two morphologic forms means, however, that experiments with either yeast cells or mycelium have inevitably given equivocal results. The availability of morphologic mutants allowed this question to be re-examined, and Shepherd (117) has shown that both the yeast and mycelial forms of *C. albicans* are pathogenic.

Paracoccidioides brasiliensis

Paracoccidioidomycosis is caused by the thermally dimorphic fungus *Paracoccidioides brasiliensis*, and the production of the yeast form in vivo is critical for pathogenesis. The disease is endemic in many parts of Latin America, and a striking feature about its epidemiology is the male/female ration for the disease of 48 : 1 (100). However, the skin test reaction indicates that the frequency of infection is the same in males and females and there is no sex-based difference in those who acquire the disease before puberty (101). These data indicate that host hormonal factors, probably sex hormones, are important in regulating the development of the disease. *Paracoccidioides brasiliensis* assumes a mycelial form at room temperature and a yeast-like form in the tissue or in culture at 37°C. After the studies of Nickerson and Edwards (89) it has been widely accepted that the dimorphic transition depends exclusively on the temperature of incubation and is independent of the nature and composition of the culture medium. More recently, Paris et al (96) have shown that the mycelium is prototrophic, and that the yeast form in vitro requires a sulphur-containing amino acid for growth. In addition, changing the source of nitrogen greatly affects the morphology of the yeast-like cells.

The yeast cells of *P. brasiliensis* vary considerably in size from less than 1 μm for recently developed blastoconidia to more than 30 μm for mature cells (109). The yeast cells are multinucleate and multiply by polar or multipolar budding. The multipolar budding is synchronous and gives rise to the important taxonomic morphologic structure, multiple budding, which has the appearance of a ship's wheel. Yeast cells develop from hyphal elements either by "rounding up" of the cell between two septa or by swelling of the hyphal tip (15).

When the temperature of growth is decreased from 37°C to 22°C, mycelial growth is initiated. The first stage in hyphal development is the formation of an elongated bud (15). It has been suggested (109) that although this is analogous to germ-tube formation, the morphology of the mycelial meristematic region originates as a consequence of deformation of the yeast cell rather than by initiation of apical growth. Indeed, there is a marked constriction at the site of emergence not dissimilar to that observed with pseudohyphal cells of *C. albicans*. True hyphae with septa and branches subsequently develop.

Coccidioides immitis

Coccidioides immitis grows as mycelium in its natural habitat of soil or on media at ambient temperatures. When soil is disturbed the conidia from the mycelium are dispersed as an aerosol. In the lungs of the host the conidia form endosporulating multinucleate spherules. Electron microscopy shows (87, 132) that endospores are formed by repeated branching and invagination of the innermost wall of the spherule. Wall ingrowth and division of the cytoplasm continues until the spherule is filled with uninucleate endospores. At maturity the spherule wall ruptures releasing packets of endospores enclosed in a membranous sac. Eventually the membrane dissolves and each endospore then produces a second generation of spherules within the host. A detailed account of the morphology and life cycle of *C. immitis* can be found in the review by Cole and Sun (28). Recent studies with scanning (87, 131) and transmission (131) electron microscopy have shown that the morphogenesis of *C. immitis* in vivo closely resembles the events observed in in vitro studies. The unusual parasitic cycle of transformation from a conidium to spherule to disseminating endospores distinguishes *C. immitis* from all other pathogenic fungi.

Sporothrix schenckii

The saprobic form of *Sporothrix schenckii* is a mycelium consisting of septate hyphae (1–2 μm in diameter) and oval conidia (approximately 2 × 4 μm). The development of lymphocutaneous sporotrichosis arises from the introduction of either hyphae or conidia into the host following trauma. Pulmonary infections result following the inhalation of the fungus. Infection then develops through the production of yeast cells. The conversion of hyphal cells to yeast cells is accomplished in vitro on glucose-cysteine blood agar at 37°C. The yeast cells are ovoid (approximately $3 \times 5\ \mu m$) and multiply by producing single or multiple blastoconidia (45).

Wangiella dermatitidis

Wangiella dermatitidis is a polymorphic fungus that exhibits a complex life cycle (134). It can exist as true septate hyphae formed by apical growth or as unicellular budding yeast cells (57, 95). In addition it forms multinucleate sclerotic bodies from enlarged yeast cells by isotropic growth, thickening of the cell walls, and finally forming internally septa. These sclerotic bodies, which are phenotypically arrested between a yeast and hyphal morphology, develop into a multicellular form with hyphae and conidia (105).

Morphologic Changes Associated with Dimorphism

A number of the general cytologic features associated with the morphogenesis of the human pathogenic fungi are described below. Light and electron microscopy have been the major techniques used to provide us with our present understanding of this process. More recently, immunoelectron microscopy has provided additional detail on the location of specific components in the cell wall.

The pathogenic fungi are typical eukaryotic cells and do not appear to possess unique cytologic features. The cell wall generally consists of several distinct layers. The outermost layer is covered with microfibrils, which appear to be rich in mannan-containing polymers because they bind to concanavalin A (17). It is postulated that these cell wall microfibrils are involved in cellular adhesion (110).

Yeast Cell Cytology

The yeast cells of dimorphic fungi reproduce by budding in which the bud cell arises as an extension of an innermost layer of the parental cell wall. Electron microscopy has revealed a number of different organelles and inclusions in the cytosol of yeast cells. For example, the nuclear apparatus consists of a nuclear membrane, nuclear pores, nucleoplasm, and nucleolus. A rough and smooth endoplasmic reticulum is scattered throughout the cytoplasm. Mitochondria also can be observed, and they are elongate with the cristae parallel to the long axis. Vacuoles appear to be much more common in older cells, and a number of lysosomal marker enzymes have been demonstrated cytochemically within the vacuoles. Glycogen and lipid bodies are also present inside the cell. A formal Golgi apparatus does not appear to be present in fungal cells, but a class of small membranous structures referred to as multivesicular bodies have been identified in yeast cells of *B. dermatitidis* (31) and *W. dermatitidis* (57).

Hyphal Cell Cytology

Generally, hyphal cytoplasm contains the same organelles and inclusions as yeast cells. The substructural components of the hyphal cell wall are poorly differentiated, but differences may be enhanced by the use of special cytochemical reactions (42, 63). The vegetative hyphae of all the pathogenic dimorphic fungi have ascomycetous-type septa (41). The septal plates are wedge-shaped and may be more electron-translucent than the cell wall proper. Gow et al (55) have shown that the hyphal septum of *C. albicans* contains a 25-nm central micropore that does not permit organelle migration but does allow cytoplasmic continuity. Woronin bodies are found in the septal area, and it is believed that these membranous bodies act as plugs regulating cytoplasmic flow between adjacent hyphal cells.

Conidial Cell Cytology

All of the pathogenic dimorphic fungi produce conidia. These propagules are characterized by elecron-opaque aggregates or particles on the outside of the cell wall. It is this area of the wall that may be responsible for coloration of the cell (47). The conidial wall of *B. dermatitidis* is thick and finely laminated varying from the inner material of low electron opacity through a gradually increasing number of fibrils to a densely packed outer layer of intense electron opacity (31).

Cytology of Dimorphism

As discussed earlier, the dimorphic change represents a wall morphogenesis and can be influenced by nutritional factors and temperature. The first event associated with germ-tube formation of *C. albicans* is the accumulation of vesicle-like bodies at the point of outgrowth (63). Then there is elongation that is accompanied by a number of structural changes in the cell wall of the developing germ-tube (18). In *P. brasiliensis*, *B. dermatitidis*, *H. capsulatum*, and *S. schenckii* the first stage of hyphal formation is the formation of a bud-like structure, which has been termed the transitional cell (46). Garrison (42) postulated that the yeast-to-mycelial transition at the ultrastructural level in most pathogenic dimorphic fungi is characterized by the presence of simple septa and associated Woronin bodies between the converting yeast and its first hyphal cell.

The Transition from Hyphal to Yeast Cells

It appears that yeast cells are formed from hyphal cells by a number of different mechanisms that include: 1) formation of budding yeast cells at the hyphal tip or on lateral branches, 2) the formation of chains of cells with subsequent fragmentation of these chains into constituent yeast cells, and 3) the direct budding of yeast cells from conidia.

The formation of swollen cells appears to be well documented for *H. capsulatum* (41) and *S. schenckii* (45). In *C. albicans* it is found that the yeast cells resulting from budding are freely dissociated from vegetative hyphae under most growing conditions. These cells then establish a yeast phase by repetative budding. In addition, chains of yeast cells may remain together in what appears to be a formal association. This is the origin of pseudomycelial growth, which is characterized by chains of elongated blastoconidia. Although dimorphism is caused by alterations in the fungal metabolism, the change in morphology is essentially a question of regulation of the temporal and spatial cell wall formation. Unfortunately there are not many cytochemical staining procedures available that allow us to visualize the fine structure of the cell walls of fungi.

Yeast and Hyphal Growth

In yeasts there is now considerable evidence for polarized secretion influencing surface growth and indeed a critical role for the cytoskeleton. During most of the cell cycle, surface growth is restricted to the site of the bud, and the mother cell shows little growth. In addition, it has been observed (36, 127, 136) that protein secretion is restricted to the growing region of the cell. These experiments were conducted with the periplasmic proteins, invertase (136) and acid phosphatase (36). In addition, a fluorescent derivative of concanavalin A was used to show that after a period of growth the regions that define sites of new growth are restricted to the bud (127). It is now believed that the actin-based cytoskeleton controls the surface growth of yeast cells. Actin is a highly conserved protein present in all eukaryotes (72). The degree of conservation of amino acid sequence is extreme and 89% of the residues are identical between *Saccharomyces* actin and mammalian actin (38). This degree of sequence conservation suggests a comparable conservation in vital cellular functions common to all eukaryotic cells. Actin polymerizes into microfilaments and together with its associated proteins it has been implicated in many aspects of the eukaryotic cell cycle (97). A fluorescence microscopy study (1) suggests several roles for yeast actin including involvement in the deposition of a ring of chitin in the neck region where the budding cell is being formed. Adams and Pringle (1) also established a correlation between the growing regions of the yeast surface and the regions showing concentrations of actin "patches." They proposed a role for actin in the localization of surface growth.

Actin appears to be absent from the yeast spindle, which suggests that it is not involved in chromosome segregation. In a phenotyic analysis of temperature-sensitive yeast actin mutants, Novick and Botstein (91) showed that at the restrictive temperature there was disruption of the actin assembly, delocalized deposition of chitin on the cell surface, partial inhibition of invertase secretion, an intracellular accumulation of secretory vesicles, and death of those cells in the budding portion of the cell cycle. These data further implicate actin in the organization and polarized growth of the yeast cell surface. It is interesting to note that in plants and yeasts, organelle transport appears to be mediated via actin where it accounts for cytoplasmic streaming and speeds of transport that can reach 100 μm/sec (114). It would appear that microtubules are not involved in yeast growth, because shifting a cold-sensitive β-tubulin mutant to its restrictive temperature or disrupting microtubules does not prevent normal polarized growth of the affected cells, nor does it result in the accumulation of vesicles (90). Unlike the reversible movement along microtubules found with mammalian cells (113), movement along actin filaments is unidirectional (116). Therefore when the flow of vesicles is reversed, as in endocystosis, the polarity of the actin filament also must be reversed.

Endocytosis is an essential feature in eukaryotic cells. It is the process or the mechanism whereby cells internalize their own plasma membrane and macromolecules from the external environment. It is a time-, temperature-, and energy-dependent process, and its functions include the provision of nutrients, internalizing hormones, and clearing unwanted or foreign proteins from the cell. The endocytic pathway may also be the infectious route for viruses and bacteria and serve as a means for the entry of toxins into cells. Riezman (103) showed, by using a fluid phase marker, that yeast cells endocytose and that several of the yeast mutants conditionally defective in secretion (90) are also defective in endocytosis.

In *S. cerevisiae* the major site for new cell wall synthesis is at the apical tip (Fig. 8-3) (reviewed in 5). Farkaš et al (35) found that incorporation of mannan into all parts of the cell wall occurred only after the bud exceeded a minimum size. In a more recent study (128) the zones of expansion on the surface of yeast and mycelial cells of *C. albicans* were monitored by the position of polylysine-coated beads. During the first two thirds of bud developments, 70% of the surface expansion was restricted to a small apical zone. When a bud reaches approximately two thirds of its final size, apical growth shuts down and the final size is accomplished through general expansion. In summary, the essential features of yeast growth are 1) organization of the cytoskeleton, particularly actin microfibrils, which defines the point of bud emergence; 2) clustering of vesicles at the site of bud emergence; 3) evagination of the mother cell wall; 4) migration of the nucleus to the bud; 5) initiation of chitin synthesis to form the chitin ring between the mother cell and bud; 6) nuclear division and the closure of the junction between the mother and daughter cells; and 7) separation of cells through secondary wall formation

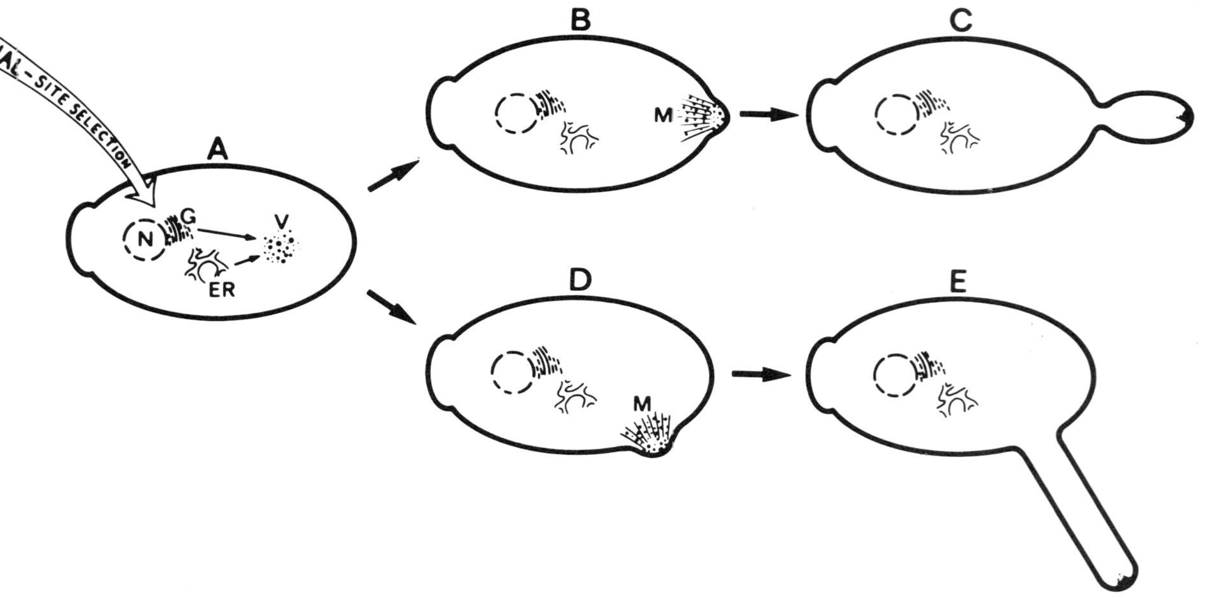

FIG. 8-3. Model for yeast-to-mycelial transformation. (A) A signal is received from the environment (temperature, pH, nutrient). The decision on yeast or mycelial growth is made and a site for evagination is selected. (B) (D) Actin fibrils move to the site of evagination and apical growth begins through the directed secretion of vesicles. (C) (E) The wall polysaccharides are synthesized through activation of the synthases in the plasma membrane. With hyphal growth (E), the rigid cylindrical shape is maintained through secondary wall formation; apical growth is continuous. In yeast cells (C), the final size of the bud is achieved through generalized (isotropic) growth. The formation of a septum occurs through the controlled activation of chitin synthase. Intracellular organelles are: N, nucleus; G, membranous assembly similar to Golgi; ER, endoplasmic reticulum; V, vesicles; and M, actin microfibrils.

producing a birth scar on the daughter cell and a bud scar on the mother cell.

Hyphae are produced by apical growth in which wall deposition is continuous, polarized, and involves little, if any, isotropism. The evidence for this is based on microscopy (106), autoradiography (6, 40, 50, 70), and fluorescent labeling (39, 64). With mycelial growth of *C. albicans* some 90% of its expansion is at the small apical growth zone, and less than 10% is due to general expansion; as long as the hyphal element is growing the apical growth zone is active (128). It would appear that the temporal and spatial regulation of these growth zones is germane to the control of yeast and mycelial growth in dimorphic fungi. In many fungi there is a cluster of tiny cytoplasmic particles at the growing tip (8, 56). These are vesicular (approximately 0.1 μm in diameter), and the dark body observed by light microscopy is a cluster of microvesicles called a Spitzenkorper (8). These transport enzymes, enzyme activators and inhibitors, and wall precursors through the cytoplasm to the plasmalemma where they fuse, discharging their contents (34). The vesicles come from the "slug" of protoplasm that moves with the extending hypha (54). Branching can only occur if new protoplasm develops within the vacuolated cell (54).

The introduction of the vesicle and its contents to the growing tip allows the development of a primary wall. Secondary wall formation, both de novo synthesis and the cross-linking of existing material, takes place in the subapical region. Hence, the topology of the cell wall dictates the formation of the rigid tubular shape characteristic of hyphae.

In *Schizophyllum commune* chitin and β-glucans are excreted from their sites of synthesis at the growing hyphal tip as individual polymers (124). They are then cross-linked in situ at a relatively slow rate. In the subapical parts of the hyphae, secondary wall development occurs giving a different kind of wall polymer. Indeed, up to 50% of the total glucan is synthesized subapically in *S. commune*. Sietsma et al (124) propose that β-1,3-linked glucan is deposited at the apex and that β-1,6-glucan residues occur in the extension zone and form the majority of subapically synthesized glucan. In *C. albicans*, the β-1,3-glucan is linked to chitin through a glycosidic linkage from the six position of N-acetylglucosamine to the one position of the terminal glucose of the glucan (Shepherd and Surarit, unpublished observations). The chitin-glucan complex is believed to provide the cell wall with the increased rigidity required for the development of hyphal morphogenesis.

The Cell Surface and Morphogenesis

It has been emphasized that fungal dimorphism is essentially a cell wall morphogenesis, and consequently the quantitative and qualitative changes in cell wall components during morphogenesis have been studied in some detail. Nevertheless, there is a paucity of information available on the architecture and fine structure of fungal walls. This is largely due to the unavailability of techniques either for visualizing details in the wall or for chemical and biochemical analysis of the wall components. The structure and mechanisms of biosynthesis of the wall carbohydrates have been particularly recalcitrant.

There is general consensus that the microfibrillar glucan and chitin provide the rigidity for fungal cell walls. This conclusion is supported by the observation that treatment of fungi with glucanases and chitinases results in the formation of protoplasts. When these are regenerated, glucans and chitin restore osmotic resistance to cells without the formation of mannoproteins (53). The shape of a β-1,3-glucan allows the molecule to form a linear twisted ribbon, one side of which contains the hydrophilic hydroxyl groups and the other side hydrophobic methine groups (5). There has been speculation that a rigid molecule is formed by two glucan chains forming a double helix with the hydrophobic surfaces in contact. This structure has been established by x-ray analysis for β-1,3-xylan (4). In any model of fungal growth, wall expansion which occurs outside the cell must be accounted for. With respect to the glucans either localized glucanases could clip the glucan molecules allowing intussusception of new polymer or the chains could slide along each other, providing primers for new helical structures from newly synthesized polymers and thus cell wall expansion.

The other molecules critical to the structure of the wall are mannoproteins and chitin. If there is extensive cross-linking of proteins by disulfide linkage (33), wall expansion would require localized protease and/or protein disulfide reductase activity. The observation that either proteases or B-mercaptoethanal enhance protoplast formation with purified glucanases (115) provides indirect evidence for disulfide cross-linking. The primary site of chitin is in a ring around the bud scar sandwiched between two layers of glucan (12). A critical feature of the yeast growth cycle is the control of chitin synthesis during septation (11). However, small amounts of chitin are dispersed around the entire cell wall (60) and a chitin-glucan complex is believed to be a critical component of secondary wall development (124). There are considerable differences between the wall components from the yeast and mycelial forms of *P. brasiliensis*. The glucan of the yeast cell wall is predominately α-1,3-linked (95%), with 5% β-1,3-linked (69). In the mycelial cell wall the glucan fraction consists predominately of two β-1,3-glucans joined through β-1,6-linkages. These differences in the wall of the two cell forms led Kanetsuna et al (68) to propose a model for dimorphism based on the assumption that the yeast shape was attained by generalized cell wall synthesis, whereas the cylindrical hyphal shape was the result of apical growth. Studies with dimorphic mutants suggest that qualitative changes in cell wall composition do not occur in the early stages of dimorphic transition. The mutant strain Pb229 is unable to complete the mycelial-to-yeast transition or to grow at 37°C (58). However, after incubating the mycelial cells at 37°C, both intercalary and terminal yeast structures are formed. Most importantly the wall glucan of these yeast structures is composed of β-1,3-glucan, not the α-1,3-glucan associated with the wall of yeast cells from wild-type cells. San-Blas and San-Blas (109) concluded from these data that 1) the α-1,3-glucan does not seem to be responsible for the yeast morphology, and 2) the α-1,3-glucan is probably essential in the liberation and autonomous replication of the yeast cells. On the basis of these and other studies with morphologic mutants, it is difficult to accept a model of dimorphism based on generalized versus apical growth. This view must be supported by studies with *S. schenckii* and *C. albicans*. The cell wall composition of the yeast, mycelium, and conidia of *S. schenkii* show only minor differences in composition (99) and it would appear that there is no single polymer responsible for alterations in the shape of cells. The glucans from all three cell types are polymers containing β-1,3-, β-1,4-, and β-1,6-linkages (98).

The cell walls of *C. albicans* yeast and mycelial cells have a similar composition, which can be summarized as: lipid 2%, protein 3–6%, chitin 0.6–2.7%, mannoprotein 20–23%, and glucan 48–60% (129). Total glucan and mannoprotein do not vary greatly with either the stage of growth or germ-tube formation. There is an increased amount of chitin in germ-tubes (129) and mycelial cells (22). An analysis of the acid-soluble and insoluble glucan fractions from yeasts, germ-tube, and hyphal forming cells of *C. albicans* has recently been completed (51). The acid-soluble fraction of each cell type consists primarily (70%) of β-1,6-glucan. In the insoluble fraction of the yeast and mycelial cells, the relative amounts of β-1,3- and β-1,6-linkages are 30% and 50%, respectively. In germ-tube forming cells β-1,3-linkages account for 67% of residues in the insoluble fraction. It appears that the newly synthesized glucan in germ-tubes consists predominantly of β-1,3-glucan.

The enzymes for cell wall assembly of *C. albicans* are located in the plasma membrane (reviewed in 121), and this is consistent with the concept of transmembrane enzymes that catalyze the vectorial synthesis of each polymer (13). The selective regulation of these membrane-bound enzymes at the growth areas (14) is critical to our understanding of dimorphism.

The major support for the concept of growth of spherical cells occurring by incorporating new cell wall material over the whole cell surface (that is, generalized growth) compared with apical growth for hyphal development comes from studies with *Mucor rouxii* (34). One interpretation of the autoradiographic data (6) is that the labeling is occurring on the cell wall during the final stages of the yeast cell maturation, leading to the conclusion of complete generalized growth.

Metabolic Changes Associated with Dimorphism

Histoplasma capsulatum yeast cells require cysteine for growth. This has prompted numerous studies which have led to a clear understanding of the metabolic events associated with morphogenesis in this organism. It is now known that cysteine and cystine are taken up equally well by both yeast and mycelial cells of *H. capsulatum* (81) and that the cysteine-stimulated respiration is due to a cytosolic cysteine oxidase found in yeast phase cells but absent in mycelium. Cysteine is also involved in the mitochondrial respiratory pathways (83). As with numerous other fungi, *H. capsulatum* respiration proceeds through two terminal oxidase systems (82): the normal cytochrome oxidase which is classically inhibited by antimycin and cyanide, and the alternate oxidase which is sensitive to salicylhydroxamic acid. There is one important difference in the respiratory systems of the yeast and mycelial cells. Whereas the yeast phase cells are completely sensitive to antimycin, the mycelial cells are only partially (approximately 50%) inhibited (82).

Kobayashi et al (71) have provided a detailed review of the changes that occur in the respiratory system of *H. capsulatum* during dimorphism. In essence there are two functions for cysteine. The first is that yeast cells have a nutritional requirement for cysteine that cannot be satisfied by other sulfhydryl-containing compounds. The second is that cysteine is required to complete the mycelial-to-yeast transition. It appears that cysteine stimulates respiration via a shunt pathway around the site of the antimycin block. Therefore, in the presence of antimycin, the mycelial cells are only partially sensitive because the shunt pathway is operative. Finally, the intracellular concentration of cysteine is high in mycelium where the shunt pathways are active and low in yeast where the shunt pathways are inactive. RNA and protein synthesis have been examined in some detail in both phases of *H. capsulatum*. RNA synthesis over an 8-hour period was 12 times higher for mycelium than for yeast cells (23). There is also increased protein synthesis and the level of cyclic AMP is about five times higher in the mycelial phase than in the yeast phase (84).

The metabolic events associated with dimorphism of *H. capsulatum* may be summarized as follows. Firstly, increasing the temperature from 25 to 37°C results in a decrease in the level of cytochromes and a cessation of respiration. RNA and protein synthesis then decrease to nondetectable levels, probably because of the absence of respiration and the consequent decrease in adenosine triphosphate (ATP) synthesis. In the presence of sulfhydryls, particularly cysteine, shunt pathways are initiated that bypass the block in respiration. The shunt pathways maintain a level of ATP that keeps the cell viable through the next stages of mycelial-to-yeast transition. Cysteine is also required for growth by the yeast phase. After the yeast cells are formed they adapt to their new environmental conditions and the cytochrome levels return to normal, resulting in higher levels of respiration. Division and growth of yeast cells then occur. A high concentration of intracellular cysteine is maintained in part by a cysteine reductase which is induced at elevated temperatures.

There are a large number of different environmental factors that are capable of effecting the yeast-to-mycelial transition in *C. albicans* (reviewed in 92). In general, the morphogenesis may be regulated by three external variables: temperature, pH, and nutrients, so that more than 90% of the yeast cells form germ-tubes in 3–4 hours. At temperatures above 35°C and at a neutral pH in an amino acid medium (77) or with N-acetylglucosamine (126) mycelial growth is favored. Low temperature and pH favor yeast growth. Despite the large number of studies on induction of germ-tube formation in *C. albicans*, it is not possible to formulate cellular roles for any of the metabolic regulators used to induce morphogenesis. It is known that *C. albicans* possesses an alternate oxidase similar to that observed with *H. capsulatum* and a number of other fungi (119). However, there is no evidence relating respiration to morpohogenesis (3, 119), and a recent study with a mycelial mutant confirms this result (Shepherd, unpublished results).

The observation of Chattaway et al (22) that there was more chitin in hyphal cells than in yeast cells has stimulated intense interest in the synthesis of this polymer. Chitin synthase is distributed all over the plasma membrane of *C. albicans* and it is an allosteric proenzyme (7, 24). The activity of the enzyme is higher in germ-tubes than in yeast cells. The enzyme exhibits positive cooperativity for its substrate UDP-N-acetylglucosamine and is activated by N-acetylglucosamine.

The proenzyme is activated in vitro by exogenous proteases (7, 24), but the proposed in vivo role for proteases is dubious (14). It is possible that activation of the chitin synthase occurs through interaction with a lipid molecule in a manner similar to that found for pyruvate oxidase (48). With pyruvate oxidase the lipid activation can only occur when both the thiamine pyrophosphate-Mg^{2+} site and the pyruvate substrate site are occupied. With enzymes such as chitin synthase it may be that the plasma membrane creates an environment for the enzyme, which renders the activation site unaccessible, and, therefore, the enzyme remains as a proenzyme. The arrival of vesicles at the site of evagination may alter the chitin synthase in the membrane so that the activation site is exposed. Chiew et al (25) demonstrated that ergosterol inhibits the chitin synthase of *C. albicans*, whereas ethanol and methanol activate the enzyme. The possible role of chitin in *C. albicans* morphogenesis lead to the discovery by Simonetti et al (126) that N-acetylglucosamine was an extracellular inducer of germ-tube formation. Shepherd et al (118) expanded these studies and showed that induction of a N-acetylglucosamine permease and the enzymes of N-acetylglucosamine catabolism occurs at both 28°C and 37°C (52, 120, 123, 130). In addition, N-acetylglucosamine derivatives (N-acetylmannosamine, N-acetylglucosamine covalently bound to agarose and colloidal chitin), which are not metabolized, gratuitously, induce both the N-acetylglucosamine permease and hyphal growth (122, 130). These data indicate that N-acetylglucosamine analogs interact with a surface receptor, which then triggers hyphal growth via an intracellular or second site messenger (19, 123). Although the metabolic events associated with morphogenesis in *C. albicans* are not known at this time a minimum model (121) would be:

$$\text{Yeast morphogenesis} \underset{2}{\overset{1}{\rightleftharpoons}} \text{Uncoupled state} \underset{4}{\overset{3}{\rightleftharpoons}} \text{Hyphal morphogenesis.}$$

In step 1 the yeast budding cycle is uncoupled by a temperature shift to 37°C. The uncoupled system may then be reorganized for either yeast growth (step 2) or hyphal growth (step 3). Hyphal growth is favored if the temperature is maintained above 37°C and the pH greater than 6.5. It would appear that the pH-regulated morphogenesis (9) must be mediated via the cell surface because the intracellular pH is similar in yeast and mycelial cells (16).

N-acetylglucosamine, proline, and other chemical inducers of germ-tube formation trigger step 3.

Morphogenesis in *Mucor* species has received considerable attention (65, 108). In early studies it was believed that there was a simple relationship between respiration (hyphal morphology) and fermentation (yeast morphology). This theory has not been sustainable, although there may be a critical role for mitochondrial functions other than in respiration. One important correlate with *Mucor* morphogenesis is cAMP: high intracellular concentrations of cAMP are found in yeast cells and low cAMP concentrations are found in hyphal cells (75). The regulation of the cAMP levels appears to be due to adenylate cyclase, not phosphodiesterase (93). The exact role cAMP plays in morphogenesis is not known at this time. In addition, nitrogen metabolism appears to differ in the two morphologic forms. Ornithine decarboxylase is the rate-limiting enzyme in polyamine biosynthesis and has been associated with cellular regulation (135). During yeast-to-hyphal development of *M. racemosus* there is a 40–60-fold increase in ornithine decarboxylase activity. Because ornithine decarboxylase may be linked to phospholipid metabolism (66), it is possible that this enzyme is associated with cell membrane changes.

Protein synthesis has been examined in some detail in *M. racemosus* (76). Changes have been found in the protein translation system, including the rate of peptide bond formation (94) and the extent of phosphorylation of ribosomal proteins (76). These data have been extended to suggest that methylation reactions are important in morphogenesis (59). In particular, the α-subunit of protein synthesis elongation factor (EF-1α) is extensively methylated (59). Fonzi et al (37) postulated that methylation increases the basicity of the lysine groups, which would enhance the ability of EF-1α to complex with the acidic aminoacyl-tRNA, ribosomes, and mRNA. This would facilitate guanosine triphosphate (GTF) hydrolysis.

Restrepo et al (102) have shown that the mycelium-to-yeast transformation of *P. brasiliensis* is inhibited in vitro by estrogen. They have found a cytosolic sterol-binding protein which has high affinity and stereospecificity for estradiol, and they postulate that this binding site is involved in the regulation of morphogenesis of the fungi. It is the inhibition of transformation by estrogen in the lungs of females at the portal of infection that would then provide an explanation for the resistance of females to the disease. A similar protein has been found in the cytosol of *C. albicans*, which binds corticosterone and progesterone with high affinity and specificity (78).

Toward a General Model for Morphogenesis

In this section I have attempted to present a model for yeast-to-mycelial transformation. In doing this I have drawn on the available cytologic and biochemical data from several dimorphic fungi.

In any discussion of the mechanism of yeast-to-mycelial morphogenesis the many points of similarity in the biochemical events associated with the growth of both forms must be accommodated. A model for the yeast-to-mycelial transition is shown in Fig. 8-3 and would include the following events:

1. The mother cell responds to a signal from the environment on whether to continue growth in the yeast or mycelial form. This signal may be presented as a change in temperature, pH, nutrient, or some combination thereof.
2. A site on the cell surface is selected for evagination. How this site is selected is not known at this time and indeed this highlights an essential, if not the essential, regulatory factor dictating which of the two forms develops. For example, in *C. albicans* germ-tubes emanate from all parts of the yeast cell surface, whereas buds tend to arise from the polar regions of the cell. This suggests that the decision to make a hyphal element or a budding cell is an early event involving the cytoskeleton.
3. The earliest cytochemical event is the development of a cytoskeletal element, particularly actin fibrils, within the growth area.
4. The wall and plasma membrane expand through apical growth. This can be accomplished by the directed secretion of vesicles along the actin fibrils to the site of wall expansion. These vesicles originate in a membranous body believed to be equivalent to the Golgi apparatus and contain new material for the plasma membrane.
5. At the plasmalemma there is accretion of the new membrane material of the vesicle into the plasma membrane. Recycling of plasma membrane occurs through endocytosis.
6. The vesicles contain membrane-bound enzymes, soluble enzymes, and perhaps polymer primers. When the membrane vesicles are incorporated into the plasma membrane the polarity of the protein is the same as it was in the vesicle.
7. In the plasma membrane the polysaccharide synthases are activated. These are transmembrane enzymes that catalyze the vectorial synthesis of polymers, that is, substrates are added to one side of the membrane and the product emerges from the other. The product now undergoes intussusception into the expanding cell wall and it is believed that lysins such as glucanases play a critical role in this process.
8. Evagination of the mother cell then occurs. For the formation of both yeast and mycelial cells the major zone of expansion appears to be in the apical tip. With yeast growth, the final size (eg, the last 30% in *C. albicans*) is achieved with generalized growth but with hyphae apical growth is continouous.
9. One important difference between yeast and hyphal growth may be in the timing of secondary wall formation, for example, if the glucan-chitin complex is formed almost immediately behind the apical tip this would give a rigid structure resulting in a hyphal element. If, however, secondary wall formation with its cross-links was delayed, a more plastic wall would result, allowing the formation of a spherical cell.

Acknowledgment

The author thanks Gillian Schep for assistance in the preparation of the manuscript.

References

1. Adams AEM, Pringle JR: Relationship of actin and tubulin distribution in wild-type and morphogenetic-mutant *Saccharomyces cerevisiae*. *J Cell Biol* 98:934–945, 1984.
2. Ainsworth GC: Pathogenicity of fungi in man and animals, in Howie JW, O'Hea AJ (eds): *Mechanisms of Microbial Pathogenicity*. Cambridge, Cambridge University Press, 1955, pp 242–262.
3. Aoki S, Ito-Kuwa S: Inhibitor suceptibility of the cyanide-resistant pathway in *Candida albicans*. *Jpn J Oral Biol* 27:737–740, 1985.
4. Atkins EDT, Parker KD, Preston RD: The helical structure of the β-1,3-linked xylan in some siphoneous green algae. *Proc R Soc Lond B* 173:209–221, 1969.
5. Ballou CE: Yeast cell wall and cell surface, in Strathern JN, Jones EW, Broach JR (eds): *The Molecular Biology of the Yeast Saccharomyces. Metabolism and Gene Expression*. Cold Spring Harbor, New York, 1982, pp 335–360.
6. Bartnicki-Garcia S, Lippman E: Fungal morphogenesis: Cell wall construction in *Mucor rouxii*. *Science* 165:302–304, 1969.
7. Braun PC, Calderone RA: Chitin synthesis in *Candida albicans*: Comparison of yeast and hyphal forms. *J Bacteriol* 133:1472–1477, 1978.
8. Brunswick H: Untersuchungen über Geschlechts und Kernverhältnisse bei der Hymenomyzetengattung *Coprinus*, in Goebel K (ed): *Botanische Abhandlungen*, Vol. 5. Jena, Gustav Fisher, 1924, pp 1–152.
9. Buffo J, Herman MA, Soll DR: A characterization of pH-regulated dimorphism in *Candida albicans*. *Mycopathologia* 85:21–30, 1984.
10. Byers B, Goetsch L: A highly ordered ring of membrane-associated filaments in budding yeast. *J Cell Biol* 69:717–721, 1976.
11. Cabib E: Molecular aspects of yeast morphogenesis. *Ann Rev Microbiol* 29:191–214, 1975.
12. Cabib E, Bowers B: Chitin and yeast budding. Localization of chitin in yeast bud scars. *J Biol Chem* 246:152–159, 1971.
13. Cabib E, Bowers B, Roberts RL: Vectorial synthesis of a polysaccharide by isolated plasma membranes. *Proc Natl Acad Sci USA* 80:3318–3321, 1983.
14. Cabib E, Roberts R, Bowers B: Synthesis of the yeast cell wall and its regulation. *Ann Rev Biochem* 51:763–793, 1982.
15. Carbonell LM: Ultrastructure of dimorphic transformation in *Paracoccidioides brasiliensis*. *J Bacteriol* 100:1076–1082, 1969.
16. Cassone A, Carpinelli G, Angiolella L, Maddaluno G, Podo F: ^{31}P nuclear magnetic reasonance study of growth and dimorphic transition in *Candida albicans*. *J Gen Microbiol* 129:1569–1575, 1983.
17. Cassone A, Mattia E, Boldrini L: Agglutination of blastospores of *Candida albicans* by concanavalin A and its relationship with the distribution of mannan polymers and the ultrastructure of the cell wall. *J Gen Microbiol* 105:263–273, 1978.
18. Cassone A, Simonetti N, Strippoli V: Ultrastructural changes in the wall during germ-tube formation from blastospores of *Candida albicans*. *J Gen Microbiol* 77:417–426, 1973.

19. Cassone A, Sullivan PA, Shepherd MG: N-acetyl-D-glucosamine-induced morphogenesis in *Candida albicans*. *Microbiologica* 8:85–99, 1985.
20. Chaffin WL: Site selection for bud and germ tube emergence in *Candida albicans*. *J Gen Microbiol* 130:431–440, 1984.
21. Chandler FW, Kaplan W, Ajello L: *A Colour Atlas and Textbook of the Histopathology of Mycotic Diseases*. London, Wolfe Medical Publications, 1980.
22. Chattaway FW, Holmes MR, Barlow AJE: Cell wall composition of the mycelial and blastospore forms of *Candida albicans*. *J Gen Microbiol* 51:367–376, 1968.
23. Cheung SC, Kobayashi GS, Schlessinger D, Medoff G: RNA metabolism during morphogenesis in *Histoplasma capsulatum*. *J Gen Microbiol* 82:301–307, 1974.
24. Chiew YY, Shepherd MG, Sullivan PA: Regulation of chitin synthesis during germ-tube formation in *Candida albicans*. *Arch Microbiol* 125:97–104, 1980.
25. Chiew YY, Sullivan PA, Shepherd MG: The effects of ergosterol and alcohols on germ-tube formation and chitin synthase in *Candida albicans*. *Can J Biochem* 60:15–20, 1982.
26. Cochrane VW: *Physiology of Fungi*. New York, Wiley & Sons, 1958.
27. Cole GT: Infectious fungal propagules, in Schlessinger D (ed): *Microbiology—1983*. Washington, D.C., American Society for Microbiology, 1983, pp 245–248.
28. Cole GT, Sun SH: Arthroconidium-spherule-endospore transformation in *Coccidioides immitis*, in Szaniszlo PJ (ed): *Fungal Dimorphism*. New York, London, Plenum Press, 1985, pp 281–333.
29. Conant NF, Howell A: The similarity of the fungus causing South American blastomycosis (paracoccidioidal granuloma) and North American blastomycosis (Gilchrist's disease). *J Invest Dermatol* 5:353–370, 1942.
30. Davis TE Jr, Domer JE, Li Y-T: Cell wall studies of *Histoplasma capsulatum* and *Blastomyces dermatitidis* using autologous and heterologous enzymes. *Infect Immun* 15:978–987, 1977.
31. Edwards GA, Edwards MR: The intracellular membranes of *Blastomyces dermatitidis*. *Am J Bot* 47:622–632, 1960.
32. Evans ZA: Tissue responses to the blastospores and hyphae of *Candida albicans* in the mouse. *J Med Microbiol* 14:307–319, 1980.
33. Falcone G, Nickerson WJ: Cell wall mannan-protein of baker's yeast. *Science* 124:272–273, 1956.
34. Farkaš V: Biosynthesis of cell walls of fungi. *Microbiol Rev* 43:117–144, 1979.
35. Farkaš V, Kovařík J, Košinová A, Bauer Š: Autoradiographic study of mannan incorporation into the growing cell walls of *Saccharomyces cerevisiae*. *J Bacteriol* 117:265–269, 1974.
36. Field C, Schekman R: Localized secretion of acid phosphatase reflects the pattern of cell surface growth in *Saccharomyces cerevisiae*. *J Cell Biol* 86:123–128, 1980.
37. Fonzi WA, Katayama C, Leathers T, Sypherd PS: Regulation of protein synthesis factor EF-1α in *Mucor racemosus*. *Mol Cell Biol* 5:1100–1103, 1985.
38. Gallwitz D, Sures I: Structure of a split yeast gene: Complete nucleotide sequence of the actin gene in *Saccharomyces cerevisiae*. *Proc Natl Acad Sci USA* 77:2546–2550, 1980.
39. Galun M, Braun A, Frensdorff A, Galun E: Hyphal walls of isolated lichen fungi. Autoradiographic localization of precursor incorporation and binding of fluorescein-conjugated lectins. *Arch Microbiol* 108:9–16, 1976.
40. Galun E: Morphogenesis of *Trichoderma*: Autoradiography of intact colonies labelled by [^{3}H]N-acetylglucosamine as a marker of new cell wall biosynthesis. *Arch Mikrobiol* 86:305–314, 1972.
41. Garrison RG: Ultrastructural cytology of the pathogenic fungi, in Howard DH (ed): *Fungi Pathogenic for Man and Animals*, Part A. New York, Marcel Dekker, 1983, pp 229–321.
42. Garrison RG: Cytological and ultrastructural aspects of dimorphism, in

Szaniszlo PJ (ed): *Fungal Dimorphism*. New York, London, Plenum Press, 1985, pp 15–47.
43. Garrison RG, Boyd KS: Electron microscopy of yeastlike cell development from the microconidium of *Histoplasma capsulatum*. *J Bacteriol* 133:345–353, 1978.
44. Garrison RG, Boyd KS: Role of the conidium in dimorphism of *Blastomyces dermatitidis*. *Mycopathologia* 64:29–33, 1978.
45. Garrison RG, Boyd KS, Mariat F: Ultrastructural studies of the mycelial-to-yeast transformation of *Sporothrix schenckii*. *J Bacteriol* 124:959–968, 1975.
46. Garrison RG, Lane JW, Johnson DR: Electron microscopy of the transitional conversion cell of *Histoplasma capsulatum*. *Mycopathol Mycol Appl* 44:121–129, 1971.
47. Garrison RG, Mariat F, Fromentin H, Mirikitani FK: Electron microscopic analysis of yeastlike cell formation from the conidia of *Sporothrix schenkii*. *Ann Microbiol (Inst Pasteur)* 133B:189–204, 1982.
48. Gennis RB, Jonas A: Protein-lipid interactions. *Ann Rev Biophys Bioeng* 6:195–238, 1977.
49. Gilardi GL: Nutrition of systemic and subcutaneous pathogenic fungi. *Bacteriol Rev* 29:406–424, 1965.
50. Gooday GW: An autoradiographic study of hyphal growth of some fungi. *J Gen Microbiol* 67:125–133, 1971.
51. Gopal PK, Shepherd MG, Sullivan PA: Analysis of wall glucans from yeast, hyphal and germ-tube forming cells of *Candida albicans*. *J Gen Microbiol* 130: 3295–3301, 1984.
52. Gopal P, Sullivan PA, Shepherd MG: Enzymes of N-acetylglucosamine metabolism during germ-tube formation in *Candida albicans*. *J Gen Microbiol* 128:2319–2326, 1982.
53. Gopal P, Sullivan PA, Shepherd MG: Metabolism of [^{14}C]glucose by regenerating spheroplasts of *Candida albicans*. *J Gen Microbiol* 130:325–335, 1984.
54. Gow NAR, Gooday GW: A model for the germ tube formation and mycelial growth form of *Candida albicans*. *Sabouraudia* 22:137–144, 1984.
55. Gow NAR, Gooday GW, Newsam RJ, Gull K: Ultrastructure of the septum in *Candida albicans*. *Curr Microbiol* 4:357–359, 1980.
56. Grove SN: The cytology of hyphal tip growth, in Smith JE, Berry DR (eds): *The Filamentous Fungi*, Vol. 3. London, Edward Arnold, 1978, pp 28–50.
57. Grove SN, Oujezdsky KB, Szaniszlo PJ: Budding in the dimorphic fungus *Phialophora dermatitidis*. *J Bacteriol* 115:323–329, 1973.
58. Hallak J, San-Blas F, San-Blas G: Isolation and wall analysis of dimorphic mutants of *Paracoccidioides brasiliensis*. *Sabouraudia* 20:51–62, 1982.
59. Hiatt WR, Garcia R, Merrick WC, Sypherd PS: Methylation of elongation factor 1α from the fungus *Mucor*. *Proc Natl Acad Sci USA* 79:3433–3437, 1982.
60. Horisberger M, Vonlanthen M: Location of mannan and chitin on thin sections of budding yeasts with gold markers: *Arch Microbiol* 115:1–7, 1977.
61. Howard DH: The morphogenesis of the parasitic forms of dimorphic fungi. A review. *Mycopathol Mycol Appl* 18:127–139, 1962.
62. Howard DH, Herndon RL: Tissue cultures of mouse peritoneal exudates inoculated with *Blastomyces dermatitidis*. *J Bacteriol* 80:522–527, 1960.
63. Hubbard MJ, Sullivan PA, Shepherd MG: Morphological studies of N-acetylglucosamine induced germ tube formation by *Candida albicans*. *Can J Microbiol* 31:696–701, 1985.
64. Hunsley D, Kay D: Wall structure of the *Neurospora* hyphal apex: Immunofluorescent localization of wall surface antigens. *J Gen Microbiol* 95:233–248, 1976.
65. Inderlied CB, Peters J, Cihlar RL: *Mucor racemosus*, in Szaniszlo PJ (ed): *Fungal Dimorphism*. New York, London, Plenum Press, 1985, pp 337–359.

66. Ito Et, Cihlar RL, Inderlied CB: Lipid synthesis during morphogenesis of *Mucor racemosus. J Bacteriol* 152:880–887, 1982.
67. Kanetsuna F, Carbonell LM: Cell wall composition of the yeastlike and mycelial forms of *Blastomyces dermatitidis. J Bacteriol* 106:946–948, 1971.
68. Kanetsuna F, Carbonell LM, Azuma I, Yamamura Y: Biochemical studies on the thermal dimorphism of *Paracoccidioides brasiliensis. J Bacteriol* 110:208–218, 1972.
69. Kanetsuna F, Carbonell LM, Moreno RE, Rodriguez J: Cell wall composition of the yeast and mycelial forms of *Paracoccidioides brasiliensis. J Bacteriol* 97: 1036–1041, 1969.
70. Katz D, Rosenberger RF: Hyphal wall synthesis in *Aspergillus nidulans*: Effect of protein synthesis inhibition and osmotic shock on chitin insertion and morphogenesis. *J Bacteriol* 108:184–190, 1971.
71. Kobayashi GS, Medoff G, Maresca B, Sacco M, Kumar BV: Studies on phase transitions in the dimorphic pathogen *Histoplasma capsulatum*, in Szaniszlo PJ (ed): *Fungal Dimorphism*. New York, London, Plenum Press, 1985, pp 69–91.
72. Korn ED: Biochemistry of actomysin-dependent cell motility (a review). *Proc Natl Acad Sci USA* 75:588–599, 1978.
73. Kown-Chung KJ: Sexual stage of *Histoplasma capsulatum. Science* 175:326, 1972.
74. Lacey J: The aerobiology of conidial fungi, in Cole GT, Kendrick B (eds): *Biology of Conidial Fungi*, Vol. 1. New York, Academic Press, 1981, pp 373–416.
75. Larsen AD, Sypherd PS: Cyclic adenosine 3′, 5′-monophosphate and morphogenesis in *Mucor racemosus. J Bacteriol* 117:432–438, 1974.
76. Larsen A, Sypherd PS: Ribosomal proteins of the dimorphic fungus, *Mucor racemosus. Mol Gen Genet* 175:99–109, 1979.
77. Lee KL, Buckley HR, Campbell CC: An amino acid liquid synthetic medium for the development of mycelial and yeast forms of *Candida albicans. Sabouraudia* 13:148–153, 1975.
78. Loose DS, Stevens DA, Schurman DJ, Feldman D: Distribution of a corticosteroid-binding protein in *Candida* and other fungal genera. *J Gen Microbiol* 129:2379–2385, 1983.
79. Mackenzie DWR: Morphogenesis of *Candida albicans* in vivo. *Sabouraudia* 3:225–232, 1964.
80. Mardon DN, Gunn, JL, Robinette E Jr: Variation in the lethal response in mice to yeast-like and pseudohyphal forms of *Candida albicans. Can J Microbiol* 21:1681–1687, 1975.
81. Maresca B, Jacobson E, Medoff G, Kobayashi G: Cystine reductase in the dimorphic fungus *Histoplasma capsulatum. J Bacteriol* 135:987–992. 1978.
82. Maresca B, Lambowitz AM, Kobayashi GS, Medoff G: Respiration in the yeast and mycelial phases of *Histoplasma capsulatum. J Bacteriol* 138:647–649, 1979.
83. Maresca B, Lambowitz AM, Kumar VB, Grant GA, Kobayashi GS, Medoff G: Role of cysteine in regulating morphogenesis and mitochondrial activity in the dimorphic fungus *Histoplasma capsulatum. Proc Natl Acad Sci USA* 78:4596–4600, 1981.
84. Maresca B, Medoff G, Schlessinger D, Kobayashi GS, Medoff J: Regulation of dimorphism in the pathogenic fungus *Histoplasma capsulatum. Nature (London)* 266:447–448, 1977.
85. Mariat F: Saprophytic and parasitic morphology of pathogenic fungi, in Smith H (ed): *Microbial Behaviour, in Vivo and in Vitro*. Cambridge, Cambridge University Press, 1964, pp 85–111.
86. Mitchell LH, Soll DR: Temporal and spatial differences in septation during synchronous mycelium and bud formation by *Candida albicans. Exp Mycol* 3:298–309, 1979.

87. Miyaji M, Nishimura K, Ajello L: Scanning electron microscope studies on the parasitic cycle of *Coccidioides immitis. Mycopathologia* 89:51–57, 1985.
88. Nickerson WJ: Enzymatic control of cell division in microorganisms. *Nature (London)* 162:241–245, 1948.
89. Nickerson WJ, Edwards GA: Studies on the physiological bases of morphogenesis in fungi. I. The respiratory metabolism of dimorphic pathogenic fungi. *J Gen Physiol* 33:41–55, 1950.
90. Novick P: Intracellular transport mutants of yeast. *Trends Biochem Sci* 10:432–434, 1985.
91. Novick P, Botstein D: Phenotypic analysis of temperature-sensitive yeast actin mutants. *Cell* 40:405–416, 1985.
92. Odds FC: Morphogenesis in *Candida albicans. CRC Crit Rev Microbiol* 12:45–93, 1985.
93. Orlowski M: Cyclic adenosine 3′,5′-monophosphate and germination of sporangiospores from the fungus *Mucor. Arch Microbiol* 126:133–140, 1980.
94. Orlowski M, Sypherd PS: Regulation of translation rate during morphogenesis in the fungus *Mucor. Biochemistry* 17:569–575, 1978.
95. Oujezdsky KB, Grove SN, Szaniszlo PJ: Morphological and structural changes during the yeast-to-mold conversion of *Phialophora dermatitidis. J Bacteriol* 113:468–477, 1973.
96. Paris S, Duran-Gonzalez S, Mariat F: Nutritional studies on *Paracoccidioides brasiliensis*: The role of organic sulfur in dimorphism. *Sabouraudia* 23:85–92, 1985.
97. Pollard TD, Selden SC, Maupin P: Interaction of actin filaments with microtubules. *J Cell Biol* 99:33s–99s, 1984.
98. Previato JO, Gorin PAJ, Haskins RH, Travassos LR: Soluble and insoluble glucans from different cell types of the human pathogen *Sporothrix schenckii. Exp Mycol* 3:92–105, 1979.
99. Previato JO, Gorin PAJ, Travassos LR: Cell wall composition in different cell types of the dimorphic species *Sporothrix schenckii. Exp Mycol* 3:83–91, 1979.
100. Restrepo A: Paracoccidioidomycosis: Actualization. *Acta Med Colombiana* 3:33–66, 1978.
101. Restrepo A: Paracoccidioidomycosis, in Feigen RD, Cherry JD (eds): *Textbook of Pediatric Infectious Disease.* Philadelphia, WB Saunders, 1981, pp 1500–1505.
102. Restrepo A, Salazar ME, Cano LE, Stover EP, Feldman D, Stevens DA: Estrogens inhibit mycelium-to-yeast transformation in the fungus *Paracoccidioides brasiliensis*: Implications for resistance of females to paracoccidioidomycosis. *Infect Immun* 47:346–353, 1984.
103. Riezman H: Endocytosis in yeast: Several of the yeast secretory mutants are defective in endocytosis. *Cell* 40:1001–1009, 1985.
104. Rippon JW: *Medical Mycology. The Pathogenic Fungi and the Pathogenic Actinomycetes.* Philadelphia, London, Toronto, WB Saunders, 1982.
105. Roberts RL, Szaniszlo PJ: Yeast-phase cell cycle of the polymorphic fungus *Wangiella dermatitidis. J Bacteriol* 144:721–731, 1980.
106. Robertson NF: The fungal hypha. *Trans Br Mycol Soc* 48:1–8, 1965.
107. Roy I, Landau JW: Protein constituents of cell walls of the dimorphic phases of *Blastomyces dermatitidis. Can J Microbiol* 18:473–478, 1972.
108. Ruiz-Herrera J: Dimorphism in *Mucor* species with emphasis on *M. rouxii* and *M. bacilliformis*, in Szaniszlo PJ (ed): *Fungal Dimorphism.* New York, London, Plenum Press, 1985, pp 361–384.
109. San-Blas F, San-Blas G: *Paracoccidioides brasiliensis*, in Szaniszlo PJ (ed): *Fungal Dimorphism.* New York, London, Plenum Press, 1985, pp 93–120.
110. Sandin RL, Rogers AL, Patterson RJ, Beneke ES: Evidence for mannose-

mediated adherence of *Candida albicans* to human buccal cells in vitro. *Infect Immun* 35:79–85, 1982.
111. Scherr GH: Studies on the dimorphism of *Histoplasma capsulatum*. I. The roles of -SH groups and incubation temperature. *Exp Cell Res* 12:92–107, 1957.
112. Scherwitz C, Martin R, Ueberberg H: Ultrastructural investigations of the formation of *Candida albicans* germ tubes and septa. *Sabouraudia* 16:115–124, 1978.
113. Schnapp BJ, Vale RD, Sheetz MP, Reese TS: Single microtubules from squid axoplasm support bidirectional movement of organelles. *Cell* 40:455–462, 1985.
114. Schroer TA, Kelly RB: In vitro translocation of organelles along microtubules. *Cell* 40:729–730, 1985.
115. Scott JH, Schekman R: Lyticase: Endoglucanase and protease activities that act together in yeast cell lysis. *J Bacteriol* 142:414–423, 1980.
116. Sheetz MP, Chasan R, Spudich JA: ATP-dependent movement of myosin in vitro: Characterization of a quantitative assay. *J Cell Biol* 99:1867–1871, 1984.
117. Shepherd MG: Pathogenicity of morphological and auxotropic mutants of *Candida albicans* in experimental infections. *Infect Immun* 50:541–544, 1985.
118. Shepherd MG, Chiew YY, Ram SP, Sullivan PA: Germ tube induction in *Candida albicans*. *Can J Microbiol* 26:21–26, 1980.
119. Shepherd MG, Chin CM, Sullivan PA: The alternate respiratory pathway of *Candida albicans*. *Arch Microbiol* 116:61–67, 1978.
120. Shepherd MG, Ghazali HM, Sullivan PA: N-acetyl-D-glucosamine kinase and germ-tube formation in *Candida albicans*. *Exp Mycol* 4:147–159, 1980.
121. Shepherd MG, Poulter RTM, Sullivan PA: *Candida albicans*: Biology, genetics, and pathogenicity. *Ann Rev Microbiol* 39:579–614, 1985.
122. Shepherd MG, Sullivan PA: *Candida albicans* germ-tube formation with immobilized GlcNAc. *FEMS Microbiol Lett* 17:167–170, 1983.
123. Shepherd MG, Sullivan PA: The control of morphogenesis in *Candida albicans*. *J Dent Res* 63:435–440, 1984.
124. Sietsma JH, Sonnenberg AMS, Wessels JGH: Localization by autoradiography of synthesis of (1→3) -β and (1→6) -β linkages in a wall glucan during hyphal growth of *Schizophyllum commune*. *J Gen Microbiol* 131:1331–1337, 1985.
125. Simonetti N, Strippoli, V: Pathogenicity of the Y form as compared to M form in experimentally induced *Candida albicans* infections. *Mycopathol Mycol Appl* 51:19–28, 1973.
126. Simonetti N, Strippoli V, Cassone A: Yeast-mycelial conversion induced by N-acetyl-D-glucosamine in *Candida albicans*. *Nature* 250:344–346, 1974.
127. Sloat BF, Pringle JR: A mutant of yeast defective in cellular morphogenesis. *Science* 200:1171–1173, 1978.
128. Staebell M, Soll DR: Temporal and spatial differences in cell wall expansion during bud and mycelium formation in *Candida albicans*. *J Gen Microbiol* 131:1467–1480, 1985.
129. Sullivan PA, Chiew YY, Molloy C, Templeton MD, Shepherd MG: An analysis of the metabolism and cell wall composition of *Candida albicans* during germ-tube formation. *Can J Microbiol* 29:1514–1525, 1983.
130. Sullivan PA, Shepherd MG: Gratuitous induction by N- acetylmannosamine of germ tube formation and enzymes for N-acetylglucosamine utilization in *Candida albicans*. *J Bacteriol* 151:1118–1122, 1982.
131. Sun SH, Cole GT, Drutz DJ, Harrison JL: Electron-microscopic observations of the *Coccidioides immitis* parasitic cycle in vivo. *J Med Vet Mycol* 24:183–192, 1986.
132. Sun SH, Sekhon SS, Huppert M: Electron microscopic studies of saprobic and parasitic forms of *Coccidioides immitis*. *Sabouraudia* 17:265–273, 1979.

133. Szaniszlo PJ (ed): *Fungal Dimorphism.* New York, London, Plenum Press, 1985.
134. Szaniszlo PJ, Geis PA, Jacobs CW, Cooper CR Jr, Harris JL: Cell wall changes associated with yeast-to-multicellular form conversion in *Wangiella dermatitidis*, in Schlessinger D (ed): *Microbiology–1983*. Washington, D.C., American Society for Microbiology, 1983, pp 239–244.
135. Tabor CW, Tabor H: 1,4-Diaminobutane (putrescine), spermidine, and spermine. *Ann Rev Biochem* 45:285–306, 1976.
136. Tkacz JS, Lampen JL: Surface distribution of invertase on growing *Saccharomyces* cells. *J Bacteriol* 113:1073–1075, 1973.

9—Epidemiology of Nosocomial Fungal Infections

DAVID J. WEBER AND WILLIAM A. RUTALA

Approximately 5% of all hospitalized patients develop a nosocomial infection. The costs associated with such infections are estimated to be more than 1 billion dollars per year. Although bacteria are the most common etiologic agents in hospital-acquired infections, fungi are also significant nosocomial pathogens.

This paper is intended as a review of the epidemiology of hospital-acquired fungal infections. It will emphasize the risk factors associated with the acquisition of nosocomial fungal infections, environmental reservoirs of nosocomial fungal pathogens, and infection control practices that may minimize such infections. Only selected information will be presented on the clinical features, diagnosis, and treatment of nosocomial fungal infections.

Incidence and Significance

It is difficult to obtain unbiased data regarding the incidence and prevalence of nosocomial fungal infections. The most representative data have been provided by the Centers for Disease Control via its National Nosocomial Infection Surveillance (NNIS) system. The 1984 data are displayed in Table 9-1 along with unpublished data from the North Carolina Memorial Hospital (NCMH), a 580-bed acute-care teaching hospital, and City of Hope National Medical Center (196), a 212-bed cancer hospital. The 1984 NNIS rates represent data collected by the Centers for Disease Control from 51 US hospitals (43). Of 26,965 infections, pathogens were identified in 84%. *Candida* spp. were the eighth most common nosocomial pathogen and accounted for 5.5% of all isolates (Table 9-1). The category of "other fungi" was ranked as the 11th most common nosocomial pathogen and accounted for 1.7% of all nosocomial isolates. The data collected at NCMH is similar to the NNIS data. Nosocomial fungal infections appear to occur most commonly on the med-

TABLE 9-1. Prevalence of Nosocomial Fungal Infections

	Relative Frequency of Isolation (% of Total Isolates)					
	NNIS (1984)		NCMH (1980–84)		Cancer Center (1979–1981)	
	Candida	Other Fungi	Yeasts*	Other Fungi†	*C. albicans*	Other Yeast
Service						
Medicine	7.0	2.3	11.6	0.7		
Surgery	4.9	1.2	6.8	0.1		
Pediatrics	7.6	1.2	4.1	0.0		
Obstetrics	1.1	0.1	ND‡	ND		
Gynecology	2.2	0.1	4.7	0.0		
Newborn	3.8	1.0	ND	ND		
Other	ND	ND	2.1	0.0		
Site						
UTI	5.4	2.2	12.8	0.0	6.9	6.4
SWI	1.7	0.4	2.3	0.0	4.1	5.5
LRI	4.0	1.4	3.7	0.8	8.0	1.3
BACT	5.6	1.3	8.7	0.0	4.7	10.7
CUT	5.8	0.9	7.8	1.0		
GI	ND	ND	16.4	0.0		
Other	14.1	2.8	7.9	0.5	3.8	1.9
Location						
ICU	ND	ND	9.7	0.1		
Non-ICU	ND	ND	6.4	0.3		

* Includes yeast, *Candida* spp., *C. albicans*, *C. parapsilosis*, *C. tropicalis*, and *Torulopsis glabrata*.
† Includes *Aspergillus* spp., *A. flavus*, *A. fumigatus*, *A. terreus*, *Cladosporium* spp., *Cryptococcus neoformans*.
‡ No data.

ical, surgical, and pediatric services, and more frequently in intensive care unit (ICU) patients compared with non-ICU patients. Fungi are infrequently the etiologic agent in surgical wound infections. Fungi are relatively more common nosocomial pathogens in cancer hospitals.

The incidence and relative frequency of *Candida* as a nosocomial pathogen appears to be increasing. NNIS data from 1980–1982 reported that *Candida* spp. accounted for 4.5% of all nosocomial pathogens (42) compared with 5.5% in 1983 (43). NNIS data have also revealed that between 1980 and 1984, candidemia increased from 0.7 to 1.5 per 10,000 discharges, and central nervous system infections increased from 0.03 to 0.05 per 10,000 discharges (51). Similar data have been reported by Morrison et al (157), who reported that *Candida* fungemia increased from 0.1 to 1.5 per 10,000 discharges from 1978 to 1984 among an average of 112 acute-care hospitals in Virginia. Possible reasons for this increasing incidence include wider use of broad spectrum antimicrobials, increased numbers of immunocompromised patients, increased numbers of premature infants and older patients, increased numbers of organ transplantation, and improved techniques of fungal isolation and treatment. However, the NNIS data have not revealed an increase in the incidence of nosocomial filamentous fungus infections (52).

Reports from hospitals specializing in oncology suggest that fungi are an increasing cause of nosocomial infections and mortality. Autopsy data from the National Cancer Institute revealed that 22% (34 of 157) of patients with acute leukemia who died between 1954 and 1958 had evidence of fungal infections compared with 43% (127 of 297) dying between 1959 and 1964 (23). Horn et al (96) analyzed 200 episodes of fungemia seen at the Memorial Sloan-Kettering Cancer Institute between 1978 and 1982, and compared them with 110 episodes of fungemia that occurred from 1974 to 1977. Overall the number of episodes of fungemia per year increased by 30.6%. Although episodes of fungemia per 100 new leukemia patients decreased by 50%, episodes per 100 new lymphoma and solid tumor patients increased by 73 and 95%, respectively.

Fungal infections have been and continue to be an important source of morbidity and mortality in oncology patients and organ transplant patients (Table 9-2). Fungal infections account for 20–30% of fatal infections in patients with acute leukemia, 10–15% of the fatal infections in patients with lymphoma, but only 5% of fatal infections in patients with solid tumors. Fungi are also an important cause of mortality in renal, cardiac, and bone marrow transplant patients.

Modes of Acquisition of Fungal Infections

The acquisition of nosocomial pathogens depends on a complex interplay of the host, pathogen, and environment. Among the host factors important in the development of a nosocomial infection are underlying medical disorders, T- and B-cell-mediated immune function, nutrition, age, and genetic factors. Microbial factors include the minimum inoculating dose sufficient to cause infection, virulence, pathogenicity, infectivity, and ability to produce a latent infection. The environment may serve as a reservoir and/or source of an infectious agent. A reservoir is defined as the place where a microorganism maintains its presence, metabolizes, and replicates. The source is the location from which the infectious agent passes to the host. Control of nosocomial fungal infections requires an understanding of the hospital as a complex ecosystem.

Nosocomial fungal infections may result from either endogenous flora (ie, fungi that are normal commensals of skin, respiratory tract, gastrointestinal tract, or genitourinary tract) or exogenous flora (ie, fungi with an environ-

TABLE 9-2. Frequency of Systemic or Invasive Fungal Infection: Autopsy Series

Reference	Years	Underlying Disease	Population	% of Population with Fungal Infections					Comments
				Candida	*Aspergillus*	Zygomycetes	*Torulopsis*	Mixed/Other	
Rifkind (193)	1962–65	Renal transplant	51	22	9.8			5.9	No. at risk = 107
Singer* (212)	1972–73	Malignancy plus sepsis	88	11	9.1			9.1	No. at risk = 300
Mirsky (152)	1968–70	Acute leukemia	65	12	15	6.2			
Myerowitz (162)	1963–70	All	2,714	0.33					
Myerowitz (162)	1971–75	All	1,325	2.3					
Bodey*§ (23)	1954–58	Acute leukemia	157	7.0	3.8	0	0	0	
Bodey*§ (23)	1959–64	Acute leukemia	297	20	11	2.0	0.67	3.4	
Pizzo* (180)	1970–75	Malignancy	132	25	8.3	0.76		14	No. at risk = 900
Pizzo* (180)	1976–79	Malignancy	88	22	2.3			2.3	No. at risk = 1200
Clift (48)	1969–80	Bone marrow transplant	266	8.6	7.1			3.3	
Schumacher (207)	1957–62	Leukemia	205	1.5	0.98			0.49	All infections in hospital
Turcotte (234)	1969–71	Renal transplant	93	0.30					Infection rate/month
Bodey*† (24)	1966–72	Acute leukemia	494	7.1	0.61	0.61		8.7	All infections in hospital
Rose (199)	1963–73	All	85,391	0.064	0.014	0.0023	0.0058	0.028	All infections in hospital
Rose (199)	1963–73	All	85,391	0.064	0.0094	0	0.0058	0	Nosocomial infections only
Sandford* (204)	1977–78	Bone marrow transplant, hematologic malignancy	89	21	2.2				All infections in hospital
Maksymiuk* (133)	1976–80	Malignancy	27,681	0.64	0.083	0.025	0.022	0.076	All infections in hospital
Robinson*‡ (196)	1979–81	Neoplasm	7,714	0.26				0.26	Nosocomial infections only
Peterson (197)§	1979–81	Bone marrow transplant	50	8.0	26	2.0	2.0		Follow-up >146 days or till death
FUNGEMIA									
Meunier-Carpentier* (148)	1974–77	Leukemia		11.9			1.0	0.50	Episodes/100 new patients
" "	1974–77	Lymphoma		1.0			0.31	0.20	Episodes/100 new patients
" "	1974–77	Solid tumor		0.13			0.06	0.007	Episodes/100 new patients
Horn* (96)	1978–82	Leukemia		6.0			0.09	0.40	Episodes/100 new patients
Horn* (96)	1978–82	Lymphoma		2.1			0.31	0.23	Episodes/100 new patients
Horn* (96)	1978–82	Solid tumor		0.33			0.06	0.005	Episodes/100 new patients

* Data from a cancer hospital.
† Includes disseminated infection or pneumonia.
‡ Nosocomial bacteremia or respiratory tract infection.

mental reservoir). Iatrogenic breaches of body integrity are a major risk factor predisposing to infection by endogenous flora. Transmission of exogenous pathogens from an environmental reservoir or source to the patient may occur by one or more of four different routes: airborne, common vehicle, contact, or vectorborne. Exogenous pathogens may directly infect or colonize the patient. Airborne transmission describes organisms that have a true airborne phase as part of their pattern of dissemination. Many fungi are primarily acquired by inhalation of airborne conidia including species of *Aspergillus*, *Blastomyces*, *Cryptococcus*, *Histoplasma*, *Paracoccidioides*, *Sporothrix*, *Absidia*, *Coccidioides*, *Pseudallescheria*, *Cunninghamella*, and *Rhizopus* (6). In common vehicle spread, a contaminated inanimate vehicle serves as the means of transmission of the infectious agent to multiple persons. Common vehicles may include the following: ingested food or water, medical instruments used for invasive procedures, implanted prosthetic devices, and infused products such as medications or intravenous fluids. In contact spread, the patient has had contact with the source that is either direct, indirect, or droplet spread. Hospital staff frequently serve as the source for direct contact spread of nosocomial pathogens, and may be important in transmission of *Candida*. Indirect contact spread requires an intermediate object, which is usually inanimate (eg, endoscopes, thermometers), in the transmission of the pathogen from the source to the patient. Droplet spread refers to the brief passage of the pathogen through the air when the source and the patient are within a few feet of each other. Vectorborne nosocomial infection have not been reported in the United States.

By far the most common nosocomial fungal pathogen is *Candida* spp. (Tables 9-2 and 9-3). Although organ and bone marrow transplant patients and oncology patients have the highest attack rate, *Candida* spp. are frequent nosocomial pathogens in a variety of settings (Table 9-2). *Aspergillus* and the Zygomycetes are also important nosocomial pathogens, which usually attack immunosuppressed hosts. Increasingly recognized as serious nosocomial fungal pathogens are *Torulopsis glabrata* (2, 4, 96, 148, 225) and *Trichosporon* spp. (9, 13, 89, 161, 184, 237). Community-acquired fungal pathogens, especially *Cryptococcus neoformans*, may cause significant mortality in immunocompromised hosts including organ transplant and oncology patients, and individuals with the acquired immunodeficiency syndrome (AIDS).

All nosocomial filamentous fungal pathogens are acquired primarily from an inanimate reservoir usually via airborne transmission. Colonization or infection of the respiratory tract may then be followed by dissemination. Contact transmission leading to colonization or primary infection of the skin is especially important for *Aspergillus* and the Zygomycetes and may also lead to disseminated disease. Although multiple outbreaks of common vehicle transmission have been noted, infection control practices have been very successful in reducing the importance of this mode of transmission.

TABLE 9-3. Relative Frequency of Fungal Isolates in Selected Settings

Reference	Young (251)	Horn (96)	Kiehn (108)	Klein (112)	Maksmiuk (133)	Meunier-Carpenter (148)
Population	Mostly tumor*	Neoplasm*	Neoplasm*	All	Neoplasm*	Neoplasm*
Source	Blood	Blood	Any site	Blood	Any site[§]	Blood
No. of episodes	?	200	?	85	232	136
No. of patients	70	188	2327	77	230	110
Study years	1962–1972	1978–1982	?	1972–1977	1976–1980	1974–1977
Data presented as	Episodes fungemia	Episodes fungemia	No. of isolates	Episodes fungemia	Episodes fungal disease	No. of patients
Candida spp.						
C. albicans	28 (22)[†]	89 (13/29)[‡]	2289	44	92	40 (13/16)[‡]
C. tropicalis	12 (9)	51 (9/14)	430	11	54	25 (8/11)
C. parapsilosis	7 (5)	23 (0/1)	122	3	7	13 (0/2)
C. krusei	1 (1)	7 (2/3)	49	—	1	3 (0/1)
C. stellatoidea	—	—	—	—	—	—
C. guilliermondii	—	—	15	—	—	—
Mixed	1	—	—	—	9	—
C. spp.	—	—	11	5	15	1 (1/1)
Other fungi						
T. glabrata	—	22 (0/4)	350	5	6	22 (0/10)
Cr. neoformans	6 (5)	1 (1/1)	10	—	8	6 (1/3)
Histoplasma capsulatum	2 (2)	—	—	—	3	—
Rhodotorula spp.	1 (0)	—	8	—	—	—
Aspergillus spp.	6 (0)	—	—	—	19	—
Penicillium spp.	6 (0)	—	—	—	—	—
Zygomycetes	—	—	—	—	7	—
Trichosporon spp.	—	1 (1/1)	15	—	4	—
Cladosporium	1 (0)	—	—	—	—	—
Multiple	1 (0)	—	—	7	4	—
Other	—	6 (0/0)	41	10	3	—

Reference	Richards (192)	Dyess (65)
Population	Burns	All
Source	Blood**	Blood**
No. of episodes	?	117
No. of patients	53	83
Study years	1954–1964	1976–1983
Data presented as	No. of patients	No. of patients
Candida spp.		
C. albicans	41	48
C. tropicalis	3	11
C. parapsilosis	2	22
C. krusei	2	—
C. stellatoidea	—	—
C. guilliermondii	2	—
Mixed	—	—
C. spp.	8	2 (*C. rugosa*)
Other fungi		
T. glabrata	—	—
Cr. neoformans	—	—
Histoplasma capsulatum	—	—
Rhodotorula spp.	—	—
Aspergillus spp.	—	—
Penicillium spp.	—	—
Zygomycetes	—	—
Trichosporon spp.	—	—
Cladosporium	—	—
Multiple	—	—
Other	—	—

* Data from a cancer hospital.
† ( ) Number of isolates associated with systemic disease.
‡ ( ) Number of cases with disseminated disease/number of autopsies performed.
§ Systemic disease.
‖ Results of fungemia: spontaneous resolution 42.8%, endophthalmitis 5.1%, requirement for antifungal therapy 36.3%, death from fungal disease 20.7%.
** Only *Candida* spp. reported.

Risk Factors for Development of Nosocomial Fungal Infections

Disseminated Candidiasis

Candida is by far the most frequent nosocomial fungal pathogen and the only fungal pathogen acquired primarily from an endogenous source. Species of *Candida* are isolated most frequently from specimen sources that are in contact with mucocutaneous tissue, specifically from the alimentary, gastrointestinal, genital, and urinary tracts. In a review of the literature, Odds (170) reported the following mean frequencies, weighted for the number of subjects, of *C. albicans* recovery from normal subjects: oral cavity, 10%; stool, 15%; vagina, 10%; and skin, less than 1%. Factors that increase carriage include hospitalization, antimicrobic therapy, older age, underlying disease, and burns (72, 170). More than 50% of hospitalized patients become colonized with potentially pathogenic *Candida* spp. (170). Investigators have been unable to isolate *Candida* spp. from air samples, even when conducted near infected patients (8, 166).

Candida spp. may cause a variety of clinical syndromes including superficial colonization, superficial cutaneous or mucus membrane infection, invasive cutaneous or mucus membrane infection, deep organ infection (especially cerebritis, ophthalmitis, myositis, pneumonitis, and endocarditis), and disseminated infections. The clinical spectrum of candidal infections has been extensively reviewed (10, 25, 26, 66). Because disseminated disease is the most serious of candidal infections, we will focus on the epidemiology of this entity.

Although more than 80 species of *Candida* have been described, only a few are frequently pathogenic for humans (Table 9-3). Medically important species include *C. albicans*, *C. tropicalis*, *C. guilliermondii*, *C. parapsilosis*, *C. krusei*, *C. pseudotropicalis*, and *C. stellatoidea*. Although *C. albicans* has been and continues to be the most frequently isolated *Candida* species isolated from invasive or disseminated infections, recent studies have highlighted the clinical and epidemiology significance of other *Candida* species. *Candida tropicalis* is the second most common species which caused disseminated or invasive infection (Table 9-3). Several reports have noted an increasing incidence of this pathogen among immunosuppressed populations, especially in patients with acute leukemia (23, 65, 96, 133, 149, 246). *Candida krusei* is also increasingly recognized as an important pathogen (147). Fungemia caused by either *C. krusei* or *C. tropicalis* is likely to indicate disseminated disease and has a mortality over 50% (96, 133). *Candida parapsilosis* has been the predominant pathogen in heroin abusers (201). Further *C. parapsilosis* appears to be the most common species associated with common source outbreaks. It has been isolated in outbreaks due to contaminated hyperalimentation fluid (181, 217), contaminated pressure monitoring devices (216), and solutions used intraoperatively (143, 224). *Torulopsis glabrata*, another yeast,

TABLE 9-4. Factors Associated with Disseminated *Candida* Infections

1. Malignancy; cytotoxic chemotherapy
2. Neutropenia
3. Antimicrobials
4. Hyperalimentation
5. Systemic adrenocortical steroids
6. Very low birth weight neonates
7. Severe burns
8. Intravenous catheters
9. Gastrointestinal surgery, especially multiple procedures
10. Gastrointestinal ulcerations
11. Repeated intravenous narcotic injections

has also emerged as an important pathogen in immunosuppressed patients (2, 4, 23).

The risk factors associated with disseminated candidiasis are outlined in Table 9-4. Serious outpatient infections occur most commonly in persons with acquired or congenital immune deficiency syndromes (111) and intraveneous drug abusers (201). Nosocomial candidiasis most commonly occurs as a complication of cytotoxic therapy for oncology patients or immunosuppressive therapy in organ transplant recipients. Although it is difficult to access the relative significance of individual risk factors in immunosuppressed patients, predisposing factors for candidiasis include neutropenia (degree and duration), chemotherapy, antimicrobics, central catheters, hyperalimentation, steroids, preceding or coexistant bacterial infection, colonization, and surgery (23, 87, 96, 112, 133, 148, 162). The spectrum of infection, diagnosis, and management of candidiasis in immunosuppressed patients has been the subject of a number of reviews (25, 26, 66).

Both antenatal and postpartum infection with *Candida* spp. are well recognized and may be increasing in frequency (35). More than 80 cases of chorioamnionitis have been described (34, 62, 95, 136, 220, 243). The most frequently isolated species is *C. albicans*, although other species have been reported (243). Risk factors appear to include use of cervical sutures for cervical incompetence and maternal use of an intrauterine device for birth control, but prolonged rupture of membranes is unnecessary (34, 62, 95, 220, 243). Amniocentesis has been implicated as a cause of chorioamnionitis (61) and suggested as a means for early diagnosis (34, 198). *Candida* chorioamnionitis may result in stillbirth of immature infants, congenital infection of the fetus, usually in low-birth-weight infants, or asymptomatic colonization of full- or near-term infants (95, 243). Congenital infection is usually manifested by cutaneous and/or pulmonary infection with positive gastric aspirates and carries a high mortality rate in low-birth-weight infants. Disseminated infection has been noted, especially in immature stillbirths (62).

Nosocomial neonatal candidiasis is a major problem in infants requiring intensive care therapy. As with congenital infection *C. albicans* is the most common pathogen, although other species may also cause disease (70, 214). Risk factors for the neonatal acquisition of *Candida* appear to include superficial colonization, gastrointestinal surgery, broad-spectrum antimicrobic therapy, umbilical vessel catheterization, central hyperalimentation, and, most importantly, very low birth weight (15, 88, 162, 214). In contrast to congenital candidiasis, neonatal disease is usually associated with disseminated infection (15, 70, 100, 106). Further, central nervous system involvement appears to occur commonly in infected infants (15, 35, 44, 70, 88, 100, 106, 163, 187). The epidemiology, clinical manifestations, and therapy of disseminated fungal infections in very-low-birth-weight infants has been reviewed (15, 16, 100).

Infection remains a major source of morbidity for the burned patient. NNIS data revealed that fungi accounted for 4.4% of microorganisms recovered from infected burns. *Candida albicans* was the most common fungal pathogen isolated (2.3%), followed by other fungi (1.2%), *Aspergillus* spp. (0.6%), and *Candida* (non-*albicans*, 0.5%). Data from other investigators also indicates that *Candida* spp. are the most commonly isolated fungi from the burn wounds, blood, and urine of burned patients (33, 127, 144, 163, 254). More than 50% of patients with extensive burns will become at least transiently colonized by *Candida* spp. (126). Risk factors for infection include depth and extent of the burn, use of mefanide acetate cream (163), broad-spectrum antimicrobials, and hyperalimentation. Although *Candida* spp. remain the major cause of septic deaths due to fungi (127), *Aspergillus* spp. and the Zygomycetes are also important nosocomial pathogens (32, 145, 163). Other fungi also have been reported to cause serious infection, including species of *Torulopsis*, *Geotrichum*, *Rhodotorula*, *Acremonium*, *Penicillium*, *Trichosporon*, *Trichophyton*, *Fusarium*, and *Fonsecaea* (33). Some of these have not been convincingly documented as pathogens. Prevention of burn wound infection has been reviewed (124, 141).

The postsurgical patient appears to be at an increased risk of invasive candidiasis. Risk factors include intraabdominal operations, multiple operations, multiple courses of antimicrobials, prolonged use of parenteral fluids, and concurrent use of cytotoxic agents or steroids (22, 75, 215, 219). Strict adherence to current guidelines may minimize postsurgical infection (76, 165, 226).

Outbreaks of candidiasis due to either common vehicle or indirect contact transmission have occasionally been reported. Two outbreaks of cutaneous candidiasis have been linked to the use of contaminated fomites (54, 134). At least 28 cases of *C. parapsilosis* pseudophakic endophthalmitis occurred after the use of a contaminated lot of irrigating solution (143, 224). Two outbreaks of *C. parapsilosis* fungemia in patients receiving hyperalimentation have been linked to the use of contaminated vacuum pumps during the preparation of the hyperalimentation fluid (181, 217). Contamination of pressure-monitoring devices due to inadequate disinfection has led to two outbreaks of *Candida* infections (216, 242).

Cross-infection with *Candida* spp. has been described in outbreaks of *C. albicans* in intensive care units (36, 178). Burnie et al (36) reported an outbreak in which 25 patients developed colonization and 13 patients developed probable or systemic infection. The epidemic strain, which was characterized by its morphology, serotype, and biotype, was isolated from the hands of two of 17 personnel immediately after direct patient care of infected patients. The authors attributed the outbreak to cross-infection via hand carriage aided in part by the epidemic strain's relative resistance to the handwashing agent used in the ICU. Control of the outbreak was achieved by prophylactic use of ketoconazole on all patients and use of a fungicidal handwashing disinfectant (37). Similarly, Phelps et al (178) described an outbreak in a neonatal ICU in which 12 infants developed infection and three colonization. Eleven of 42 hand samples were positive for the epidemic strain. In neither of these two outbreaks was an environmental reservoir discovered despite vigorous investigation. Hand carriage of *Candida* spp. may be important in the nosocomial transmission of these organisms (38).

Typing schemes of *Candida* spp. and other fungi have been devised to aid in elucidating the epidemiology of these organisms and evaluating the source of epidemics (171, 239). Control of nosocomial candidiasis depends on reducing or eliminating factors that promote colonization and minimizing therapeutic interventions that lead to disruption of skin or mucosal surfaces.

Invasive and Disseminated *Aspergillus* Infection

Aspergillus spp. are soil-dwelling organisms that contribute to the decay of organic debris and are widely distributed in nature (93). The concentration of *A. fumigatus* conidia in outside air has been reported to show seasonal and geographic variation and reach high concentrations in special circumstances such as near compost heaps and in hay barns (160, 191). The recovery of *Aspergillus* spp. or the Zygomycetes within hospitals has been variable, but commonly at least small numbers can be isolated from the air, accumulated dust, and environmental surfaces (93, 167, 218).

Although approximately 200 species of *Aspergillus* have been described, only a few are pathogenic for humans (194). Major human pathogens include *A. fumigatus* , *A. flavus*, and *A. niger*. Occasional disease may be caused by *A. terreus*, *A. nidulans*, *A. niveus*, *A. clavatus*, and *A. restrictus*. Major clinical syndromes include allergic aspergillosis, aspergilloma, and invasive disease (118, 194, 197, 251). Further discussion will focus on invasive and disseminated disease.

Invasive infection caused by *Aspergillus* species include hemorrhagic bronchopneumonia, pulmonary infarction, pulmonary cavitation and fungus ball, rhinocerebral infection, pansinusitis, myocardial infarction, cerebral hemorrhage or infarction, and cutaneous infection (27, 92, 194). Risk factors for the development of invasive *Aspergillus* infections include: corticosteroid

TABLE 9-5. Factors Associated with Invasive/Disseminated *Aspergillus* Infection

1. Contaminated hospital air supply
2. Hematologic malignancy; cytotoxic chemotherapy, especially with profound neutropenia
3. Organ transplantation with immunosuppression
4. Skin damage due to adhesive tape or arm boards in immunosuppressed patients
5. Severe burns
6. Corticosteroid therapy, especially high-dose therapy
7. Broad spectrum antimicrobial therapy?

therapy, especially when given in high doses (84, 151, 251); cytotoxic chemotherapy, especially when associated with profound leukopenia (WBC < $500/mm^3$) (71, 151, 251); transplantation, especially during acute rejection when immunosuppressive therapy is often increased (39, 84, 241); and possible broad-spectrum antimicrobial therapy (80) (Table 9-5). In patients receiving immunosuppression after organ transplantation or cytotoxic therapy for malignancy, the risk of invasive aspergillosis appears most related to the duration and degree of neutropenia (79, 80) and the intensity of immunosuppression (241). *Aspergillus* infection in transplant patients is unusual within the first 30 days of transplantation (200).

Uncommonly, invasive aspergillosis may occur in patients apparently immunocompetent, or only mildly to moderately immunocompromised, such as those with hepatic failure, influenza, and diabetic ketoacidosis (103, 118) Nosocomial aspergillosis may be associated with environmental reservoirs, including contaminated air supplies, bandages, and arm boards.

Invasive Zygomycete Infection

The phyllum Zygomycetes includes several genera of fungi which are important nosocomial human pathogens: *Rhizopus*, and, rarely, *Absidia*. The epidemiology of these fungi is similar to that of *Aspergillus* spp.. Acquisition is primarily via inhalation, although the levels of zygomycete spores in hospital air have not been well defined. Cutaneous inoculation may also occur resulting in nosocomial infection (137). Major infectious syndromes include: rhinocerebral, rhinoorbital, and paranasal infection; pulmonary infection; cutaneous infection; disseminated disease; and gastrointestinal infection (116, 137, 149, 175). Major risk factors for acquisition of invasive zygomycete infection (Table 9-6) include: leukemia and lymphoma, especially when associated with leukopenia from cytotoxic therapy (116, 137, 150, 175); diabetes, especially when associated with ketoacidosis (116, 137, 150, 175); organ transplantation, especially when associated with profound immunosuppression (116, 137, 155, 175); and intensive care therapy or a prolonged postoperative course (1). Other less significant risk factors include renal failure, cirrhosis, malnutrition, gastrointestinal disorders, and congenital heart disease (116,

137, 175). As with *Aspergillus*, occasionally nonimmunocompromised hosts may develop serious infection.

Airborne Transmission of Nosocomial Fungal Infections

Inhalation of airborne filamentous fungal conidia or spores by immunocompromised patients appears to be the most important factor for nosocomial filamentous fungal disease, especially aspergillosis (191). This statement is supported by studies of endemic and epidemic nosocomial aspergillosis and success in reducing this infection by controlling the purity of hospital air. Colonization of the nose and upper airways appears to precede either dissemination or lower respiratory infection (5). Whereas a variety of fungal species may cause invasive disease in immunocompromised patients, detailed studies of environmental correlates of nosocomial disease are largely restricted to *A. flavus* and *A. fumigatus*. However, it is probably reasonable to extrapolate from *Aspergillus* to other fungal species. Human infection is related to the virulence of these organisms, their ubiquitous nature, and an appropriate conidium or spore size, which favors deposition into alveoli (191).

Epidemics of Airborne Fungal Infections

Contamination of the hospital air supply by fungi has led to several well-documented epidemics. The fungi involved in these outbreaks have included *A. fumigatus* (11, 74, 115), *A. flavus* (4, 205), *Aspergillus* spp. (117, 129, 173), *Rhizopus indicus* (114), and *Rhizomucor pusillus* (94). Sources of airborne fungi in these hospital outbreaks have included the following: 1) dust associated with hospital renovation (11, 114, 173); 2) outside construction with an inadequate (117) or malfunctioning hospital ventilation system (205); 3) contaminated cellulose fireproofing material (3); 4) contamination of the hospital air supply by pigeon droppings (74, 115) or malfunctioning hospital ventilation system (129); and 5) an inadequate filtration system

TABLE 9-6. Factors Associated with Invasive Zygomycete Infection

1. Diabetes mellitus, espeically with ketoacidosis
2. Severe underlying diseases
3. Hematologic malignancy
4. Elasticized adhesive tape used to bind wound dressings
5. Wounds, especially extensive burns
6. Site of adhesive tape or arm board contact in immunocompromised host
7. Organ transplantation, especially in the setting of profound immunosuppression
8. Contaminated hospital air supply

coupled with location of the outside air intake vent near a refuse container (94). In most cases contamination of the air supply to the patients' rooms has been noted. However, Gage et al (74) linked three cases of *A. fumigatus* endocarditis to contamination of the operating room air supply by pigeon excreta; Hopkins et al (personal communication) linked a cluster of six cases of *A. fumigatus* to renovation in a radiology department; and England et al (68) linked two cases of *Rhizopus arrhizus* infection to a contaminated air conditioner filter in a physician's office building. A recent report described an outburst of airborne *Penicillium* conidia (5.5×10^5 CFU per hour), which was traced to rotting wood in a cabinet under a sink with leaking plumming in a medication room (227).

Prevention

Hospital air should be nearly free of *Aspergillus* and other fungal conidia and spores. This can be achieved by use of a central ventilation system with ultra high-efficiency air filters (HEPA) in critical areas, such as transplant units, and the use of at least 90–95% efficient filters in less critical patient areas (191). The use of a central ventilation system with an adequate filtration system has been shown to decrease levels of fungi isolated from the air and reduce nosocomial fungal infections (173, 191, 205). For a central ventilation system to be effective, the hospital must be airtight (ie, all windows and doors must be kept closed). Further, routine maintenance must assure that all fans are operative, clean filters are in place, and pigeons are excluded from air intake and discharge ducts.

General guidelines when hospital construction is being considered include the following (52): 1) where possible, seal off patient care areas from the construction activity with impermeable plastic barriers; 2) visually evaluate the ceilings in the wards below and adjacent to the construction/renovation area as potential sources of airborne pathogens; 3) remove seriously compromised patients from floors adjacent to construction activity when contamination of their rooms with dust is likely; 4) ensure that the ventilation system is producing the proper air pressure and number of air exchanges in critical areas near the construction; 5) ensure that the ventilation system is not circulating contaminated air from construction areas into other hospital areas; 6) contact hospital engineers about special maintenance and cleaning of the ventilation system and sealing doors and windows near excavation sites; and 7) thoroughly clean renovated wards before admitting patients.

Although routine air sampling is not indicated, it would be appropriate to monitor hospital air quality when an increase in fungal conidia or spores in the hospital air is anticipated. Vacuuming should be avoided in rooms occupied by patients vulnerable to aspergillosis, and vacuum exhausts should be filtered. In new construction, all wet potentially nutritive material should be treated with a fungicide. If surveillance reveals an increase in airborne-transmitted fungal infection, careful culturing of the environment and possibly nasal cultures of immunocompromised patients may prove useful in defining the source of infection and extent of patient colonization.

Marijuana

Marijuana is widely used in today's society by both normal and immunodeficient individuals. It also has been used therapeutically in hospitals to control chemotherapy-induced nausea. Cultures of marijauna cigarettes frequently result in the isolation of *Aspergillus* spp. (46, 102, 122), and have been linked to invasive pulmonary, sinusitis, and allergic bronchopulmonary aspergillosis (46, 102, 122, 208, 230). If marijuana is used in the hospital setting it should be rendered sterile before use.

Procedure-Related Fungal Infections

Infusion Related

More than 50% of hospitalized patients in the United States receive infusion therapy for administration of fluid and electrolytes, blood products, medications, total parenteral nutrition, or hemodynamic monitoring (132). Up to one third of all outbreaks of nosocomial bacteremia, up to one third of all endemic nosocomial bacteremia, and the majority of candidemia are infusion related (132).

Fungal infection associated with an intravascular line may occur due to colonization or infection of the cannula site, or contamination of the infusate. Cannula-associated colonization or infection may lead to local wound infection, septic phlebitis, transient fungemia, prolonged fungemia, or distal systemic infection. The pathogenesis and epidemiology of infusion-related infections has been comprehensively reviewed (86, 130, 132). Although *Candida* spp. are the most common fungal pathogens related to infusion therapy, intravascular lines may become seeded by other fungi during an episode of fungemia and later serve as a nidus for remote infection. Unusual pathogens described include *C. neoformans*, *Fusarium chlamydosporum*, *C. rugosa*, *T. candida*, and other yeasts (18, 104, 109, 190, 225).

Hamory (86) reviewed the results of 11 studies that used semiquantitative cannula cultures to evaluate the frequency of colonization and subsequent bacteremia from peripheral intravenous cannulas. Overall, 4.27% of 5,690 devices were positive on culture. However, only 3.7% of positive peripheral cannulas were associated with positive blood cultures (overall incidence of positive blood cultures, 0.16%). Only 0.18% of peripheral venous cannulas yielded isolates of *Candida*. The risk of candidemia after catheter colonization was 10%. Prospective studies of central venous catheters have revealed much higher rates of colonization and subsequent sepsis (50, 86, 97, 121, 183). The colonization by *Candida* has ranged from 2–8%, with 18% of these being associated with fungemia (50, 97, 183). *Candida* colonization and/or infection may be a complication of pulmonary artery catheters, Hickman-Broviac indwelling catheters, and arterial pressure monitoring systems (86).

Cannula wound infections may result in local abscesses or suppurative phlebitis of peripheral veins. Occasionally exit site infections or local abscesses may lead to remote infection or disseminated disease (47, 90, 231). The microorganisms most frequently implicated in suppurative phlebitis are the same organisms that cause uncomplicated cannula-related septicemia: *Staphylococcus aureus* and aerobic gram-negative bacilli (132). *Candida* spp. are an important cause of septic thrombophlebitis, especially in patients who are predisposed to this organism as a result of burn injury (172), immunosuppression (131), parenteral nutrition (60), or prior antimicrobial therapy (20, 101, 233). Although *Candida* was not the etiologic agent in any of 100 cases of septic thrombophlebitis recently reported from a general hospital (14), *Candida* spp. constituted up to 17% of the causative agents in high-risk burn patients (185). Although most cases of *Candida* thrombophlebitis result only in local infection, dissemination infection may occur (135, 233). The recognition, prevention, and management of candidal suppurative peripheral thrombophlebitis recently has been reviewed (236, see also 248). Factors associated with infection in this series of seven patients included concomitant or preceding bacterial infections, multiple antimicrobic administered for at least 2 weeks, preceding *Candida* colonization in five of seven patients, deficient local catheter site care, and lack of rotation of infusion sites every 48 hours (236). All patients were febrile (38.1–40.0°C); six of seven patients had an elevated white blood cell count; and in four of seven pus could be expressed at the catheter entrance site. Pathogens included *C. albicans* (5), *C. lipolytica* (1), and *C. tropicalis* (1).

Septic thrombophlebitis of central veins by *Candida* spp. also may occur, most commonly in the setting of hyperalimentation (21, 99, 228). The clinical features and management of this entity have been reviewed (228).

Contamination of the infusate may occur during manufacture or during manipulation by pharmacy personnel or floor nurses. Plouffe et al (181) described an outbreak in which 103 patients received fluids contaminated with *C. parapsilosis* leading to 22 infections. An epidemiologic investigation revealed that the source of the epidemic organism was a contaminated vacuum system used in the intravenous additive preparation room; organisms apparently refluxed into intravenous bottles when aliquots were removed to accommodate additives. Solomon et al (217) described an outbreak of five patients with fungemia or colonization of an intravascular cannula by *C. parapsilosis*, also due to the use of a contaminated vacuum pump for the preparation of hyperalimentation fluids.

Individual infusates may become contaminated with fungi. Although clinical infection may result, notable adverse affects have not been noted in most patients (57, 140, 195). In most cases careful examination will reveal defects in the infusate container, such as hairline fractures. Pathogens isolated from cases reported in the literature have included: *Sporothrix schenckii* (one), *Trichoderma* sp. (one), *Penicillium* spp. (six), *Aspergillus* spp. (four), *Cunninghamella* sp. (one), *Alternaria* sp. (one), *T. glabrata* (one), *C. tropicalis* (one), *Cladosporium* (one), and an algae (one). In several cases multiple fungi were isolated.

Hyperalimentation

Commercial 10% lipid emulsions are able to support the growth of bacteria and fungi. Whereas bacteria may multiply more readily, *Candida* spp. (*C. tropicalis* and *C. albicans*) are able to reach levels of 10^5 CFU/ml by 24 hours (55, 110). Further, even very low innocula (2 CFU/ml), such as would be consistent with touch contamination during preparation or administration, resulted in increases in concentrations of 1–3 logs by 24 hours (105).

Candida spp. have been reported to be the most common pathogen associated with total parenteral nutrition. However, the use of intravenous fat emulsions may permit sepsis with unusual lipophilic fungi such as *Malassezia furfur* (123, 182, 188). Investigators in the 1970s reported rates of candidal retinal lesions and/or sepsis of up to 23% in patients receiving parenteral nutrition (12, 56, 153). Implementation of infection control guidelines developed by the Centers for Disease Control and use of "hyperalimentation teams" has been reported to have decreased the incidence of candidemia to between 1.4 and 2.5% (164, 189). However, some reports in the 1980s have noted a high incidence of retinal lesions (9.9%) and candidemia (6.9%) in patients receiving hyperalimentation (91).

Implantable Foreign Bodies

Foreign bodies may be colonized before the time of insertion due to a breakdown of normal sterilization procedures at the time of insertion, airborne contamination in the operating room or contact with the skin, or infection during an episode of transient or prolonged fungemia. Infection of foreign bodies may lead to prolonged local invasive disease or serve as a nidus for disseminated infection. Fungal infection of implantable bodies frequently requires surgical removal for cure, leading to high morbidity and mortality. *Candida* spp. have been the usual causative organisms. Prevention of infections involving implantable foreign bodies requires treating all implantable devices as critical items which must be sterilized before insertion (202). Current guidelines designed to prevent wound infections should be used (76, 165, 229). All attempts should be made to eliminate risk factors for fungemia in these patients.

Prosthetic valve endocarditis (PVE) is a well-recognized complication of valve replacement. It has been reported to occur in approximately 3% of patients within 12 months of surgery and 4–5% of patients by 48 months postsurgery (40, 98). A compilation of major series yielded 348 patients who developed PVE out of a total patient population of 12,164 (2.9%) (40, 64, 98, 140, 213, 245). Twenty-one episodes of PVE in 20 patients were caused by fungi (5.7%). Fungi were responsible for 9.8% of PVE occurring within 60 days of surgery, and 4.4% of PVE occurring later than 60 days postsurgery. This suggests that most cases of fungal PVE may be due to seeding of the valve at the time of surgery. Pathogens included *C. albicans* (seven), *Candida* spp. (four), *C. parapsilosis* (three), *Aspergillus* spp. (three) *Scopulariopsis brevicaulis* (one), *C. tropicalis* plus *C. parapsilosis* (one), and unspecified fungus (one). Only one of 14 patients for whom mortality could be determined survived his fungal infection, but he died 5 months later with a relapse of *C. parapsilosis* endocarditis. The evaluation and management of fungal endocarditis has been reviewed (201).

Infectious complications of permanent implanted pacemakers occur in 1–3% of insertions. Infection may involve the pacer pocket, the generator, or the transvenous pacer wire. Fungal infection of these devices has only occasionally been reported. Pathogens have included *C. albicans* (49), *Candida* spp. (58), *A. flavus* (154), *Pseudallescheria boydii* (59), and *Aspergillus* spp. (113). All five patients were older than 60 years of age and had underlying diseases that may have predisposed them to fungal infection or had recently undergone surgical procedures. Complications of the fungal infection included disseminated fungal infection (59, 113), pulmonary emboli (49), and tricuspid endocarditis (58, 59, 154). All five patients died of their infection.

Infections complicate 1–5% of all prosthetic joint replacements. Only rarely have fungi been reported as infecting a prosthetic joint. Pathogens have included *C. parapsilosis* (119, 120, 125, 253), *T. glabrata* (82), *C. tropicalis* (82), and *C. albicans* (120), and involved joints have included the shoulder (119, 120), the hip (82, 253), and the knee (82, 120, 125). Infection was believed to be secondary to arthrocentesis (125), intravenous use of heroin (119), or introduction of the pathogen at the time of surgery (82, 253).

Vascular grafts may become seeded by fungi leading to disseminated and/or locally invasive disease (30). Other devices reportedly infected by fungi include artificial urethral sphincters in two children (*C. albicans*) (238) and voice prostheses (*Candida* spp.) (128).

Intraocular Lens Implantation

The incidence of postoperative infectious endophthalmitis after cataract surgery or implantation of an intraocular lens has been reported to be approximately 0.1% (7, 45, 221). Bacteria, especially coagulase negative staphylococci and *Staphylococcus aureus*, are the most common etiologic agents reported in the literature (240). However, both sporadic and epidemic fungal pseudophakic endophthalmitis have been reported. Pathogens isolated from sporadic cases have included *Candida* spp., *Aspergillus* spp., *P. boydii*, *S. schenckii*, *Penicillium* spp., *Acremonium* spp., and others (81, 232, 235). Multiple epidemics of postoperative endophthalmitis have resulted from the intraoperative use of contaminated solutions. Thirteen cases of *Paecilomyces lilacinus* endophthalmitis resulted from the use of a contaminated batch of neutralizing solution (177), three cases of *Volutella* resulted from the use of a contaminated cocaine solutions (232), and at least 28 cases of *C. parapsilosis* resulted from the use of a contaminated irrigating solution (143, 224). Environmental standards for intraocular lens implantation have been published and the value of a centralized surveillance system during epidemics of endophthalmitis stressed (53, 169). The presentation and treatment of fungal endophthalmitis have been reviewed (73, 232, 240).

Peritoneal Dialysis

Since the introduction of the permanent indwelling Tenckhoff catheter, peritoneal dialysis has become a widely used alternative to chronic hemodialysis for patients with endstage renal disease. It is safe, effective, practical, and relatively inexpensive. Infection remains the major complication of peritoneal dialysis. A recent review of the literature reported that the incidence of peritonitis in patients undergoing chronic ambulatory peritoneal dialysis ranged from 0.4–6.3 episodes per patient-year, with an average incidence of 2.1 episodes per patient-year. Fungi were reported as the causative pathogen in 33 of 422 episodes of peritonitis in 14 reports (222).

The subject of fungal peritonitis in patients receiving peritoneal dialysis has recently been reviewed (67). Fungi causing peritonitis in 88 patients reported in the literature included (number of cases): *C. albicans* (37), *C. tropicalis* (12), *Candida* spp. (7), *Fusarium* spp. (6), *C. parapsilosis* (3), *Rhodotorula rubra* (3), *C. guilliermondii* (3), *Bipolaris spicifera* (2), and *T. glabrata* (2). Single cases were reported due to *C. krusei*, *Mucor* sp., *A. flavus*, *A. fumigatus*, *Bipolaris australiensis*, *Trichoderma viride*, *Exophiala jeanselmei*, *Acremonium* sp., and an unidentified fungus. No single predominating cause of underlying renal disease was apparent. Potential risk factors for the development of fungal peritonitis included previous bacterial peritonitis within 1 month (51%), antimicrobic use within 1 month (69%), hospitalization within 10 days (33%), extraperitoneal site of infection (18%), bowel perforation or peritoneal-vaginal communication (15%), and use of immunosuppressive agents (7%). No possible risk factor was identified in 27% of patients. Fungal peritonitis was hospital-acquired in 18 patients, of whom only two had neither a recent episode of bacterial peritonitis nor received antimicrobials. Sixteen of these patients had early fungal peritonitis acquired while the patients were receiving dialysis on an emergency basis for acute renal failure.

Bronchoscopes

Flexible bronchoscopy has proven to be an invaluable and safe diagnostic procedure. Serious infection as a result of bronchoscopy is rare (202). However, pseudoepidemics with clusters of positive cultures of respiratory tract secretions obtained bronchoscopically have been linked to use of contaminated bronchoscopes or fluids used during bronchscopy (202). Schleupner and Hamilton (206) reported a pseudoepidemic of fungal infections in which *Trichosporon beigelii* and a *Penicillium* species were obtained from bronchial washings and sputa obtained after fiberoptic bronchoscopy on eight clinically uninfected patients. Investigation revealed contamination of the cocaine solutions used for topical anesthesia during bronchoscopy.

Proper sterilization or disinfection of all instruments used for invasive procedures is important to prevent nosocomial infection (202). Further, the recognition of a cluster of unusual organisms from presumed sterile sites, especially if the clinical condition does not suggest infection, should lead to an evaluation for a "pseudoepidemic."

Contact

Bandages

Although the fact is not commonly appreciated, many products that are used as bandages or in the preparation of plaster casts are not sterile and may lead to nosocomial infections. Outbreaks of cutaneous zygomycosis, sometimes with deep tissue invasion, have resulted from the use of elasticized bandages contaminated with these fungi. Pathogens have included *Rhizopus rhizopodiformis* (28, 77, 221) and *R. arrhizus* (63, 85, 107, 146). The majority of the reported patients were neither on immunosuppressive medication nor immunodeficient. Despite the lack of immunosuppression, most patients died from invasive zygomycete infection.

Cutaneous aspergillosis has been reported in at least 20 immunocompromised patients (17, 41, 69, 83, 142, 186, 247). Cutaneous manifestations were characterized by erythematous to violaceous, edematous, indurated plaques that progressed to necrotic bullae. Pathogens have included *A. flavus* (11 cases), *A. fumigatus* (three cases), *A. niger* (one case), *A. flavipes* (one case), *A. flavus*/*A. terreus* (two cases), *A. terreus*/*A. niger* (one case), and *Aspergillus* spp. (one case). In most cases the initial lesion developed at a site of insertion of an intravenous cannula or at points of contact with adhesive tape or arm boards securing intravenous infusion sets. Epidemiologic investigations conducted by Grossman et al (83) discovered *Aspergillus* contamination of adhesive tape and arm board covers, which had been stored in a room with a false ceiling that had recently been repaired for a water leak. McCarty et al (142) described two definite and two probable cases of cutaneous aspergillosis occurring at the site of skin contact with an arm board. Although the arm board filling, the plastic covering, and the cloth tape were all culture negative, the wrapping gauze from the manufacturer's containers grew *A. terreus*, *A. niger*, *A. fumigatus*, and *Rhizopus*. sp.. Other investigators (17) have been unable to demonstrate *Aspergillus* contamination of intravenous supplies, suggesting that cutaneous lesions could have arisen via airborne conidia or localization of *Aspergillus* during fungemia in areas of stasis/local damage resulting from point contact with the arm board of adhesive tape. Colonization or infection with *C. albicans* (138), *C. tropicalis* (247), *R. pusillus* (203), *Saksenaea vasiformis* (168), and *Rhizopus* sp. (247) has also been noted at the site of insertion of an intravenous cannula or at points of contact with adhesive tape or arm boards securing intravenous infusion sets. Other devices which abrade the skin also may lead to invasive and/or disseminated fungal disease, such as condom catheters (*C. tropicalis*) (158) and nasal prongs (*C. parapsilosis*) (209).

Preventive measures include the following. Only sterile bandage material should be used in immunocompromised patients or to cover damaged cutaneous areas in noncompromised hosts. The use of adhesive tape and the number of intravenous lines should be minimized in immunocompromised hosts. Store intravenous supplies in "clean utility rooms." Enclose areas of construction or renovation by barriers with monitoring for fungal conidia and spores in affected areas of the hospital.

The differential diagnosis and therapy of skin lesions in immunocompromised hosts has been reviewed (179, 247). With prompt institution of amphotericin B and when indicated, local debridement, many patients will survive.

Plaster Casts

Nosocomial infections underneath plaster casts may occur (202). Sources of infection have included intrinsically contaminated plaster of Paris, intrinsically contaminated cast padding, and the residual water in a plaster bucket used to immerse the plaster. Boyce et al (29) reported a case of *Cunninghamella bertholletiae* wound infection in a diabetic man and suggested it was acquired from nonsterile cast padding (29). Whereas cultures of unopened packages of cast padding did not yield *C. bertholletiae*, they did reveal *Bacillus* sp. and at least six genera of fungi, including *Fusarium*, *Rhizopus*, *Aspergillus*, *Chrysosporium*, and *Acremonium*.

Contact Lenses

Use of hydrophilic contact lenses has led to "an alarming increase in reports of serious contact lens-related infectious ulcerative keratitis" (223). Although most lens-related infections are due to bacteria, fungal and amoebic infections have also been recognized. Hydrophilic soft contact lenses have been reported to become contaminated by a variety of fungi, including *Alternaria alternata* (31), *Penicillium* spp. (156, 210), *Aspergillus* spp. (19, 244), *Candida* spp. (78, 244), Ascomycetes (174), *Acremonium* sp. (249), *Cladosporium* spp. (244), *Fusarium* spp. (244), *Dermatophilus congolensis* (19), and others (244). Case reports and studies in rabbits suggest that wearing contaminated lenses may lead to inflammatory keratitis but only rarely to fungal keratitis. However, keratitis and corneal ulcers may occur (244, 249). Patients should rigidly adhere to a daily cleaning and disinfection regimen (223). Failure to adhere to such guidelines will lead to a high incidence of contaminated solutions in which lenses are stored and colonized lenses.

Nosocomial Spread of Dermatophytes

Nosocomial spread of dermatophytes has rarely been reported. Mossovitch et al (159) reported an outbreak of *Microsporum canis* skin infection involving the left forearm of seven nurses and occiput of an infant. The authors hypothesized that transmission occurred via contact during bottle feeding of the infected infant. After the introduction of long sleeves for all nurses, no further cases occurred.

References

1. Agger WA, Maki DG: Mucormycosis: A complication of critical care. *Arch Intern Med* 138:925–927, 1978.
2. Aisner J, Schimpff SC, Sutherland JC, Young VM, Wiernik PH: *Torulopsis glabrata* infections in patients with cancer. *Am J Med* 61:23–28, 1976.
3. Aisner J, Schimpff SC, Bennett JE, Young VM, Wiernik PH: *Aspergillus* infections in cancer patients: Association with fireproofing materials in a new hospital. *JAMA* 235:411–412, 1976.
4. Aisner J, Sickles EA, Schimpff SC, Young VM, Greene WH, Wiernik PH: *Torulopsis glabrata* pneumonitis in patients with cancer. *JAMA* 230:584–585, 1974.
5. Aisner J, Murillo J, Schimpff SC, Steere AC: Invasive aspergillosis in acute leukemia: Correlation with nose cultures and antibiotic use. *Ann Intern Med* 90:4–9, 1979.
6. Ajello L: Natural habitats of the fungi that cause pulmonary mycoses. *Med Mycol*, Zbl. Bakt. 8 (suppl):31–42, 1980.
7. Allen HF, Mangiaracine AB: Bacterial endophthalmitis after cataract extraction. II. Incidence in 36,000 consecutive operations with special reference to preoperative topical antibiotics. *Arch Ophthalmol* 91:3–7, 1974.
8. Anderson NA, Sage DN, Spaulding EH: Oral moniliasis in newborn infants. *Am J Dis Child* 67:450–456, 1944.
9. Apaliski SJ, Moore MD, Reiner BJ, Wald ER: Disseminated *Trichosporon beigelii* in an immunocompromised child. *Ped Infect Dis* 3:451–454, 1984.
10. Armstrong D: Fungal infections in the compromised host, in Rubin RH, Young LS (eds): *Clinical Approach to Infection in the Compromised Host*. New York, Plenum, 1981.

11. Arnow PM, Andersen RL, Mainous PD, Smith EJ: Pulmonary aspergillosis during hospital renovation. *Am Rev Respir Dis* 118:49–53, 1978.
12. Ashcraft KW, Leape LL: *Candida* sepsis complicating parenteral feeding. *JAMA* 212:454–456, 1970.
13. Baird DR, Harris M, Menon R, Stoddart RW: Systemic infection with *Trichosporon capitatum* in two patients with acute leukaemia. *Eur J Clin Microbiol* 4:62–64, 1985.
14. Baker CC, Peterson SR, Sheldon GF: Septic phlebitis: A neglected disease. *Am J Surg* 138:97–102, 1979.
15. Baley JE, Kliegman RM, Fanaroff AA: Disseminated fungal infections in very-low-birth weight infants: Clinical manifestations and epidemiology. *Pediatrics* 73:144–152, 1984.
16. Baley JE, Kliegman RM, Fanaroff AA: Disseminated fungal infections in very low-birth-weight infants: Therapeutic toxicity. *Pediatrics* 73:153–157, 1984.
17. Barson WJ, Ruymann FB: Palmar aspergillosis in immunocompromised children. *Pediatr Infect Dis* 5:264–268, 1986.
18. Begala JE, Maher K, Cherry JD: Risk of infection associated with the use of Broviac and Hickman catheters. *Am J Infect Control* 10:17–23, 1982.
19. Berger RO, Streeten BW: Fungal growth in aphakic soft contact lenses. *Am J Ophthalmol* 91:630–633, 1981.
20. Berkowitz FE, Argent AC, Baise T: Suppurative thrombophlebitis: A serious nosocomial infection. *Pediatr Infect Dis* 6:64–67, 1987.
21. Bernard RW, Stahl WM, Chase RM: Subclavian vein catheterizations: A prospective stuty. II. Infectious complications. *Ann Surg* 173:191–200, 1971.
22. Bernhardt HE, Orlando JC, Benfield JR, Hirose FM, Foos RY: Disseminated candidiasis in surgical patients. *Surg Gynecol Obstet* 134:819–825, 1972.
23. Bodey GP: Fungal infections complicating acute leukemia. *J Chron Dis* 19:667–687, 1966.
24. Bodey GP, Rodriguez V, Chang H-Y, Narboni G: Fever and infection in leukemic patients. *Cancer* 41:1610–1622, 1978.
25. Bodey GP: Candidiasis in cancer patients. *Am J Med* 77 (suppl): 13–19, 1984.
26. Bodey GP, Fainstein V: *Candidiasis*. New York, Raven Press, 1985.
27. Bodey GP: Fungal infection and fever of unknown origin in neutropenic patients. *Am J Med* 80 (suppl): 112–119, 1986.
28. Bottone EJ, Weitzman I, Hanna BA: *Rhizopus rhizopodiformis*: Emerging etiological agent of mucormycosis. *J Clin Microbiol* 9:530–537, 1979.
29. Boyce JM, Lawson LA, Lockwood WR, Hughes JL: *Cunninghamella bertholletiae* wound infection of probable nosocomial origin. *South Med J* 74:1132–1135, 1981.
30. Brandt SJ, Thompson RL, Wenzel RP: Mycotic pseudoaneurysm of an aortic bypass graft and contiguous vertebral osteomyelitis due to *Aspergillus fumigatus*. *Am J Med* 79:259–261, 1985.
31. Brooks AMV, Lazarus MG, Weiner JM: Soft contact lens contamination by *Alternaria alternata*. *Med J Aust* 140:490–491, 1984.
32. Bruck HM, Nash G, Foley FD, Pruitt BA Jr: Opportunistic fungal infection of the burn wound with Phycomycetes and *Aspergillus*. *Arch Surg* 102:476–482, 1971.
33. Bruck HM, Nash NG, Stein JM, Lindberg RB: Studies on the occurrence and significance of yeasts and fungi in the burn wound. *Ann Surg* 176:108–110, 1972.
34. Bruner JP, Elliott JP, Kilbride HW, Garite TJ, Knox GE: *Candida* chorioaminionitis diagnosed by amniocentesis with subsequent fetal infection. *Am J Perinatol* 3:213–318, 1986.
35. Buchs S: *Candida* meningitis: A growing threat to premature and fullterm infants. *Pediatr Infect Dis* 4:122–123, 1985.

36. Burnie JP, Odds FC, Lee W, Webster C, Williams JD: Outbreak of systemic *Candida albicans* in intensive care unit caused by cross infection. *Br Med J* 290:746–748, 1985.
37. Burnie JP, Lee W, Williams JD, Matthews RC, Odds FC: Control of an outbreak of systemic *Candida albicans*. *Br Med J* 291:1092–1093, 1985.
38. Burnie JP. *Candida* and hands. *J Hosp Infect* 8:1–4, 1986.
39. Burton JR, Zachery JB, Bessin R, Rathbun HK, Greenough III WB, Sterioff S, Wright JR, Slavin RE, Williams GM: Aspergillosis in four renal transplant recipients: Diagnosis and effective treatment with amphotericin B. *Ann Intern Med* 77:383–388, 1972.
40. Calderwood SB, Swinski LA, Waternaux CM, Karchmer AW, Buckley MJ: Risk factors for the development of prosthetic valve endocarditis. *Circulation* 1985: 31–37, 72.
41. Carlile JR, Millet RE, Cho CT, Vats TS: Primary cutaneous aspergillosis in a leukemic child. *Arch Dermatol* 114:78–80, 1978.
42. Centers for Disease Control: CDC surveillance summaries. Nosocomial infection surveillance, 1980–1982. 32:1–16SS. 1983.
43. Centers for Disease Control: Nosocomial infection surveillance, 35:17–29SS, 1984.
44. Chesney PJ, Justman RA, Bogdanowicz WM: *Candida* meningitis in newborn infants: A review and report of combined amphotericin B-flucytosine therapy. *Johns Hopkins Med J* 142:155–160, 1978.
45. Christy NE, Lall P: Postoperative endophthalmitis following cataract surgery. *Arch Ophthalmol* 90:361–366, 1973.
46. Chusid MJ, Gelfand JA, Nutter C, Fauci AS: Pulmonary aspergillosis, inhalation of contaminated marijuana smoke, chronic granulomatous disease. *Ann Intern Med* 82:682–683, 1975.
47. Clancy M-T, Gad-al-Rab J, Keane CT: Venous catheter associated *Candida albicans* septicaemia. *Ir J Med Sci* 145:348–349, 1976.
48. Clift RA: Candidiasis in the renal transplant patient. *Am J Med* 77 (suppl): 34–38, 1984.
49. Cole WJ, Slater J, Kronzon I, Galler M, Trehan N, Cohen M, Gargiulo A: *Candida albicans* infected transvenous pacemaker wire: Detection by two-dimensional echocardiography. *Am Heart J* 111:417–418, 1986.
50. Collignon PJ, Soni N, Pearson IY, Woods WP, Munro R, Sorrell TC: Is semi-quantitative culture of central vein catheter tips useful in the diagnosis of catheter-associated bacteremia? *J Clin Microbiol* 24:532–535, 1986.
51. Conversations in Infection Control: Severe nosocomial yeast infections. *Stuart Pharmaceuticals* 6:1–12, 1985.
52. Conversations in Infection Control: Invasive Fungal Disease. *Stuart Pharmaceuticals* 6:1–12, 1985.
53. Crawford BA, Kaufman DV: Environmental standards for intraocular lens implantation. *Aust J Ophthalmol* 12:49–55, 1984.
54. Cremer G, DeGroot WP: An epidemic of thrush in a premature nursery. *Dermatologica* 135:107–114, 1967.
55. Crocker KS, Noga R, Filibeck DJ, Krey SM, Markovic M, Steffee WP: Microbial growth comparisons of five commercial parenteral lipid emulsions. *J Parenteral Enteral Nutr* 8:391–395, 1984.
56. Curry CR, Quie PG: Fungal septicemia in patients receiving parenteral hyperalimentation. *New Engl J Med* 285:1221–1225, 1971.
57. Daisy JA, Abrutyn EA, MacGregor RR: Inadvertent administration of intravenous fluids contaminated with fungus. *Ann Intern Med* 91:563–565, 1979.
58. Davis JM, Moss AJ, Schenk EA: Tricuspid *Candida* endocarditis complicating a permanently implanted transvenous pacemaker. *Am Heart J* 77:818–821, 1969.

59. Davis WA, Isner JM, Bracey AW, Roberts WC, Garagusi VF: Disseminated *Petriellidium boydii* and pacemaker endocarditis. *Am J Med* 69:929–932, 1980.
60. Deitch EA, Marini JJ, Huseby JS: Suppurative *Candida* phlebitis of a peripheral vein. *J Trauma* 20:618–620, 1980.
61. Delaplane D, Wiringa KS, Shulman ST, Yogev R: Congenital mucocutaneous candidiasis following diagnostic amniocentesis. *Am J Obstet Gynecol* 147:342–343, 1983.
62. Delprado WJ, Baird PJ, Russell P: Placental candidiasis: Report of three cases with a review of the literature. *Pathology* 14:191–195, 1982.
63. Dennis JE, Rhodes KH, Cooney DR, Roberts GD: Nosocomial *Rhizopus* infection (zygomycosis) in children. *J Pediatr* 96:824–828, 1980.
64. Dismukes WE, Karchmer AW, Buckley MJ, Austen WG, Swartz MN: Prosthetic valve endocarditis: Analysis of 38 cases. *Circulation* 48:365–377, 1973.
65. Dyess DL, Garrison N, Fry DE: *Candida* sepsis: Implications of polymicrobial blood-borne infection. *Arch Surg* 120:345–348, 1985.
66. Edwards JE, Lehrer RI, Stiehm ER, Fischer TJ, Young LS: Severe candidal infections: Clinical perspective, immune defense mechanisms, and current concepts of therapy. *Ann Intern Med* 89:91–106, 1978.
67. Eisenberg ES, Leviton I, Soeiro R: Fungal peritonitis in patients receiving peritoneal dialysis: Experience with 11 patients and review of the literature. *Rev Infect Dis* 8:309–321, 1986.
68. England AC III, Weinstein M, Ellner JJ, Ajello L: Two cases of rhinocerebral zygomycosis (mucormycosis) with common epidemiologic and environmental features. *Am Rev Respir Dis* 124:497–498, 1981.
69. Estes SA, Hendricks AA, Merz WG, Prystowsky SD: Primary cutaneous aspergillosis. *J Am Acad Dermatol* 3:397–400, 1980.
70. Faix RG: Systemic *Candida* infections in infants in intensive care nurseries: High incidence of central nervous system involvement. *J Pediatr* 105:616–622, 1984.
71. Fisher BD, Armstrong D, Yu B, Gold JWM: Invasive aspergillosis: Progress in early diagnosis and treatment. *Am J Med* 71:571–577, 1981.
72. Fitzpatrick JJ, Topley HE: Ampicillin therapy and *Candida* outgrowth. *Am J Med Sci* 252:310–313, 1966.
73. Forster RK, Abbott RL, Gelender H: Management of infectious endophthalmitis. *Ophthalmology* 87:313–318, 1980.
74. Gage AA, Dean DC, Schimert G, Minsley N: *Aspergillus* infection after cardiac surgery. *Arch Surg* 101:384–387, 1970.
75. Gaines JD, Remington JS: Disseminated candidiasis in the surgical patient. *Surgery* 72:730–736, 1972.
76. Garner JS: Guidelines for prevention of surgical wound infections. Centers for Disease Control, Atlanta, GA, 1985.
77. Gartenberg G, Battone EJ, Keusch GT, Weitzman I: Hospital-acquired mucormycosis (*Rhizopus rhizopodiformis*) of skin and subcutaneous tissue. *N Engl J Med* 299:1115–1118, 1978.
78. Gasset AR, Mattingly TP, Hood I: Source of fungus contamination of hydrophilic soft contact lenses. *Ann Ophthalmol* 11:1295–1298, 1979.
79. Gerson SL, Talbot GH, Hurwitz S, Strom BL, Lusk EJ, Cassileth PA: Prolonged granulocytopenia: The major risk factor for invasive pulmonary aspergillosis in patients with acute leukemia. *Ann Intern Med* 100:345–351, 1984.
80. Gerson SL, Talbot GH, Lusk E, Hurwitz S, Strom BL, Cassileth PA: Invasive pulmonary aspergillosis in adult acute leukemia: Clinical clues to its diagnosis. *J Clin Oncol* 3:1109–1115, 1985.
81. Gilbert CM, Novak MA: Successful treatment of postoperative *Candida* endophthalmitis in an eye with an intraocular lens implant. *Am J Ophthalmol* 97: 593–595, 1984.

82. Goodman JS, Seibert DG, Reahl GE Jr, Geckler R: Fungal infection of prosthetic joints: A report of two cases. *J Rheumatol* 10:494–495, 1983.
83. Grossman ME, Fithian EC, Behrens C, Bissinger J, Fracaro M, Neu HC: Primary cutaneous aspergillosis in six leukemic children. *J Am Acad Dermatol* 12:313–318, 1985.
84. Gustafson TL, Schaffner W, Lavely GB, Stratton CW, Johnson HK, Hutcheson RH Jr: Invasive aspergillosis in renal transplant recipients: Correlation with corticosteroid therapy. *J Infect Dis* 148:230–237, 1983.
85. Hammond DE, Winkelmann RK: Cutaneous phycomycosis: Report of three cases with identification of *Rhizopus*. *Arch Dermatol* 115:990–992, 1979.
86. Hamory BH: Nosocomial bloodstream and intravascular device-related infections, in RP Wenzel (ed): *Prevention and Control of Nosocomial Infections*. Baltimore, MD, Williams & Wilkins, 1985, pp 283–319.
87. Hart PD, Russel E Jr, Remington JS: The compromised host and infection. II. Deep fungal infection. *J Infect Dis* 120:169–191, 1969.
88. Haruda F, Bergman MA, Headings D: Unrecognized *Candida* brain abscess in infancy: Two cases and a review of the literature. *Johns Hopkins Med J* 147: 182–185, 1980.
89. Haupt HM, Merz WG, Beschorner WE, Vaughan WP, Saral R: Colonization and infection with *Trichosporon* species in the immunosuppressed host. *J Infect Dis* 147:199–203, 1983.
90. Helton WS, Carrico CJ, Zaveruha PA, Schaller R: Diagnosis and treatment of splenic fungal abscesses in thc immune-suppressed patient. *Arch Surg* 121: 580–586, 1986.
91. Henderson DK, Edwards JE Jr, Montgomerie JZ: Hematogenous *Candida* endophthalmitis in patients receiving parenteral hyperalimentation fluids. *J Infect Dis* 143:655–661, 1981.
92. Herbert PA, Bayer AS: Fungal pneumonia (part 4): Invasive pulmonary aspergillosis. *Chest* 80:220–225, 1981.
93. Herman LG: *Aspergillus* in patient case areas. *Ann NY Acad Sci* 353:140–146, 1980.
94. Hernanz AP, Fereres J, Garraus SL, Rodriguez-Noriega A, Sanz AS: Nosocomial infection by *Rhizomucor pusillus* in a clinical haematology unit. *J Hosp Infect* 4:45–49, 1983.
95. Honore LH: Placental candidiasis: Report of two cases, one associated with an IUCD in situ. *Contraception* 30:555–560, 1984.
96. Horn R, Wong B, Kiehn T, Armstrong D: Fungemia in a cancer hospital: Changing frequency, earlier onset and results of therapy. *Rev Infect Dis* 7:646–655, 1985.
97. Hoshal VL Jr: Intravenous catheters and infection. *Surg Clin North Am* 52: 1407–1417, 1972.
98. Ivert TSA, Dismukes WE, Cobbs CG, Blackstone EH, Kirklin JW, Bergdahl LAL: Prosthetic valve endocarditis. *Circulation* 69:223–232, 1984.
99. Jarrett F, Maki DG, Chan C-K: Management of septic thrombosis of the inferior vena cava caused by *Candida*. *Arch Surg* 113:637–639, 1978.
100. Johnson DE, Thompson TR, Green TP, Ferrieri P: Systemic candidiasis in very low-birth-weight infants (<1,500 grams). *Pediatrics* 73:138–143, 1984.
101. Johnson RA, Zajac RA, Evans ME: Suppurative thrombophlebitis: Correlation between pathogen and underlying disease. *Infect Control* 7:582–585, 1986.
102. Kagen SL: *Aspergillus*: An inhalable contaminant of marijuana. *N Engl J Med* 304:483–484, 1981.
103. Karam GH, Griffin FM Jr: Invasive pulmonary aspergillosis in nonimmunocompromised, nonneutropenic hosts. *Rev Infect Dis* 8:357–363, 1986.

104. Kauffman CA, Severance PJ: Nosocomial cryptococcal infection. *South Med J* 73:267, 1980.
105. Keammerer D, Mayhall CG, Hall GO, Pesko LJ, Thomas RB: Microbial growth patterns in intravenous fat emulsions. *Am J Hosp Pharmacol* 40:1650–1653, 1983.
106. Keller MA, Sellers BB Jr, Melish ME, Kaplan GW, Miller KE, Mendoza SA: Systemic candidiasis in infants: A case presentation and literature review. *Am J Dis Child* 131:1260–1263, 1977.
107. Keys TF, Haldorson AM, Rhodes KH, Roberts GD, Fifer EZ: Nosocomial outbreaks of *Rhizopus* infections associated with Elastoplast wound dressing-Minnisota. *MMWR* 27:33–34, 1978.
108. Kiehn TE, Edwards FF, Armstrong D: The prevalence of yeasts in clinical specimens from cancer patients. *Am J Clin Pathol* 73:518–521, 1980.
109. Kiehn TE, Nelson PE, Bernard EM, Edwards FF, Koziner B, Armstrong D: Catheter-associated fungemia caused by *Fusarium chlamydosporum* in a patient with lymphoctic lymphoma. *J Clin Microbiol* 21:501–504, 1985.
110. Kim CH, Lewis DE, Kumar A: Bacterial and fungal growth in intravenous fat emulsions. *Am J Hosp Pharmacol* 40:2159–2161, 1983.
111. Kirkpatrick CH: Host factors in defense against fungal infections. *Am J Med* 77 (suppl): 1–12, 1984.
112. Klein JJ, Watanakunakorn C: Hospital-acquired fungemia: Its natural course and clinical significance. *Am J Med* 67:51–58, 1979.
113. Kramer L, Rojas-Corona RR, Sheff D, Eisenberg ES: Disseminated aspergillosis and pacemaker endocarditis. *PACE* 8:225–229, 1985.
114. Krasinski K, Holzman RS, Hanna B, Greco MA, Graff M, Bhogal M: Nosocomial fungal infection during hospital renovation. *Infect Control* 6:278–282, 1985.
115. Kyriakides GK, Zinneman HH, Hall WH, Arora VK, Lifton J, DeWolf WC, Miller J: Immunologic monitoring and aspergillosis in renal transplant patients. *Am J Surg* 131:246–252, 1976.
116. Lehrer RI, Howard DH, Sypherd PS, Edwards JE, Segal GP, Winston DJ: Mucormycosis. *Ann Intern Med* 93:93–108, 1980.
117. Lentino JR, Rosenkranz MA, Michaels JA, Kurup VP, Rose HD, Rytel MW: Nosocomial aspergillosis: A retrospective review of airborne disease secondary to road construction and contaminated air conditioners. *Am J Epidemiol* 116: 430–437, 1982.
118. Levitz SM, Diamond RD: Changing patterns of aspergillosis infections. *Adv Int Med* 30:153–174, 1984.
119. Lichtman EA: *Candida* infection of a prosthetic shoulder joint. *Skel Radiol* 10:176–177, 1983.
120. Lim EVA, Stern PJ: *Candida* infection after implant arthroplasty. *J Bone Joint Surg* 68-A: 143–145, 1986.
121. Linares J, Sitges-Serra A, Garau J, Perez JL, Martin R: Pathogenesis of catheter sepsis: A prospective study with quantitative and semiquantitative cultures of catheter hub and segments. *J Clin Microbiol* 21:357–360, 1985.
122. Llamas R, Hart R, Schneider NS: Allergic bronchopulmonary aspergillosis associated with smoking moldy marijuana. *Chest* 6:871–872, 1978.
123. Long JG, Keyserling HL: Catheter-related infection in infants due to an unusual lipophilic yeast-*Malassezia furfur*. *Pediatrics* 76:896–900, 1985.
124. Luterman A, Dacso CC, Curreri PW: Infections in burn patients. *Am J Med* 81 (suppl): 45–52, 1986.
125. MacGregor RR, Schimmer BM, Steinberg ME: Results of combined amphotericin B-5-fluorcytosine therapy for prosthetic knee joint infected with *Candida parapsilosis*. *J Rheumatol* 6:451–455, 1979.

126. MacMillan BG, Law EJ, Holder IA: Experience with *Candida* infections in the burn patient. *Arch Surg* 104:509–514, 1972.
127. MacMillan BG: Infections following burn injury. *Surg Clin North Am* 60:185–196, 1980.
128. Mahieu HF, Rosingh HJ, Saene RKFV, Schutte HK: Deterioration of voice prostheses caused by fungal vegetations. *Arch Otolaryngol* 111:280, 1985.
129. Mahoney DH, Steuber CP, Starling KA, Barrett FF, Goldberg J, Fernbach DJ: An outbreak of aspergillosis in children with acute leukemia. *J Pediatr* 95:70–72, 1979.
130. Maki DG, Goldman DA, Rhame FS: Infection control in intravenous therapy. *Ann Intern Med* 79:867–887, 1973.
131. Maki DG, Drinka PJ, Davis TE: Suppurative phlebitis of arm vein from a "scalp-vein needle." *N Engl J Med* 292:1116–1117, 1975.
132. Maki DG: Infections due to infusion therapy, in Bennett JV, Brachman PS (eds): Hospital Infections. Boston, Little, Brown and Company, 1986, pp 561–580.
133. Maksymiuk AW, Thongprasert S, Hopfer R, Luna M, Fainstein V, Bodey GP: Systemic candidiasis in cancer patients. *Am J Med* 77 (suppl): 20–27, 1984.
134. Malamatinis JE, Mattmiller ED, Westfall JN: Cutaneous moniliasis affecting varsity athletes. *J Am Coll Health Assoc* 16:294–295, 1968.
135. Malfroot A, Verboven M, Levy J, Dab I, Naessens A, Delree M, Ziekenhuis A: Suppurative thrombophlebitis with sepsis due to *Candida albicans* an unusual complication of intravenous therapy in cystic fibrosis. *Pediatr Infect Dis* 5: 376–377, 1986.
136. Mamlok RJ, Richardson CJ, Mamlok V, Nichols MM, Goldblum RM: A case of intrauterine pulmonary candidiasis. *Pediatr Infect Dis* 4:692–693, 1985.
137. Marchevsky AM, Bottone EJ, Geller SA, Giger DK: The changing spectrum of disease, etiology, and diagnosis of mucormycosis. *Hum Pathol* 11:457–464, 1980.
138. Marples RR, Richardson JF, Seal DV, Cooke EM: Adhesive tapes in the special care baby unit. *J Hosp Infect* 6:398–403, 1985.
139. Mayhall CG: Surgical infections including burns, Wenzel RP (ed): in *Prevention and Control of Nosocomial Infections*. Baltimore, Williams & Wilkins, 1987, pp 335–384.
140. Masur H, Johnson WD: Prosthetic valve endocarditis. *J Thorac Cardiovasc Surg* 80:31–37, 1980.
141. Matlow AG, Goldman CB, Mucklow MG, Kane J: Contamination of intravenous fluid with *Sporothrix schenckii*. *J Infect* 10:169–171, 1985.
142. McCarty JM, Flam MS, Pullen G, Jones R, Kassel: Outbreak of primary cutaneous aspergillosis related to intravenous arm boards. *J Pediatr* 108:721–724, 1986.
143. McCray E, Rampell N, Solomon SL, Bond WW, Martone WJ, O'Day D: Outbreak of *Candida parapsilosis* endophthalmitis after cataract extraction and intraocular lens implantation. *J Clin Microbiol* 24:625–628, 1986.
144. McManus WF, Goodwin CW, Mason AD Jr, Pruitt BA Jr: Burn wound infection. *J Trauma* 21:753–756, 1981.
145. McManus AT, McManus WF, Mason AD Jr, Aitcheson AR, Pruitt BA Jr: Microbial colonization in a new intensive care burn unit. *Arch Surg* 120:217–223, 1985.
146. Mead JH, Lupton GP, Dillavou CL, Odom RB: Cutaneous *Rhizopus* infection: Occurrence as a postoperative complication associated with an elasticized adhesive dressing. *JAMA* 242:272–274, 1979.
147. Merz WG, Karp JE, Schron D, Saral R: Increased incidence of fungemia caused by *Candida krusei*. *J Clin Microbiol* 24:581–584, 1986.
148. Meunier-Carpentier F, Kiehn TE, Armstrong D: Fungemia in the immuno-

compromised host: Changing patterns, antigenemia, high mortality. *Am J Med* 71:363–370, 1981.
149. Meyer RD, Rosen P, Armstrong D: Phycomycosis complicating leukemia and lymphoma. *Ann Intern Med* 77:871–879, 1972.
150. Meyer RD, Young LS, Armstrong D, Yu B: Aspergillosis complicating neoplastic disease. *Am J Med* 54:6–15, 1973.
151. Meyer RD, Armstrong D: Mucormycosis-changing status. *CRC Crit Rev Clin Lab Sci* 4:421–451, 1973.
152. Mirsky H, Cuttner J: Fungal infection in acute leukemia. *Cancer* 30:348–352, 1972.
153. Mongomerie JZ, Edwards JE Jr: Association of infection due to *Candida albicans* with intravenous hyperalimentation. *J Infect Dis* 137:197–201, 1978.
154. Moorman JR, Steenbergen C, Durack DT: *Aspergillus* infection of a permanent ventricular pacing lead. *PACE* 7:361–366, 1984.
155. Morduchowicz G, Shmueli D, Shapira Z, Cohen SL, Yussim A, Block CS, Rosenfeld JB, Pitlik SD: Rhinocerebral mucormycosis in renal transplant recipients: Report of three cases and review of the literature. *Rev Infect Dis* 8:441–446, 1986.
156. Morgan JF: Complications associated with contact lens solutions. *Ophthalmology* 86:1107–1119, 1979.
157. Morrison AJ Jr, Freer CV, Searcy MA, Landry SM, Wenzel RP: Nosocomial bloodstream infections: Secular trends in a statewide surveillance program in Virginia (abstract 452), in *Program and Abstracts of the Twenty-Fifth Interscience Conference on Antimicrobial Agents and Chemotherapy*, September 29–October 2, 1985, Minneapolis, Minnesota.
158. Morrissey R, Xavier A, Nguyen N, Webb DW: Invasive candidal balanitis due to a condom catheter in a neutropenic patient. *South Med J* 78:1247–1248, 1985.
159. Mossovitch M, Mossovitch B, Alkan M: Nosocomial dermatophytosis caused by *Microsporum canis* in a newborn department. *Infect Control* 7:593–595, 1986.
160. Mullins J, Hutcheson PS, Slavin RG: *Aspergillus fumigatus* spore concentration in outside air: Cardiff and St Louis compared. *Clin Allergy* 14:351–354, 1984.
161. Murray-Leisure KA, Aber RC, Rowley LJ, Applebaum PC, Wisman CB, Pennock JL, Pierce WS: Disseminated *Trichosporon beigelii* (*cutaneum*) infection in an artificial heart recipient. *JAMA* 256:2995–2998, 1986.
162. Myerowitz RL, Pazin GJ, Allen CM: Disseminated candidiasis: Changes in incidence, underlying diseases, and pathology. *Am J Clin Pathol* 68:29–38, 1977.
163. Nash G, Foley FD, Goodwin MN Jr, Bruck HM, Greenwald KA, Pruitt BA Jr: Fungal burn wound infection. *JAMA* 215:1664–1666, 1971.
164. Nehme AE: Nutritional support of the hospitalized patient: The team concept. *JAMA* 243:1906–1908, 1980.
165. Nichols RL: Techniques known to prevent post-operative wound infection. *Infect Control* 3:6–9, 1982.
166. Nilsby I, Norden A: Studies of the occurrence of *Candida albicans*. *Acta Med Scand* 133:340–345, 1949.
167. Noble WC, Clayton YM: Fungi in the air of hospital wards. *J Gen Microbiol* 32:397–402, 1963.
168. Oberle AD, Penn RL: Nosocomial Invasive *Saksenaea vasiformis* infection. *Am J Clin Pathol* 80:885–888, 1983.
169. O'Day DM: Value of a centralized surveillance system during a national epidemic of endophthalmitis. *Ophthalmology* 92:309–315, 1985.
170. Odds FC: *Candida and Candidosis*. Baltimore, University Park Press, 1979, pp 50–74.
171. Odds FC: Biotyping of medically important fungi, in McGinnis MR (ed): *Current Topics in Medical Mycology*, New York, Springer-Verlag, 1985, pp 155–171.

172. O'Neill JA Jr, Pruitt BA Jr, Foley FD, Moncrief JA: Suppurative thrombophlebitis—a lethal complication of intravenous therapy. *J Trauma* 8:256–266, 1968.
173. Opal SM, Asp AA, Cannady PB, Morse PL, Burton LJ, Hammer PG II: Efficacy of infection control measures during a nosocomial outbreak of disseminated *Aspergillus* associated with hospital construction. *J Infect Dis* 153:634–637, 1986.
174. Palmer E, Ferry AP, Safir A: Fungal invasion of a soft (Griffin Bionite) contact lens. *Arch Ophthalmol* 93:278–280, 1975.
175. Parfrey NA: Improved diagnosis and prognosis of mucormycosis: A clinicopathologic study of 33 cases. *Medicine* 65:113–122, 1986.
176. Peterson PK, McGlave P, Ramsay NKC, Rhame F, Cohen E, Perry GS III, Goldman AI, Kersey J: A prospective study of infections disease following bone marrow transplantation: Emergence of *Aspergillus* and cytomegalovirus as the major causes of mortality. *Infect Control* 4:81–89, 1983.
177. Pettit TH, Olson RJ, Foos RY, Martin WJ: Fungal endophtalmitis following intraocular lens implantation: A surgical epidemic. *Arch Ophthalmol* 98:1025–1039, 1980.
178. Phelps M, Ayliffe AJ, Babb JR: An outbreak of candidiasis in a special care baby unit: The use of a resistogram typing method. *J Hosp Infect* 7:13–20, 1986.
179. Pizzo PA: Infectious complications in the child with cancer. II. Management of specific infectious organisms. *J Pediatr* 98:513–523, 1981.
180. Pizzo PA, Robichaud KJ, Gill FA, Witebsky FG: Empiric antibiotic and antifungal therapy for cancer patients with prolonged fever and granulocytopenia. *Am J Med* 72:101–111, 1982.
181. Plouffe JF, Brown DG, Silva J Jr, Eck T, Stricof RL, Fekety FR Jr: Nosocomial outbreak of *Candida parapsilosis* fungemia related to intravenous infusions. *Arch Intern Med* 137:1686–1689, 1977.
182. Powell DA, Aungst J, Snedden S, Hansen N, Brady M: Broviac catheter-related *Malassezia furfur* sepsis in five infants receiving intravenous fat emulsions. *J Pediatr* 105:987–990, 1984.
183. Prager RL, Silva J Jr: Colonization of central venous catheters. *South Med J* 77:458–461, 1984.
184. Pritchard RC, Muir DB: *Trichosporon beigelii*: Survey of isolates from clinical material. *Pathology* 17:20–23, 1985.
185. Pruitt BA Jr, Stein JM, Foley FD, Moncrief JA, O'Neill JA Jr: Intravenous therapy in burn patients. *Arch Surg* 100:399–404, 1970.
186. Prystowsky SD, Vogelstein B, Ettinger DS, Merz WG, Kaizer H, Sulica VI, Zinkham WH: Invasive aspergillosis. *N Engl J Med* 295:655–658, 1976.
187. Rao HKM, Myers GJ: *Candida* meningitis in the newborn. *South Med J* 72:1468–1471, 1979.
188. Redline RW, Dahms BB: *Malassezia* pulmonary vasculitis in an infant on long-term intralipid therapy. *N Engl J Med* 305:1395–1398, 1981.
189. Reinhardt GF, Gelbart SM, Greenlee HB: Catheter infection factors affecting total parenteral nutrition. *Am Surg* 44:401–405, 1978.
190. Reinhardt JF, Ruane PJ, Walker LJ, George WL: Intravenous catheter-associated fungemia due to *Candida rugosa*. *J Clin Microbiol* 22:1056–1057, 1985.
191. Rhame FS, Streifel AJ, Kersey JH Jr, McGlave PB: Extrinsic risk factors for pneumonia in the patient at high risk of infection. *Am J Med* 76 (suppl):42–52, 1984.
192. Richards KE, Pierson CL, Bucciarelli L, Feller I: Monilial sepsis in the surgical patient. *Surg Clin North Am* 52:1399–1406, 1972.
193. Rifkind D, Marchioro TL, Schneck SA, Hill RB Jr: Systemic fungal infections

complicating renal transplantation and immunosuppressive therapy. *Am J Med* 43:28–38, 1967.
194. Rinaldi MG: Invasive aspergillosis. *Rev Infect Dis* 5:1061–1077, 1983.
195. Robertson MH: Fungi in fluids—a hazard of intravenous therapy. *J Med Microbiol* 3:99–102, 1970.
196. Robinson GV, Tegtmeier BR, Zaia JA: Brief report: nosocomial infection rates in a cancer treatment center. *Infect Control* 5:289–294, 1984.
197. Rohatgi PK, Rohatgi NB: Clinical spectrum of pulmonary aspergillosis. *South Med J* 77:1291–1301, 1984.
198. Romero R, Reece EA, Duff GW, Coultrip L, Hobbins JC: Prenatal diagnosis of *Candida albicans* chorioamnionitis. *Am J Perinatol* 2:121–122, 1985.
199. Rose HD, Varkey KB: Deep mycotic infection in the hospitalized adult: A study of 123 patients. *Medicine* 54:499–507, 1975.
200. Rubin RH, Wolfson JS, Cosimi AB: Infection in the renal transplant patient. *Am J Med* 70:405–411, 1981.
201. Rubinstein E, Noriega ER, Simberkoff MS, Holzman R, Rahal JJ Jr: Fungal endocarditis: Analysis of 24 cases and review of the literature. *Medicine* 54: 331–344, 1975.
202. Rutala WA, Weber DJ: Environmental issues and nosocomial infections, in Farber BF (ed): *Infection Control in Intensive Care*. New York, Churchill Livingston pp 131–171, 1987.
203. Ryan ME, Ochs J: Primary cutaneous mucormycosis: Superficial and gangrenous infection. *Pediatr Infect Dis* 1:110–114, 1982.
204. Sandford GR, Merr WG, Wingard JR, Charache P, Saral R: The value of fungal surveillance cultures as predictors of systemic fungal infections. *J Infect Dis* 142:503–509, 1980.
205. Sarubbi FA Jr, Kopf HB, Wilson MB, McGinnis MR, Rutala WA: Increased recovery of *Aspergillus flavus* from respiratory specimens during hospital construction. *Am Rev Respir Dis* 125:33–38, 1982.
206. Schleupner CJ, Hamilton JR: A pseudoepidemic of pulmonary fungal infections related to fiberoptic bronchoscopy. *Infect Control* 1:38–42, 1980.
207. Schumacher HR, Ginns DA, Warren WJ: Fungus infection complicating leukemia. *Am J Med Sci* 247:313–323, 1964.
208. Schwartz IS: Marijuana and fungal infection. *Am J Clin Pathol* 84:256, 1985.
209. Shaikh BS, Appelbaum PC, Jones JM, Christiansen D: Colonization of nasal ulcers as a source of *Candida parapsilosis* fungemia. *Arch Otolaryngol* 106: 434–436, 1980.
210. Shapiro I: *Penicillium* species fungus growth on a Bionite hydrophilic contact. *Minn Med* 57:943–944, 1974.
211. Sheldon DL, Johnson WC: Cutaneous mucormycosis: Two documented cases of suspected nosocomial cause. *JAMA* 241:1032–1033, 1979.
212. Singer C, Kaplan MH, Armstrong D: Bacteremia and fungemia complicating neoplastic disease. *Am J Med* 62:731–742, 1977.
213. Slaughter L, Morris JE, Starr A: Prosthetic valvular endocarditis. *Circulation* 47:1319–1326, 1973.
214. Smith H, Congdon P: Neonatal systemic candidiasis. *Arch Dis Child* 60:365–369, 1985.
215. Solomon SL, Alexander H, Eley JW, Anderson RL, Goodpasture HC, Smart S, Furman RM, Martone WJ: Nosocomial fungemia in neonates associated with intravascular pressure-monitoring devices. *Pediatr Infect Dis* 5:680–685, 1986.
216. Solomon SL, Khabbaz RF, Parker RH, Anderson RL, Geraghty MA, Furman RM, Martone WJ: An outbreak of *Candida parapsilosis* bloodstream infections in patients receiving parenteral nutrition. *J Infect Dis* 149:98–102, 1984.

217. Solomon WR, Burge HP, Boise JR: Airborne *Aspergillus fumigatus* levels outside and within a large clinical center. *J Allergy Clin Immunol* 62:56–60, 1978.
218. Solomkin JS, Flohr AM, Simmons RL: Indications for therapy for fungemia in postoperative patients. *Arch Surg* 117:1272–1275, 1982.
219. Soutter DI, Todd TRJ: Systemic candidiasis in a surgical intensive care unit. *Can J Surg* 29:197–199, 1986.
220. Spaun E, Klunder K: *Candida* chorioaminionitis and intrauterine contraceptive device. *Acta Obstet Gynecol Scand* 65:183–184, 1986.
221. Stark WJ, Worthen DM, Holladay JT, Bath PE, Jacobs ME, Murray GC, McGhee ET, Talbott MW, Shipp MD, Thomas NE, Barnes RW, Brown DWC, Buxton JN, Reinecke RD, Lao C-S, Fisher S: The FDA report on intraocular lenses. *Ophthalmology* 90:311–331, 1983.
222. Steigbigel RT, Cross AS: Infections associated with hemodialysis and chronic peritoneal dialysis, in Remington JS, Swartz MN (eds): *Current Clinical Topics in Infectious Disease*. New York, McGraw-Hill, 1984, pp 124–145.
223. Stenson S: Soft contact lenses and corneal infection. *Arch Ophthalmol* 104: 1287–1289, 1986.
224. Stern WH, Tamura E, Jacobs RA, Pons VG, Stone RD, O'Day DM, Irvine AR: Epidemic postsurgical *Candida parapsilosis* endophthalmitis. *Ophthalmology* 92:1701–1709, 1985.
225. St.-Germain G, Laverdiere M: *Torulopsis candida*, a new opportunistic pathogen. *J Clin Microbiol* 24:884–885, 1986.
226. Stone HH: Infection in postoperative patients. *Am J Med* 81 (suppl): 39–44, 1986.
227. Streifel AJ, Stevens PP, Rhame FS: In-hospital source of airborne *Penicillium* species spores. *J Clin Microbiol* 25:1–4, 1987.
228. Strinden WD, Helgerson RB, Maki DG: *Candida* septic thrombosis of the great central veins associated with central catheters. *Ann Surg* 202:653–657, 1985.
229. Sugarman B: Infections and prosthetic devices. *Am J Med* 81 (suppl): 78–84, 1986.
230. Sutton S, Lum BL, Torti FM: Possible risk of invasive pulmonary aspergillosis with marijuana use during chemotherapy for small cell lung cancer. *Drug Intell Clin Pharmacol* 20:289–291, 1986.
231. Tchekmedyian NS, Newman K, Moody MR, Costerton JW, Aisner J, Schimpff SC, Reed WP: Case report: Special studies of the Hickman catheter of a patient with recurrent bacteremia and candidemia. *Am J Med Sci* 291:419–424, 1986.
232. Theodore FH: Etiology and diagnosis of fungal postoperative endophthalmitis. *Ophthalmology* 85:327–340, 1978.
233. Torres-Rojas JR, Stratton CW, Sanders CV, Horsman TA, Hawley HB, Dascomb HE, Vial LJ Jr: Candidal suppurative peripheral thrombophlebitis. *Ann Intern Med* 96:431–435, 1982.
234. Turcotte JG: Infection and renal transplantation. *Surg Clin North Am* 52: 1501–1512, 1972.
235. Verbraeken H, Mendoza A, Van Oye R: Pseudophakic endophthalmitis. *Bull Soc Belg Ophthalmol* 206:55–59, 1983.
236. Walsh TJ, Bustamente CI, Vlahov D, Standiford HC: Candidal suppurative peripheral thrombophlebitis: Recognition, prevention, and management. *Infect Control* 7:16–22, 1986.
237. Walsh TJ, Newman KR, Moody M, Wharton RC, Wade JC: Trichosporonosis in patients with neoplastic disease. *Medicine* 65:268–279, 1986.
238. Walterspiel JN, Kaplan SL, Fishman I, Scott FB: Fungal infection associated with artificial urethral sphincters in children. *J Urol* 135:1245–1246, 1986.
239. Warnock DW: Typing of *Candida albicans*. *J Hosp Infect* 5:244–252, 1984.
240. Weber DJ, Hoffman KL, Thoft RA, Baker AS: Endophthalmitis following

intraocular lens implantation: Report of 30 cases and review of the literature. *Rev Infect Dis* 8:12–20, 1986.
241. Weiland D, Ferguson RM, Peterson PK, Snover DC, Simmons RL, Najarian JS: Aspergillosis in 25 renal transplant patients. *Ann Surg* 198:622–629, 1983.
242. Weinstein RA, Stamm WE, Kramer L, Corey L: Pressure monitoring devices. *JAMA* 236:936–938, 1976.
243. Whyte RK, Hussain Z, deSA D: Antenatal infections with Candida species. *Arch Dis Child* 57:528–535, 1982.
244. Wilson LA, Ahearn DG: Association of fungi with extended-wear soft contact lenses. *Am J Ophthalmol* 101:434–436, 1986.
245. Wilson WR, Jaumin PM, Danielson GK, Giuliani ER, Washington JA II, Geraci JE: Prosthetic valve endocarditis. *Ann Intern Med* 82:751–756, 1975.
246. Wingard JR, Merz WB, Saral R: *Candida tropicalis*: A major pathogen in immunocompromised patients. *Ann Intern Med* 91:539–545, 1979.
247. Wolfson JS, Sober AJ, Rubin RH: Dermatologic manifestation of infections in immunocompromised patients. *Medicine* 64:115–133, 1985.
248. Yackee JM, Topiel MS, Simon GL: Septic phlebitis caused by *Candida albicans* and diagnosed by needle biopsy. *South Med J* 78:1262–1263, 1985.
249. Yamamoto GK, Pavan-Langston D, Stowe GC III, Albert DM: Fungal invasion of a therapeutic soft contact lens and cornea. *Ann Ophthalmol*: 1731–1735, 1979.
250. Younkin S, Evarts CM, Steigbigel RT: *Candida parapsilosis* infection of a total hip-joint replacement: Successful reimplantation after treatment with amphotericin B and 5-fluorocytosine. *J Bone Joint Surg* 66-A: 142–143, 1984.
251. Young RC, Bennett JE, Geelhoed GW, Levine AS: Fungemia with compromised host resistance. *Ann Intern Med* 80:605–612, 1974.
252. Young RC, Bennett JE, Vogel CL, Carbone PP, DeVita VT: Aspergillosis. *Medicine* 49:147–173, 1970.
253. Zapata-Sirvent RL, Wang X-W, Miller G, Davies JWL, Sun Y-H, Zhang M-L, Cao D-X, Ma R-L: *Candida* infection in severe burns. *Burns* 11:330–336, 1985.

10—Melanins and Their Importance in Pathogenic Fungi

MICHAEL H. WHEELER and ALOIS A. BELL

Melanins are generally described as dark brown or black pigments of high molecular weight formed by oxidative polymerization of phenolic compounds. Certain yellow, red, green, purple, or blue pigments have similar chemical structures and occasionally are referred to as types of melanins. Melanins are found in humans and various other warm- and cold-blooded vertebrates; invertebrates, including insects; higher plants; fungi; and bacteria, including actinomycetes. Most animal melanins are synthesized by tyrosinase, whereas a number of less specific polyphenol oxidases may form melanins in various cellular and extracellular environments of other organisms. In some cases melanins are autoxidative products made in the absence of enzymes.

The black melanins in humans and other animals have been most widely studied and are described in a number of reviews (21, 22, 63, 188, 256, 288). They are derived from tyrosine via 3,4-dihydroxyphenylalanine (DOPA) and are commonly called eumelanins. The reddish pigments of hair and feathers are called phaeomelanins because of structural similarity to eumelanins; cysteine is copolymerized with DOPA to form the red pigment. The synthesis of eumelanins and phaeomelanins from tyrosine by the action of tyrosinase (22, 63, 188) takes place in specialized cells of higher animals.

Tyrosinase also occurs in the common mushroom, *Agaricus brunnescens* (as *A. bisporus*), and in *Neurospora crassa* (144). Thus, some researchers concluded that fungal melanins in these and other fungi are also derived from tyrosine. A number of other phenolic metabolites, for example, 1,8-dihydroxynaphthalene (DHN) (31, 74, 279, 282, 290), catechol (175, 190), γ-glutaminyl-3,4,-dihydroxybenzene (GDHB) (209, 253), and catecholamines (193) also have been proposed as natural precursors. Fungal melanins occur in cell walls and as extracellular polymers formed enzymically or autoxidatively in the medium around cell walls.

The melanins are important for survival and longevity of fungal propagules (53, 141, 254). They also function as defense systems in a number of ways. In humans and a number of vertebrates and invertebrates, they serve as important sources of camouflage (172, 206) as well as protectants against sunlight. For example the "ink" released by squid and octopus is protective and consists of a fine suspension of DOPA melanin granules, acting as a screen against predators.

Fungal melanins are important for virulence at least in certain plant pathogens (15). Thus, fungal diseases potentially can be controlled by inhibiting melanin synthesis. Several compounds prevent direct fungal penetration of plant tissue by inhibiting melanin synthesis in appressorial cells of fungal pathogens (240, 241), and tricyclazole, fthalide and pyroquilon (Fig. 10-4) are used now commercially to prevent rice blast disease caused by *Pyricularia oryzae*. The treated appressoria still produce germ pegs, but these are unable to penetrate through the plants outer epidermal layer.

Tricyclazole also inhibits melanin biosynthesis in a number of fungi that cause human disease (Table 10-1). Melanin in these fungi is synthesized via the

TABLE 10-1. Results of Tricyclazole and Homogenate Studies to Show 1,8-Dihydroxynaphthalene (DHN) Melanin*

Ascomycotina
- *Aspergillus nidulans*, —, HP (U)
- *Cochliobolus carbonum*, TI, EA, PP (279)
- *C. miyabeanus*, TI, EA, PP (279)
- *Pleospora infectoria*, TI, EA, PP (279)
- *Sclerotinia minor*, EA, PP (279)
- *S. trifoliorum*, EA, PP (279)
- *Wetzelinia sclerotiorum*, TI, EA, PP (26, 279)

Fungi Imperfecti
- *Alternaria alternata*, TI, PP, HP (279)
- *A. brassicicola*, TI, EA, PP (279)
- *A. eichhorniae*, TI, EA, PP (U)
- *A. solani*, TI, PP (133)
- *Aspergillus niger*, —, HP (279)
- *A.* sp., — (U)[†]
- *Aureobasidium pullulans*, TI (237)
- *Bipolaris sorokiniana*, TI, EA, PP (279)
- *Botrytis cinerea*, TI, PP (300)
- *Cladosporium carrionii*, TI, HP (259)
- *Colletotrichum gossypii*, TI, PP (279)
- *C. lagenarium*, TI, PP (123)
- *C. lindemuthianum*, TI, PP (242, 287)
- *Curvularia protuberata*, TI, EA, PP (279)
- *Diplodia gossypina*, TI, EA, PP (279)
- *D. natalensis*, TI, EA, PP (279)
- *Epicoccum nigrum*, — (U)
- *Exophiala jeanselmei*, TI, HP (259)
- *Fonsecaea compacta*, TI, HP (259)
- *F. pedrosoi*, TI, HP (259)
- *Hendersonula toruloidea*, TI, EA, PP, HP (U)
- *Macrophomina phaseoli*, TI, PP (279)
- *Microdochium bolleyi*, TI, PP (47)
- *Monilinia fructicola*, TI, PP (18)
- *Phaeoannellomyces werneckii*, TI, HP (259)
- *Phaeococcomyces* sp., TI (32)
- *Phialophora richardsiae*, TI, HP (259)
- *P. verrucosa*, TI, HP (259)
- *Pyricularia oryzae*, TI, EA, PP (277, 290)
- *Rhizoctonia leguminicola*, TI, EA, PP (279)
- *Sclerotium cepivorum*, EA, PP (279)
- *Thielaviopsis basicola*, TI, PP (280)
- *Verticillium albo-atrum*, TI, EA, PP (279)
- *V. dahliae*, TI, EA, PP (266, 278)
- *V. nigrescens*, TI, PP (262, 279)
- *V. tricorpus*, TI, EA, PP (262, 279)
- *Wangiella dermatitidis*, TI, EA, HP (281)
- *Xylohypha bantiana*, TI, HP (259)

Basidiomycotina
- *Thanatephorus cucumeris*, —, PP (279)
- *Sphacelotheca reiliana*, —, PP (279)
- *Sclerotium rolfsii*, —, PP (279)
- *Typhula idahoensis*, —, PP (279)
- *T. ishikariensis*, —, PP (279)
- *Ustilago maydis*, —, PP (279)

Mastigomycotina
- *Allomyces macrogynus*, — (U)
- *Blastocladiella emersonii*, — (U)

Zygomycotina
- *Mucor rouxii*, — (U)

*EA = DHN melanin pathway demonstrated by enzyme assay; HP = accepted as human pathogen (160); PP = plant pathogen; TI = DHN melanin pathway demonstrated by tricyclazole inhibition; U = M.H. Wheeler and A.A. Bell, unpublished; and — = no effect with tricyclazole inhibition or enzyme assay.
[†]Member of *Aspergillus glaucus* group. Isolate provided by Dr. K Haider.

pentaketide pathway and is identical to melanin previously reported in the plant pathogens *Verticillium dahliae* (13, 263, 266) and *P. oryzae* (290). The human pathogens affected by tricyclazole include causative agents of chromoblastomycosis, phaeohyphomycosis, and related diseases (38, 214, 259, 274, 282, 298). Melanin formed from pentaketides also occurs in several genera of plant pathogens and other fungi that occasionally cause opportunistic infections in humans. These infections caused by *Alternaria* spp., *Bipolaris* spp. *Curvularia* spp., *Exserohilum* spp. and other fungi have been reviewed by Rippon (214) and others (158a, 161a). These fungi usually attack debilitated or compromised patients with suppressed immune systems. The numbers of such cases have increased over the last few years with the development and accelerated use of antimicrobics, steroids, and other improved medical treatments. Other melanins described in animal and plant pathogens are also discussed in this review. Emphasis is placed on their classification, biosynthesis, cytology, properties, and functions.

Properties, Classification, and Biosynthesis of Melanins

Melanins in fungi have been categorized in a number of ways based on their biosynthesis from various phenolic compounds and on their chemical composition and properties. Swan (256) stated that "conclusions drawn regarding the structure of natural melanins can in no case be accepted without question." This is especially true of fungal melanins. In this section the properties and chemical characterization of melanins that have been reported in the fungi are described.

Chemical and Physical Properties

Melanins and related pigments are difficult to study and characterize because of their polymeric, inert nature. They are generally insoluble in water, aqueous acids, and common organic solvents, and often are poorly soluble in alkali. Occasionally, however, they are conjugated with carbohydrates or proteins, and consequently are soluble in water. Aspergillin, a black melanin from conidia of *Aspergillus niger* (210), for example, is water soluble and present in cytoplasmic homogenates prepared by cell fractionation. It also differs from other melanins because its synthesis is inhibited by dimethylsulfoxide (36). When hydrolyzed, aspergillin yields sugars and amino acids (256), apparently from carbohydrates and proteins associated with the chromophore.

Melanins are usually purified by methods involving their dissolution in alkali and reprecipitation in acid. Proteins, carbohydrates, and lipids associated with melanins are removed by prolonged hydrolysis in aqueous acid.

Additional purification is achieved by using alternating cycles of organic solvents and hot acids.

Melanins derived from DOPA, catechol, GDHB, and DHN are made from similar phenolic and quinone precursors. These melanins apparently have similar chemical and physical properties, but most studies on the properties of melanin have used DOPA melanin purified from animals, synthesized by autoxidation, or synthesized by enzymic oxidation with mushroom tyrosinase (21, 135). Catechol melanin has also been studied as a pure compound obtained from *Ustilago maydis* (191). Natural GDHB and DHN fungal melanins have not been studied in purified form. Infrared (IR) spectra of the melanins are similar (21, 27, 55, 58, 220, 253). This shows that the polymers have identical functional groups and helps to explain why their properties are similar.

The structure of melanins, especially the combination of quinones and hydroquinones, allows them to exist as free radicals that are easily formed under various conditions, that is, irradiation with ultraviolet (UV) or γ rays (166, 168, 244, 303), incubation at increased temperature (302), or reaction with chemical reductants (21). Melanins also act as either proton donors or receivers (21, 135). Thus, they are oxidized by H_2O_2 or sodium hypochlorite and reduced by silver ions or hydrosulfite.

DOPA melanin (and probably other melanins) converts light to heat (172) and is an excellent sound-absorbing material (203). It has been described as a battery (cf, 203) and an amorphous semiconductor (158), and may be used as an amorphous semiconductor threshold switch (157). It has superoxide dismutase activity (77, 168), is a cation exchange material (286), and binds with aromatic and cyclic compounds (23), including a number of drugs (103, 276). These diverse properties may explain how DOPA melanin functions in diverse organs, for example, the skin, eye, midbrain, and inner ear, and why it and other melanins interfere with the actions of a number of therapeutic drugs (103, 276).

DOPA Melanins

Dark pigments in many fungi have been reported to be DOPA (or indolic) melanins, suggesting that they are chemically identical to those made in humans and other animals. Bourquelot and Bertrand, according to Swan (256), reported in 1895 that an enzyme present in the mushroom *Russula nigricans* could transform tyrosine into a black insoluble pigment. Similar enzyme activity was later reported in preparations from a number of other fungi, including *Neurospora crassa* (97, 225), *Aspergillus nidulans* (30), and the mushroom *A. brunnescens* (as *A. campestris*) (114), which produce melanin in cell walls. The tyrosinases have been purified and thoroughly characterized from *N. crassa* (66, 134) and *A. brunnescens* (as *A. bisporus*) (52, 174).

The occurrence, composition, and biosynthesis of melanins made from

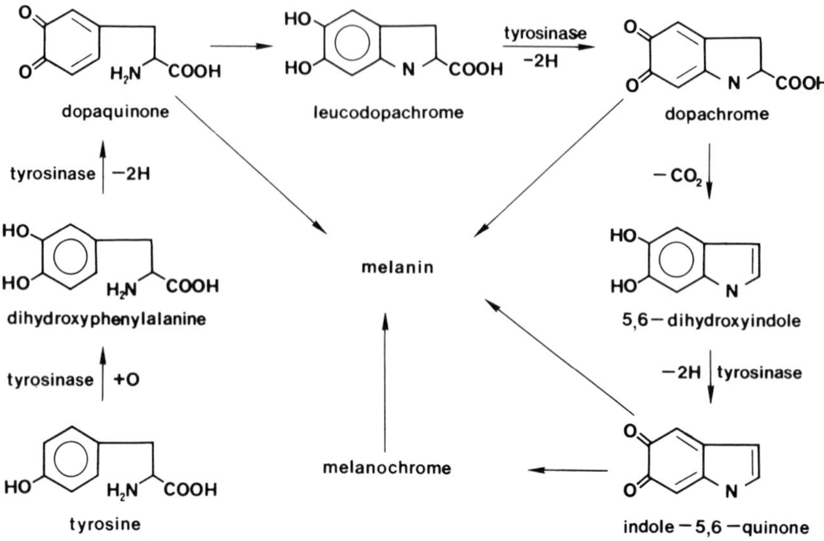

FIG. 10-1. Biosynthesis of melanin from tyrosine (188). DOPA melanin is believed to be a heteropolymer made from a number of quinone intermediates. It was earlier thought to be a homopolymer derived solely from indole-5,6-quinone.

tyrosine and DOPA have been reviewed (21, 22, 175, 188, 256); there is good evidence that these melanins are heteropolymers made from a number of different compounds derived from tyrosine as shown in Fig. 10-1. This heteropolymer scheme of melanin biosynthesis is similar to the Raper-Mason scheme (154) derived earlier, but is less restrictive and indicates that melanin is not a homopolymer derived solely from 5,6-dihydroxyquinone.

The role of tyrosinase in the oxidation of tyrosine to DOPA and DOPA to dopaquinone has been confirmed in many laboratories. These conversions occur via cresolase and catecholase reactions that oxidize monophenols and *o*-diphenols, respectively. The reactions leading from dopaquinone to melanin occur spontaneously. In addition, tyrosinase, purified from murine melanoma and skin of brown mice, catalyzes the conversion of 5,6-dihydroxyindole to melanochrome (117).

To be classified as a tyrosinase, a fungal or plant polyphenoloxidase should be able to convert tyrosine to DOPA. Marr (146, 147) reported that most investigations during the past four decades confirm that L-tyrosine is a specific substrate of tyrosinase. Other polyphenoloxidases that do not oxidize tyrosine should be referred to in a more general sense as catecholases or laccases (*o*- or *p*-diphenoloxidases, respectively). This can be a problem because the cresolase activity required to oxidize tyrosine to DOPA is often labile and lost during purification of tyrosinase enzymes (156). Also tyrosine is poorly soluble and can be difficult to use as a substrate (147). Thus, a tyrosinase can be confused with a less specific catecholase or a laccase.

Tyrosinase from animal tissues is relatively specific for tyrosine and DOPA, whereas the tyrosinases from fungi and higher plants act on a wide range of mono- and *o*-diphenols (156). Also, the specificity for optical isomers, that is, L-tyrosine, which is well-defined in the mammalian enzyme, is less evident in the enzymes from fungi or higher plants.

The cytology of DOPA melanin synthesis in animals has been studied in detail (64, 229). In vertebrates, melanins are synthesized in the melanosomes, which are subcellular granules in pigment cells known as "melanocytes" in warm-blooded vertebrates (64, 177, 288) and "melanophores" in cold-blooded vertebrates (43). Melanosomes have a limiting membrane and regular internal lamellar structures (188). They form from unmelanized granules known as premelanosomes and when fully melanized are called melanin granules. These generally remain dispersed in the cytoplasm and retain the melanosome membrane. Some melanocytes retain their melanin granules and are referred to as "continent" melanocytes (64), whereas others the "secretory" melanocytes transfer their granules to receptor cells, known as keratinocytes or melanophages in mammalian tissues.

DOPA melanins in animals are synthesized and maintained almost totally in melanosomes. Fungal melanins, in contrast, occur either in cell walls, a fibrillar network surrounding the walls, or as extracellular polymers formed in the medium around cells. Melanin generally does not occur in fungal cytoplasm, although structures resembling premelanosomes have been reported (87, 118, 189). In our opinion, the ultrastructural findings of "premelanosomes" in fungal cells probably are not correct, because the resemblance of any of the observed structures to premelanosomes of animals is slight, and there is no evidence that the structures are actually involved in melanin synthesis or accumulation. Nevertheless, we believe that certain types of cytoplasmic organelles probably are involved in the biosynthesis of fungal melanin precursors. The final enzymic polymerization of the precursors apparently occurs in other locations, for example, cell walls and the medium surrounding cells.

A number of fungi, including *A. nidulans* (27), *Aureobasidium pullulans* (258), *Oidiodendron cerealis* (236), *Phomopsis* sp. (56), *Amorphotheca resinae*, *Epicoccum nigrum*, *Humicola grisea*, *Colletotrichum coccodes*, and *V. dahliae* (55) have been reported to contain DOPA melanin in their cell walls. However, we do not believe there is conclusive proof that this type of melanin occurs in any fungal cell wall. In fact there is strong proof that *A. pullulans* (237), *Colletotrichum* spp. (122, 279, 287), *H. grisea* (MH Wheeler and AA Bell, unpublished), and *V. dahliae* (13) make melanin from the pentaketide derivative DHN.

There has been a tendency to report DOPA melanin from fungi because the amino acid tyrosine occurs universally in living organisms, and the enzyme tyrosinase has been documented in a few fungi. Tyrosinase has not been conclusively found in the outer cell wall where melanin is synthesized; however, laccase has been reported to occur and oxidize DOPA to melanin in cell walls of *Leptosphaerulina briosiana* (238). This fungus does not make melanin from the monophenols tyrosine and *p*-cresol, which are metabolized by fungal tyrosinases. Also, albino mutants of *Thielaviopsis basicola* (280) and *V. dahliae* (284), that synthesize normal appearing melanin in their outer cell walls from scytalone and DHN, are unable to convert DOPA to normal appearing pigments.

Albinos of *V. dahliae* convert 1-naphthol to a purple pigment in the outer cell wall in patterns resembling those of melanin deposition (MH Wheeler and AA Bell, unpublished). Although mushroom tyrosinase has been shown to metabolize 1-naphthol to 1,2-naphthoquinone and 1,4-naphthoquinone (51), 1-naphthol is a more specific substrate for laccase than for tyrosinase (146). This further suggests that laccase is a common wall bound enzyme associated with melanin synthesis in fungi. Laccase enzymes have been reported to cause green pigment production in conidial cell walls of *Penicillium cyclopium* (11), and laccases have been shown to participate in the synthesis of green conidial (46, 125, 126) and red cleistothecial pigments (89) in *A. nidulans*. The work with *A. nidulans* further shows that tyrosinase is not necessarily associated with pigmentation, even when the enzyme is produced by the fungus.

DHN Melanin

A number of imperfect and ascomycetous fungi, including several human and plant pathogens, make brown to black melanin from DHN and related pentaketide metabolites (Table 10-1). The human pathogens include *Wangiella dermatitidis* (74, 259, 281) and seven other soil-inhabiting dematiaceous fungi (259) that cause chromoblastomycosis, phaeohyphomycosis, and related dermal, systemic, and neurotropic diseases. A related fungus, *Phaeoannellomyces werneckii* (*Exophiala werneckii*), that causes a superficial infection (tinea nigra) of the stratum corneum also makes DHN melanin (259).

The DHN pathway, shown in Fig. 10-2, was discovered in *V. dahliae* (13) by using mutants that produce melanin-deficient resting structures known as microsclerotia. These overwintering propagules are normally black in wild-type isolates. Cultures of brown mutants accumulate two types of metabolites: 1) intermediates in the direct pathway to melanin, that is, scytalone and DHN; and 2) products in branch pathways made by oxidation and subsequent reactions of unstable intermediates in the melanin pathway. The mutants and their characteristics are summarized in Table 10-2.

The mutation *brm-1* eliminates the ability to dehydrate scytalone to 1,3,8 trihydroxynaphthalene (1,3,8-THN) and vermelone to DHN. Thus, scytalone, a stable metabolite, accumulates in cultures as a consequence of this mutation, and can be isolated in appreciable yields (14). Cultures of the mutant also accumulate flaviolin and *cis*-4-hydroxyscytalone (4-HS), which are formed as shunt products from 1,3,6,8-tetrahydroxynaphthalene (1,3,6,8-

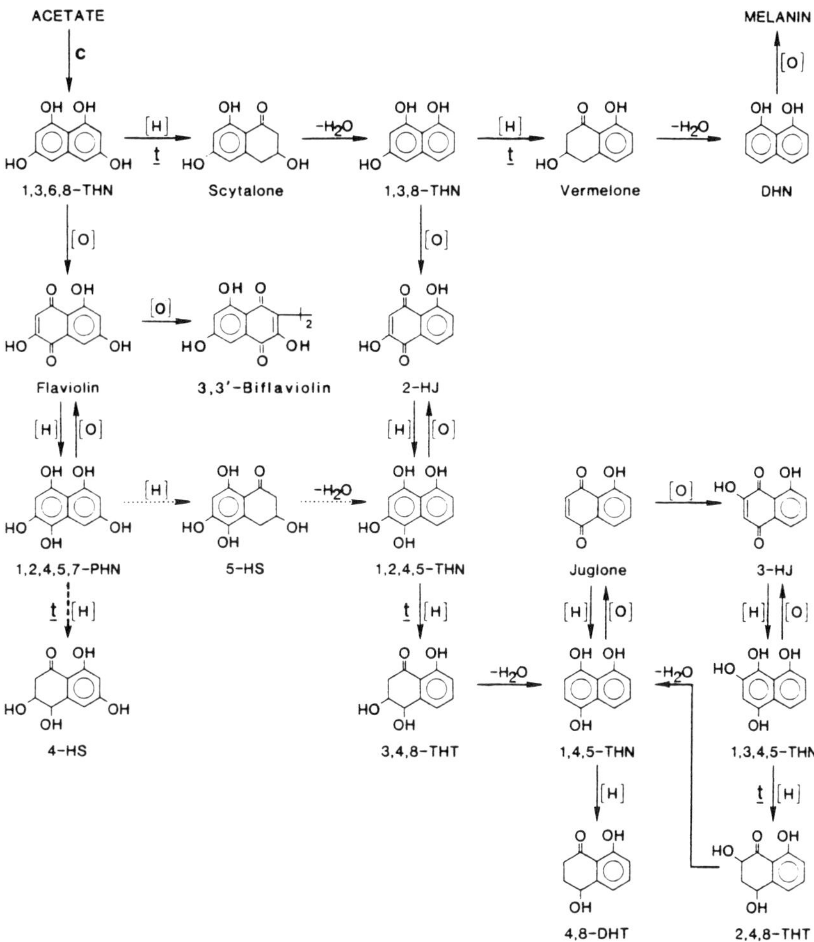

FIG. 10-2. Biosynthesis of DHN melanin from acetate via scytalone and DHN. Also shown are branch products produced because of mutations eliminating reductase (H) or dehydratase (-H_2O) enzymes or because of tricyclazole (t) inhibition. Cerulenin (C) inhibition occurs early in polyketide synthesis and prevents production of cyclized compounds. Scheme taken from Wheeler and Stipanovic (280) and amended to show 3,3'-biflaviolin (250).

THN). Flaviolin is an oxidation product of 1,3,6,8-THN (14), and 4-HS is a reduction product of flaviolin. Vermelone is produced by feeding exogenous 1,3,8-THN to cultures of *brm-1* (248), because the reduction of 1,3,8-THN occurs downstream from the block between scytalone and 1,3,8-THN.

The mutation *brm-2* blocks the reduction of 1,3,8-THN to vermelone and causes the accumulation of 1,3,8-THN and its oxidized shunt product 2-hydroxyjuglone (2-HJ) in cultures (249). This mutation also causes the accu-

TABLE 10-2. Characteristics of Melanin-Deficiency Mutations in *Verticillium dahliae*, *Wangiella dermatitidis*, and *Pyricularia oryzae*

Fungus	Mutation US Strain	Designation Russian Strain*	Enzyme Deficiency†	Major Product Accumulated‡
V. dahliae	*alm-1*	*alm-A*	Unknown	None
	alm-2		"	"
	alm-3		"	"
	brm-1	*chm-1*	Dehydratase	Scytalone, flaviolin, 4-HS
	brm-3		"	" " "
	brm-2	*brm*	Reductase	2-HJ, 3,4,8-THT, 4,8-DHT
	brm-4	*chm-2*	"	Flaviolin
	gym-1		Oxidase	DHN, 2,2′-dimer of DHN
		olim	"	DHN
W. dermatitidis	*mel-1*		Dehydratase	Scytalone, flaviolin
	mel-2		Oxidase	DHN
	mel-3		Unknown	None
P. oryzae	CP-412		Unknown	None
	P-2m-1		Reductase	2-HJ, 3,4,8-THT
	P-2m-20		"	" "
	P-2m-23		"	" "

*Symbols: *alm* = albino microsclerotia, *brm* = brown microsclerotia, *chm* = cherry microsclererotia, *CP-412* = albino, *gym* = gray microsclerotia, *mel* = melanin deficient, *olim* = olive microsclerotia, and *P-2m* = buff (13, 74, 204, 233, 234, 290).

†Function of enzymes in melanin synthesis shown in Fig. 10-2.

‡Shunt products that accumulated as a result of the mutation were isolated and identified from culture media (14, 204, 234, 263); structures are shown in Fig. 10-2.

mulation of several other metabolites. These include 3-hydroxyjuglone (3-HJ), juglone, 4,8-dihydroxytetralone (4,8-DHT), and 3,4,8-trihydroxytetralone (3,4,8-THT). The *brm-2* mutation only partially inhibits the reduction of 1,3,6,8-THN under culture conditions. Thus, cultures of *brm-2* accumulate mainly 2-HJ and branch products from 2-HJ, with only traces of flaviolin or 4-HS (249).

The mutations *alm-1*, *-2*, or *-3* block the synthesis of 1,3,6,8-THN, but allow metabolism of scytalone, vermelone, and DHN to melanin like that in wild-type isolates (13, 248, 284). The albinos also produce normal melanins when paired together in genetic complementation tests (13). This suggests that their mutations affect different enzymic sites in the pathway before 1,3,6,8-THN.

The mutation *brm-3* causes accumulation of the same metabolites as *brm-1*, but complements with *brm-1* producing natural appearing melanin. The mutation *brm-4* complements with *brm-2*, but lacks both types of reductase activity and only accumulates flaviolin. The selectivity of the *brm-2* mutation for preventing the reaction between 1,3,8-THN and vermelone indicates that if a single enzyme carries out both reductions, it probably has a greater binding affinity for 1,3,6,8-THN than 1,3,8-THN at its active site.

Analogous lesions to those in *brm-1*, *-2*, *-3*, or *-4* and *alm-1*, *-2*, or *-3* have been reported in Russian strains of *V. dahliae* (233, 234, 263). They are summarized in Table 10-2. Similar mutations have been obtained in other plant and animal pathogenic fungi, including *W. dermatitidis* and *P. oryzae* (Table 10-2) and *V. nigrescens* and *V. tricorpus* (235). This indicates that these fungi contain DHN melanin biosynthesized via the identical pathway present in *V. dahliae*.

Mutations in *V. dahliae* that cause the accumulation of DHN and the 2,2′-dimer of DHN (Fig. 10-3) have been obtained and named *olim* (233, 234) and *gym-1* (204), respectively. Both of these mutations cause deficiences in the oxidase (probably laccase) that polymerizes and oxidizes DHN into melanin. A similar mutation that causes the accumulation of DHN in cultures of *W. dermatitidis* has been reported (74). The 1,1′-dimer of DHN has been isolated from wild-type *Daldinia concentrica* and has been suggested as a dimeric intermediate in the synthesis of melanin (31). We have fed both DHN dimers to albino mutants of *V. dahliae* (AA Bell and MH Wheeler, unpublished). Both are converted to black melanin granules, but the oxidation of the 2,2′-dimer proceeds through olive-black intermediates, whereas oxidation of the 1,1′-dimer proceeds through red to red-brown intermediates. In our experience, the olive-colored intermediates are normally observed in the wild type, suggesting that 2,2′-dimerization is most frequent at least in *V. dahliae*.

The 1,1′-dimer of DHN is also converted to 4,9-dihydroxyperylene-3,10-quinone in *D. concentrica* (4, 31) and *Bulgaria inquinans* (cf. 269). It or a similar 1,1′-dimer containing one or more subunits from 1,3,8-THN (239) is metabolized to similar compounds in certain *Alternaria* spp. (181, 216) and *Stemphylium botryosum* (7) (Fig. 10-3). The synthesis of two of these compounds, alteichin and anhydroalteichin, was recently found to be blocked by tricyclazole in *Alternaria eichhorniae* (MH Wheeler and R Beier, unpublished). This also indicates these compounds are biosynthesized by reactions in the melanin pathway.

Tricyclazole and other compounds (Fig. 10-4) that inhibit DHN melanin synthesis in *V. dahliae* and *P. oryzae* mimic the *brm-2* and *brm-4* mutations (266, 290). Thus, these inhibitors can be used to cause shunt-product accumulation and to demonstrate the presence of DHN melanin in various fungi (259, 279). The minimum concentration of tricyclazole required to inhibit reductase activity varies from less than 0.1–10 μg/ml for different species. Tricyclazole inhibits the reduction of 1,3,8-THN (Fig. 10-2) at 1.0 μg/ml in cultures of *V. dahliae* (266) and causes the accumulation of 2-HJ, thus mimicking the *brm-2* mutation. At higher concentrations, that is, 30 μg/ml, tricyclazole mimics the *brm-4* mutation and inhibits the melanin pathway between 1,3,6,8-THN and scytalone (Fig. 10-2). The latter inhibitory effect is not seen with all fungi but has been reported for *A. solani* (133), *P. oryzae* (290), *V. dahliae* (266), and *W. dermatitidis* (281). The results with tricyclazole suggest that the same reductase enzyme may carry out the two reactions but has a different binding affinity for substrates or inhibitors. The reductase

A

DHN 2,2′-Dimer
MELANIN
alteichin
DHN
DHN 1,1′-Dimer
4,9-dihydroxy-perylene-3,10-quinone
anhydroalteichin

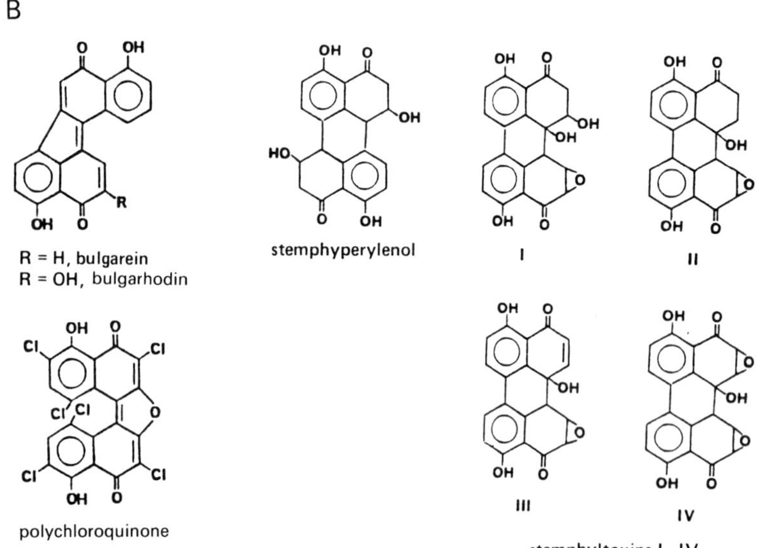

FIG. 10-3. (A-B) Structures and synthesis of compounds that appear to be products of 1,3,8-trihydroxynaphthalene and/or 1,8-dihydroxynaphthalene (4, 7, 31, 33, 181, 204, 216, 269).

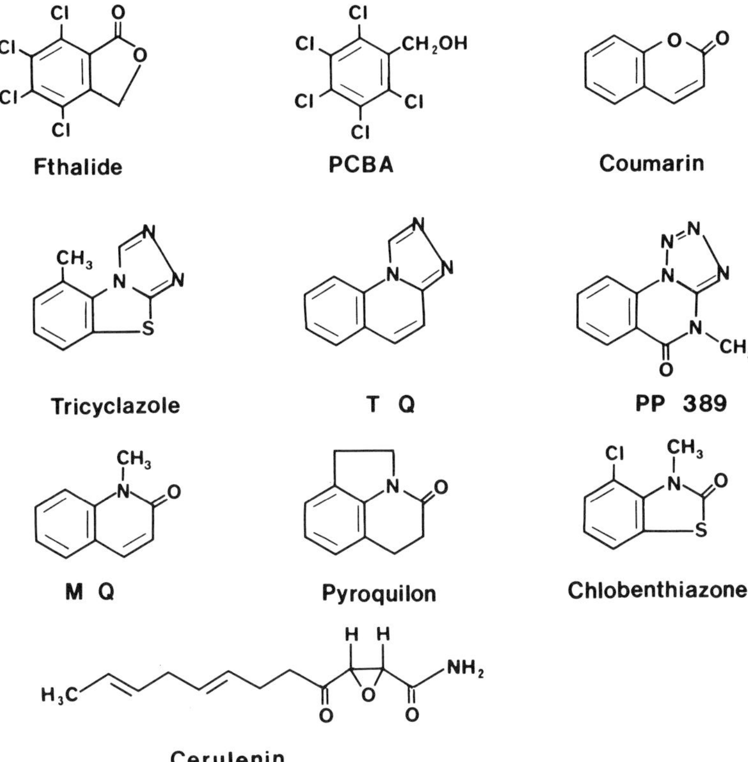

FIG. 10-4. Antipenetrant fungicides that inhibit DHN melanin biosynthesis. Cerulenin acts at an earlier site in the melanin pathway than tricyclazole and the other compounds.

probably helps reduce flaviolin, 2-HJ, and other naphthoquinones in the branch pathways. The reactions involve similar naphtholic substrates as in the main melanin pathway (281) and are inhibited by tricyclazole (Fig. 10-2).

A technique to demonstrate reductase and dehydratase activities in cell-free homogenates has been developed (278, 279). Various intermediates in melanin synthesis or the branch pathways and NADPH are used as substrates, and subsequent products in the pathways are measured at time intervals to gauge enzyme activity. Effective studies of tricyclazole inhibition and enzyme assays require measurements of melanin intermediates and shunt metabolites. A technique for measuring these compounds using high-performance liquid chromatography has been developed (80) and will facilitate future studies.

Tricyclazole inhibition of melanin synthesis and demonstration of reductase and dehydratase activity in cell-free homogenates alone or in combination have been used to demonstate DHN melanin in most of the imperfect and ascomycetous fungi listed in Table 10-1. Tricyclazole at 42 μM, for example, prevents normal dark brown to black pigmentation in cell walls of the human pathogenic fungi *Cladosporium carrionii*, *Exophiala jeanselmei*, *Fonsecaea compacta*, *F. pedrosoi*, *P. werneckii*, *Phialophora richardsiae*, *P. verrucosa*, and *Xylohypha bantiana* (*Cladosporium bantianum*) (259, 282). Inhibition of the melanin pathway causes the accumulation of 2-HJ and flaviolin in cultures. Melanin biosynthesis in these eight pathogens is similar to that in the human pathogen *W. dermatitidis* and the plant pathogens *P. oryzae* and *V. dahliae*. Fungi that did not show evidence of DHN melanin with tricyclazole or homogenates include *Aspergillus glaucus* (an *Aspergillus* sp. belonging to the *A. glaucus* group), *A. nidulans*, *A. niger*, *E. nigrum*, and *Stachybotrys chartarum* of the Fungi Imperfecti and related Ascomycotina, and all of the fungi tested in the Basidiomycotina, Mastigomycotina, and Zygomycotina (Table 10-1).

Intermediates and shunt products from DHN melanin synthesis (Fig. 10-2) have been isolated in small quantities from several wild-type fungal isolates. Because these compounds appear to be uniquely derived from the DHN melanin pathway, their presence indicates this type of melanin. The intermediate scytalone has been isolated from wild-type cultures of *Ceratocystis minor* (88, 164), *Phialophora lagerbergii* (3, 10, 223, 224, 231), *Scytalidium* spp. (62), *Penicillium carneolutescens* (cf, 269), and *V. dahliae* (264); the intermediate DHN has been isolated from *D. concentrica* in its mono- and dimethyl ether forms (4). The shunt product flaviolin or its methylated derivative has been isolated from *A. niger* (163) (also referred to as *A. citricus* (9, 50)), *Macrophomina phaseoli* (MH Wheeler and AA Bell, unpublished), *Phoma wasabiae* (245), *Streptomyces* sp. (76, 163), and *P. lagerbergii* (3). The tetralone shunt products 3,4,8-THT or 4,8-DHT have been isolated from *Scytalidium* spp. (61), *P. oryzae* (109, 110), *Whetzelinia sclerotiorum* (173), and *Achaetormium cristalliferum* (cf, 269). As mentioned earlier, compounds that appear to be dimeric shunt derivatives of DHN (and/or 1,3,8-THN) have been isolated from *Alternaria* spp. (181, 216), *S. botryosum* (7), and *B. inquinans* (cf, 269). Thus, evidence now exists for DHN melanin in more than 50 species of the Ascomycotina and related Fungi Imperfecti. Of the various species studied in these groups, only four, *A. nidulans*, *A. glaucus* group, *E. nigrum*, and *S. chartarum*, have not given evidence of DHN melanin. The results shows that a large number of fungi belonging to the Ascomycotina and related Fungi Imperfecti produce DHN melanin. This suggests that many other human pathogens that are pigmented, for example, *A. fumigatus*, *Madurella grisea*, *M. mycetomatis*, *Piedraia hortae*, *Pseudallescheria boydii*, *Sporothrix schenckii*, and *Stenella araguata*, may also produce DHN melanin in their saprophytic or pathogenic forms.

The synthesis of scytalone and flaviolin from 1,3,6,8-THN produced via polyketide biosynthesis (Fig. 10-2) has been confirmed using ^{2}H-, ^{13}C- and ^{14}C-labeled acetate in feeding experiments (163, 223, 224, 231). The labeling studies did not unequivocally distinguish between true pentaketides and naphthalenes derived from larger chains, such as a hexaketides, by degradation (10). Thus, the polyketide precursor of 1,3,6,8-THN and related melanin metabolites needs to be better defined.

Three lines of evidence indicate that the electron-dense materials in fungal cell walls are melanins. First, only walls of melanized cells show electron-dense granules; walls of hyaline cells are electron translucent (280, 284, 285). Second, walls that are melanized and electron dense in wild-type isolates are electron translucent in corresponding albino mutants, but normal patterns of electron-dense melanin appear when melanin precursors are fed to the albinos (280, 281, 283–285). Finally, adding nontoxic concentrations of tricyclazole, a melanin synthesis inhibitor, to the culture medium eliminates or greatly diminishes the appearance of electron-dense granules in chlamydospore walls of *T. basicola* (280) and in walls of rind cells of sclerotia of *Botrytis cinerea* (300) and *W. sclerotiorum* (26), with no other apparent change in treated cells. Collectively, these observations show that electron-dense granules in and on fungal walls are melanins.

Melanin of wild-type *V. dahliae* occurs as granules in the outer layer of microsclerotial cell walls and in a fibrillar network encapsulating the walls. Albino microsclerotial strains of the wild type do not make melanin in the absence of melanin precursors but turn black when treated with scytalone or DHN (284, 285). The melanin granules in albinos are similar in appearance and distribution to those in the wild type. These observations agree with genetic and biochemical findings and suggest that scytalone and DHN are natural intermediates of melanin synthesis in *V. dahliae*. An albino of *W. dermatitidis* also metabolizes scytalone to a wall-bound pigment indistinguishable from melanin in wild-type cell walls (Fig. 10-5). DHN darkens cell walls of the albino but has not been used in ultrastructural studies because of its autoxidation to extracellular products (284). Albino mutants of *T. basicola* (280), and *C. protuberata*, *Bipolaris sorokiniana*, and *P. infectoria* (283) have also been shown to make normal appearing melanin from scytalone and DHN.

The oxidase involved in producing the final melanin polymer has not been characterized. However, several observations indicate that it is a wall-bound laccase. The enzyme polymerizes DHN (or its dimeric products) to melanin in cell walls. It also oxidizes a number of other substrates, including catechol and DOPA (280, 284) and 1-naphthol (Wheeler and Bell, unpublished) to cell wall-bounded polymers. Melanins formed from catechol, DOPA, or 1-naphthol in albinos of *V. dahliae* are ultrastructurally different from wild-type melanins. Catechol and DOPA melanins are deposited in the outer cell wall and on microfibrils, but cause only slight increases in the electron density of walls. These melanins do not occur in the form of granules like those in cell walls of the wild type or DHN-treated albinos. The melanin from 1-naphthol is purple and under the electron microscope has the appearance of circular bodies that differ from granules of the wild type.

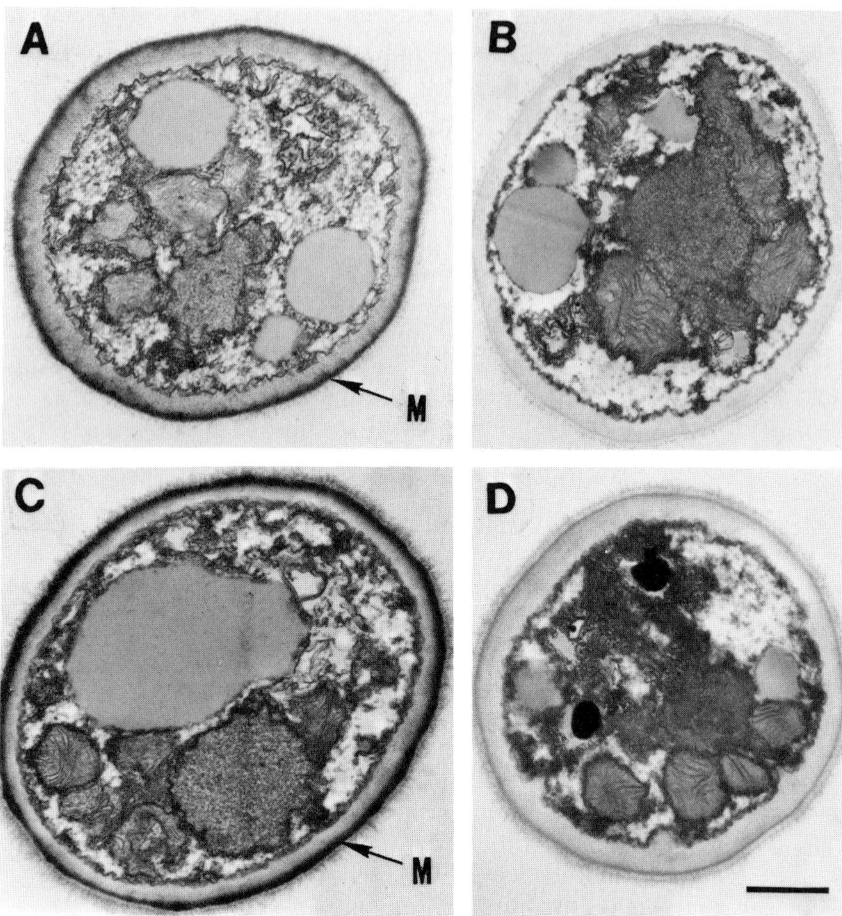

FIG. 10-5. (A-D) Electron micrographs comparing the cell walls of a wild-type isolate of *W. dermatitidis* and an albino (*mel-3*) and a brown (*mel-1*) mutant. The albino mutant (B) is hyaline but metabolizes scytalone to wall-bound DHN melanin (C) like that in the wild type (A). The brown mutant (D) makes scytalone but does not convert it to melanin. Bar = 0.5 μm (for all panels).

The biochemical and ultrastructural studies described in this section show that DHN melanin is common in species of the Ascomycotina and related Fungi Imperfecti. Thus, reports of other types of brown to black melanins in these fungi should be carefully evaluated. Reports of DOPA melanin in a number of imperfect and ascomycetous fungi; catechol melanin in *P. verrucosa* (211), and *V. albo-atrum* and *V. dahliae* (71, 85); and mixed melanins in *Cochlioboulus miyabeanus* (105, 106) and *Alternaria* sp. (202) should be reinvestigated because the same or similar species more recently have been shown to produce DHN melanin.

Melanin-Like Pigment in *Penicillium* and *Trichoderma* Species

Green pigments in conidia of *Penicillium* spp. and *Trichoderma* spp. have not been identified, but are reported to be polyphenolic in nature (11, 16, 19, 82). They are electron dense under the electron microscope and appear in the outer layer of the spore wall. The melanins in *T. viride* (19) and *P. cyclopium* (82) have been partially characterized. These melanins are believed to be nonindolic based on their nitrogen content (82) and negative reaction with Ehrlich's reagent (19).

We (MH Wheeler and AA Bell, unpublished) have found that the appearance of green melanins in *T. viride* and *T. harzianum* is not affected by tricyclazole or related melanin inhibitors. In contrast synthesis of the green pigments in various *Penicillium* species, for example, *P. italicum* and *P. digitatum*, is blocked by tricyclazole. The inhibitors prevent the development of normal green pigment and give the fungi a tan appearance. We have not observed the accumulation of flaviolin, 2-HJ, or other metabolites in the presence of the melanin inhibitors. Our results suggest that the pigment pathway in the genus *Penicillium* has some enzymes common to the DHN melanin pathway. If so, analogous intermediates are possibly produced in both pathways; some of these may be converted by reduction reactions similar to those that reduce 1,3,6,8-THN and 1,3,8-THN.

GDHB Melanin

The nitrogenous melanins in cell walls of basidiospores from *A. brunnescens* (as *A. bisporus* and *A. campestris*) (167) appear to be synthesized from γ-glutaminyl-4-hydroxybenzene (GHB) (209, 253) instead of tyrosine or DOPA. GHB is a product of the shikimic acid pathway (253) and is apparently oxidized sequentially to γ-glutaminyl-3,4-dihydroxybenzene (GDHB) and γ-glutaminyl-3,4-benzoquinone (GBQ) on the way to melanin (Fig. 10-6). Details of the enzymic oxidation of GHB to GBQ have been described by Boekelheide et al (25).

An alternate pathway to this melanin possibly involves 4-aminocatechol produced by the loss of the γ-glutamyl residue from GHB or GDHB (209). The mushroom fruiting body contains a γ-glutamyltransferase that has the ability to transfer the γ-glutamyl residue to a variety of acceptors. As indicated in Fig. 10-6, GHB melanin may be a mixed polymer from GDHB and 4-aminocatechol.

A granular melanin has been synthesized in vitro from GHB (87, 209, 253) using a crude commercial preparation of *A. brunnescens* (as *A. bisporus*) tyrosinase (with some peroxidase activity). It has ultrastructural and chemical properties that are almost identical to those of the granular melanin obtained

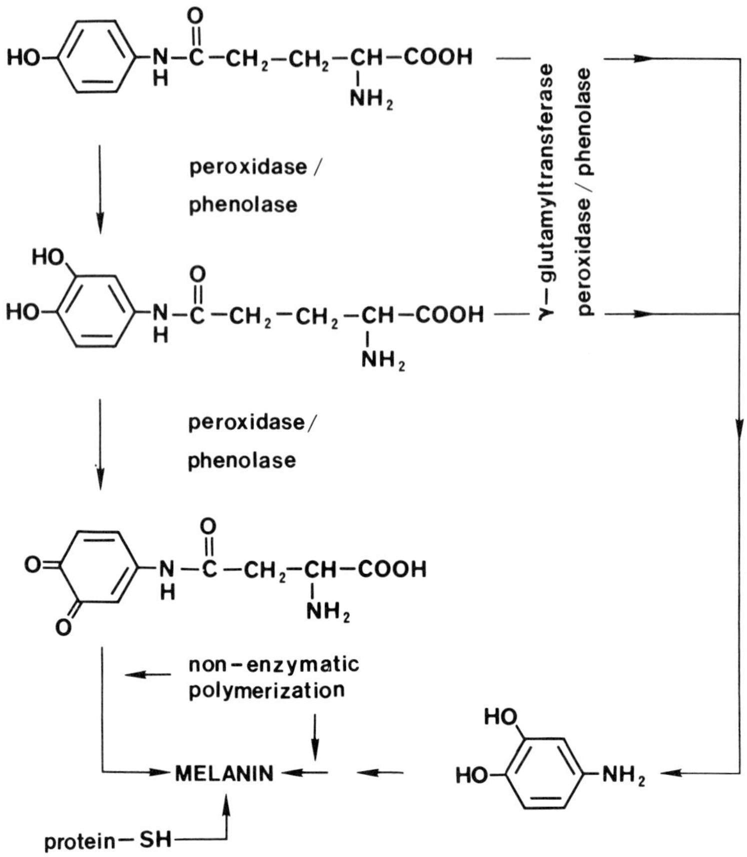

FIG. 10-6. Biosynthesis of γ-glutaminyl-3,4-dihydroxybenzene (GDHB) melanin from γ-glutaminyl-4-hydroxybenzene (209).

from the outer layer of basidiospore cell walls. The synthetic GHB melanin and *A. brunnescens* melanins have similar elemental composition (including nitrogen percentage), almost the same IR spectra, and identical solubility properties.

The above studies strongly suggest that GDHB melanin is the natural melanin in *A. brunnescens*. GHB and GDHB also occur in other mushroom species (269). Thus, these metabolites may be natural precursors to melanin in many other species of Basidiomycotina that produce tyrosinases as their major phenol oxidases. GHB occurs in the mycelium as well as the fruiting body, but GDHB is restricted to the reproductive hyphae, which form the melanized spores. Traces of GHB have been found in spores, but GDHB has not been found, presumably because it is oxidized to melanin (209, 253).

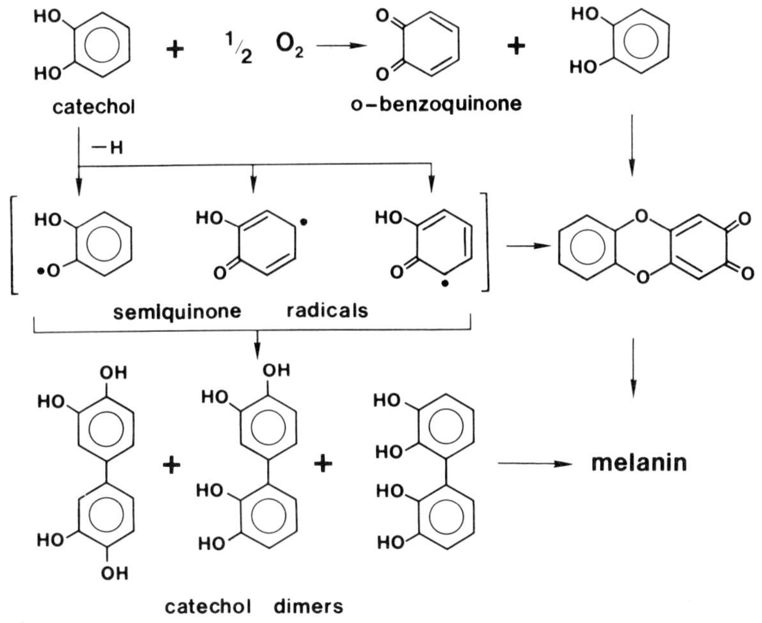

FIG. 10-7. Biosynthesis of catechol melanin from catechol (256).

Catechol Melanin

There is chemical evidence that the melanin deposited in cell walls of teliospores of *U. maydis* (207) is made from catechol. Ethanol extracts from the spores contain catechol, and degradation of melanin isolated from the spores gives products that could be derived from it (175, 176, 190, 191). The percentages of nitrogen, carbon, hydrogen, and carboxyl groups in melanin from *U. maydis* are nearly identical with those in catechol melanin formed by oxidation of catechol with mushroom tyrosinase. Also, reducing the natural melanin with sodium in pyridine or heating it at a high temperature in nitrogen yields small amounts of catechol; reduction at 200°C with palladium-carbon gives catechol and 3,3′4,4′-tetrahydroxybiphenyl (a dimer); and fusion with alkali produces catechol, 3,4-dihydroxybenzoic acid, and 2-hydroxybenzoic acid.

The biosynthesis of the catechol melanin polymer probably proceeds through free radicals or quinone-catechol adducts (Fig. 10-7). All of these dimeric products occur among the enzymic oxidation products of catechol (256). The degradation products obtained from *Ustilago* melanin indicate that both carbon-carbon and carbon-oxygen bonds occur in the natural melanin polymer. The biosynthetic origin of catechol is unknown, but the shikimic acid pathway is suspected. Likewise, the nature of the phenol oxidase in *U. maydis* spore walls has not been determined.

The report of catechol melanin in *U. maydis* led many investigators to look for this melanin in other fungi. The work was stimulated by the fact that purified fungal melanins often contain less nitrogen than DOPA melanins and produce catechol-related compounds, for example, protocatechuic acid, when subjected to alkali fusion and other degradative procedures. Also, the interest in catechol as a melanin substrate has been stimulated by its use as a substrate with enzymes associated with melanin production (35, 71, 211).

The presence of catechol melanin has been suggested in other fungi besides *U. maydis*, including *V. albo-atrum* and *V. dahliae* (71, 85), and *P. verrucosa* (211). The two *Verticillium* species and *P. verrucosa* are now known to produce DHN melanin, not catechol melanin, but *U. maydis* and other fungi such as *Blastocladiella emersonii*, that convert catechol to pigments (35), may produce catechol melanins. The basidiomycetous fungi rarely produce polyketide metabolites (268) and may use other metabolites such as catechol and GHB as melanin substrates.

Extracellular Melanins

Many studies have been carried out on heterogenous melanins that are extracellular in nature. We define extracellular melanins as melanins synthesized completely apart from cell walls. Melanin granules in the fibrillar matrix surrounding many cells are sometimes referred to as extracellular melanin (70, 137, 219). However, we prefer to call these wall-bound melanins because the fibrils are an extension of the wall. Thus, melanin granules broken off from fibrils into shake culture media should also be considered wall-bound melanin.

Extracellular melanins appear to be derived from two mechanisms: 1) secretion of phenol oxidases, that is, tyrosinase, laccase, or peroxidase into the external environment to oxidize phenolic compounds of various origins; and 2) secretion of phenols into the external environment, where they are autoxidized or are oxidized by enzymes later released from the fungus (often during autolysis). In shake cultures, extracellular melanin formed by autoxidation may adhere to the fungal wall (or matrix) surface, giving a false impression of wall-bound melanin (284).

Fungi or bacteria that secrete tyrosinase often cause dark discoloration of media containing hydrolyzed proteins such as peptone or casein hydrolysate. The discoloration can be accentuated by adding tyrosine to the medium (94, 187, 227). The production of such extracellular melanin has been observed frequently in bacteria, including actinomycetes, and fungi pathogenic to humans.

Adding appropriate substrates (eg, hydroquinone, *p*-phenylenediamine, 1-naphthol, or syringaldazine) to culture media allows detection of extracellular laccases or peroxidases. *Rhizoctonia* and many wood-rotting species of the Basidiomycotina secrete laccases that polymerize phenols in plant tissues degraded by the fungi (156). Secretion of peroxidase and hydrogen peroxide occurs only rarely in fungi (115).

Wood-rot fungi and fungi that decompose plant tissue use extracellular laccase and tyrosinase in combination with other enzymes both to decompose plant phenols and to oxidize the phenolic metabolites into new polymers (81, 150–152). Plant phenols that are oxidized into black pigments (melanins) include catechol, DOPA, dopamine, tannic acid, gallic acid, and quinol (*p*-dihydroxybenzene) (267). The plant phenols catechin, chlorogenic acid, and caffeic acid are oxidized to dark brown pigments. The catecholamines (eg, epinephrine and norepinephrine) from animals are also oxidized to melanins (148, 267). In addition, breakdown products of some pesticides are converted to dark pigments by extracellular phenol oxidases: examples are 1-naphthol from the insecticide Carbaryl (243) and chlorinated catechol derivatives from the herbicide 2,4-D (251).

Some fungi, normally saprophytes, accumulate large amounts of dark brown pigments in the culture medium These pigments may be entirely distinct from the wall-bound melanins, because albino mutants of *C. protuberata*, *B sorokiniana*, *P. infectoria*, and *Ulocladium* sp. that are devoid of wall-bound melanins still form the extracellular brown pigments (AA Bell and MH Wheeler, unpublished data). Similar brown pigments have been referred to both as melanins and as "fungal humic acids" (83, 149, 226). They have solubility properties similar to humic acid extracted from soil with dilute alkali. These pigments are complex in structure, being derived from various phenols, amino acids, proteins, carbohydrates, and lipids (139, 150, 222, 226). Synthesis of these melanins requires secretion of phenols into the medium, and melanization is usually triggered by alkaline conditions, which cause autoxidation of phenols and complexing of oxidation products with other phenols and compounds such as proteins. Secretion of phenols by fungi may not discolor media for a few weeks, but after several months the medium around certain fungi becomes darkly pigmented, especially at pH levels above 7. In some cases, delayed release of a polyphenoloxidase (PPO), possibly from autolysing hyphae, may be involved in synthesis of heterogeneous melanins (218).

Fungi that form considerable amounts of extracellular melanins from secreted phenols include *A. glaucus* group (140), *A. nidulans* (37, 218), *E. nigrum* (83, 149). *Eurotium echinulatum* (221), *Hendersonula toruloidea* (153), *Stachybotrys atra* (149), and *S. chartarum* (149). These fungi accumulate a large number of phenols derived from tetraketides in culture media. *Aspergillus glaucus* group and *E. echinulatum* also accumulate anthraquinones derived from octaketides; these are also incorporated into the autoxidized polymer (140, 221). Enzyme-catalyzed polymers of these phenols have been prepared by reaction with commercial peroxidase (140). Polyphenoloxidases that may cause similar oxidation have been found in some fungi that produce extracellular melanin (83, 153). As much as 10–30% of the biomass synthesized by certain fungi is extracellular heterogenous melanin, which is considered an important source of soil humus (138–140, 221). This type of melanin may also be obtained by extracting the fungal cells with dilute NaOH (149, 218). Thus part of autoxidized melanin is apparently encrusted onto the mycelium. Many species of *Aspergillus*, *Penicillium*, and related genera other than those studied also synthesize polyphenols from polyketides, secrete appreciable amounts of the phenols into the media (269), and probably form heterogeneous melanins. Heterogeneous melanins, likewise, are formed in media by many actinomycetes (299).

Melanins of *Cryptococcus neoformans*

Cryptococcus neoformans is the anamorphic yeast stage of the basidiomycete *Filobasidiella neoformans* (127). It is a human pathogen that causes chronic, subacute or, less often, acute pulmonary, systemic, or meningeal infection in humans and other animals. Opportunistic infection by the fungus often arises as a complication of other diseases in debilitated patients and may become rapidly systemic. The fungus has a high predilection for infecting the central nervous system, and infection of the brain and related tissue is the most frequently diagnosed form of the disease.

Colonies of *C. neoformans* are lightly pigmented (cream to brown in color) on Sabouraud glucose agar. However, the fungus oxidizes a large number of exogenous compounds, including *o*- and *p*-diphenols (40, 54, 205, 232); aminophenols and diaminobenzene compounds (41); indoles (130); catecholamines (193); and tryptophan and anthranilic acid (42) to melanins and pigments of various colors. The melanins are generally described as intracellular or extracellular and have been found in cell walls (128, 178, 232). The ability to form melanin has been used to differentiate *C. neoformans* from similar appearing fungi (40, 96, 160, 232). The ability to produce melanin reportedly enhances virulence (128, 193, 213), thus playing a role in disease.

Staib (247) first discovered that colonies of *C. neoformans* become distinctively brown when grown on agar medium containing a hot water extract of *Guizotia abyssinica* seed (nigerseed). This medium and subsequent media and tests developed from it have been used for selective isolation and identification of *C. neoformans*. Most of the differential media and tests use nigerseed extract (185, 247), caffeic acid (3,4-dihydroxycinnamic acid) (65, 86, 95, 96, 112, 132, 160), or DOPA (39, 112, 185). Occasionally, other members of the genus *Cryptococcus*, that is, *C albidus*, *C. laurentii*, *C. luteolus*, and *C. terreus*, may make pigments (160, 275), but this generally occurs after a prolonged incubation time of 10 or more days. Final identification should include morphologic examination and biochemical tests.

Strachen et al (252) isolated caffeic acid from nigerseed and observed that it and a number of other *o*-diphenols are metabolized to brown pigment in *C. neoformans*. Tyrosine and nine other phenolic compounds did not induce coloration. They concluded that the coloration was dependent on the hydroxyl groups in the 3,4 position of the phenyl ring. Pulverer and Korth (205) reported that *C. neoformans* produces pigments not only from *o*-diphenols (ie, DOPA or caffeic acid) or *o*-triphenols, but also from *p*-diphenols. Only one of three *m*-diphenols tested was metabolized to a melanin pigment, and its conversion occurred only in the presence of iron. They also discovered that iron generally enhances pigment production with other diphenols. As a result, ferric citrate has since been used in many caffeic acid and DOPA tests for the identification of *C. neoformans* (86, 96, 112, 185).

Chaskes and Tyndall (40) found that *o*- and *p*-diphenols often produce intracellular pigments that are insoluble in common organic solvents. More strains of *C. neoformans* produced intracellular pigments with *o*-diphenols as substrates, than with *p*-diphenols. Extracellular pigments also were often made from *p*-diphenols by *C. neoformans*. These pigments are water soluble and diffuse into the surrounding medium. Although other *Cryptococcus* species are able to use hydroquinone as a substrate, pigment formation from *o*- and *p*-diphenols occurs almost exclusively with *C. neoformans*.

Melanin production from aminophenols and diaminobenzenes in *C. neoformans* appears similar to that from diphenols (41). There are obvious structural similarities of the three types of substrates, and intracellular pigments made from any of them are difficult to extract. In contrast to most diphenols, the aminophenols and diaminobenzenes are not highly specific as substrates for *C. neoformans* and are converted to melanin pigments by other *Cryptococcus* and *Candida* species.

Indoles with a hydroxyl or an amino group on the phenyl ring also serve as melanin precursors for *C. neoformans* (130). This shows that PPO activity in *C. neoformans* is not entirely limited to substrates with two reactive moieties on the same phenyl ring as suggested with other substrates. Indoles with methoxy, nitro, methyl, and fluorine substituents on the phenyl ring or a hydroxyl group at the 2 position are not precursors.

Only limited studies have been carried out on PPO from *C. neoformans*. Shaw and Kapica (232) showed that *o*-diphenols are converted to pigments by an $(NH_4)_2SO_4$ fraction from cell-free extracts of *C. neoformans*. The pigments are also produced by cultures and whole cells. The "phenoloxidase" was not further purified and could have contained a number of enzymes with oxidative activity. Unlike plant and mushroom tyrosinase that use tyrosine and other monophenols, the "phenoloxidase" preparations from *C. neoformans* only oxidized diphenolic compounds. Thus, tyrosine is not a substrate for the enzyme. The "phenoloxidase" activity is inhibited by the copper chelators phenylthiourea and diethyldithiocarbamate, but is not affected by catalase. This indicates that the enzymatic preparation does not contain peroxidative activity and is similar to catecholase or laccase preparations from other fungi and plants (156).

Polacheck et al (193) cautioned that the extracts used by Shaw and Kapica (232) were obtained by low-speed centrifugation and may have contained membraneous debris. They (193) discovered PPO activity associated with membranes of protoplasts and with a soluble fraction obtained from membranes by digitonin treatment. The PPO did not appear to be bound to cell walls, because the protoplasts were liberated through a localized opening rather than by complete digestion of the wall. Copper chelators did not inhibit the PPO preparations, but iron-chelating agents, such as hydroximide derivatives or 8-hydroxyquinoline, were effective inhibitors. This was in contrast to the findings of Shaw and Kapica (232), and suggests that the PPO in *C. neoformans* might be an iron rather than a copper containing enzyme. The two reports on PPO in *C. neoformans* dealt with crude preparations and did not adequately describe the enzyme(s), substrates, and cofactors associated with pigment production. For a better understanding of melanin synthesis in *C. neoformans*, the PPO enzymes need to be purified and tested with the various substrates and metal chelating agents.

Certain substrates are converted to melanins that appear in the cell walls of *C. neoformans*. Nurudeen and Ahearn (178), using light microscopy, found that cell walls of the fungus contained melanin pigments after treatment with DOPA and three aminophenols and diaminobenzenes. Similar results were obtained by Kwon-Chung et al (128), who concluded that cells of *C. neoformans*, grown on media containing DOPA, manifest the pigment in part of the cell wall and not in the cytoplasm. Electron micrographs of cells incubated in DOPA show deposition of melanin in the cell wall (128, 232). This suggests that some of the PPO in *C. neoformans* is wall bound. PPO enzymes apparently exist in the cell walls of a large number of other fungi that normally produce wall-bound melanins. Thus, albino mutants of *Phaeococcomyces* sp. (32), *T. basicola* (280), *V. dahliae* (267, 284, 285), *W. dermatitidis* (281), and a number of other normally dark brown to black fungi are able to convert phenolic substrates to wall-bound melanins (283).

Melanins produced by PPO may protect *C. neoformans* in the host. Mutants that lack the ability to produce melanins from *o*-diphenolic compounds, that is, catecholamines, have decreased virulence and lack PPO activity (129, 193, 213). Revertants to wild-type characteristics regain the ability to produce PPO activity, melanins, and disease. These relationship will be discussed in the next section.

Pathogenicity and Virulence in Humans and Animals

Mutant strains of *C. neoformans*, that lacked PPO activity and the ability to produce melanin from various diphenols, had a diminished capacity for colonizing organs, that is, brain, liver, or spleen, when injected into mice (128, 129, 213). Revertant strains with wild-type characteristics were obtained from mice inoculated with PPO-deficient mutants. The revertants were virulent when injected into other mice, had higher levels of PPO activity than their related PPO-deficient mutants, and produced melanin in agar medium containing DOPA, nigerseed extract, or catecholamines (129, 213). The mice inoculated with the revertants died at about the same time as mice infected with wild-type strains. This showed that revertants were similar to wild types in pathogenicity, and the ability to make melanin was constantly associated with virulence.

Cryptococcus neoformans produces a thick capsular sheath (2). Heavily encapsulated strains of the fungus resist phagocytosis by neutrophils and macrophages, and the capsule is believed to play an important role in the pathogenicity of the fungus in humans and animals (68, 101). Capsule formation (129) and temperature (128) independently affected virulence in studies dealing with PPO in *C. neoformans*. Strains with PPO activity had to grow at 37°C on agar medium and produce capsular material to be highly virulent. Strains having capsular material but no PPO activity also were much less virulent than those with capsular material and PPO activity (129). Thus, both the production of the polysaccharide capsule and PPO were essential factors for virulence in *C. neoformans*.

The previous studies of *C. neoformans* involved only two different wild types, mutant strains derived from them, and progeny from backcrosses between the mutants and wild types. The wild types (a- and α- mating types) are closely related and derived from a cross between two isolates derived from the type of *Filobasidiella neoformans*, the teleomorphic state for *C. neoformans* (212). Kwon-Chung and Rhodes (129) also described finding "rare isolates" from clinical specimens that produced encapsulated cells but failed to form melanin on either nigerseed or dopamine agar. These isolates lacked PPO activity but were virulent in mice. Thus, additional studies of other wild-type isolates of *C. neoformans* are needed to determine the extent of the relationship between PPO activity and virulence.

The leprosy bacterium, *Mycobacterium leprae*, also produces a PPO that may be important in virulence (196, 197, 198, 199). The purified bacillus and preparations of its PPO convert a wide range of phenolic compounds to quinones and melanins but show no PPO activity with monophenols, that is, L-tyrosine (199). Compounds that bind copper are good inhibitors of the enzyme in vitro, and diethyldithiocarbamate completely suppresses PPO activity at concentrations as low as 0.5 mM (197). A number of compounds that inhibit PPO suppress multiplication of *M. leprae* in mice (198).

The PPO of *M. leprae* is consistently found and remains unaltered through repeated passages of the bacterium in mice and armadillos (196). The enzyme has not been detected in other mycobacteria, including *M. lepraemurium* separated from mouse tissues or cultivable mycobacteria derived from tissues of feral armadillos (196, 201). For this reason DOPA oxidation is now being widely used as a rapid identification of the bacterium (196, 200).

M. leprae multiplies in sites in the human body such as the skin, eye, leptomeninges, peripheral nerves, mucosal membranes, and endothelium of blood vessels where metabolism of DOPA or catecholamines is important

(196, 198, 199). Also, hypopigmentation of skin lesions is a characteristic feature of leprosy. Prabhakaran et al (199) reported that the bacillic occur at the spreading outer margins of lesions that become hypopigmented, whereas the healing middle regions often regain pigment. They also showed that suspensions of the bacilli suppressed normal pigment formation in cultures of melanocytes, whereas heat-killed bacilli did not prevent the development of normal pigment. Thus, use of DOPA and catecholamines by *M. leprae* may account for its affinity for certain tissues and for the loss of normal pigmentation in skin lesions of leprosy.

Polacheck et al (193) did not work with *M. leprae* but have summarized the similarities and differences of PPO from *C. neoformans* and *M. leprae* and suggested that the enzymes are different. They reported that *Cryptococcus* PPO is distinct from the bacterial enzyme in several respects. First, *M. leprae* appears to oxidize DOPA only to indole-5,6-quinone, whereas the enzyme of *C. neoformans* follows the conventional DOPA melanin pathway, yielding dopachrome (Fig. 10-1). It has been proposed that the PPO in *M. leprae* may be associated with a decarboxylase that allows the direct conversion of DOPA to indole-5,6-quinone (198). Second, the enzyme from *C. neoformans* is completely inhibited by mimosine and cyanide which do not affect the bacterial enzyme; in fact, mimosine, a substrate analogue of DOPA, is a substrate rather than an inhibitor for the *M. leprae* enzyme (197). Finally, copper-binding compounds are ineffective inhibitors for PPO from *C. neoformans.* On the other hand, Polacheck et al (193) emphasized that the enzymes are similar in several respects. They are membrane bound, use the same range of substrates, and are neurotropic.

The ability to produce melanin has been associated with human infections caused by *Basidiobolus* spp. Cutler and Swatek (49) reported that nine of 29 isolates of *Basidiobolus* spp. produced a black pigment when grown on agar or broth media, containing only L-tyrosine as a carbon source. The nine isolates were obtained from humans and the other 20 isolates were from nonhuman sources. For some reason the human isolates were lumped together and not given species names, whereas the nonhuman isolates were divided into five groups and classified according to species. The ability to produce pigment was a stable characteristic of the nine human isolates; it was not affected by multiple transfers on nutrient media or passages through the gut of toads and frogs, which are asymptomatic carriers of *Basidiobolus* spp. Cutler and Swatek (49) did not attempt to characterize the pigment and were unable to reproduce the disease in mice with the human isolates. Since this work was published in 1969, there apparently have been no follow-up reports on melanins or melanin-like pigments produced by species of *Basidiobolus*.

Melanin production also has been associated with elevated enterotoxin prodution by the pathogenic bacterium *Vibrio cholerae* (107, 108). A mutant, *Htx-3*, obtained from a wild type of the bacterium produced elevated levels of enterotoxins and made a dark brown melanin not produced by the wild type (107). Ivins and Holmes (108) used labeling studies to show that L-tyrosine and L-cysteine stimulated production of this melanin when incorporated in the media, and were retained as part of the "phaeomelanin" after partial purification. They cautioned that the tyrosinase in the mutant has not been shown to convert DOPA to dopaquinone and may only convert tyrosine to DOPA which can be autoxidized to melanin.

Ivins and Holmes (107) also looked at 28 other mutants derived from wild-type *V. cholerae*, and concluded that the induction of mutations regulating melanin formation were correlated with mutations affecting enterotoxin production as well as other phenotypic traits. However, their studies did not show a consistent pattern between the ability to produce melanin and other traits, that is, enterotoxin production, motility, or growth on a minimal medium; in many cases, melanin-producing mutants made far less enterotoxin than the nonmelanin-producing wild type from which they were derived. This was true even on the medium originally used to describe *Htx-3* as a hypervirulent mutant of the wild type. Also, *Htx-3* produced less enterotoxin on various media than the wild type, although the mutant was still able to produce melanin. In strain *Htx-3*, the genes responsible for hypertoxinogenicity and for pigment production are distinct and occur at different loci (165). The results with the other mutant strains suggest the strains probably contain multiple gene mutations.

Extracellular melanin production by *Madurella mycetomatis*, a causative agent of black grain mycetoma in humans, has been studied chemically and ultrastructurally (59, 60). The diffusible pigment appears to combine with host proteins and tissue debris to form dark colored grains 0.5–1 mm in diameter. The fungus within the grain is apparently sheltered to some extent. Drugs and antibodies of large molecular weight are quite possibly kept out of reach by the grain, because the disease is difficult to treat with antimycotic agents (59). Successful treatment of the disease might require inhibition of pigment production or low molecular weight fungicides. At the present time amputation is often the final action in treatment if ketoconazole is ineffective.

M. mycetomatis also produces gray and brownish melanin pigments associated with the hyphae on agar media (214); it and certain other fungi causing mycetoma, that is, *Madurella grisea* and *Pseudallescheria boydii*, might produce DHN melanin. *Exophiala jeanselmei* occasionally is found as the cause of black grain mycetoma (214). It produces an extracellular melanin that has been described as similar (but not identical) to that extracted from cell walls (67). Synthesis of the wall-bound melanin is inhibited by tricyclazole in culture causing the accumulation of flaviolin and 2-HJ. Thus, the melanin appears to be made from DHN (259). The effect of tricyclazole on the extracellular melanin has not been studied. This melanin is of particular interest because it appears to be of low molecular weight and apparently anchors to extracellular proteins (67). In this respect the extracellular melanin appears to be similar to that from *M. mycetomatis* and might help form the cement in typical black grains.

The role of melanin in diseases caused by heavily pigmented fungi is not known. However, many pathogenic fungi produce DHN melanin and are affected by tricyclazole and other compounds that inhibit normal pigmentation (Fig. 10-4). Phaeohyphomycosis (160, 214) is a clinical entity that includes various invasive infectious processes for which the etiologic agent is a brown pigmented, dematiaceous fungus in culture and the form found in tissue consists of melanized mycelial or yeastlike cells (158a). These characteristics separate phaeohyphomycosis from other types of disease involving brown pigmented fungi, in which the tissue morphology is a grain as previously discussed (mycetoma) or a sclerotic body (chromoblastomycosis). In some cases a fungus can cause more than one of these disease entities at the same time.

Certain fungi, for example, *W. dermatitidis* (50b, 154a) and *X. bantiana* (160a), occasionally cause phaeohyphomycosis in brain and other tissues. Phaeohyphomycosis is also caused by other fungi known to produce DHN melanin, that is, *Alternaria alternata* (57), the *Alternaria* anamorph of *Pleospora infectoria* (72), *Aureobasidium pullulans* (222a, 273), and *E. jeanselmei* (158a). According to McGinnis (160) *P. infectoria* is a questionable agent of the disease and should have been better documented. The phaeohyphomycotic agents have been reviewed by Rippon (214) and include a number of other dematiaceous fungi including *Dactylaria constricta* (50c) and species of *Bipolaris* (69, 159, 161a), *Curvularia* (113, 131, 217), *Exophiala* (162, 214), *Exserohilum* (1, 161a), *Phialophora* (170, 296), *Phoma* (79, 297), and possibly fungi originally identified as *Helminthosporium* (84, 119, 159). Fungi in these or closely related genera produce DHN melanin (Table 10-1). The fungi causing phaeohyphomycotic infections are opportunistic and less likely to infect humans than the primary pathogens, for example, *Histoplasma capsulatum* or *Coccidioides immitis*. They are widespread in nature and capable of multiplying in animal tissues at typical body temperatures, but usually undergo little change in morphology from their saprophytic form when grown in animals. They generally are not serious pathogens unless they infect hosts that are diseased or debilitated in some way.

Hendersonula toruloidea and *Scytalidium hyalinum* are also fungi that can cause human infections. They occasionally attack skin and nails and are considered weak pathogens (34, 75, 145, 160). *H. toruloidea* may cause a dermatophyte-like disease in patients living in tropical regions (214). It produces DHN melanin in cell walls (Table 10-1) and makes extracellular humic acid-like polymers in various media (138, 153). *Scytalidium* is a synanamorph associated with *Hendersonula* (160, 214), and was the first genus from which the DHN melanin precursor scytalone was isolated.

DHN melanin has been demonstrated (259, 282) in *P. verrucosa* and a number of other fungi that cause chromoblastomycosis and related dermal disease in humans. Geis and Szaniszlo (73) have reported that the melanin and carotenoids in *W. dermatitidis* have a "shielding effect" against UV irradiation and may confer resistance to photo-induced damage. They also found that the sclerotic form of *W. dermatitidis* has five times more melanin in its cell wall than does the yeast form (257). Thus, the heavily melanized wall in *W. dermatitidis* and related chromoblastomycotic fungi may be protecting the fungi from host defense mechanisms.

Wild-type *W. dermatitidis* and a melanin-deficient albino strain derived from it have been compared for pathogenic and virulent effects in albino mice following intravenous infection (50b). Parameters examined were mouse survival, signs of infection of the central nervous system, and time of appearance of the fungus in various organs (including the brain). Over a range of concentrations the wild type produced 100% mortality, whereas the albino strain produced no mortality by 21 days after inoculation. In chronic infections with the albino, mice developed ataxia and torticollis. These signs of disease were indistinguishable from those produced by low concentrations of the wild type. Histologic responses to the two strains appeared to be indistinguishable in host tissues. However, the mutant did not form the invasive hyphal forms of growth that were associated with the acute, fatal infections caused by the wild type. Although the absence of melanin was associated with decreased mortality in mice, the chronic neurologic signs of mouse phaeohyphomycosis were unrelated to melanin.

Additional experiments are need to confirm whether melanin-deficient mutants or melanin inhibitors change the pathogenicity of *W. dermatitidis* and other fungi in animals. For example, studies should be carried out with the albino strain of *W. dermatitidis* treated with scytalone and the wild type treated with tricyclazole or cerulenin. The melanized albino will not produce melanized cells in tissues, but it might stand a better chance of overcoming host defense mechanisms than the unmelanized albino. Conversely, the tricyclazole- or cerulenin-treated wild type might be less pathogenic than normal due to the loss of melanin.

The fungi causing phaeohyphomycosis and chromoblastomycosis are resistant to most antimycotic drugs, including amphotericin B and the imidazoles (48, 214, 274, 298). This does not necessarily mean that DHN melanin has a protective effect against antimicrobics, but most unmelanized pathogens are more susceptible to the drugs. The combined effects of melanin inhibitors, that is, tricyclazole or pyroquilon (Fig. 10-4), with antibiotics should be tested in vitro and in vivo to see if the efficiency of amphotericin B and other antimycotic drugs can be improved. Presently, the most success with antimycotic drugs against fungi causing chromoblastomycosis and phaeohyphomycosis is achieved with 5-fluorocytosine by itself or in combination with other drugs such as amphotericin B or ketoconazole (48, 50a, 214).

The dermatophytes (*Trichophyton* spp., *Microsporum* spp., and *Epidermophyton floccosum*) produce a variety of colored pigments, many of which are used for identification of the fungi on Sabouraud glucose agar and other media (17, 160, 214). A few of the pigments have been partially characterized (93, 169, 309). The genetics of pigmentation in *Arthroderma benhamiae*, the teleomorph of *T. mentagrophytes*, also has been studied and reviewed (78, 98).

In general, however, little has been learned about the pigments, including their biochemical origin, chemical structures, or functions. *T. rubrum*, a common and widely distributed dermatophyte in humans, produces an intense, non-diffusing red pigment in agar media. The color of media may be yellow at first, turning green, and finally becoming red. Zussman et al (309) found that several water-insoluble pigments are formed by *T. rubrum*, differing in quantities at different times. Because ^{14}C-labeled tyrosine is incorporated into the pigments, they suggested that the pigments were made from this substrate. However, the pigments in their studies were not highly purified and contained low levels (approximately 4%) of nitrogen. Thus, their preparation might have included a nonnitrogenous pigment chromophore complexed with protein.

Diffusible brown to black melanin-like pigments exude into culture media of various dermatophytes, that is, *E. floccosum*, *T. mentagrophytes*, and *T. rubrum* (93, 227, 228). Schonborn (227) reported that, although only a small percentage of strains representative of each species produce these pigments, the "melanoid" strains retain their ability to produce the pigments at fairly constant concentrations. The amount of pigment produced depends on the particular strain and the type of nutrient media used in the studies. Tyrosine and phenylalanine, when incorporated into media, stimulate pigment production, suggesting that the pigment is a DOPA melanin. The strongest pigment producers are among the strains of *T. rubrum*, and all strains of *T. verrucosum* are devoid of melanin-producing capacity. Strains of *T. rubrum* that produce the brown to black pigments on tyrosine-ammended media also produce the reddish pigment characteristic of *T. rubrum* of cornmeal-glucose agar. Schonborn (227) suggested that the reddish and brown to black pigments might be biosynthesized from a common pathway, but was unable to isolate a PPO responsible for melanin formation, and offered no enzymic proof for his suggestion.

Strains of *T. rubrum* that produce dark brown to black pigments are often called *T. rubrum* var. *nigricans*. The other characteristics of these strains are the same as typical isolates of *T. rubrum* (93, 214). Schonborn and Schuhmann (228) reported antimicrobic activity of the brown to black pigments from *T. rubrum* against *T. mentagrophytes* and *Staphylococcus aureus*, and mentioned the pigments do not prevent normal growth of *Candida albicans*, *Escherichia coli*, and *Microsporum gypseum*. They spread the test organisms over media on which *T. rubrum* had been grown and did not isolate the inhibiting compounds. Although the inhibitory activity appeared to be proportional to the amount of melanin produced, other compounds with antibiotic activity might have been present to cause the inhibition.

Different colored strains of other human pathogens apparently exist in nature. McGinnis et al (161) for example reported an "albino variant" of *A. fumigatus* var. *ellipticus* as the cause of an unusual case of paranasal aspergilloma. The original culture of this fungus used for comparison was lily green in color and was isolated from a case of chronic emphysema (208).

Terreni et al (265) obtained several red pigmented isolates of *Histoplasma capsulatum* from a canebrake which served as a blackbird roost. Typically the fungus is tan in color. The unnatural looking isolates of *A. fumigatus var. ellipticus* and *H. capsulatum* are possibly mutant strains that were able to survive in nature. The red pigmented isolate of *H. capsulatum* should be tested for flaviolin or 2-HJ production, because tan isolates of the fungus may produce DHN melanin.

Pathogenicity and Virulence in Plants

Studies with inhibitors of melanin synthesis and melanin-deficient strains have shown that DHN melanin is required for penetration of rice, cucumber, and bean by appressoria of *Pyricularia oryzae*, *Colletotrichum lagenarium*, and *C. lindemuthianium*, respectively. The melanin inhibitor tricyclazole (Fig. 10-4), at concentrations that inhibit melanization, but not mycelial growth, conidial germination, and appressorial formation, prevents penetration of host epidermis by all three species (31a, 104, 121, 123, 155, 179, 180, 241, 242, 287, 290, 291, 293). The same concentrations of tricyclazole also inhibit penetration of *Bryophyllum pinnatum* epidermal cell walls and Formvar polyvinyl plastic membranes by *P. oryzae* (291) and *C. lindemuthianium* (242, 287) as well as penetration of cellulose, cellophane, or nitrocellulose membranes by *P. oryzae* (5, 180) and *C. lagenarium* (121).

Cerulenin (Fig. 10-4), an inhibitor of fatty acid and polyketide biosynthesis (184), also inhibits DHN melanin synthesis in *P. oryzae* (45). It acts at an earlier site in the melanin pathway than tricyclazole (Fig. 10-2) and prevents the formation of cyclized intermediates of the melanin pathway in appressoria of wild types. It causes the formation of hyaline appressoria that are unable to penetrate epidermal walls. Melanized appressoria of untreated wild types penetrate walls directly to gain access to host tissue.

Adding vermelone or DHN, both of which occur beyond the tricyclazole and cerulenin blocks in melanin synthesis, restores melanization of appressoria of the *Pyricularia* and *Colletotrichum* species. This allows penetration of synthetic membranes and epidermis of *B. pinnatum* and onion (45, 123, 180, 242, 294). Scytalone, which occurs before the tricyclazole block in melanin synthesis, restores melanization and pentration with cerulenin as an inhibitor (45) but not with tricyclazole (123, 180). The restoration of penetration by vermelone and DHN in the presence of tricyclazole is only partial, probably because these compounds are fungitoxic at concentrations above 0.1 mM (294). DOPA, which is nontoxic at low concentrations, also forms a melanin in tricyclazole-inhibited appressoria of *P. oryzae* and restores penetration (180), even though it is not a natural melanin intermediate in this fungus. Wounding host plants or applying tricyclazole after penetration allows normal disease development (121, 291). Similar results have been obtained with eight other chemicals (Fig. 10-4) that selectively inhibit melanin synthesis at the same enzymic sites as tricyclazole (5, 104, 123, 287, 289, 292–294).

Studies with mutants confirm the critical need for melanization in the development of penetration pegs from appressoria. Buff (reductase-deficient) mutations of *P. oryzae* (180, 241, 290, 291) and albino mutations of *C. lagenarium* (121, 122, 255) and *P. oryzae* (45) prevent penetration of host plants, epidermal strips, or cellulose membranes. On cucumber cotyledons and nitrocellulose membranes, *C. lagenarium* albino appressoria germinate laterally to form secondary appressoria but do not penetrate these membranes (122, 255). Wounding allows infection of rice by the buff mutants, indicating that penetration is the major pathogenic character affected by the mutation (291). DOPA and DHN partially restore melanization and penetration of cellulose membranes by the buff mutant of *P. oryzae* (180, 290), and DOPA and scytalone restore melanization and penetration of cucumber cell walls and cellulose membranes by the albino mutant of *C. lagenarium* (120, 122, 123). Scytalone and DHN restore melanization and penetration of onion epidermal strips by the ablino, *CP-412*, of *P. oryzae* (45) and an albino, *AL-3*, of a similar pathogen, *Pyricularia grisea* (31a). These behavioral patterns are similar to those of tricyclazole-treated appressoria (31a, 123).

Melanized appressoria of *P. oryzae* are impermeable to sucrose and various solutes, whereas nonmelanized appressoria are freely permeable (291). Melanized appressoria are also conical and have only a relatively small nonmelanized pore centered against the cuticle, whereas albino or tricyclazole-treated appressoria have a large, flat basal area with no focus on the cuticle (287, 291). Therefore, normal melanization appears to give both the necessary rigidity to appressoria and the direction for penetration-peg development.

The melanin shunt-product 2-HJ (Fig. 10-2) accumulates after tricyclazole treatment and is toxic to protoplasts of *P. oryzae* (293, 295). Consequently, 2-HJ has been suggested as a cause of aborted penetration. However, several observations are not in agreement with this suggestion. In the normal sequence of shunt reactions (Fig. 10-2), 2-HJ is converted at least partially to 3,4,8-THT and other nontoxic metabolites, preventing accumulation of high concentrations of 2-HJ (249, 266, 290). More importantly, albino mutants of *P. oryzae* (45) and *C. lagenarium* (122, 255) and the cerulenin-treated wild type of *P. oryzae* (45) do not synthesize 2-HJ and still completely lack the ability to penetrate host epidermis. Thus, inhibition of melanization appears to be the primary, if not the only, reason for the antipenetrant action of the melanin inhibitors.

Shunt products from DHN melanins also have been reported to have phytotoxic activity that may contribute to pathogenicity. Alteichin, a phytotoxin from *Alternaria eichhorniae* (216), has a structure that resembles the DHN 1,1′-dimer (Fig. 10-3). The synthesis of this toxin is blocked by tricyclazole (MH Wheeler and RC Beier, unpublished), indicating that it is derived from 1,3,6,8-THN. The phytotoxin cercosporin and the closely related compounds isocercosporin, phleichrome, and isophleichrome have the dihydroxyperylene quinone nucleus as well, but they contain six additional carbons (6, 8), indicating that they are formed from heptaketide rather than from pentaketide pathways (269).

A phytotoxin isolated from *V. dahliae* has been identified as a peptide conjugate of flaviolin (261). Production of this toxin (PKZh-1) in culture was correlated with virulence among six isolates of *V. dahliae* (264). The shunt-product 4,8-DHT (Fig. 10-2) and related tetralones inhibit rice-root elongation at 500 μg/ml but stimulate root and shoot growth at lower concentrations (109, 110). More detailed studies using melanin-deficient mutants or melanin inhibitors are needed to evaluate the importance of these phytotoxins in disease development.

Pure melanins and melanoproteins also have been implicated in disease. A purified melanin from *Stachybotrys alternans* shows allelopathic action against root growth of wheat, rye, and cress (230). However, its mode of action is unclear. Likewise, a melanoprotein from *Venturia inaequalis* increases lesion number and size when added to inoculated leaves (90, 91). However, two low-virulent mutants contain comparatively large amounts of melanin (92). Therefore, the importance of melanin in the melanoprotein is unclear.

Resistance to Environmental and Microbial Stresses

Although fungal melanins and related pigments function in a variety of ways in diseases of animals and plants, they are probably most important for protecting fungi against environmental and microbial stresses. A high proportion of melanin-producing microorganisms has been associated with environmentally stressed areas such as the desert (53), the alpine regions (171), and the upper biosphere (102). Melanins also contribute residual materials, that is, humic acids, to soils.

Fungi with melanized conidia are more resistant to killing by UV light (53, 271, 301) or solar radiation (307) than those with hyaline conidia. The degree of protection is proportional to the melanin concentration in conidial walls (53, 304, 307). Repressing melanin synthesis by adding hexachloroacetone to cultures increases killing of fungal cells by UV light (53). Similarly, the resistance of melanized conidia to γ irradiation (171, 272, 301) and x-rays (142) is greater than that of hyaline conidia, and the degree of protection is directly proportional to melanin concentrations, as measured by ESR (272, 305). Damage by UV light and γ irradiation is increased in melanin-deficient mutants (305); conversely, it is decreased by suspending various conidia in melanin suspensions prepared from fungal cell walls (236, 306). The effects of melanins on fungal resistance to desiccation and high temperatures have received little attention. However, Zhdanova et al (302) have reported that the thermostability of *Cladosporium transchelii*, *Humicola lanuginosa*, *Stemphylium ilicis*, and three melanin-altered mutants of *C. transchelii* is not related to the degree of pigmentation. More studies are needed before any general conclusions can be reached on the importance of melanins for resistance to drought or heat.

Melanins in insects and other invertebrates are also formed as part of the immune response to microorganisms (192, 260, 270, 308). The products associated with melanins in defense reactions, however, can be damaging to animal cells as well as to the parasite (20). A comparable defense role is postulated for melanins in plants (12). Melanins in fungi also appear to be important for resistance to microbial attack. Hyaline conidia or hyphae in soils are quickly killed and lysed, whereas melanized cells may survive several years (136, 141, 246, 254). Accordingly, most of the fungal biomass found in soils is melanized (99).

The most important role of melanin may be its ability to protect against hydrolytic enzymes. Most antagonists that cause lysis of fungal cells also produce chitinase, and β-1,3- and β-1,6-glucanase (24, 111, 124). Generally, the ability of this mixture of enzymes to hydrolyze fungal cell walls is inversely related to the melanin content of the walls (24, 28, 100, 124, 143, 190, 195). Melanin-deficient mutants of *A. nidulans* (124) and *Cochliobolus sativus* (182) were highly susceptible to digestion by the enzyme mixture. Besides melanin, the *A. nidulans* mutant lacked α-(1,3)-glucan, which also resists hydrolysis by the enzyme mixture (194). Treatments with EDTA that decrease melanization of walls also enhance digestibility by the enzymes (44), whereas treatments with polyoxin that increase melanization decrease digestibility (116). When melanized sclerotia or cell walls are attacked by microorganisms, the nonmelanized cells of the sclerotia and the nonmelanized portions of cell walls are generally lysed, whereas the melanized cells or portions of walls remain intact (24, 183). Thus, melanins inhibit various enzyme mixtures used by antagonists to digest fungal cell walls. The inhibition of glucanase, chitinase, or cellulase by *A. nidulans* melanin is a time-dependent, noncompetitive type, resulting in an irreversible enzyme-melanin complex (28, 29).

Summary and Comments

Fungal melanins are produced from a variety of natural precursors, for example, catechol, DHN, and GDHB. The melanins are usually wall bound or extracellular in nature, although a few, such as aspergillin in *A. niger*, are cytoplasmic. Colored pigments also may be formed in either the cell wall or cytoplasm when exogenous phenols or aromatic amines are added to media of certain fungi, such as *C. neoformans*. Fungal melanins have many chemical properties in common with the cytoplasmic eumelanins and phaeomelanins produced by animals, probably because both contain phenol and quinone moieties in the polymer. Fungal melanins, like animal melanins, also are difficult to degrade and study chemically. Nevertheless, advances have been made in their characterization during the past few years because of improved biochemical and ultrastructural techniques.

The wall-bound melanin in many ascomycetous and imperfect fungi, including animal and plant pathogens, is made from DHN via pentaketide biosynthesis. Many chemical intermediates of this melanin pathway have been purified and identified. Related branch pathways and metabolites activated by mutations or chemical inhibitors also have been described. Some branch pathways metabolize naphthoquinones to less toxic compounds, whereas others dimerize naphthols, for example, 1,3,8-THN and DHN, and convert the dimers to various products which are known to be toxic or highly reactive. DHN melanin has not been found in basidiomycetous, zygomycetous, or chytridomycetous fungi, which apparently produce other melanins. For example, the basidiomycetes *U. maydis* and *A. brunnescens* apparently produce melanins from catechol and GDHB, respectively.

Advances also have been made in understanding the enzymology of melanin synthesis. Reductase and dehydratase enzymes that carry out reactions in the DHN melanin and DHN melanin branch pathways have been identified; these enzymes are soluble and cytoplasmic in nature. The terminal oxidative enzyme that produces the final melanin polymer from DHN, or related metabolites, is localized and bound in cell walls. The oxidative enzymes that produce catechol and GDHB melanins also apparently are localized in cell walls, where the two melanins are formed. The oxidative enzyme that make the three types of melanins have specificities similar to laccase but have not been identified. These enzymes need to be isolated from cell walls and more thoroughly characterized.

The functions of fungal melanins vary, depending on the fungus and its ecologic niche. Melanins protect fungi against environmental and microbial stress, but the role of melanins in pathogenicity and virulence of fungi to plants and animals generally has not been clarified. An exception is the effect of DHN melanin on pathogenicity by the plant pathogens *Pyricularia oryzae*, *Colletotrichum lagenarium*, and *C. lindemuthianum*. These fungi use melanized appressoria to penetrate the surface of host plants. DHN melanin inhibitors, for example, tricyclazole and pyroquilon, prevent infection, by inhibiting enzymes in the melanin pathway and thus aborting penetration. Melanin synthesis and pathogenicity is restored by adding melanin precursors that are produced beyond the enzyme affected by the inhibitors.

Many dematiaceous fungi pathogenic to humans and animals also produce DHN melanin. These include fungi that cause phaeohyphomycosis, chromoblastomycosis, and mycetoma. Although these fungi do not infect hosts by means of appressoria, melanin may affect their virulence or degree of resistance to antimycotic agents. Additional studies should be carried out to determine the effects of melanin on diseases caused by *W. dermatitidis* and other fungi by experimentally infecting animals with normal (melanized) and melanin-deficient strains. Melanin-deficient strains of many dematiaceous fungi are easily produced by UV irradiation or chemical means (13, 74). Model systems also could be used to search for chemicals that inhibit fungal melanin synthesis in animals. These inhibitors might reduce virulence or lower resistance to amphotericin B or other antifungal agents.

Melanin (or PPO) synthesis appears to be related to virulence in the fungus *C. neoformans* and the bacterium *M. leprae*, but these relationships need to be investigated in greater detail. In both cases the PPO involved in melanin synthesis should be purified and studied with different substrates and chelating agents. Additional work also is needed to determine whether or not the two pathogens use PPO to produce protective melanins or smaller, related compounds in humans and animals. Both pathogens have an affinity for tissues that are known to produce DOPA and catecholamines, and *C. neoformans* produces wall-bound melanins from DOPA added to cultures. This specificity for DOPA and catecholamines suggests that the normal metabolism of catecholamines in humans and animals may be disrupted by these pathogens.

Continued research in areas dealing with fungal melanins is needed because these pigments are often abundant in cell walls and are important for the survival of fungi. The role of fungal melanins in pathogenicity and virulence in animals and plants has not been adequately studied and is poorly understood in most cases.

References

1. Ajello L, Iger M, Wybel R, Vigil FJ: *Drechslera rostrata* as an agent of phaeohyphomycosis. *Mycologia* 82:1094–1102, 1980.
2. Al-Doory Y: The ultrastructure of *Cryptococcus neoformans*. *Sabouraudia* 9:113–118, 1971.
3. Aldridge DC, Davies AB, Jackson, MR, Turner WB: Pentaketide metabolites of the fungus *Phialophora lagerbergii*. *J Chem Soc Perkin Trans* I:1540–1541, 1974.
4. Allport DC, Bu'Lock JD: Biosynthetic pathways in *Daldinia concentrica*. *J Chem Soc* Part I, pp 654–662, 1960.
5. Araki F, Miyagi Y: Effects of fungicides on penetration by *Pyricularia oryzae* as evaluated by an improved cellophane method. *J Pesticide Sci* 2:457–461, 1977.
6. Arnone A, Camarda L, Nasini G: Secondary mould metabolites. Part 13. Fungal perylenequinones: Phleichrome, isophleichrome, and their endoperoxides. *J Chem Soc Perkin Trans* I:1387–1392, 1985.
7. Arnone A, Nasini G, Merlini L, Assante G: Secondary mould metabolites. Part 16. Stemphylotoxins. New reduced perylenequinone metabolites from *Stemphylium botryosum* var. *lactucum*. *J Chem Soc Perkin Trans* I:525–530, 1986.
8. Assante G, Locci R, Camarda L, Merlini L, Nasini G: Screening of the genus *Cercospora* for secondary metabolites. *Phytochemistry* 16:243–247, 1977.
9. Astill BD, Roberts JC: Studies in mycological chemistry. Part I. Flaviolin, 2 (or 3):5:7-trihydroxy-1:4-naphthaquinone, a metabolic product of *Aspergillus citricus* (Wehmer) Mosseray. *J Chem Soc* Part 3, pp 3302–3307, 1953.

10. Bardshiri E, Simpson TJ: ^{13}C and ^{2}H labelling studies on the biosynthesis of scytalone in *Phialophora lagerbergii*. *Tetrahedron* 39: 3539–3542, 1983.
11. Bartsch E, Lerbs W, Luckner M: Phenol oxidase activity and pigment synthesis in conidiospores of *Pencillium cuclopium*. *Z Allg Mikrobiol* 19: 75–82, 1979.
12. Bell AA: Biochemical mechanisms of disease resistance. *Ann Rev Plant Physiol* 32: 21–81, 1981.
13. Bell AA, Puhalla, JE, Tolmsoff WJ, Stipanovic RD: Use of mutants to establish (+)-scytalone as an intermediate in melanin biosynthesis by *Verticillium dahliae*. *Can J Microbiol* 22: 787–799, 1976.
14. Bell AA, Stipanovic RD, Puhalla JE: Pentaketide metabolites of *Verticillium dahliae*: Identification of (+)-scytalone as a natural precursor to melanin. *Tetrahedron* 32: 1353–1356, 1976.
15. Bell AA, Wheeler MH: Biosynthesis and functions of fungal melanins. *Ann Rev Phytopathol* 24: 411–451, 1986.
16. Bellinck C: Chemical study of *Penicillium* and *Trichoderma* pigments. *Ann Microbiol* 2: 131–142, 1975.
17. Beneke ES, Rogers AL: *Medical Mycology Manual with Human Mycoses Monograph*, (4th ed). Minneapolis, Burgess Publishing, 1980.
18. Benes SE, Ritchie DF: Evidence for increased malanin content in dicarboximide-resistant strains of *Monilinia fructicola*. *Phytopathology* 74 (abstract A697): 877, 1984.
19. Benitez T, Villa TG, Acha IG: Some chemical and structural features of the conidial wall of *Trichoderma viride*. *Can J Microbiol* 22: 318–321, 1976.
20. Beresky MA, Hall DW: The influence of phenylthiourea on encapsulation, melanization, and survival in larvae of the mosquito *Aedes aegypti* parasitized by the nematode *Neoaplectana carpocapsae*. *J Invert Pathol* 29: 74–80, 1977.
21. Blois MS Jr: Physical studies of the melanins, in Kawamura T, Fitzpatrick TB, Seiji M (eds): *Biology of Normal and Abnormal Melanocytes*. Tokyo, University of Tokyo Press, 1971, pp 125–139.
22. Blois MS Jr: The melanins: Their synthesis and structure. *Photochem Photobiol Rev* 3: 115–134, 1978.
23. Blois MS Jr, Taskovich L: The reversible binding of some aromatic and cyclic compounds to biopolymers in vitro. *J Invest Dermatol* 53: 344–350, 1969.
24. Bloomfield BJ, Alexander M: Melanins and resistance of fungi to lysis. *J Bacteriol* 93: 1276–1280, 1967.
25. Boekelheide K, Graham DG, Mize PD, Anderson CW, Jeffs PW: Synthesis of γ-L-Glutaminyl-[3,5-^{3}H] 4-hydroxybenzene and the study of reactions catalyzed by the tyrosinase of *Agaricus bisporus*. *J Biol Chem* 254: 12185–12191, 1979.
26. Buchenauer H, Zeun R, Schinzer U: Effect of tricyclazole on mycelium growth as well as on development and pigmentation of scelorotia of *Sclerotinia sclerotiorum*. *Z Pflanzenkr Pflanzenschutz* 92: 17–26, 1985.
27. Bull AT: Chemical composition of wild-type and mutant *Aspergillus nidulans* cell walls. The nature of polysaccharide and melanin constituents. *J Gen Microbiol* 63: 75–94, 1970.
28. Bull AT: Kinetics of cellulase inactivation by melanin. *Enzymologia* 39: 333–347, 1970.
29. Bull AT: Inhibition of polysaccharases by melanin: Enzyme inhibition in relation to mycolysis. *Arch Biochem Biophys* 137: 345–356, 1970.
30. Bull AT, Carter BLA: The isolation of tyrosinase from *Aspergillus nidulans*, its kinetic and molecular properties and some consideration of its activity in vivo. *J Gen Microbiol* 75: 61–73, 1973.
31. Bu'Lock, J: *Essays in Biosynthesis and Microbial Development*. New York, Wiley and Sons, 1967.

31a. Bustamam M, Sisler HD: Effect of pentachloronitrobenzene, pentachloroaniline and albinism on epidermal penetration of appressoria of *Pyricularia*. *Pestic Biochem Physiol* (in press).
32. Butler MJ, Lachance M-A: Quantitative binding of azure A to melanin of the black yeast *Phaeococcomyces*. *Exp Mycol* 10:166–170, 1986.
33. Cameron DW, Sidell MD: 1,3,6,8,11,13-Hexachloro-4,10-dihydroxydinaphtho [2,1-*b*:1 2′-*d*] furan-5,9-dione. A polychloro quinone from green soils. *Aust J Chem* 31:1323–1333, 1978.
34. Campbell CK, Mulder JL: Skin and nail infection by *Scytalidium hyalinum* sp. nov. *Sabouraudia* 15:161–166, 1977.
35. Cantino EC, Horenstein EA: The role of ketoglutarate and polyphenol oxidase in the synthesis of melanin during morphogenesis in *Blastocladiella emersonii*. *Physiol Plant* 8:189–221, 1955.
36. Carley HE, Watson RD, Huber DM: Inhibition of pigmentation in *Aspergillus niger* by dimethylsulfoxide. *Can J Bot* 45:1451–1453, 1967.
37. Carter BLA, Bull AT: Studies of fungal growth and intermediary carbon metabolism under steady and non-steady state conditions. *Biotechnol Bioeng* 11:785–804, 1969.
38. Chantarakul N: Subcutaneous cystic granuloma due to brown pigmented fungi (subcutaneous chromoblastomycosis) Report of 6 cases. *J Med Assoc Thailand* 54:953–958, 1971.
39. Chaskes S, Edberg SC, Singer JM: A DL-DOPA drop test for the identification of *Cryptococcus neoformans*. *Mycopathologia* 74:143–148, 1981.
40. Chaskes S, Tyndall RL: Pigment production by *Cryptococcus neoformans* from *para*- and *ortho*-diphenols: Effect of the nitrogen source. *J Clin Microbiol* 1:509–514, 1975.
41. Chaskes S, Tyndall RL: Pigment production by *Cryptococcus neofomans* and other *Cryptococcus* species from aminophenols and diaminobenzenes. *J Clin Microbiol* 7:146–152, 1978.
42. Chaskes S, Tyndall RL: Pigmentation and autofluorescence of *Cryptococcus* species after growth on tryptophan and anthranilic acid media. *Mycopathologia* 64:105–112, 1978.
43. Chavin W: Mechanisms in the control of dermal pigment in fishes, in Fitzpatrick TB, Kukita A, Morikawa A, Seiji M, Sober AJ, Toda K (eds): *Biology and Disease of Dermal Pigmentation*. Tokyo, University of Tokyo Press, 1981, pp 345–362.
44. Chet I, Henis Y: Effect of catechol and disodium EDTA on melanin content of hyphal and sclerotial walls of *Sclerotium rolfsii* Sacc. and the role of melanin in the susceptibility of these walls to β-(1,3)-glucanase and chitinase. *Soil Biol Biochem* 1:131–138, 1969.
45. Chida T, Sisler HD: Restoration of appressorial penetration ability with melanin precursors in *Pyricularia oryzae* treated with antipenetrants and in melanin-deficient mutants. *J Pesticide Sci* 12:49–55, 1987.
46. Clutterbuck AJ: Absence of laccase from yellow-spored mutants of *Aspergillus nidulans*. *J Gen Microbiol* 70:423–435, 1972.
47. Cooper LA, Gadd GM: Differentiation and melanin production in hyaline and pigmented strains of *Microdochium bolleyi*. *Antonie van Leeuwenhoek* 50:53–62, 1984.
48. Corrado ML, Kramer M, Cummings M, Eng RH: Susceptibility of dematiaceous fungi to amphotericin B, miconazole, ketoconazole, flucytosine and rifampin alone and in combination. *Sabouraudia* 20:109–113, 1982.
49. Cutler JE, Swatek FE: Pigment production by *Basidiobolus* in the presence of tyrosine. *Mycologia* 61:130–135, 1969.

50. Davies JE, King FE, Roberts JC: The structure of flaviolin. *Chem Ind* No. 36, pp 1110–1111, 1954.
50a. Dixon DM, Polak A: In vitro and in vivo drug studies with three agents of central nervous system phaeohyphomycosis. *Chemotherapy* 33:129–140, 1987.
50b. Dixon DM, Polak A, Szaniszlo PJ: Pathogenicity and virulence of wild-type and melanin-deficient *Wangiella dermatitidis*. *J Med Vet Mycol* 25:97–106, 1987.
50c. Dixon DM, Walsh TJ, Salkin IF, Polak A: *Dactylaria constricta*: Another dematiaceous fungus with neurotropic potential in mammals. *J Med Vet Mycol* 25:55–58, 1986.
51. Doherty MD, Cohen GM, Gant TW, Naish S, Riley PA: Metabolism of 1-naphthol by tyrosinase. *Biochem Pharmacol* 34:3167–3172, 1985.
52. Duckworth HW, Coleman JE: Physicochemical and kinetic properties of mushroom tyrosinase. *J Biol Chem* 245:1613–1625, 1970.
53. Durrell LW: The composition and structure of walls of dark fungus spores. *Mycopathol Mycol Appl* 23:339–345, 1964.
54. Edberg SC, Chaskes SJ, Alture-Werber E, Singer JM: Esculin-based medium for isolation and identification of *Cryptococcus neoformans*. *J Clin Microbiol* 12:332–335, 1980.
55. Ellis DH, Griffiths DA: The location and analysis of melanins in the cell walls of some soil fungi. *Can J Microbiol* 20:1379–1386, 1974.
56. Ellis DH, Griffiths DA: Melanin deposition in the hyphae of a species of *Phomopsis*. *Can J Microbiol* 21:442–452, 1975.
57. Farmer SG, Komorowski RA: Cutaneous microabscess formation from *Alternaria alternata*. *Am J Clin Pathol* 66:565–569, 1976.
58. Filip Z, Haider K, Beutelspacher H, Martin JP: Comparisons of IR-spectra from melanins of microscopc soil fungi, humic acids and model phenol polymers. *Geoderma* 11:37–52, 1974.
59. Findlay GH, Vismer HF: Black grain mycetoma. A study of the chemistry, formation and significance of the tissue grain in *Madurella mycetomi* infection. *Br J Dermatol* 91:297–303, 1974.
60. Findlay GH, Vismer HF, Liebenberg NvdW: Black grain mycetoma: The ultrastructure of *Madurella mycetomi*. *Mycopathologia* 67:51–54, 1979.
61. Findlay JA, Kwan D: Metabolites from a *Scytalidium* species. *Can J Chem* 51:3299–3301, 1973.
62. Findlay JA, Kwan D: Scytalone (3,6,8-trihydroxytetralone), a metabolite from a *Scytalidium* species. *Can J Chem* 51:1617–1619, 1973.
63. Fitzpatrick TB, Kukita A, Morikawa F, Seiji M, Sober AJ, Toda K, (eds): *Biology and Diseases of Dermal Pigmentation*. Tokyo, University of Tokyo Press, 1981.
64. Fitzpatrick TB, Lerner AB, Nordlund JJ, Anderson RR, Szabo G, et al: Introduction to dermal pigment biology and dermal pigmentary disorders (Ceruloderma): Significance, physical basis, cytologic and biochemical basis, in Fitzpatrick TB et al (eds): *Biology and Diseases of Dermal Pigmentation*. Tokyo, University of Tokyo Press, 1981, pp 3–18.
65. Fleming WH, Hopkins JM, Land GA: New culture medium for the presumptive identification of *Candida albicans* and *Cryptococcus neoformans*. *J Clin Microbiol* 5:236–243, 1977.
66. Fling M, Horowitz NH, Heinemann SF: The isolation and properties of crystalline tyrosinase from *Neurospora*. *J Biol Chem* 238:2045–2052, 1963.
67. Friis J, Ottolenghi P: Pigment formation by the "black yeast" *Phialophora jeanselmii*. *Antonie van Leeuwenhoek Yeast Symp* 35(suppl):H13–14, 1969.
68. Fromtling RA, Shadomy HJ, Jacobson ES: Decreased virulence in stable,

acapsular mutants of *Cryptococcus neoformans*. *Mycopathologia* 79:23–29, 1982.

69. Fuste FJ, Ajello L, Threlkeld R, Henry JE Jr: *Drechslera hawaiiensis*: Causative agent of a fatal fungal meningo-encephalitis. *Sabouraudia* 11:59–63, 1973.
70. Gadd GM: Melanin production and differentiation in batch cultures of the polymorphic fungus, *Aureobasidium pullulans*. *FEMS Microbiol Lett* 9:237–240, 1980.
71. Gafoor A, Heale JB: Melanin formation and peroxidase activity in *Verticillium*. *Microbios* 3:87–95, 1971.
72. Garau J, Diamond RD, Lagrotteria LB, Kabins SA: *Alternaria* osteomyelitis. *Ann Intern Med* 86:747–748, 1977.
73. Geis PA, Szaniszlo PJ: Carotenoid pigments of the dematiaceous fungus *Wangiella dermatitidis*. *Mycologia* 76:268–273, 1984.
74. Geis PA, Wheeler MH, Szaniszlo PJ: Pentaketide metabolites of melanin synthesis in the dematiaceous fungus *Wangiella dermatitidis*. *Arch Microbiol* 137:324–328, 1984.
75. Gentles JC, Evans EG: Infection of the feet and nails with *Hendersonula toruloidea*. *Sabouraudia* 8:72–75, 1970.
76. Gerber NN, Wieclawek B: The structures of two naphthoquinone pigments from an actinomycete. *J Org Chem* 31:1496–1498, 1966.
77. Geremia E, Corsaro C, Bonomo R: Eumelanins as free radicals trap and superoxide dismutase activities in amphibia. *Comp Biochem Physiol* 79:67–69, 1984.
78. Ghani HM, Lancaster JH, Larsh HW: Genetic analysis of pigmentation in *Arthroderma benhamiae*. *J Gen Microbiol* 84:205–208, 1974.
79. Gordon MA, Salkin IF, Stone WB: *Phoma* (*Peyronellaea*) as zoopathogen. *Sabouraudia* 13:329–333, 1975.
80. Greenblatt GA, Wheeler MH: HPLC analysis of fungal melanin intermediates and related metabolites. *J Liquid Chromatogr* 9:971–981, 1986.
81. Haars A, Huttermann A: Function of laccase in the white-rot fungus *Fomes annosus*. *Arch Microbiol* 125:233–237, 1980.
82. Ha-Huy-Ke, Luckner M: Structure and function of the conidiospore pigments of *Pencillium cyclopium*. *Z Allg Mikrobiol* 19:117–122, 1979.
83. Haider K, Martin JP: Synthesis and transformation of phenolic compounds by *Epicoccum nigrum* in relation to humic acid formation. *Soil Sci Soc Am Proc* 31:766–771, 1967.
84. Harris R, Smith RE, Wood TR, Biddle M: *Helminthosporium* corneal ulcers. *Ann Ophthalmol* 10:729–733, 1978.
85. Heale JB, Isaac I: Dark pigment formation in *Verticillium albo-atrum*. *Nature* 202:412–413, 1964.
86. Healy ME, Dillavou CL, Taylor GE: Diagnostic medium containing inositol, urea, and caffeic acid for selective growth of *Cryptococcus neformans*. *J Clin Microbiol* 6:387–391, 1977.
87. Hegnauer H, Nyhlen LE, Rast DM: Ultrastructure of native and synthetic *Agaricus bisporus* melanins—implications as to the compartmentation of melanogenesis in fungi. *Exp Mycol* 9:221–229, 1985.
88. Hemingway RW, McGraw GW, Barras SJ: Polyphenols in *Ceratocystis minor* infected *Pinus taeda*: Fungal metabolites, phloem and xylem phenols. *J Agric Food Chem* 25:717–722, 1977.
89. Hermann TE, Kurtz MB, Champe SP: Laccase localized in hulle cells and cleistothecial primordia of *Aspergillus nidulans*. *J Bacteriol* 154:955–964, 1983.
90. Hignett RC, Kirkham DS: The role of extracellular melanoproteins of *Venturia inaequalis* in host susceptability. *J Gen Microbiol* 48:269–275, 1967.

91. Hignett RC, Roberts AL, Carder JH: The properties of extracellular enzymes of *Venturia inaequalis* and their association with loss of virulence of the fungus in culture. *J Gen Microbiol* 110:67–75, 1979.
92. Hignett RC, Roberts AL, Carder JH: Melanoprotein and virulence determinants of *Venturia inaequalis*. *Physiol Plant Pathol* 24:321–330, 1984.
93. Hironaga M, Watanabe S: Studies on the genera *Arthroderma-Trichophyton*. *Jpn J Med Mycol* 18:161–168, 1977.
94. Hollis JP: Studies on *Streptomyces scabies*. I. Variability in a melanin-indicator medium. *Phytopathology* 42:273–276, 1952.
95. Hopfer RL, Blank F: Caffeic acid-containing medium for identification of *Cryptococcus neoformans*. *J Clin Microbiol* 2:115–120, 1975.
96. Hopfer RL, Groschel D: Six-hour pigmentation test for the identification of *Cryptococcus neoformans*. *J Clin Microbiol* 2:96–98, 1975.
97. Horowitz NH, Fling M, Macleod HL, Watanabe Y: Structural and regulative genes controlling tyrosinase synthesis in *Neurospora*. *Cold Spring Harbor Symp Quant Biol* 26:233–238, 1961.
98. Howard DH, Dabrowa N: Mutants of *Arthroderma benhamiae*. *Sabouraudia* 17:35–50, 1979.
99. Hunt GA, Fogel R: Fungal hyphal dynamics in a western Oregon Douglas-fir stand. *Soil Biol Biochem* 15:641–649, 1983.
100. Hurst HM, Wagner GH: Decomposition of ^{14}C-labeled cell wall and cytoplasmic fractions rom hyaline and melanic fungi. *Soil Sci Soc Am Proc* 33:707–711, 1969.
101. Ikeda R, Shinoda T, Kagaya K, Fukazawa Y: Role of serum factors in the phagocytosis of weakly or heavily encapsulated *Cryptococcus neoformans* strains by guinea pig peripheral blood leukocytes. *Microbiol Immunol* 28:51–61, 1984.
102. Imshenetsky AA, Lysenko SV, Kazokov GA: Upper boundary of the biosphere. *Appl Environ Microbiol* 35:1–5, 1978.
103. Ings RMJ: The melanin binding of drugs and its implications. *Drug Metab Rev* 15:1183–1212, 1984.
104. Inoue S, Maeda K, Uematsu T, Kato T: Comparison of tetrachlorophthalide and pentachlorobenzyl alcohol with chlobenthiazone and other melanin inhibitors in the mechanism of rice blast control, *J Pesticide Sci* 9:731–761, 1984.
105. Ito Y, Nanba H, Kuroda H: Melanin produced by *Cochliobolus miyabeanus* I. The physical and chemical properties. *Yakugaku Zasshi* 99:1027–1030, 1979.
106. Ito Y, Nanba H, Kuroda, H: Melanin produced by *Cohliobolus miyabeanus*. II. Gas chromatographic-mass spectrometric analysis of the degradation products by alkaline fusion. *Yakugaku Zasshi* 99:971–975, 1979.
107. Ivins BE, Holmes RK: Isolation and characterization of melanin-producing (*mel*) mutants of *Vibrio cholerae*. *Infect Immun* 27:721–736, 1980.
108. Ivins BE, Holmes RK: Factors affecting phaeomelanin production by a melanin-producing (*mel*) mutant of *Vibrio cholerae*. *Infect Immun* 34:895–899, 1981.
109. Iwasaki S, Muro H, Nozoe S, Okuda S: Isolation of 3,4-dihydro-3,4,8-trihydroxy-1(2*H*)-naphthalenone and tenuazonic acid from *Pyricularia oryzae* Cavara. *Tetrahedron Lett* No. 1, pp 13–16, 1972.
110. Iwasaki S, Muro H, Sasaki K, Nozoe S, Okuda S: Isolations of phytotoxic substances produced by *Pyricularia oryzae* Cavara. *Tetrahedron Lett* No. 37, pp 3537–3542, 1973.
111. Jackson GVH, Gay JL: Perennation of *Sphaerotheca mors-uvae* as cleistothecia with particular reference to microbiol activity. *Trans Br Mycol Soc* 66:463–471, 1976.
112. Kaufmann CS, Merz WG: Two rapid pigmentation tests for identification of *Cryptococcus neoformans*. *J Clin Microbiol* 15:339–341, 1982.

113. Kaufman SM: *Curvularia* endocarditis following cardiac surgery. *Am J Clin Pathol* 56:466–470, 1971.
114. Keilin D, Mann T: Polyphenol oxidase: purification, nature and properties. *Proc Roy Soc B* 125:187–204, 1938.
115. Koenigs JW: Production of extracellular hydrogen peroxide and peroxidase by wood-rotting fungi. *Phytopathology* 62:100–110, 1972.
116. Kohno M, Ishizaki H, Lin P-H, Yamamori K, Kunoh H: Effect of polyoxin on fungi. (IX). Ultrastructural and cytochemical analyses of polyoxin-treated hyphae of *Alternaria kikuchiana* Tanaka. *Ann Phytopathol Soc Jpn* 49:38–46, 1983.
117. Korner A, Pawelek J: Mammalian tyrosinase catalyzes three reactions in the biosynthesis of melanin. *Science* 217:1163–1165, 1982.
118. Kozlova TM, Lyakh SP: Morphological and ultrastructural features of the black yeast *Nadsoniella nigra* var. *psychrophilica*. *Microbiology USSR* 50:198–202, 1981.
119. Krachmer JH, Anderson RL, Binder PS, Waring GO, Rowsey JJ, Meek ES: *Helminthosporium* corneal ulcers. *Am J Ophthalmol* 85:666–670, 1978.
120. Kubo Y, Furusawa I: Localization of melanin in appressoria of *Colletotrichum lagenarium*. *Can J Microbiol* 32:280–283, 1986.
121. Kubo Y, Suzuki K, Furusawa I, Yamamoto M: Effect of tricyclazole on appressorial pigmentation and penetration from appressoria of *Colletotrichum lagenarium*. *Phytopathology* 72:1198–1200, 1982.
122. Kubo Y, Suzuki K, Furusawa I, Yamamoto M: Scytalone as a natural intermediate of melanin biosynthesis in appressoria of *Colletotrichum lagenarium*. *Exp Mycol* 7:208–215, 1983.
123. Kubo Y, Suzuki K, Furusawa I, Yamamoto M: Melanin biosynthesis as a prerequisite for penetration by appressoria of *Colletotrichum lagenarium*: Site of inhibition by melanin-inhibiting fungicides and their action on appressoria. *Pestic Biochem Physiol* 23:47–55, 1985.
124. Kuo M-J, Alexander M: Inhibition of the lysis of fungi by melanins. *J Bacteriol* 94:624–629, 1967.
125. Kurtz MB, Champe SP: Dominant spore color mutants of *Aspergillus nidulans* defective in germination and sexual development. *J Bacteriol* 148:629–638, 1981.
126. Kurtz MB, Champe SP: Purification and characterization of the conidial laccase of *Aspergillus nidulans*. *J Bacteriol* 151:1338–1345, 1982.
127. Kwon-Chung KJ, Bennett JE, Rhodes JC: Taxonomic studies on *Filobasidiella* species and their anamorphs. *Antonie van Leeuwenhoek* 48:25–38, 1982.
128. Kwon-Chung KH, Polacheck I, Popkin TJ: Melanin-lacking mutants of *Cryptococcus neoformans* and their virulence for mice. *J Bacteriol* 150:1414–1421, 1982.
129. Kwon-Chung KH, Rhodes JC: Encapsulation and melanin formation as indicators of virulence in *Cryptococcus neoformans*. *Infect Immun* 51:218–223, 1986.
130. Kwon-Chung KJ, Tom WK, Costa JL: Utilization of indole compounds by *Cryptococcus neoformans* to produce a melanin-like pigment. *J Clin Microbiol* 18:1419–1421, 1983.
131. Lampert RP, Hutto JH, Donnelly WH, Shulman ST: Pulmonary and cerebral mycetoma caused by *Curvularia pallescens*. *J Pediatr* 91:603–605, 1977.
132. Land GA, Dorn GL, Fleming WH, Beadles TA, Foxworth JH: Isolation and rapid identification of yeasts from compromised hosts. *Mycopathologia* 65:123–131, 1978.
133. Lazarovits G, Stoessl A: Tricyclazole inhibition of melanin and altersolanol A formation in *Alternaria solani*. *Abst 6th Internat Cong of Pestic Chem*, Ottawa,

1986, P 2F-14.
134. Lerch K: *Neurospora* tyrosinase: Structural, spectroscopic and catalytic properties. *Mol Cell Biochem* 52:125–138, 1983.
135. Lillie RD: Histochemistry of melanins, in Wolman M (ed): *Pigments in Pathology*. New York, Academic Press, 1969, pp 327–351.
136. Linderman RG, Toussoun TA: Behavior of albino chlamydospores of *Thielaviopsis basicola*. *Phytopathology* 56:887, 1966.
137. Lingappa Y, Sussman AS, Bernstein IA: Effect of light and media upon growth and melanin formation in *Aureobasidium pullulans* (DeBary) Arn. (= *Pullularia pullulans*). *Mycopathol Mycol Appl* 20:109–128, 1963.
138. Linhares LF, Martin JP: Decomposition in soil of the humic acid-type polymers (melanins) of *Eurotium echinulatum*, *Aspergillus glaucus* sp. and other fungi. *Soil Sci Soc Am J* 43:738–743, 1978.
139. Linhares LF, Martin JP: Carbohydrate content of fungal humic acid-type polymers (melanins). *Soil Sci Soc Am J* 43:313–318, 1979.
140. Linhares LF, Martin JP: Decomposition in soil of emodin, chrysophanic acid, and a mixture of anthraquinones synthesized by an *Aspergillus glaucus* isolate. *Soil Sci Soc Am J* 43:940–945, 1979.
141. Lockwood JL: Lysis of mycelium of plant-pathogenic fungi by natural soil. *Phytopathology* 50:787–789, 1960.
142. Lukiewicz S, Ablewicz E: EPR studies on the radioprotective role of melanins. *Radiat Res* 59:220–221, 1974.
143. Luther JP, Lipke H: Degradation of melanin by *Aspergillus fumigatus*. *Appl Environ Microbiol* 40:145–155, 1980.
144. Malmstrom BG, Ryden L: The copper-containing oxidases, in Singer TP (ed): *Biological Oxidations*, New York, Interscience, 1968, pp 415–438.
145. Mariat F, Liautaud B, Liautaud M, Marill F-G: *Hendersonula toruloidea*, agent d'une dermatite verruqueuse mycosique observee en Algerie. *Sabouraudia* 16:133–140, 1978.
146. Marr CD: Laccase and tyrosinase oxidation of spot test reagents. *Mycotaxon* 9:244–276, 1979.
147. Marr CD: Spot tests for detection of tyrosinase. *Mycotaxon* 19:299–305, 1984.
148. Marsden CD: Brain melanin, in Wolman M (ed): *Pigments in Pathology*. New York, Academic Press, pp 395–420.
149. Martin JP, Haider K: Phenolic polymers of *Stachybotrys atra*, *Stachybotrys chartarum*, and *Epicoccum nigrum* in relation to humic acid formation. *Soil Sci* 107:260–270, 1969.
150. Martin JP, Haider K: A comparison of the use of phenolase and peroxidase for the synthesis of model humic acid-type polymers. *Soil Sci Soc Am J* 44:983–988, 1980.
151. Martin JP, Haider K, Bondietti E: Properties of model humic acids synthesized by phenoloxidase and autoxidation of phenols and other compounds formed by soil fungi in *Proc Int Meet Humic Substances*. Pudoc, Nieuwersluis, 1972, pp 171–186.
152. Martin JP, Haider K, Linhares LF: Decomposition and stabilization of ring-^{14}C-labeled catechol in soil. *Soil Sci Soc Am J* 43:100–104, 1979.
153. Martin JP, Haider K, Wolf D: Synthesis of phenols and phenolic polymers by *Hendersonula toruloidea* in relation to humic acid formation. *Soil Sci Soc Am Proc* 36:311–315, 1972.
154. Mason HS: The chemistry of melanin. III. Mechanism of the oxidation of dihydroxyphenylalanine by tyrosinase. *J Biol Chem* 172:83–99, 1948.
154a. Matsumoto T, Padhye AA, Ajello L, Standard PG, McGinnis MR: Critical review of human isolates of *Wangiella dermatitidis*. *Mycologia* 76:232–249, 1984.
155. Matsuura K: Effect of melanin synthesis inhibitors on appressorial function in plant pathogenic fungi. *J Pesticide Sci* 8:379–383, 1983.

156. Mayer AM, Harel E: Polyphenol oxidases in plants. *Phytochemistry* 18:193–215, 1979.
157. McGinness J, Corry P, Proctor P: Amorphous semiconductor switching in melanins. *Science* 183:854–855, 1974.
158. McGinness JE: Mobility gaps: A mechanism for band gaps in melanins. *Science* 177:896–897, 1972.
158a. McGinnis MR: Chromoblastomycosis and phaeohyphomycosis: New concepts, diagnosis, and mycology. *J Am Acad Dermatol* 8:1–16, 1983.
159. McGinnis MR: *Helminthosporium* corneal ulcers. *Am J Opthalmol* 86:853, 1978.
160. McGinnis MR: *Laboratory Handbook of Medical Mycology*. New York, Academic Press, 1980.
160a. McGinnis MR, Borelli D, Padhye AA, Ajello L: Reclassification of *Cladosporium bantianum* in the genus *Xylohypha*. *J Clin Microbiol* 23:1148–1151, 1986.
161. McGinnis MR, Buck DL, Katz B: Paranasal aspergilloma caused by an albino variant of *Aspergillus fumigatus*. *South Med J* 70:886–888, 1977.
161a. McGinnis MR, Rinaldi MG, Winn RE: Emerging agents of phaeohyphomycosis: Pathogenic species of *Bipolaris* and *Exserohilum*. *J Clin Microbiol* 24:250–259, 1986.
162. McGinnis MR, Sorell DF, Miller RL, Kaminski GW: Subcutaneous phaeohyphomycosis caused by *Exophiala moniliae*. *Mycopathologia* 73:69–72, 1981.
163. McGovern EP, Bentley R: Biosynthesis of flaviolin and 5,8-dihydroxy-2,7-dimethoxy-1,4-napthoquinone. *Biochemistry* 14:3138–3143, 1975.
164. McGraw GW, Hemingway RW: 6,8-Dihydroxy-3-hydroxymethyl-isocoumarin, and other phenolic metabolites of *Ceratocystis minor*. *Phytochemistry* 16:1315–1316, 1977.
165. Mekalanos JJ, Sublett RD, Ronig WR: Genetic mapping of toxin regulatory mutations in *Vibrio cholerae*. *J Bacteriol* 139:859–865, 1979.
166. Melezhik AV: Electron tunneling between photo-induced paramagnetic centres in melanin pigment. *Biophysics* 25:247–251, 1980.
167. Mendoza CG, Leal JA, Novaes-Ledieu M: Studies of the spore walls of *Agaricus bisporus* and *Agaricus campestris*. *Can J Microbiol* 25:32–39, 1979.
168. Menon IA, Persad S, Ranadive NS, Haberman HF: Role of superoxide and hydrogen peroxide in cell lysis during irradiation in vitro of Ehrlich ascitic carcinoma cells in the presence of melanin. *Can J Biochem Cell Biol* 63:278–283, 1985.
169. Merz WG, Lloyd KO, Silva-Hunter M: Characterization of a *Trichophyton mentagrophytes* and its diffusible pigment. *Sabouraudia* 10:86–93, 1972.
170. Meyers WM, Dooley JR, Kwon-Chung KJ: Mycotic granuloma caused by *Phialophora repens*. *Am J Clin Pathol* 64:549–555, 1975.
171. Mirchink TG, Kashkina GB, Abatwrov YuD: The resistance of fungi with various pigments to γ-radiation. *Microbiology USSR* 41:67–69, 1972.
172. Morison WL: What is the function of melanin? *Arch Dermatol* 121:1160–1163, 1985.
173. Morita T, Aoki H: Isosclerone, a new metabolite of *Sclerotinia sclerotiorum* (Lib.) De Bary. *Agr Biol Chem* 38:1501–1505, 1974.
174. Nelson RM, Mason HS: Tyrosinase (mushroom), in Tabor H and Tabor CW (eds): *Methods in Enzymology*, Vol XVIIA. New York, Academic Press, 1970, pp 626–632.
175. Nicolaus RA, Piattelli M: Progress in the Chemistry of natural black pigments. *Rend Acad Sci Fis Mat Naples Ser* 32:83–97, 1965.
176. Nicolaus RA, Piattelli M, Fattorusso E: The structure of melanins and melanogenesis-IV: On some natural melanins. *Tetrahedron* 20:1163–1172, 1964.

177. Niebauer G: Dendritic cells of human skin, in *Experimental and Biological Medicine*, Vol. 2. Basel, Karger, 1968.
178. Nurudeen TA, Ahearn DG: Regulation of melanin production by *Cryptococcus neoformans*. *J Clin Microbiol* 10:724–729, 1979.
179. Okuno T, Kitamura Y, Matsuura K: Mechanism of inhibitory effect of tricyclazole on secondary infection by spores of *Pyricularia oryzae*. *J Pesticide Sci* 8:361–362, 1983.
180. Okuno T, Matsuura K, Furusawa I: Recovery of appressorial penetration by some melanin precursors in *Pyricularia oryzae* treated with tricyclazole and in a melanin deficient mutant. *J Pesticide Sci* 8:357–360, 1983.
181. Okuno T, Natsume I, Sawai K, Sawamura K, Furusaki A, Matsumato T: Structure of antifungal and phytotoxic pigments produced by *Alternaria* spp. *Tetrahedron Lett* 24:5653–5656, 1983.
182. Old KM, Robertson WM: Effects of lytic enzymes and natural soil on the fine structure of conidia of *Cochliobolus sativus*. *Trans Br Mycol Soc* 54:343–350, 1970.
183. Old KM, Robertson WM: Growth of bacteria within lysing fungal conidia in soil. *Trans Br Mycol Soc* 54:337–341, 1970.
184. Omura S: The antibiotic cerulenin, a novel tool for biochemistry as an inhibitor of fatty acid synthesis. *Bacteriol Rev* 40:681–697, 1976.
185. Paliwal DK, Randhawa HS: A rapid pigmentation test for identification of *Cryptococcus neoformans*. *Antonie van Leeuwenhoek* 44:243–246, 1978.
186. Paliwal DK, Randhawa HS: Evaluation of a simplified *Guizotia abyssinica* seed medium for differentiation of *Cryptococcus neoformans*. *J Clin Microbiol* 7:346–348, 1978.
187. Pavlenko GV, Loitsyanskaya MS, Nemirovskaya NI: Melanin pigment of *Gluconobacter oxydans*. *Microbiology USSR* 50:539–542, 1982.
188. Pawelek JM, Korner AM: The biosynthesis of mammalian melanin. *Am Sci* 70:136–145, 1982.
189. Pechak DG, Crang RE: Observations on melanin synthesis in the black yeast *Aureobasidium pullulans*. *Micron* 10:207–208, 1979.
190. Piattelli M, Fattorusso E, Magno S, Nicolaus RA: *Ustilago* melanin, a naturally occurring catechol melanin. *Tetrahedron Lett* No. 15, pp 997–998, 1963.
191. Piattelli M, Fattorusso E, Nicolaus RA, Magno S: The structure of melanins and melanogensis-V. Ustilagomelanin. *Tetrahedron* 21:3229–3236, 1965.
192. Poinar GO: Arthropod immunity to worms, in Jackson GJ, Herman RA, Singer I (eds): *Immunity to Parasitic Animals*. New York, Appleton-Century-Crofts, 1969, pp 173–210.
193. Polacheck I, Hearing VJ, Kwon-Chung KJ: Biochemical studies of phenoloxidase and utilization of catecholamines in *Cryptococcus neoformans*. *J Bacteriol* 150:1212–1220, 1982.
194. Polacheck I, Rosenberger RF: *Aspergillus nidulans* mutant lacking α-(1,3)-glucan, melanin, and cleistothecia. *J Bacteriol* 132:650–656, 1977.
195. Potgieter HJ, Alexander M: Susceptibility and resistance of several fungi to microbial lysis. *J Bacteriol* 91:1526–1532, 1966.
196. Prabhakaran K: Biochemical studies on *Mycobacterium leprae*. *J Basic Microbiol* 26:2:117–126, 1986.
197. Prabhakaran K, Harris EB, Kirchheimer WF: Effect of inhibitors on phenoloxidase of *Mycobacterium leprae*. *J Bacteriol* 100:935–938, 1969.
198. Prabhakaran K, Harris EB, Kirchheimer WF: The nature of the phenolase enzyme in *Mycobacterium leprae*: Structure-activity relationships of substrates and comparison with other copper proteins and enzymes. *Microbios* 5:273–281, 1972.
199. Prabhakaran K, Harris EB, Kirchheimer WF: Hypopigmentation of skin

lesions in leprosy and occurrence of *o*-diphenoloxidase in *Mycobacterium leprae*, in Biley V (ed): *Pigment Cell*, Vol. 3. Basel, Karger, 1976, pp 152–164.
200. Prabhakaran K, Harris EB, Kirchheimer WF: Confirmation of the spot test for the identification of *Mycobacterium leprae* and occurrence of tissue inhibitors of DOPA oxidation. *Lepr Rev* 48:49–52, 1977.
201. Prabhakaran K, Harris EB, Kirchheimer WF: Failure to detect *o*-diphenoloxidase in cultivable mycobacteria obtained from feral armadillos. *Lepr Rev* 51:341–349, 1980.
202. Pridham JB, Woodhead S: The biosynthesis of melanin in *Alternaria. Phytochemistry* 16:903–906, 1977.
203. Proctor PH, McGinness JE: The function of melanin. *Arch Dermatol* 122:507–508, 1986.
204. Puhalla JE, Bell AA: Genetics and biochemistry of wilt pathogens, in Mace ME, Bell AA, Beckman CH (eds): *Fungal Wilt Disease of Plants.* New York, Academic, 1981, pp 145–192.
205. Pulverer G, Korth H: *Cryptococcus neoformans*: Pigmentbildung aus verschiedenen polyphenolen. *Med Microbiol Immunol* 157:46–51, 1971.
206. Quevedo WC: Physiology of vertebrate pigmentation, in Fitzpatrick TB, et al (eds): *Biology and Diseases of Dermal Pigmentation.* Tokyo, University of Tokyo Press, 1981, pp 39–50.
207. Ramberg JE, McLaughlin DJ: Ultrastructural study of promycelial development and basidiospore initiation in *Ustilago maydis. Can J Bot* 58:1548–1561, 1980.
208. Raper KB, Fennell DI: *The Genus Aspergillus.* Baltimore, Williams and Wilkins, 1965, p 686.
209. Rast DM, Stussi H, Hegnauer H, Nyhlen LE: Melanins, in Turian G, Hohl HR (eds): *The Fungal Spore: Morphogenetic Controls.* New York, Academic Press, 1981, pp 507–531.
210. Ray AC, Eakin RE: Studies on the biosynthesis of aspergillin by *Aspergillus niger. Appl Microbiol* 30:909–915, 1975.
211. Reiss E, Nickerson WJ: Characterization of two melanins produced by *Phialophora verrucosa. Sabouraudia* 12:193–201, 1971.
212. Rhodes JC, Howard DH: Isolation and characterization of arginine auxotrophs of *Cryptococcus neoformans. Infect Immun* 27:910–914, 1980.
213. Rhodes JC, Polacheck I, Kwon-Chung KJ: Phenoloxidase activity and virulence in isogenic strains of *Cryptococcus neoformans. Infect Immun* 36:1175–1184, 1982.
214. Rippon JW: *Medical Mycology. The Pathogenic Fungi and the Pathogenic Actinomycetes*, (2nd ed). Philadelphia, WB Saunders, 1982.
215. Rippon JW, Garber D: Dermatophyte infection as a function of mating type and associated enzymes. *J Invest Dermatol* 53:445–448, 1969.
216. Robeson D, Strobel G, Matusumoto GK, Fisher EL, Chen MH, Clardy J: Alteichin: An unusual phytotoxin from *Alternaria eichorniae*, a fungal pathogen of water hyacinth. *Experientia* 40:1248–1250, 1984.
217. Rohwedder JJ, Simmons JL, Colfer H, Gatmaitan B: Disseminated *Curvularia lunata* infection in a football player. *Arch Intern Med* 139:940–941, 1979.
218. Rowley BI, Bull AT: Influence of growth rate history on production of melanin by *Aspergillus nidulans. Trans Br Mycol Soc* 70:453–455, 1978.
219. Ruban EL, Liakh SP, Volkova-Kozlova TM: *Nadsoniella nigra* mutant synthesizing extracell melanin. *Biol Bull Acad Sci USSR* 2:283–285, 1969.
220. Russell JD, Vaughan D, Jones D, Fraser AR: An IR spectroscopic study of soil humin and its relationship to other soil humic substances and fungal pigments. *Geoderma* 29:1–12, 1983.
221. Saiz-Jimenez C, Haider K, Martin JP: Anthraquinones and phenols as inter-

mediates in the formation of dark colored, humic acid-like pigments by *Eurotium echinulatum*. *Soil Sci Soc Am Proc* 39:649–653, 1975.

222. Saiz-Jimenez C, Martin F, Cert A: Low bioling-point compounds produced by pyrolysis of fungal melanins and model phenolic polymers. *Soil Biol Biochem* 11:305–310, 1979.

222a. Salkin IF, Martinez JA, Kemna ME: Opportunistic infection of the spleen caused by *Aureobasidium pullulans*. *J Clin Microbiol* 23:828–831, 1986.

223. Sankawa U, Shimada H, Sato T, Kinoshita T, Yamasaki K: Biosynthesis of scytalone. *Tetrahedron Lett* 1977, pp 483–486.

224. Sankawa U, Shimada H, Sato T, Kinoshita T, Yamasaki K: Biosynthesis of scytalone. *Chem Pharm Bull* 29:3536–3542, 1981.

225. Schaeffer P: A black mutant of *Neurospora crassa*. Mode of action of the mutant allele and action of light on melanogenesis. *Arch Biochem Biophys* 47:359–379, 1953.

226. Schnitzer M, Neyroud JA: Further investigations on the chemistry of fungal "humic acids." *Soil Biol Biochem* 7:365–371, 1975.

227. Schonborn C: Dermatophytes with melanoid pigment. 1. Communication: Investigation on the frequency of pigment-forming fungal stains and the intensity of their pigment production. *Z Gesamte Hyg Grenzgeb* 17:773–778, 1971.

228. Schonborn C, Schuhmann P: Dermatophytes with melanoid pigment 2. Communication: contribution on biology of pigment-forming fungal strains. *Z Gesamte Hyg Grenzgeb* 17:779–784, 1971.

229. Seiji M: Biology of dermal melanin, in Fitzpatrick TB, et al (eds): *Biology and Diseases of Dermal Pigmentation*. Tokyo, Tokyo University Press, 1981, pp 21–38.

230. Seredyuk LS, Yurchak LD: Allelopathic effect of melanins of *Stachybotrys alternans*. *Prikl Biokhim Mikrobiol* 7:174–177, 1971.

231. Seto H, Yonehara H: Utilization of ^{13}C-^{13}C coupling in structural and biosynthetic studies. VIII. The cyclization pattern of a fungal metabolite, scytalone. *Tetrahedron Lett* No. 5, pp 487–488, 1977.

232. Shaw CE, Kapica L: Production of diagnostic pigment by phenoloxidase activity of *Cryptococcus neoformans*. *Appl Microbiol* 24:824–830, 1972.

233. Shevtsova VM: Genetics of the cotton wilt pathogen *Verticillium dahliae* Kleb IV. Complementation analysis of the melanin-deficient mutants of *Verticillium dahliae* Kleb. *Sov Genet* 18:1500–1505, 1982.

234. Shevtsova VM, Kas'yaneko AG, Ten LN, Stepanichenko NN, Samoilov GG: Genetics of the cotton wilt pathogen, *Verticillium dahliae* Kleb III. Use of biochemical genetic methods to study melanin synthesis in *Verticillium dahliae*. *Sov Genet* 18:1391–1401, 1982.

235. Shevtsova, VM, Ten LN, Stepanichenko NN: Genetical and biochemical studies of melanogenesis in *Verticillium tricorpus* and *Verticillium nigrescens*. *Genetika* 20:1968–1973, 1984.

236. Shmyun MP, Zhdanova NM, Svyshchuk AA: Affinity of dark pigment of *Oidiodendron cerealis* to melanins. *Mikrobiol Zh Kiev* 37:700–702, 1975.

237. Siehr DJ: Melanin biosynthesis in *Aureobasidium pullulans*. *J Coat Tech* 53:23–25, 1981.

238. Simon LT, Bishop DS, Hooper GR: Ultrastructure and cytochemical localization of laccase in two strains of *Leptosphaerulina briosiana* (Pollaci) Graham and Luttrell. *J Bacteriol* 137:537–544, 1979.

239. Simpson TJ: The biosynthesis of polyketides. *Nat Prod Rep* 7:321–349, 1985.

240. Sisler HD: Control of fungal diseases by compounds acting as antipenetrants. *Crop Prot* 5:306–313, 1986.

241. Sisler HD, Woloshuk CP, Wolkow PM: Studies on the mode of action of

tricyclazole and related compounds, in Lyr H, Polter C (eds): *Systemische Fungizide und Antifungale Verbindungen.* Berlin, Akademie-Verlag, 1983, pp 171–176.

242. Sisler HD, Woloshuk CP, Wolkow PM: Specific chemical regulation of appressorial function. Tagungsber Akad Landwirtschaftswiss. *DDR* 222:17–28, 1984.
243. Sjoblad RD, Minard RD, Bollag JM: Polymerization of 1-naphthol and related phenolic compounds by an extracellular fungal enzyme. *Pestic Biochem Physiol* 6:457–463, 1976.
244. Slawinska D, Slawinski J, Sarna T: Photoinduced luminescence and EPR signals of polyphenol and quinone polymers. *Photochem Photobiol* 21:393–396, 1975.
245. Soga O: Stimulative production of flaviolin by *Phoma wasabiae. Agric Biol Chem* 46:1061–1063, 1982.
246. Sorokin DYu, Bab'eva IP: Lysis of natural yeast populations by soil microorganisms. *Microbiology USSR* 51:275–278, 1982.
247. Staib F: *Cryptococcus neoformans* and *Guizotia abyssinica* (Syn *G. oleifera*). *Z Hyg Infektionskr* 148:466–475, 1962.
248. Stipanovic RD, Bell AA: Pentaketide metabolites of *Verticillium dahliae.* 3. Identification of (−)-3,4-dihydro-3,8-dihydroxy-1(2*H*)-naphthalenone [(−)-vermelone] as a precursor to melanin. *J Org Chem* 41:2468–2469, 1976.
249. Stipanovic RD, Bell AA: Pentaketide metabolites of *Verticillium dahliae.* II. Accumulation of naphthol derivatives by the aberrant-melanin mutant *brm-2. Mycologia* 69:164–172, 1977.
250. Stipanovic RD, Wheeler MH: Accumulation of 3,3′-biflaviolin, a melanin shunt product, by tricyclazole-treated *Thielaviopsis basicola. Pestic Biochem Physiol* 13:198–201, 1980.
251. Stott DE, Martin JP, Focht DD, Haider K: Biodegradation, stabilization in humus, and incorporation into soil biomass of 2,4-D and chlorocatechol carbons. *Soil Sci Soc Am J* 47:66–70, 1983.
252. Strachan AA, Yu RJ, Blank F: Pigment production of *Cryptococcus neoformans* grown with extracts of *Guizotia abyssinica. Appl Microbiol* 22:478–479, 1971.
253. Stussi H, Rast DM: The biosynthesis and possible function of γ-glutaminyl-4-hydroxybenzene in *Agaricus bisporus. Phytochemistry* 20:2347–2352, 1981.
254. Sussman AS: Longevity and survivability of fungi, in Ainsworth GC, Sussman AS (eds): *The Fungi*, Vol. 3. New York, Academic Press, 1968, pp 447–486.
255. Suzuki K, Kubo Y, Furusawa I, Ishida N, Yamamoto M: Behavior of colorless appressoria in an albino mutant of *Colletotrichum lagenarium. Can J Microbiol* 28:1210–1213, 1982.
256. Swan GA: Structure, chemistry, and biosynthesis of the melanins. *Fortschr Chem Organ Natur* 31:521–582, 1973.
257. Szaniszlo PJ, Geis PA, Jacobs CW, Cooper CR, Harris JL: Cell wall changes associated with yeast-to-multicellular form conversion in *Wangiella dermatitidis*, in Schlessinger D (ed): *Microbiology*, Vol. 83. Washington, American Society for Microbiology, 1983, pp 239–244.
258. Tarasov BP, Yurlova NA, Elinov NP: Melanins formed by a culture of *Aureobasidium* (*Pullularia*) *pullulans* Arnaud (DeBary), 1910. *Chem Nat Comp* (*Engl Transl*) 216–221, 1977.
259. Taylor BE, Wheeler MH, Szaniszlo PJ: Evidence for pentaketide melanin biosynthesis in dematiaceous human pathogenic fungi. *Mycologia* 79:320–322, 1987.
260. Taylor RL: A suggested role for the polyphenol-phenoloxidase system in invertebrate immunity. *J Invertebr Pathol* 14:427–428, 1969.
261. Ten LN, Otroshchenko OS, Stepanichenko NN, Inoyatova DA: Metabolites of

the pathogenic fungus *Verticillium dahliae*. VII. The phytotoxic pigment PKZh-1 from the culture liquid. *Chem Nat Comp (Engl Transl)* 572–574, 1977.

262. Ten LN, Stepanichenko NN, Mukhamedzhanov SZ, Khotyanovich AV: Action of tricyclazole on the biosynthesis of melanin in some fungi of the genus *Verticillium*. *Chem Nat Comp (Engl Transl)* 384–385, 1983.
263. Ten LN, Stepanichenko NN, Shevtsova VM, Mukhamedzhanov SZ, Kas'yanenko AG, Otroshckenko OS: Metabolites of the pathogenic fungus *Verticillium dahliae*. IX. Pentaketides of mutants and their role in the biosynthesis of melanin. *Chem Nat Comp (Engl Transl)* 298–302, 1980.
264. Ten LN, Tyshchenko AA, Stepanichenko NN, Gusakova SD, Mukhamedzhanov SZ, et al: Metabolites of the pathogenic fungus *Verticillium dahliae*. VI. Pentaketide metabolites and neutral lipids of virulent and avirulent strains. *Chem Nat Comp (Engl Transl)* 524–527, 1978.
265. Terreni AA, Morris PR, Di Salvo AF: A red-pigmented strain of *Histoplasma capsulatum*. *Abst 1985 Am Soc Microbiol Ann Meet*, p 369.
266. Tokousbalides MC, Sisler HD: Site of inhibition by tricyclazole in the melanin biosynthetic pathway of *Verticillium dahliae*. *Pestic Biochem Physiol* 11:64–73, 1979.
267. Tolmsoff WJ, Bell AA, Wheeler MH: Pigment formation from artificial substrates by albino microsclerotia of *Verticillium dahliae* in relation to melanin synthesis. *Proc Beltwide Cotton Prod Res Conf*, 1975, pp 27–28.
268. Turner WB: *Fungal Metabolites*. New York, Academic Press, 1971.
269. Turner WB, Aldridge DC: *Fungal Metabolites II*. New York, Academic Press, 1983.
270. Unestam T: Defense reactions in and susceptibility of Australian and New-Guinean fresh water crayfish to European crayfish plague fungus. *Aust J Exp Biol Med Sci* 53:349–359, 1975.
271. Uspenskaya GD, Reshetnikova IA, Kozlenko TN: Some characteristics of the pycnidial mucus of fungi from the genera *Ascochyta* and *Phoma*. *Mikol Fitopatol* 14:21–23, 1980.
272. Vasilevskaya AI, Zhdanova NM, Pokhodenko VD: Character of survival of some gamma irradiated species of dark-colored Hyphomycetes. *Mikrobiol Zh* 33:438–441, 1970.
273. Vermeil C, Grodeff A: *Blastomycose cheloidienne*, a *Aureobasidium pullulans*. *Mycopathologia* 43:35–39, 1971.
274. Vollum DI: Chromomycosis: A review. *Br J Dermatol* 96:454–458, 1977.
275. Wang HS, Zeimis RT, Roberts GD: Evaluation of a caffeic acid-ferric citrate test for rapid identification of *Cryptococcus neoformans*. *J Clin Microbiol* 6:445–449, 1977.
276. Wasterstrom S-A: Accumulation of drugs on inner ear melanin. Therapeutic and ototoxic mechanisms. *Scand Audiol Suppl 23*. Stockholm, Almquist & Wiksell, 1984.
277. Wheeler MH: Melanin biosynthetic enzymes in cell-free homogenates of *Verticillium dahliae* and *Pyricularia oryzae*. *Phytopathology* 71:912, 1981.
278. Wheeler MH: Melanin biosynthesis in *Verticillium dahliae*: Dehydration and reduction reactions in cell-free homogenates. *Exp Mycol* 6:171–179, 1982.
279. Wheeler MH: Comparisons of fungal melanin biosynthesis in ascomycetous, imperfect and basidiomycetous fungi. *Trans Br Mycol Soc* 81:29–36, 1983.
280. Wheeler MH, Stipanovic RD: Melanin biosynthesis in *Thielaviopsis basicola*. *Exp Mycol* 3:340–350, 1979.
281. Wheeler MH, Stipanovic RD: Melanin biosynthesis and the metabolism of flaviolin and 2-hydroxyjuglone in *Wangiella dermatitidis*. *Arch Microbiol* 142:234–241, 1985.
282. Wheeler MH, Taylor BE, Szaniszlo PJ: Evidence for pentaketide melanin

biosynthesis in dematiaceous pathogenic fungi. *Abst 1986 Am Soc Microbiol Ann Meet*, p 410.
283. Wheeler MH, Tolmsoff WJ, Bell AA: Ultrastructure of melanin formation in *Curvularia* sp., *Alternaria* sp., and *Drechslera sorokiniana. Proc 35th Ann Meet Electron Microsc Soc Am*, 1977, pp 398–399.
284. Wheeler MH, Tolmsoff WJ, Bell AA: Ultrastructural and chemical distinction of melanins formed by *Verticillium dahliae* from (+)-scytalone, 1,8-dihydroxynaphthanlene, catechol, and L-3,4-dihydroxyphenylalanine. *Can J Microbiol* 24:289–97, 1978.
285. Wheeler MH, Tolmsoff WJ, Meola S: Ultrastructure of melanin formation in *Verticillium dahliae* with (+)-scytalone as a biosynthetic intermediate. *Can J Microbiol* 22:702–711, 1976.
286. White LP: Melanin: A naturally occurring cation exchange material. *Nature* 182:1427–1428, 1958.
287. Wolkow PM, Sisler HD, Vigil EL: Effect of inhibitors of melanin biosynthesis on structure and function of appressoria of *Colletotrichum lindemuthianum. Physiol Plant Pathol* 23:55–72, 1983.
288. Wolman M (ed): *Pigments in Pathology*, New York, Academic Press, 1969.
289. Woloshuk CP, Sisler HD: Tricyclazole, pyroquilon, tetrachlorophthalide, PCBA, coumarin and related compounds inhibit melanization and epidermal penetration by *Pyricularia oryzae. J Pestic Sci* 7:161–166, 1982.
290. Woloshuk CP, Sisler HD, Tokousbalides MC, Dutky SR: Melanin biosynthesis in *Pyricularia oryzae*: Site of tricyclazole inhibition and pathogenicity of melanin deficient mutants. *Pestic Biochem Physiol* 14:256–264, 1980.
291. Woloshuk CP, Sisler HD, Vigil EL: Action of the antipenetrant, tricyclazole, on appressoria of *Pyricularia oryzae. Physiol Plant Pathol* 22:245–259, 1983.
292. Woloshuk CP, Wolkow PM, Sisler HD: The effect of three fungicides, specific for the control of rice blast disease, on the growth and melanin biosynthesis by *Pyricularia oryzae* Cav. *Pestic Sci* 12:86–90, 1981.
293. Yamaguchi I, Sekido S, Misato T: The effect of non-fungicidal antiblast chemicals on the melanin biosynthesis and infection by *Pyricularia oryzae. J Pestic Sci* 7:523–529, 1982.
294. Yamaguchi I, Sekido S, Misato T: Inhibition of appressorial melanization in *Pyricularia oryzae* by non-fungicidal anti-blast chemicals. *J Pestic Sci* 8:229–232, 1983.
295. Yamaguchi I, Sekido S, Seto H, Misato T: Cytotoxic effect of 2-hydroxyjuglone, a metabolite in the branched pathway of melanin biosynthesis in *Pyricularia oryzae. J Pestic Sci* 8:545–550, 1983.
296. Yangco BG, TeStrake D, Okafor J: *Phialophora richardsiae* isolated from infected human bone: Morphological, physiological and antifungal susceptibility studies. *Mycopathologia* 86:103–111, 1984.
297. Young NA, Kwon-Chung KJ, Freeman J: Subcutaneous abcess caused by *Phoma* sp. resembling *Pyrenochaeta romeroi*: Unique fungal infection occurring in immunosuppressed recipient of renal allograft. *Am J Clin Pathol* 59:810–816, 1973.
298. Zaias N: Chromomycosis. *J Cut Pathol* 5:155–164, 1978.
299. Zenova GM: Melanoid pigments of nonchromogenic actinomycetes. *Microbiology USSR* 37:367–371, 1968.
300. Zeun R, Buchenauer H: Effect of tricyclazole on production and melanin contents of sclerotia of *Botrytis cinerea. Phytopathol Z* 112:259–267, 1985.
301. Zhdanova NN, Gauryushina AI, Vasilevskaya AI: Effect of γ- and UV-irradiation on survival of *Cladosporium* sp. and *Oidiodendron cerealis. Mikrobiol Zh Kiev* 35:449–452, 1973.

302. Zhdanova NN, Melezhik AV, Vasilevskaya AI: Thermostability of some melanin-containing fungi. *Biol Bull Acad Sci USSR* 7:305–310, 1980.
303. Zhdanova NN, Melezhik AV, Vasilevskaya AI, Pokhodendo VD: Formation and destruction of photoinduced paramagnetic centers in melanin containing fungi. *Biol Bull Acad Sci USSR* 5:453–458, 1978.
304. Zhdanova NN, Pokhodenko VD: The possible participation of a melanin pigment in the protection of the fungus cell from desiccation. *Microbiology USSR* 42:753–757, 1973.
305. Zhdanova NN, Pokhodenko VD: The protective properties of fungal melanin pigment of some soil Dematiaceae. *Radiat Res* 59:221, 1974.
306. Zhdanova NN, Svishchuk AA, Shmygun MP, Bondar AI: The protective effect of the pigment isolated from the fungus *Cladosporium* sp. *Microbiology USSR* 39:520–524, 1970.
307. Zhdanova NN, Vasilevskaya AI, Antonenko AL, Udobenko VF: Resistance of some melanin-containing hyphal fungi to artificial solar light. *Mikrobiol Zh Kiev* 43:178–182, 1981.
308. Ziprin R, Hartman PA: Toxicity of *Pseudomonas aeruginosa* bacterins and cell walls to the greater wax moth, *Galleria mellonella*. *J Invert Pathol* 17:265–269, 1971.
309. Zussman RA, Lyon L, Vicher EE: Melanoid pigment production in a strain of *Trichophyton rubrum*. *J Bacteriol* 80:708–713, 1960.

11—Cytochrome P450 of Fungi: Primary Target for Azole Antifungal Agents

YUZO YOSHIDA

Numerous azole compounds have been developed as potent antifungal agents. These compounds inhibit the growth of fungi by disturbing membrane and membrane-bound enzyme systems. Such disturbance is caused by the depletion of ergosterol and the accumulation of 14-methylsterols such as lanosterol, 24-methylene-24,25-dihydrolanosterol, obtusifoliol, and 14-methylfecosterol in the membrane. Ergosterol is synthesized from lanosterol with the 14-methylsterols appearing as intermediates in the metabolic pathway. The azole antifungal agents inhibit the 14α-demethylation of methylsterols. The 14α-demethylation is a cytochrome P450-dependent reaction, and the cytochrome P450 that catalyzes removal of the 14α-methyl group of 14-methylsterols is believed to be the primary target for azole antifungal agents [for a review, see (101)].

Recent knowledge of fungal cytochrome P450 has become indispensable in understanding the mechanism of action of azole antifungal agents and for the development of more effective and safe antifungal agents. The purpose of this review is to summarize current knowledge of fungal cytochrome P450 and how this cytochrome fits into the classification scheme of cytochromes. To appreciate the importance of cytochrome P450, a brief introduction to fungal cytochromes and related electron transport systems is necessary. In addition, molecular mechanisms of interaction between azole antifungal agents and purified $P450_{14DM}$ will be discussed in the last section of this contribution.

General Consideration of the Cytochromes and Related Electron Transport Systems of Fungi

Cytochrome is the collective name for a distinct group of hemoproteins functioning in biologic redox systems as electron carriers or terminal oxidases (51). Functionally, the cytochromes occurring in fungi are classified into two categories. The first group consists of cytochromes participating in oxidative energy metabolism, and the second group includes those functioning in the redox metabolism of cellular constituents.

Cytochromes Participating in Respiration and Energy Metabolism

In aerobically grown respiring fungi, cytochromes *a*, *b*, *c*, and c_1 predominate in the cells (26, 27). It has been established that these cytochromes are localized in mitochondria, constitute an electron transport system called the respiratory chain, and contribute to oxidative energy metabolism (Fig. 11-1). The purpose of the respiratory chain is to transfer electrons from substrates such as succinate and reduced nicotinamide adenine dinucleotide (NADH) to molecular oxygen. Electron transport couples with the phosphorylation of adenosine diphosphate (ADP) to adenosine triphosphate (ATP), which is

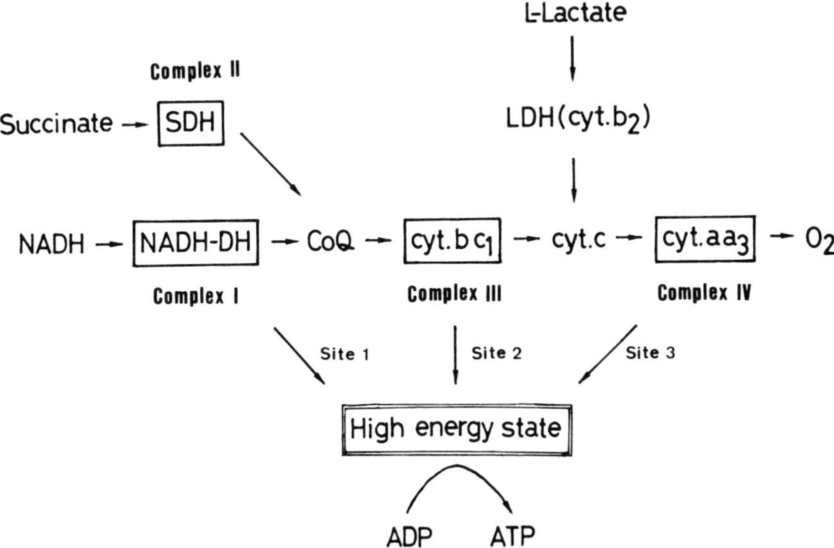

FIG. 11-1. The respiratory chain and the oxidative phosphorylation system of yeast mitochondria. Cytochromes *a*, a_3, *b*, and c_1 are integrated in the inner membrane of mitochondria together with various factors functioning in the oxidative phosphorylation, whereas cytochrome *c* interacts loosely with the membrane. Complex I is NADH-coenzyme Q reductase, consisting of NADH-dehydrogenase (NADH-DH) and an iron-sulphur complex. Complex II is succinate-coenzyme Q reductase, containing succinate dehydrogenase (SDH) and an iron-sulphur complex. Complex III is the cytochrome bc_1 complex acting as reduced coenzyme Q-cytochrome *c* reductase. Complex IV is cytochrome *c* oxidase, consisting of cytochrome aa_3. LDH is L-lactate dehydrogenase, containing cytochrome b_2. Sites 1, 2, and 3 indicate the sites where redox potential couples with the energy conservation by the phosphorylation of ADP. Construction of this energy-generating system is essentially identical with that of mammals, but the phosphorylation at site 1 is uncertain in *Saccharomyces cerevisiae* (71).

known as oxidative phosphorylation (71, 72). The phosphorylation occurs at three points called sites 1, 2, and 3 in the respiratory chain. As shown in Fig. 11-1, sites 1, 2, and 3 correspond to NADH-CoQ reductase complex (complex I), cytochrome bc_1 complex (complex III), and cytochrome *c* oxidase (cytochrome aa_3) complex (complex IV), respectively. The organization and function of the respiratory chain, as well as the oxidative phosphorylation system of fungi are essentially identical with those of higher eukaryotes. The phosphorylation process at site 1 is not clearly established in *Saccharomyces cerevisiae* (72).

Yeasts contain another cytochrome that may contribute to the oxidation of substrates. This cytochrome is called cytochrome b_2 (15), which is a lactate dehydrogenase [EC 1.1.2.3] consisting of a flavoheme protein containing flavin mononucleotide (FMN) and protoheme as the prosthetic group (39). This enzyme mediates the electron transfer from L-lactate to ferricytochrome *c*. This fact suggests that cytochrome b_2 supplies electrons from L-lactate to the respiratory chain at the level of cytochrome *c* (Fig. 11-1). It has been shown that L-lactate can support the aerobic growth of *S. cerevisiae* when oxidative phosphorylation at sites 1 and 2 is inhibited by antimycin A (39). However, the function of this cytochrome in actively growing aerobic yeasts has not been established.

Cytochromes and Electron Transport System of Endoplasmic Reticulum

Another group of important cytochromes, cytochromes P450 and b_5, are located in the endoplasmic reticulum (109, 110, 111) and constitute an electron transport system called the "microsomal electron transport system" in conjunction with other electron-transferring components such as NADH-cytochrome b_5 reductase (55), reduced nicotinamide adenine dinucleotide phosphate (NADPH)-cytochrome P450(*c*) reductase (5, 56), cyanide-sensitive factor (CSF) (70, 93), and squalene-2,3,-epoxidase (81). Fig. 11-2 shows the organization and function of the microsomal electron transport system of yeasts. The microsomal electron transport system contributes to the oxidative metabolism of lipophilic small molecules such as sterols and fatty acids. Although these reactions simply appear to be desaturation or demethylation processes, they actually consist of monooxygenation requiring both NAD(P)H and molecular oxygen, following dehydration, decarboxylation, or deformilation. It is evident that the microsomal electron transport system is a multifunctional complex monooxygenase system.

As shown in Fig 11-2, terminal oxidases of the electron transport system are multiple, which supports the functional multiplicity of this system. Cytochrome P450, the subject of this review, is the principal terminal oxidase of the microsomal electron transport system.

The microsomal electron transport system contains several nonheme ter-

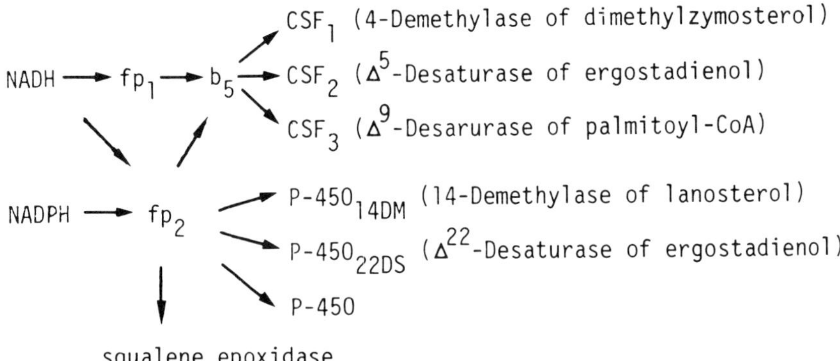

FIG. 11-2. Construction and function of the microsomal electron transport system of yeast. The abbreviations fp_1, fp_2, and b_5 represent NADH-cytochrome b_5 reductse, NADPH-cytochrome P450 (*c*) reductase, and cytochrome b_5, respectively. NADPH-cytochrome P450 (*c*) reductase (fp_2) transfers electrons from NADPH not only to cytochrome P450, but also to other electron acceptors in this system. This flavoprotein acts as a multifunctional electron distributor in the electron transport system.

minal oxidases. One group of these oxidases is CSF. As shown in Fig. 11-2, at least three functionally different CSFs may occur in yeast microsomes (9, 70, 78, 93). However, none of them have yet been isolated and little is known on their molecular properties. Two CSFs catalyzing oxidative desaturation of long-chain fatty acyl-CoAs have been purified from rat liver microsomes and characterized as iron-sulphur proteins (73, 87).

The microsomal electron transport system contains one additional non-heme terminal oxidase, squalene-2,3-epoxidase (81). Purification of this enzyme obtained from fungi has not yet been accomplished. However, a similar enzyme has been isolated from rat liver microsomes and reported to be a FAD-requiring monooxygenase (77, 89). Recently, Ryder and Dupont (81) reported that squalene epoxidase of *Candida albicans* requires FAD for its maximum activity. It is, therefore, likely that fungal squalene epoxidase is also a FAD-dependent flavin monooxygenase. Epoxidation of squalene is the initial reaction of the squalene cyclization to form lanosterol and is an important step in sterol biosynthesis. Recently, it was demonstrated that fungal squalene-2,3-epoxidase was strongly and specifically inhibited by the antifungal agents naftifine and its derivative SF 86-327 (Sandoz) (82). Squalene epoxidase is another important target for antifungal agents that inhibit ergosterol biosynthesis. Extensive studies on this enzyme are expected.

Cytochrome b_5 (110, 115), which is another cytochrome of the microsomal electron transport system, serves as an electron carrier between a flavoprotein, NADH-cytochrome b_5 reductase (55), and CSFs (9, 78, 93) (Fig. 11-2). Cytochrome b_5 in yeast microsomes is readily reduced by NADPH (109), and purified NADPH-cytochrome P450 reductase mediates the reduction of the cytochrome by NADPH (5). Cytochrome b_5 is considered to act as an electron carrier between the P450 reductase and CSFs (Fig. 11-2). In addition, it was reported that the cytochrome P450-dependent alkane hydroxylase activity of petroleum-assimilating yeast microsomes reached its maximum when both NADPH and NADH were present in the reaction medium (24, 67). It is well established that the phenomenon described above is due to the supply of the second electron necessary for the monooxygenation from NAD(P)H via cytochrome b_5 (18, 44, and Fig. 11-3). Accordingly, cytochrome b_5 may serve as the second electron carrier of the cytochrome P450 system in the fungal cell.

Effects of Growth Conditions on Cytochrome Composition

At the beginning of the investigation of yeast cytochromes by pioneers like Keilin and Fink, it was found that cytochrome components of aerobically grown baker's yeast and anaerobically grown brewer's yeast were different from each other (29). Baker's yeast contains cytochromes *a*, *b*, and *c*, and brewer's yeast contains cytochromes a_1 and b_1. Later, it was found that the cytochrome constitution of brewer's yeast was converted to that of baker's yeast by sufficient aeration (26, 27, 58, 59).

The cytochromes found by Keilin (51) in aerobically grown baker's yeast correspond to those of the respiratory chain (71), and the conversion of cytochrome upon aeration reflects the adaptive formation of functional mitochondria for the aerobic life cycle. In addition to typical mitochondrial cytochromes, cytochrome b_2 (15) is also formed upon aerobic adaptation (39). In facultative aerobic yeasts, the mitochondrial cytochromes are formed only when the cells are grown under aerobic and respiring conditions.

Cytochromes a_1 and b_1 (27) found by Fink (29), which are characteristically found in anaerobically grown yeasts, are now designated as cytochrome *c* peroxidase (46, 108) and cytochrome b_5 (109, 110), respectively. These two cytochromes are found also in yeast cells grown under aerobic conditions (Yoshida Y, unpublished result). However, their detection in whole cell suspensions or crude cell-free preparations of respiring yeasts by conventional spectrophotometry is difficult because of the presence of large amounts of mitochondrial cytochromes in these preparations. This may be the reason why cytochromes a_1 and b_1 were originally considered to be specific components of anaerobic yeasts when yeast cytochromes were first being characterized (26, 27, 29).

Cytochrome P450 also was found as a characteristic component of anaerobically grown yeasts (59). The content of cytochrome P450 is significantly decreased by aerobic adaptation (45, 88) and the cytochrome becomes undetectable by spectroscopy. However, aerobically grown yeast cells contain a sufficient amount of cytochrome P450 to support their growth (8). Alkane assimilating yeasts such as *Candida* spp. contain a specific cytochrome P450 which converts *n*-alkanes to the corresponding alkanols (32, 57). This cytochrome is formed adaptively when the yeast is grown aerobically and supplied *n*-alkanes as a sole carbon source (64, 90, 91). In addition to these conditions, growth phase of the yeast and glucose concentration in the growth medium are known to affect the cytochrome P450 content in the yeast (54, 64, 83). The role of cyclic AMP on induction of cytochrome P450 has been described (104). Thus, the cellular content of cytochrome P450 is affected by various growth conditions. Routinely, we use yeast cells grown semianaerobically in late logarithmic phase on 3% glucose as the most suitable material for studying cytochrome P450, which catalyzes lanosterol 14α-demethylation.

Properties and Function of Fungal Cytochrome P450

General Aspects of Cytochrome P450

Definition

Cytochrome P450 is the collective name given for a special class of protoheme proteins which show their Soret absorption band at approximately 450 nm in their reduced CO complexes. This unique spectrophotometric characteristic of cytochrome P450 is now recognized to be due to the coordination of the thiolate anion (S^-) of a cysteine residue in the apoprotein to the heme iron (see Fig. 11-4). Cytochrome P450 acts as a monooxygenase, although there may be a few exceptions. It can thus be said that cytochrome P450 is a group of monooxygenases having thiolate-ligated iron protoporphyrin IX as the prosthetic group.

Molecular Multiplicity

Cytochrome P450 has been found in most eukaryotes and in a few bacteria (76, 84). Cytochrome P450 catalyzes monooxygenation of a great variety of compounds (76, 84). Substrates metabolized by cytochrome P450 include physiologically important endogenous compounds such as steroids, fatty acids, prostanoids, secondary metabolites of higher plants, and molds, etc. Miscellaneous xenobiotics such as drugs, pesticides, plant-protecting agents, food additives, and environmental pollutants are also important substrates for cytochrome P450. To metabolize such diverse substrates, cytochrome P450 shows considerable molecular multiplicity (60, 76, 84). For example, more than 20 species of cytochrome P450 have been isolated from mammals. In recent years, the primary structure of several species of cytochrome P450 have been determined (30, 31, 34, 36, 40, 50, 66, 107, 123). It believed that the multiple forms of cytochrome P450 may have been derived from a common ancestor by gene duplication and mutation during evolution.

Reaction Mechanism of the Cytochrome P450-Catalyzed Monooxygenation

Upon monooxygenation, cytochrome P450 requires NADPH and molecular oxygen. The catalytic cycle of the cytochrome is illustrated in Fig. 11-3. At the first step a substrate (AH) combines with the oxidized form, $P450^{3+}$. Then the substrate complex $P450^{3+}$-AH is reduced to $P450^{2+}$-AH by the first electron and reacts with O_2 to form the $P450^{2+}$-AH-O_2 ternary complex. Carbon monoxide interferes with binding of O_2 to $P450^{2+}$-AH and inhibits the catalytic cycle at this step. The second electron is introduced into the ternary complex. The oxygen is activated, and one atom attacks the substrate to form a oxygenated product (AOH) and the other is reduced to H_2O with $P450^{3+}$ being restored. Two electrons consumed during the catalytic cycle are generally supplied from NADPH, and the overall reaction is expressed as follows:

$$AH + NADPH + H^+ + O_2 \rightarrow AOH + NADP^+ + H_2O$$

Cytochrome P450 does not react directly with NADPH. The flavoprotein NADPH-cytochrome P450(*c*) reductase, mediates the electron transfer from NADPH to the cytochrome. This flavoprotein can transfer both the first and the second electrons to the cytochrome. However, in many cases, the second electron is transferred via cytochrome b_5 from NADH or NADPH (18, 44).

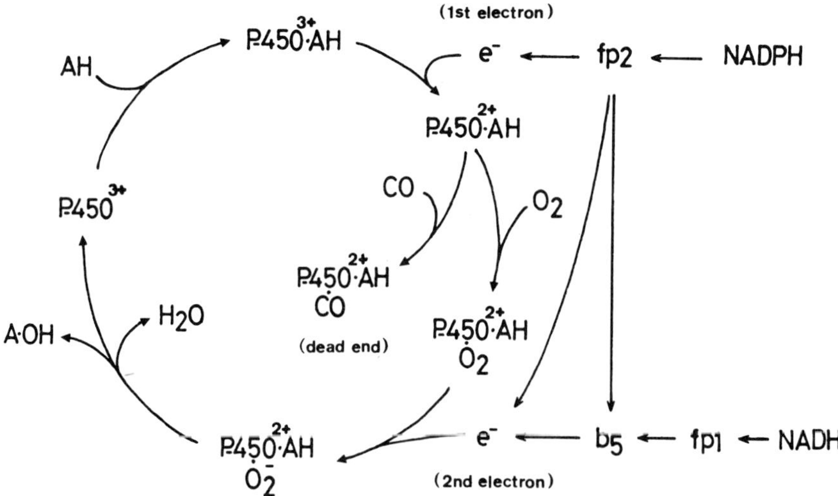

FIG. 11-3. Catalytic cycle of cytochrome P450. For the abbreviations fp_1, fp_2, and b_5, see Fig. 11-2. The catalytic cycle is started by binding the substrate (AH) to the oxidized cytochrome ($P450^{3+}$). For further details, see text.

Substrate-Induced Spectral Change and the Spin-State Equilibrium

Binding of a substrate to oxidized cytochrome P450 usually causes certain spectral change of the cytochrome called "substrate-induced spectral change" (42, 85). The substrate-induced spectral change is classified into two categories, types I and II (85), which are based on the shape of the resulting spectra (substrate-induced difference spectra, Fig. 11-4).

The substrate-induced spectral change is caused by removal or exchange of the sixth ligand of oxidized cytochrome P450 concomitant with the binding of a substrate (112). Although there are a few exceptions, the substrate-free

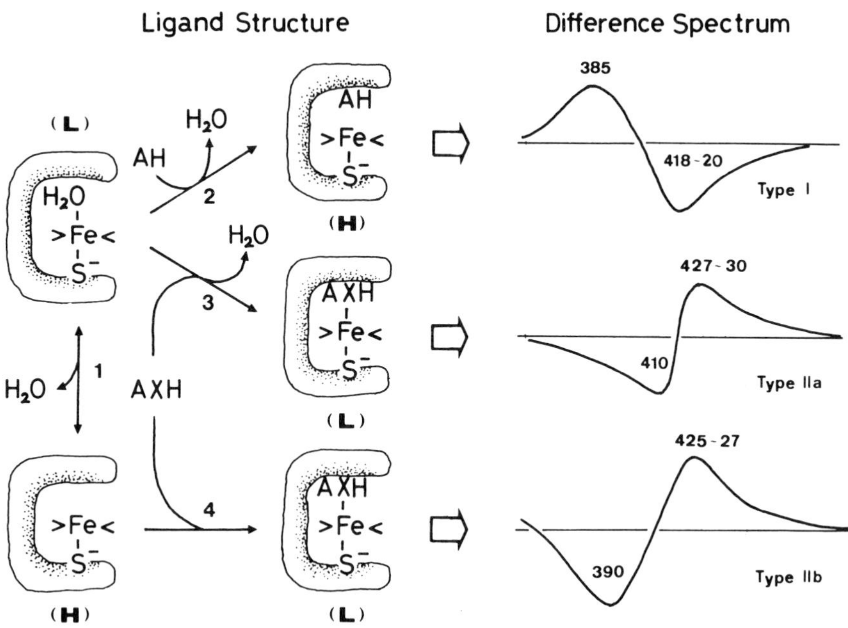

FIG. 11-4. Spin-state equilibrium, substrate binding, and the substrate-induced spectral change of cytochrome P450 in relation to ligand structure of the cytochrome. S^- represents the thiolate fifth ligand characterizing the cytochrome. Spin state of each structure is represented by H (high spin) or L (low spin). The substrate-free resting form is in equilibrium between the high-spin (penta-coordinate) and the low-spin (water-ligated) forms (reaction 1). Reaction 2 indicates binding of a substrate that has no coordinating group (AH) to the low-spin form. This interaction converts the water-ligated low-spin form to the penta-coordinate high-spin form and induces the type I spectral change. Reactions 3 and 4 represent binding of another type of substrate (AXH), which contains a coordinating atom (X), to the low-spin and high-spin forms, respectively. In these cases, X coordinates to the heme-iron, an artificial low-spin complex is formed, and the type II spectral change is induced. The shape of the type II difference spectrum is affected by the spin state of the substrate-free form, and they are discriminated as type IIa and type IIb in this figure.

resting form of the cytochrome is in the ferric low-spin state, which shows a Soret absorption band at 416–418 nm. As shown in Fig. 11-4, the native sixth ligand of the ferric low-spin form of the cytochrome is probably a water molecule, which may equilibrate with bulk solvent water (22, 35, 103, 104, 114, 117). This equilibrium (reaction 1 of Fig. 11-4) is dependent on hydrophobicity and steric hinderance of the heme pocket. If a lipophilic substrate (AH) binds to the substrate site near the sixth coordination position, which is the oxygen activating site, accessibility of a water molecule to the heme is reduced, and the cytochrome moves to the penta-coordinated high-spin configuration, showing the Soret band at approximately 393 nm (117). The type I spectral change represents the low- to high-spin state transition (reaction 2 of Fig. 11-4).

In contrast, if a substrate that can act as a heme ligand (AXH) is bound to the substrate site, the substrate may interact with the heme as an external sixth ligand instead of the water molecule (22, 104, 114, 117). In this case, the cytochrome is converted to an artificial hexa-coordinated low-spin complex (reaction 3 or 4 of Fig. 11-4). The type II spectral change is induced by this type of substrate binding. The absorption maximum of the Soret band of a low-spin complex of cytochrome P450 is dependent on the nature of the sixth ligand (22, 104, 114). In addition, cytochrome P450 found in intact microsomes occurs in a mixture of high- and low-spin states (48, 112). Accordingly, difference spectra relating to the type II spectral change (type II difference spectra) are different from one another depending on the nature of the coordinating groups of the substrates and the spin states of the cytochrome (types IIa and IIb of Fig. 11-4). The type II spectral change can be induced by any compound that interacts with the cytochrome as a sixth ligand. For example, heterocycles such as pyridine and the imidazoles can induce the type II spectral change in most cytochromes P450. Thus, the type II spectral change is not a hallmark of binding of a compound to the substrate site of the cytochrome.

The substrate-induced spectral change thus provides some information on the mode of interaction of a substrate with the cytochrome. As a matter of cause, the substrate-induced spectral change is induced by inhibitors that can interact with the cytochrome at the active site. Therefore, the substrate-induced spectral change is useful for studying cytochrome P450 inhibitors.

Short History of Fungal Cytochrome P450

Fungal cytochrome P450 was first found in anaerobically grown cells of *S. cerevisiae* by Lindenmayer and Smith (59). In 1969, Ishidate et al (45, 46) reported that cytochrome P450 of *S. cerevisiae* was located in a particular fraction of semianaerobically grown cells and disappeared upon their aerobic adaptation. At that time, cytochrome P450 was considered to be a hemoprotein characteristic of nonrespiring cells. The function of the cytochrome was believed to be involved with oxidative metabolism occurring under a low oxygen tension (88).

In the latter half of the 1970s, the presence of the microsomal electron transport system in semianaerobically grown cells of *S. cerevisiae* was established by Yoshida and co-workers (5, 55, 56, 93, 109, 110, 111, 113). Cytochrome P450 included in this electron transport system was purified (113, 116) and characterized in detail (12, 116). This cytochrome was identified as lanosterol 14α-demethylase (6, 7, 12) and named $P450_{14DM}$ (116). They also found that $P450_{14DM}$ was present in aerobically grown respiring cells of *S. cerevisiae* (8). Although the content of the cytochrome in these cells was low, the level was enough to support ergosterol synthesis (8). This finding demonstrated that cytochrome P450 was not a restricted component of nonrespiring yeasts but was an important constitutive enzyme functioning in ergosterol biosynthesis.

In the meantime, another cytochrome P450, which participated in *n*-alkane hydroxylation was found in petroleum-assimilating yeasts (32, 57). This cytochrome was isolated by Duppel et al (24) and by Bertrand et al (17) from *Candida tropicalis*, later being purified by Riege et al (80) from *Lodderomyces elongisporus* [recently they reidentified this strain as *C. maltosa* (Muller, H-G, personal communication)]. An additional cytochrome P450, which had an arylhydrocarbon hydroxylase activity (106), was isolated from aerobically grown glucose-repressed cells (52) of *S. cerevisiae* by Azari and Wiseman (14, 53). In addition, Hata et al (37, 38) suggested that the Δ^{22}-desaturation of 22,23-dihydroergosterol was a cytochrome P450-dependent reaction and this cytochrome P450 must be different from $P450_{14DM}$. Based on these findings, it is now clear that the yeasts have multiple species of cytochrome P450 as do mammals.

Studies on cytochromes P450 of other fungi are not as extensive. Occurrence of cytochrome P450 has been suggested in various molds such as *Aspergillus ochraceus* (25, 33, 47), *Cunninghamella* sp. (20, 21, 28), *Nectria haematococca* (63), *Rhizopus stolonifera* (19), and *Penicillium patulinum* (69) based on monooxygenase activities observed in these organisms. In addition, the presence of cytochrome P450, which catalyzes 14α-demethylation of 14-methylsterols in molds, can be assumed from the inhibitory effects of azole antifungal agents on sterol metabolism (101). However, attempts to isolate cytochrome P450 from mold cells and their detailed spectrophotometric and enzymologic analysis have not yet been made.

Cytochrome P450 that Catalyzes Lanosterol 14α-Demethylation ($P450_{14DM}$): Target for Azole Antifungal Agents

Purification and Molecular Properties of $P450_{14DM}$ of S. cerevisiae

As described by Lindenmayer and Smith (59) and by Ishidate et al (45), the cellular content of cytochrome P450 in *S. cerevisiae* reaches its maximum when the yeast is cultivated under a low oxygen tension and a high glucose concentration. Under these conditions, the content of cytochrome P450 in *S. cerevisiae* microsomes is usually in a range of 0.03–0.1 nmol/mg protein (109, 116). $P450_{14DM}$ can be purified from the microsomes by the following procedure (116). The microsomes are solubilized with sodium cholate in the presence of 20% glycerol, and the solubilized cytochrome $P450_{14DM}$ is precipitated with ammonium sulfate between 35 and 60% saturation. The concentrated cytochrome is chromatographed with an aminohexyl-Sepharose 4B (AH-Sepharose 4B, Pharmacia) column. The partially purified preparation (specific content, 5–7 nmol/mg protein) of the cytochrome obtained is further purified by successive column chromatography with hydroxyapatite and CM-Sephadex C-50 to give a purified preparation (specific content, 13–15 nmol/mg protein) (113, 116). The overall yield of the cytochrome from the microsomes is 30–40% (113, 116), indicating that $P450_{14DM}$ is the predominant cytochrome P450 of microsomes. The purified preparation does not lose its catalytic activity for more than 1 year when it is stored at −70°C in the presence of 20% glycerol (116).

A monomeric molecular weight for $P450_{14DM}$ is estimated to be 58,000 by polyacrylamide gel electrophoresis in the presence of sodium dodecylsulfate (116). Oxidized $P450_{14DM}$ shows the Soret band at 417 nm and no absorption band at 650 nm (Fig. 11-5) (113, 116). These spectral characteristics indicate that the oxidized form is in a low-spin state. The low-spin nature of ferric $P450_{14DM}$ is further confirmed by the electron paramagnetic resonance spec-

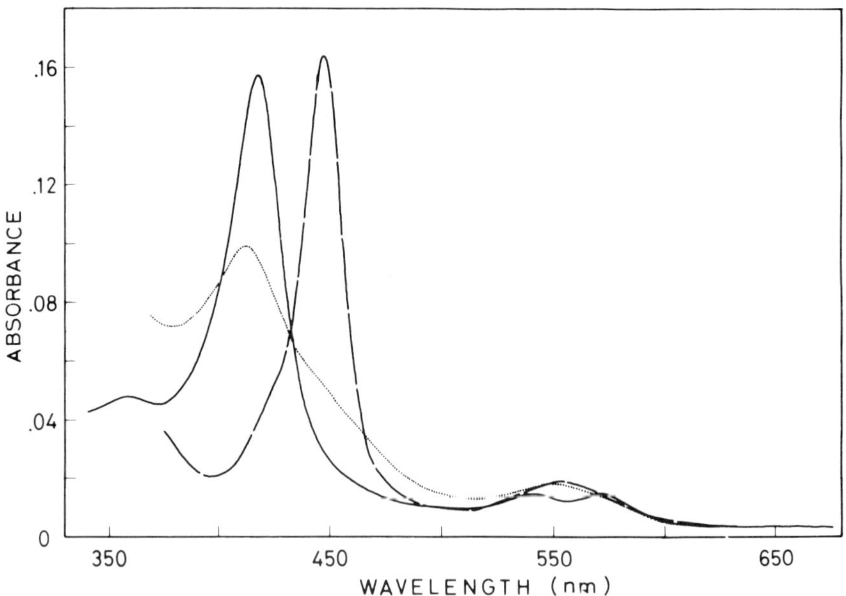

FIG. 11-5. Absorption spectra of purified $P450_{14DM}$ (113). Oxidized form (*solid line*), reduced form by sodium dithionite (*dotted line*), and reduced CO complex (*dashed line*).

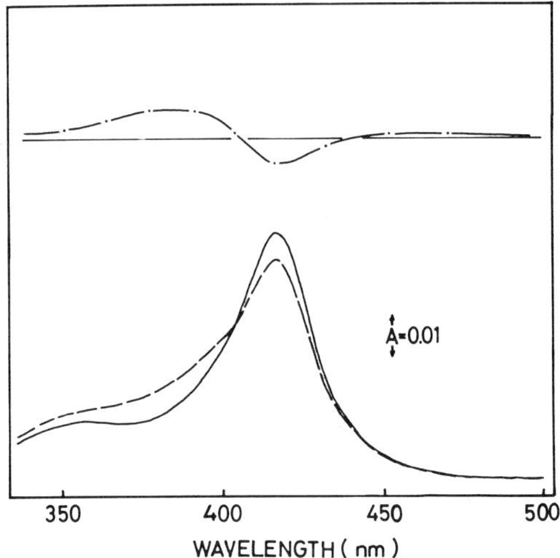

FIG. 11-6. The spectral change of $P450_{14DM}$ induced by lanosterol (121). Substrate-free oxidized form before addition of lanosterol (*solid line*) (A), absorption spectrum observed in the presence of excess lanosterol (*dashed line*) (B), and the type I difference spectrum induced by lanosteol depicted by subtracting spectrum A from B (*dotted/dashed line*).

trum showing three characteristic signals at $g = 1.92, 2.27$, and 2.45 (116). The Soret band of the reduced CO complex that is characteristic of cytochrome P450 is observed at 447 nm (Fig. 11-5) (113, 116).

Lanosterol induces the type I spectral change on ferric $P450_{14DM}$ (Fig. 11-6), indicating that it is binding to the active site near the heme molecule (7, 116). Lanosterol is the only compound that induces the type I spectral change for $P450_{14DM}$ (7). However, the spectral change is incomplete (Fig. 11-6) and the spectrophotometrically determined high-spin content in the presence of excess lanosterol does not exceed 20% (116). This fact indicates that the lanosterol-bound form of $P450_{14DM}$ is in an equilibrium between high- and low-spin states. An apparent dissociation constant of lanosterol determined by the spectral titration is 7 μM (116), which is comparable to the Km of lanosterol (see below). Basic amines which induce the type II spectral change of many cytochromes P450 induce the type II spectral change for $P450_{14DM}$ (111). They include metyrapone, imidazole, pyridine, and their derivatives. Among them, metyrapone acts as a moderate inhibitor for $P450_{14DM}$ (12). Azole antifungal agents, the potent inhibitors for $P450_{14DM}$, also induce the type II spectral change (121). This will be discussed later.

Cytochrome P450 is known to be denatured by treatment with chaotropic salts, mercurials, and bile acids (43). This denaturation converts the cytochrome into the denatured form called "P420," which shows the Soret peak of the reduced CO complex at 420 nm (74, 75). $P450_{14DM}$ is relatively resistant to such denaturation. For example, complete conversion of $P450_{14DM}$ to the

P420 form in the presence of 1 M potassium thiocyanate requires 150 minutes at room temperature (111, 113, 116).

Catalytic Properties

A reconstituted system consisting of $P450_{14DM}$ and NADPH-cytochrome P450 reductase purified from yeast microsomes catalyzes the conversion of lanosterol to 4,4-dimethy-5α-cholesta-8,14,24-trien-3β-ol (6, 12). This activity is dependent upon both the cytochrome and the reductase; it also requires NADPH and molecular oxygen (12). It is thus clear that $P450_{14DM}$ constitutes an electron transport system together with the reductase and catalyzes 14α-demethylation of lanosterol. Under standard assay conditions, the system converts lanosterol to the corresponding metabolite at a rate of 8–10 nmol/minute/nmol $P450_{14DM}$ (12), with an apparent Km for lanosterol of 6 μM (13). 24,25-Dihydrolanosterol can also serve as a substrate and is converted to the corresponding 14-demethylated product. However, an apparent Km for 24,25-dihydrolanosterol (20 μM) is more than three times larger than that for lanosterol (13).

It was reported by Mitropoulos, Akhtar, and their colleagues (1, 4, 65, 102) that the 14α-methyl group (C-32) of lanosterol was removed as formic acid

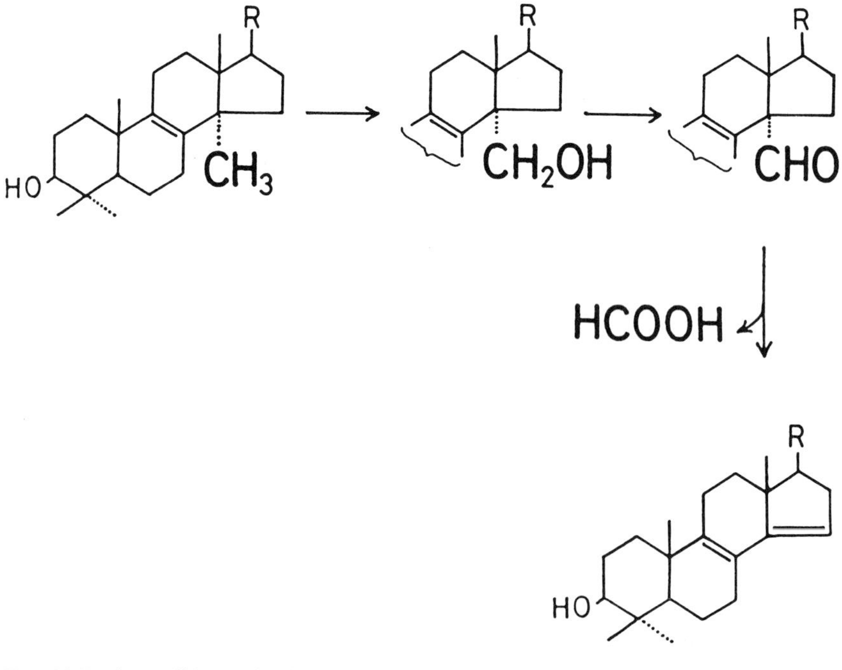

Fig. 11-7. A possible mechanism for the removal of C-32 from lanosterol catalyzed by $P450_{14DM}$ (12).

and the sterol was converted to 4,4-dimethyl-5α-cholesta-8,14,24-trien-3β-ol upon incubation with yeast or liver microsomes in the presence of NADPH and molecular oxygen. Judging from the chemical structure of the products, the demethylation probably occurs as illustrated in Fig. 11-7 (2, 3, 12). The cytochrome must catalyze the entire process of the demethylation, which consists of three oxygenation reactions (12). Recently, we found that 32-hydroxy-24,25-dihydrolanosterol was converted to 4,4-dimethyl-5α-cholesta-8,14-dien-3β-ol by the reconstituted system, and the rate of this conversion was considerably higher than that of 24,25-dihydrolanosterol to the same metabolite (13). It can thus be concluded that the rate-limiting step of the demethylation is the initial hydroxylation of the 14-methyl group. This is consistent with the observation that intermediates do not accumulate during the metabolism of lanosterol or 24,25-dihydrolanosterol by the reconstituted system (12).

$P450_{14DM}$ is readily reduced by NADPH in the reconstituted system (Fig. 11-8, curve B) (12). However, the rate of reduction is markedly decreased

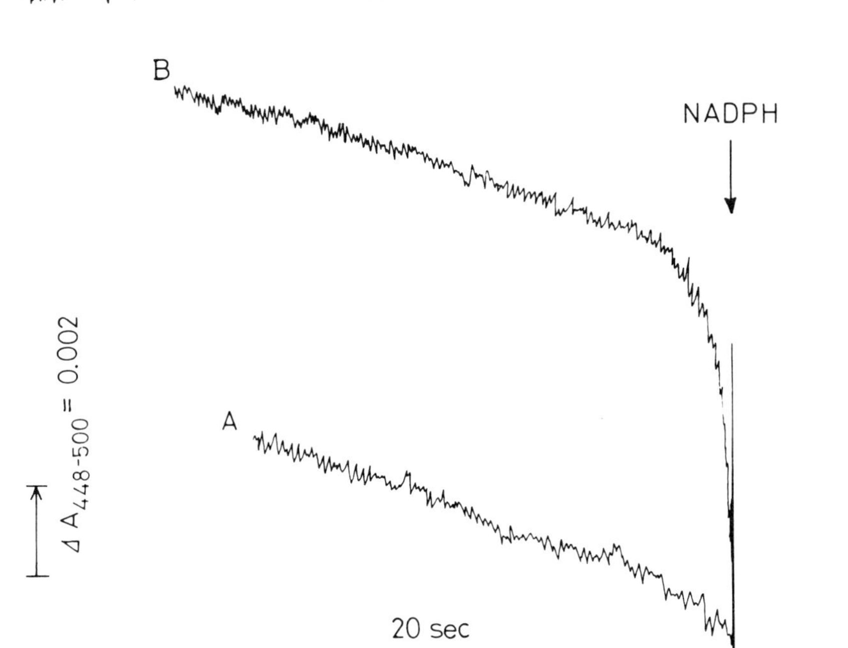

FIG. 11-8. Reduction kinetics of $P450_{14DM}$ in the reconstituted system (12). $P450_{14DM}$ in the reconstituted system was reduced by NADPH under CO atmosphere. Reduction of the cytochrome was recorded by increments of absorption difference between 448 and 500 nm due to the formation of the reduced CO complex. Trace A = lanosterol was omitted from the reaction system. Trace B = lanosterol was added to the reaction system.

when lanosterol or dihydrolanosterol is omitted from the reaction system (Fig. 11-8, curve A) (12). This fact indicates that $P450_{14DM}$ has a regulatory mechanism to repress idling of the redox cycle in the absence of the substrate.

$P450_{14DM}$ of a Mutant Yeast that is Defective in Lanosterol 14α-Demethylation

Recently, Yoshida et al (118, 119) purified a cytochrome P450 ($P450_{SG1}$) from a nystatin-resistant mutant, *S. cerevisiae* SG1, which was defective in lanosterol 14α-demethylation (10, 94, 95). $P450_{SG1}$ is immunochemically the same protein as $P450_{14DM}$, and peptide maps of $P450_{SG1}$ are superimposable on those of $P450_{14DM}$ (10, 119). This indicates that $P450_{SG1}$ is essentially the same protein as $P450_{14DM}$. However, $P450_{SG1}$ can not catalyze lanosterol 14α-demetylation (10, 119) and spectrophotometric characteristics of $P450_{SG1}$ are slightly but clearly different from those of $P450_{14DM}$ (118). The absorption spectrum of ferric $P450_{SG1}$ indicates that an imidazole group of a histidine residue in the apoprotein binds to the heme-iron at the sixth coordination position. The sixth coordination position of the native ferric $P450_{14DM}$ must be occupied by a water molecule as believed for other low-spin cytochromes P450 (22, 35, 104, 114, 117, and Fig. 11-4). $P450_{SG1}$ is thus considered as an altered molecule of $P450_{14DM}$ which loses catalytic activity. $P450_{SG1}$ can not interact with buthiobate (10), a compound which interacts specifically with $P450_{14DM}$ (11). Thus, the reactivity of $P450_{14DM}$ with the antifungal agent is closely related to its catalytic ability.

$P450_{14DM}$ of Other Fungi

Removal of C-32 from lanosterol or 24,25-dihydrolanosterol is indispensable for ergosterol biosynthesis by fungi. The same reaction occurs during cholesterol biosynthesis by mammals, and a cytochrome P450 corresponding to $P450_{14DM}$ has been found in rat liver microsomes (86, 96, 97). Accordingly, $P450_{14DM}$ is considered to be distributed widely in eukaryotes and apparently occurs in fungi which possess de novo synthesis of ergosterol. Actually, we have found that lanosterol 14α-demethylase activity of several yeasts was inhibited by buthiobate, one of the potent inhibitors for $P450_{14DM}$, as well as CO (Aoyama Y, and Yoshida Y, unpublished result). We also found that rabbit antibodies to $P450_{14DM}$ of *S. cerevisiae* (12) inhibited the demethylase activity of some yeasts, although the inhibition was weaker than that observed with *S. cerevisiae* microsomes (Aoyama Y, and Yoshida Y, unpublished results). Furthermore there are many studies (16, 41, 49, 62, 79, 92, 99) describing accumulation of 14-methylsterols in pathogenic fungi treated with antifungal agents known to inhibit $P450_{14DM}$. However, no attempt has been made to isolate and characterize the $P450_{14DM}$.

The initial step of lanosterol metabolism in yeasts is the 14α-demethylation by $P450_{14DM}$. A large amount of the sterol is known to accumulate in a mutant yeast, *S. cerevisiae* SG1 (94, 95), which is defective in $P450_{14DM}$ (10). In contrast, there are some studies (16, 41, 49, 62, 92, 99, 101) describing the observation that many fungi treated with an antifungal agent known to inhibit $P450_{14DM}$ will result in the accumulation of 24-methylene-24,25-dihydrolanosterol rather than lanosterol. This suggests that lanosterol is first methylated at C-24 and then 24-methylene-24, 25-dihydrolanosterol undergoes 14α-demethylation (Fig. 11-9). Accordingly, the substrate specificity of *S. cerevisiae* $P450_{14DM}$ is somewhat different from that of the cytochrome of other fungi.

Other Cytochromes P450 Found in Fungi

P450 that Catalyzes 22-Desaturation of 22,23-Dihydroergosterol ($P450_{22DS}$)

Desaturation at C-22 during ergosterol biosynthesis (Fig. 11-9) by *S. cerevisiae* is catalyzed by a cytochrome P450 known as $P450_{22DS}$ (37, 38). Although this cytochrome has not yet been isolated, several lines of evidence indicate that $P450_{22DS}$ is different from $P450_{14DM}$ (38). For example, rabbit antibodies to $P450_{14DM}$ (12) do not inhibit the 22-desaturation catalyzed by *S. cerevisiae* microsomes. The 22-desaturation is insensitive to buthiobate and N-substituted azoles, which are potent inhibitors of $P450_{14DM}$ (12, 101). Furthermore, a yeast mutant, *S. cerevisiae* SG1, that is defective in lanosterol 14α-demethylation (see the preceding section) has 22-desaturase activity. In contrast, another mutant *S. cerevisiae* N22, which is defective in the 22-desaturase, can convert lanosterol to 4,4-dimethylzymosterol (38).

$P450_{22DS}$ is the first example of cytochrome P450 which catalyzes a desaturation reaction, and the 22-desaturation of 22,23-dihydroergosterol is the first example of a cytochrome P450-dependent desaturation reaction. As described in the preceding section, other desaturations occurring in microsomes of yeast and mammals are mediated by another type of terminal oxidase (Fig. 11-2).

Recently, Takano et al (92) reported that a newly developed triazole antifungal agent, diniconazole (S-3308), inhibited 22-desaturation as well as lanosterol 14α-demethylation. $P450_{22DS}$ is thus considered to be a new target for azole antifungal agents. The cytochrome is not always the target for antifungal agents which inhibit $P450_{14DM}$ because of its insensitivity for buthiobate (38).

Cytochrome P450 that Catalyzes Alkane Hydroxylation

The initial step of alkane metabolism by petroleum-assimilating yeasts is a cytochrome P450-dependent hydroxylation of *n*-alkanes. The cytochrome

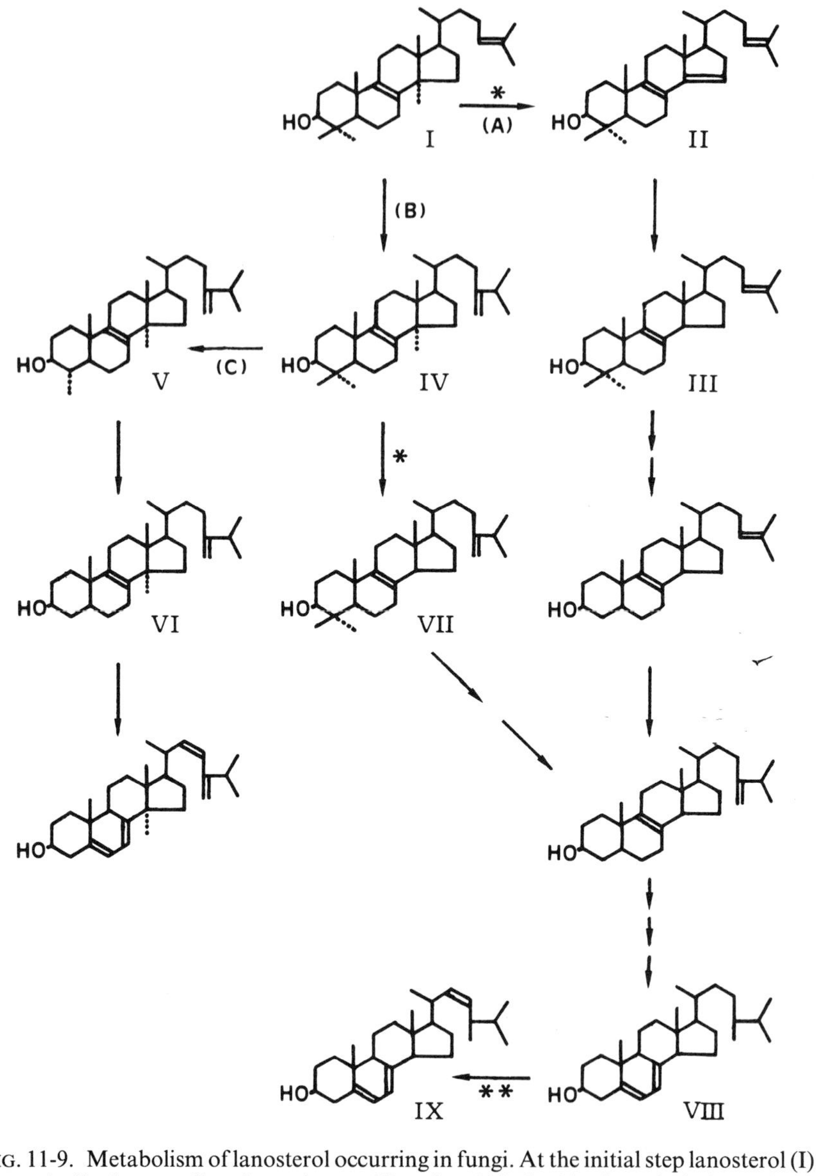

FIG. 11-9. Metabolism of lanosterol occurring in fungi. At the initial step lanosterol (I) is metabolized to two directions; the one (direction A) is the 14α-demethylation to form 4,4-dimethyl-5α-cholesta-8,14,24-trien-3β-ol (II), and the other (direction B) is the transmethylation at C-24 to form 24-methylene-24,25-dihydrolanosterol (IV). In yeasts, direction A is predominant and I is metabolized to ergosterol via II and 4,4-dimethylzymosterol (III), whereas direction B must be the main pathway for molds, and ergosterol is synthesized from I via IV and 4,4-dimethylfecosterol (VII). $P450_{14DM}$ mediates the conversion of I to II and IV to VII as indicated by asterisks. If $P450_{14DM}$ is inhibited or deficient, I may be metabolized to direction C, and 14-methylsterols such as obtusifoliol (V) and 14-methylfecosterol (VI) are accumulated together with I (yeasts) or IV (molds). The 22-desaturation of 22,23-dihydroergosterol (VIII) to ergosterol (IX) indicated by a double asterisk is catalyzed by another cytochrome P450 ($P450_{22DS}$).

P450 participating in this metabolism is induced when the yeast is grown aerobically on *n*-alkanes (64, 90, 91). The molecular and catalytic properties of the cytochrome described below clearly indicate that the alkane-metabolizing cytochrome P450 is a unique species of cytochrome P450 that is different from either $P450_{14DM}$ or $P450_{22DS}$. Attempts to isolate this cytochrome from alkane-grown *C. tropicalis* were made by Duppel et al (24) and by Bertrand et al (17). A homogenous preparation of this cytochrome was isolated by Riege et al (80) from alkane-grown *Lodderomyces elongisporus*.

Cytochrome P450 purified from *L. elongisporus* catalyzes hydroxylation of long-chain alkanes in the presence of NADPH-cytochrome P450 reductase, NADPH, and molecular oxygen (80). Hexadecane, a physiologic substrate for the cytochrome, induces the type I spectral change of the cytochrome, and basic amines such as imidazole and aniline induce the type II spectral change (68).

The alkane-hydroxylating cytochrome P450 of *C. tropicalis* catalyzes hydroxylation of long-chain alkanes and fatty acids (17, 24) in essentially the same manner as in the *L. elongisporus* system. Duppel et al (24) also reported that the *C. tropicalis* system catalyzed oxidative metabolism of some drug substances. However, such activity was not observed with the *L. elongisporus* system (68) and the cytochrome preparations from *C. tropicalis* still contained considerable impurities. Consequently, it has not been confirmed whether or not the hydroxylation of alkanes and drugs are catalyzed by the same cytochrome P450.

Cytochrome P450 that Catalyzes Hydroxylation of Carcinogens

In 1982, Azari et al (14) isolated a cytochrome P450 (P448) which catalyzed hydroxylation of benzo[a]pyrene from *S. cerevisiae* cells cultivated aerobically using a high concentration of glucose for a long duration. This cytochrome shows the type I spectral change upon addition of benzo[a]pyrene (14, 53, 106). Judging from the yield, this cytochrome appears to be the major cytochrome P450 component of these cells. As described in the preceding section, the major component of cytochrome P450 of *S. cerevisiae* grown on glucose under semianaerobic conditions is $P450_{14DM}$. $P450_{14DM}$ does not react with benzo[a]pyrene (Aoyama and Yoshida, unpublished observation). Therefore, the cytochrome P450 purified by Azari et al (14, 53) may be different from $P450_{14DM}$, although both of them are considered to be major cytochrome P450 components of *S. cerevisiae*. The cultivation conditions used by Azari et al (14) and by us (109, 116) are considerably different. Thus, *S. cerevisiae* may change its major cytochrome P450 component in response to growth conditions such as glucose concentration, oxygen tension, and the duration of cultivation. At the present time, however, a possibility that the cytochrome P450 purified by Azari et al (14, 53) is the same molecular species as $P450_{14DM}$ can not be completely ruled out.

Effects of Azole Antifungal Agents on Purified $P450_{14DM}$

Inhibition of Lanosterol 14α-Demethylation

$P450_{14DM}$ is proposed to be a target for azole antifungal agents (101). In fact, azole antifungal agents such as ketoconazole, itraconazole, triadimefon, and triadimenol inhibited lanosterol 14α-demethylation by the reconstituted system consisting of $P450_{14DM}$ and NADPH-cytochrome P450 reductase (121, 122). These compounds also inhibited the enzymatic reduction of $P450_{14DM}$ by NADPH in the reconstituted system (121). However, they do not inhibit NADPH-cytochrome *c* reductase activity catalyzed by the P450 reductase itself (121). These antifungal agents induce marked spectral changes of $P450_{14DM}$ at low concentrations (121, 122). Consequently, it can be concluded that azole antifungal agents interact with $P450_{14DM}$ and inhibit the activity of the cytochrome. Fig. 11-10 represents dose-response profiles of the inhibition experiments with ketoconazole, itraconazole, and triadimefon. The concentration of these antifungal agents necessary to inhibit the demethylase activity is extremely low, and the complete inhibition by ketoconazole or itraconazole is observed when they are added at an equal concentration to $P450_{14DM}$. This suggests that these antifungal agents inhibit the demethylase activity by forming stoichiometric complexes with $P450_{14DM}$. Their affinity for the cytochrome is extremely high.

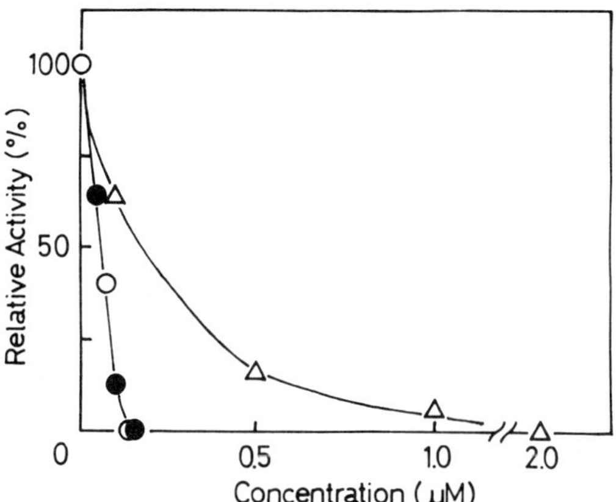

FIG. 11-10. Inhibition of $P450_{14DM}$-catalyzed lanosterol 14α-demethylation by azole antifungal agents (122). Effects of ketoconazole (*open circles*), itraconazole (*closed circles*), and triadimefon (*open triangles*) on lanosterol 14α-demethylation by the reconstituted system containing 0.14 μM of $P450_{14DM}$ were assayed. Inhibition by ketoconazole (*open circles*) or itraconazole (*closed circles*) reached 100% when they were added at the concentration equivalent to $P450_{14DM}$.

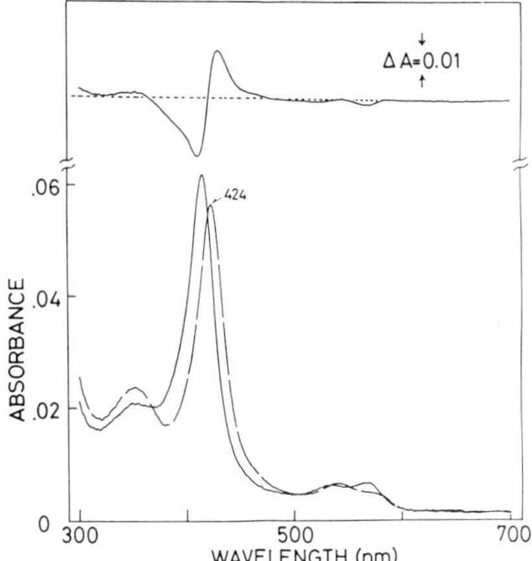

FIG. 11-11. Spectrophotometric detection of interaction of ketoconazole with ferric $P450_{14DM}$ (121). Ferric $P450_{14DM}$ (*solid line*) was converted to the ketoconazole complex (*dashed line*) by the addition of stoichiometric amount of the antifungal agent. The upper spectrum represents ketoconazole-induced type II spectrum.

Spectrophotometric Analysis of the Interaction Between Azole Antifungal Agents and Purified $P450_{14DM}$

Azole antifungal agents form one-to-one complexes with oxidized $P450_{14DM}$ and induce a type II spectral change of the cytochrome (100, 121, 122). Fig. 11-11 represents the ketoconazole-induced spectral change of $P450_{14DM}$, and Fig. 11-12 shows spectral titration of the cytochrome with the antifungal agent. Essentially the same results are obtained with other antifungal agents such as itraconazole, triadimefon, and triadimenol. Absorption spectra of azole antifungal agent complexes of ferric $P450_{14DM}$ show their Soret band at 420–424 nm, suggesting that the azole groups of these compounds interact with the heme-iron of the cytochrome. As described in the previous section, the type II spectral change of various cytochrome P450 species is induced by many nitrogen-containing heterocycles, and $P450_{14DM}$ shows the type II spectral change upon binding with pyridine, imidazole, and so forth. Affinity of these ligands for $P450_{14DM}$ is not too high (apparent Kd values of 0.5 mM or more). In contrast, the cytochrome shows high affinity for azole antifungal agents. For example, binding of ketoconazole to the cytochrome is quantitative (Fig. 11-12) and the Kd is assumed to be less than 0.01 μM. This suggests that azole antifungal agents interact with $P450_{14DM}$ not only at the heme-iron, but also at some region in the apoprotein. The latter interaction may determine their affinity for the cytochrome.

Azole antifungal agents interact with reduced $P450_{14DM}$. Fig. 11-13 represents spectral change caused by reduction of the itraconazole com-

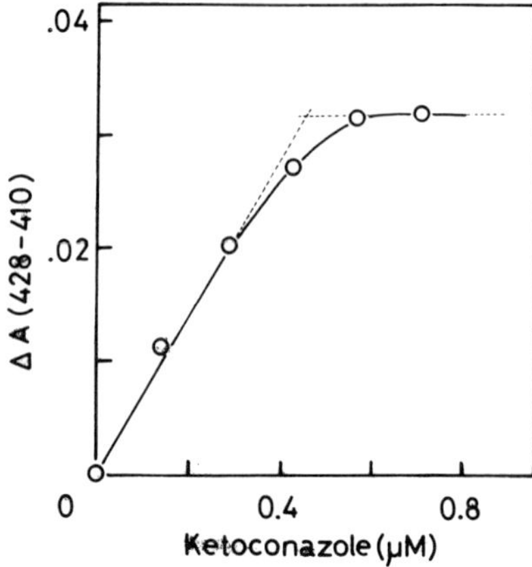

FIG. 11-12. Spectral titration of ferric $P450_{14DM}$ with ketoconazole (121). Ferric $P450_{14DM}$ (0.42 μM) was titrated with ketoconazole by means of the spectral change shown in Fig. 11-11. Ketoconazole binds to the cytochrome with a one-to-one stoichiometry.

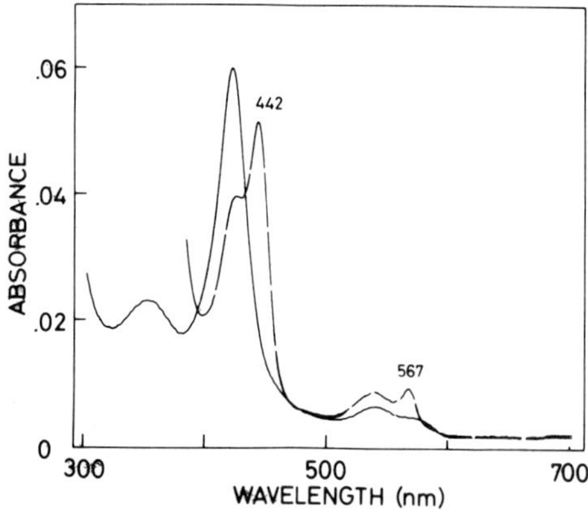

FIG. 11-13. Spectral change of itraconazole complex of ferric $P450_{14DM}$ caused by reduction with sodium dithionite (121). The itraconazole complex of ferric $P450_{14DM}$ (*solid line*) was reduced to the ferrous complex (*dashed line*) by the addition of sodium dithionite. The ferrous complex can be formed only by the reduction of the ferric complex and it can not be formed by the addition of the antifungal agent to ferrous $P450_{14DM}$.

plex of ferric $P450_{14DM}$ with sodium dithionite. The absorption spectrum of the reduced complex shows the characteristics of a hexa-coordinated ferrous low-spin complex (23), indicating the binding of the triazole group to the reduced heme-iron (121, 122). All azole antifungal agents so far tested can interact with the reduced heme-iron of $P450_{14DM}$ (121, 122). However, the absorption spectra of these complexes are different from one another, indicating that the mode of interaction of each compound is different (121, 122).

It is well known that the reduced form of cytochrome P450 combines avidly with CO and forms the reduced CO complex having the Soret band at approximately 450 nm. Vanden Bossche and associates (98, 100) reported that ketoconazole and itraconazole interfer with the appearance of the Soret band at 448 nm in the reduced CO difference spectrum of yeast microsomes. The absorption spectrum for the itraconazole complex of reduced $P450_{14DM}$ shown in Fig. 11-13 was not affected by the addition of CO. Similarly, the ketoconazole complex of ferrous $P450_{14DM}$ reacted with CO at a very low rate. These observations clearly indicate that itraconazole and ketoconazole, which have large substituents at N-1 of their azole groups, interfere with binding of CO to the ferrous $P450_{14DM}$. It is well known that CO inhibits oxygen activation by the cytochrome (see Fig. 11-13). It can be assumed that these antifungal agents can inhibit oxygen activation by $P450_{14DM}$. In contrast, the triadimefon complex of the reduced $P450_{14DM}$ is readily converted to the reduced CO complex upon addition of CO (Fig. 11-14). The same phenomenon has been observed with the buthiobate and triadimenol complexes of the cytochrome (11). These facts indicate that an antifungal agent that has a relatively small substituent at the N-1 of its azole group shows practically no interference with the binding of CO to $P450_{14DM}$, although it inhibits the activity of the cytochrome. Accordingly, interference of CO binding or oxygen activation may not be essential for the inhibitory action of azole antifungal agents on $P450_{14DM}$.

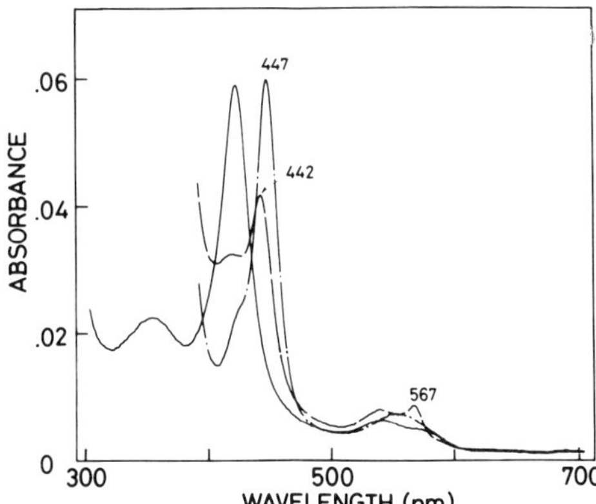

FIG. 11-14. Spectral change of the triadimefon complex of ferric $P450_{14DM}$ caused by the reduction with sodium dithionite after addition of CO (121). The ferric and ferrous complexes of $P450_{14DM}$ with triadimefon are expressed by the *solid line* and *dashed line*, respectively. Addition of CO to the ferrous complex immediately converted it to the ferrous CO-complex (*dashed/dotted line*).

Possible Mechanism of Interaction Between Azole Antifungal Agents and $P450_{14DM}$

As described above, an azole antifungal agent combines with $P450_{14DM}$ both in oxidized and reduced states with a one-to-one stoichiometry (120, 121, 122). An azole antifungal agent interacts with the cytochrome at two sites; the azole moiety coordinates to the heme-iron and the substituent at N-1 of the azole moiety interacts with the apoprotein near the heme (Fig. 11-15) (121, 122).

Interaction of the N-1 substituent of an azole antifungal agent with the cytochrome is believed to occur at the substrate-binding site or a site closely linked to this site near the sixth coordination position of the heme. Affinity of an azole antifungal agent for the cytochrome may be determined by this interaction. This interaction must inhibit the binding or access of a substrate to the active site and play the predominant role in the inhibition. Steric hinderance is not important for determining the affinity of an azole antifungal agent for the cytochrome because itraconazole, which has the largest substituent, shows the highest affinity. In other words, some stereospecific interaction of the N-1 substituents with the apoprotein must be important.

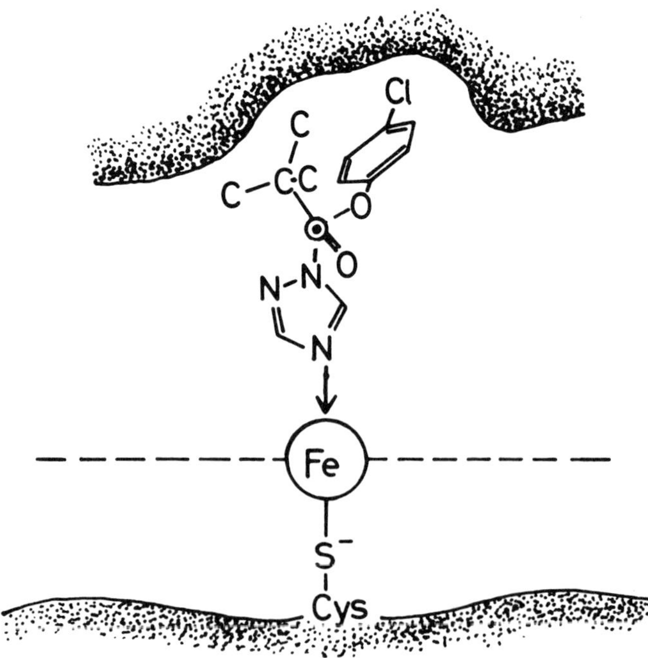

Fig. 11-15. Schematic representation of a possible interaction of triadimefon with the active site of $P450_{14DM}$ (122). Azole antifungal agents interact with $P450_{14DM}$ at two sites; the one is the sixth coordination position of the heme and the other at a site in the apoprotein above the sixth coordination position.

Recently, we found that $P450_{14DM}$ could discriminate the enantiomers of diniconazole (S-3308) (120). This finding provides further support for the importance of the stereospecific interaction between the N-1 substituent and the apoprotein.

The azole group is essential for the antifungal activity of azole antifungal agents (61). As shown in Fig. 11-15, the azole group binds to the sixth coordination position of the heme-iron, which is the oxygen-activating site of the cytochrome. However, many small azole antifungal agents may not inhibit oxygen activation at the heme-iron because they are readily replaced by CO; ferrous $P450_{14DM}$ bound with them is highly autooxidizable. Accordingly, interference of oxygen activation by binding of an azole group to the heme-iron is not essential for the inhibition of lanosterol 14α-demethylation by azole antifungal agents. Another possible role of binding of the azole group to the heme iron as part of the inhibitory mechanism, may involve modifications of the reducibility of $P450_{14DM}$. Actually, all azole antifungal agents so far tested inhibit enzymatic reduction of $P450_{14DM}$ by NADPH. This possibility is still speculative because effects of azole antifungal agents on the redox potential of $P450_{14DM}$ have not yet been determined. Furthermore, there is another explanation for the inhibition of $P450_{14DM}$ reduction by azole antifungal agents; the inhibition results from the interference of binding of lanosterol to the substrate site of the cytochrome because the rate of reduction of $P450_{14DM}$ is slow unless it binds with lanosterol or 24,25-dihydrolanosterol (see Fig. 11-8) (12). Finally, it is noteworthy that azole groups may have some potent synergistic effect that increases the affinity of antifungal agents for the cytochrome, because azole antifungal agents interact with the cytochrome both at the heme-iron with their azole groups and at the apoprotein with the N-1 substituents. In any case, the role of azole groups on the inhibitory effect of azole antifungal agents has yet to be clarified.

Summary

Cytochromes of fungi are essentially similar to those of animals. Cytochromes of fungi constitute two electron transport systems occurring in mitochondria and the endoplasmic reticulum. The former system, called the respiratory chain, contributes to cellular respiration and ATP generation, whereas the latter system, named the microsomal electron transport system, is responsible for biosynthesis of several cellular components.

The oxidative metabolism of lanosterol, that is included in the biosynthetic pathway of ergosterol, is one of the important functions of the microsomal electron transport system, which is catalyzed by $P450_{14DM}$. Many azole antifungal agents avidly combine with $P450_{14DM}$ and inhibit the oxidative removal of C-32 (the 14α-demethylation) of lanosterol. This inhibition causes depletion of ergosterol and accumulation of 14-methylsterols in the membrane of fungal cells. Such change in sterol composition disturbs membrane function and results in growth inhibition and death of the fungal cells. Accordingly, $P450_{14DM}$ is considered as the primary target for azole antifungal agents.

Cytochrome P450, which mediates the 14α-demethylation of lanosterol, is also present in mammalian cells. Mammalian cells contain various species of cytochrome P450 which are responsible for many important cellular metabolic functions. If azole antifungal agents inhibit mammalian cytochrome P450 too, their systemic use may result in potentially significant adverse reactions. The high selectivity of azole antifungal agents for fungal $P450_{14DM}$ will be necessary for their systemic application. Binding ability of an azole antifungal agent to $P450_{14DM}$ is predominantly determined by the substituent at N-1 of the azole group, and the substituent must interact with the substrate site of the cytochrome. Extensive modification of the N-1 substituents and the screening of newly developed compounds with respect to the selectivity to fungal $P450_{14DM}$ with some conventional methods will be necessary. For this project, a biochemical understanding of cytochrome P450 and other cytochromes is important.

References

1. Akhtar M, Watkinson IA, Rahimtula AD, Wilton DC, Munday KA: The role of a cholesta-8,14-dien-3β-ol system in cholesterol biosynthesis. *Biochem J* 111: 757–761, 1969.
2. Akhtar M, Freeman CW, Wilton DC, Boar RB, Copsey DB: The pathway for the removal of the 14α-methyl group of lanosterol. The role of lanost-8-ene-3β,32-diol in cholesterol biosynthesis. *Bioorg Chem* 6:473–481, 1977.
3. Akhtar M, Alexander K, Boar RB, McGhie JF, Barton DHR: Chemical and enzymatic studies on the characterization of intermediates during the removal of the 14α-methyl group in cholesterol biosynthesis. The use of 32-functionalized lanosterol derivatives. *Biochem J* 169:449–463, 1978.
4. Alexander K, Akhtar M, Boar RB, McGhie JF, Barton DHR: The removal of the 32-carbon atom as formic acid in cholesterol biosynthesis. *J Chem Soc Chem Commun* 1972:383–385, 1972.
5. Aoyama Y, Yoshida Y, Kubota S, Kumaoka H, Furumichi A: NADPH-cytochrome P450 reductase of yeast microsomes. *Arch Biochem Biophys* 185: 362–369, 1978.
6. Aoyama Y, Yoshida Y: The 14α-demethylation of lanosterol by a reconstituted cytochrome P450 system from yeast microsomes. *Biochem Biophys Res Commun* 85:28–34, 1978.
7. Aoyama Y, Yoshida Y: Interaction of lanosterol to cytochrome P450 purified from yeast microsomes: Evidence for contribution of cytochrome P450 to lanosterol metabolism. *Biochem Biophys Res Commun* 82:33–38, 1978.
8. Aoyama Y, Okikawa T, Yoshida Y: Evidence for the presence of cytochrome P450 functional in lanosterol demethylation in microsomes of aerobically grown respiring yeast. *Biochim Biophys Acta* 665:596–601, 1981.
9. Aoyama Y, Yoshida Y, Sato R, Susani M, Ruis H: Involvement of cytochrome b_5 and a cyanide-sensitive monooxygenase in the 4-demethylation of 4,4-dimethylzymosterol by yeast microsomes. *Biochim Biophys Acta* 663:194–202, 1981.

10. Aoyama Y, Yoshida Y, Hata S, Nishino T, Katsuki H, Maitra US, Mohan VP, Sprinson DB: Altered cytochrome P450 in a yeast mutant blocked in demethylating C-32 of lanosterol. *J Biol Chem* 258:9040–9042, 1983.
11. Aoyama Y, Yoshida Y, Hata S, Nishino T, Katsuki H: Buthiobate: A potent inhibitor for yeast cytochrome P450 catalyzing 14α-demethylation of lanosterol. *Biochem Biophys Res Commun* 115:642–647, 1983.
12. Aoyama Y, Yoshida Y, Sato R: Yeast cytochrome P450 catalyzing lanosterol 14α-demethylation. II. Lanosterol metabolism by purified $P450_{14DM}$ and by intact microsomes. *J Biol Chem* 259:1661–1666, 1984.
13. Aoyama Y, Yoshida Y, Sonoda Y, Sato Y: Metabolism of 32-hydroxy-24,25-dihydrolanosterol by purified cytochrome $P450_{14DM}$ from yeast. Evidence for contribution of the cytochrome to whole process of lanosterol 14α-demethylation. *J Biol Chem* 262:1239–1243, 1987.
14. Azari MR, Wiseman A: Purification and characterization of the cytochrome P448 component of a benzo[a]pyrene hydroxylase from *Saccharomyces cerevisiae*. *Anal Biochem* 122:129–138, 1982.
15. Bach SJ, Dixon M, Keilin D: A new soluble cytochrome component from yeast. *Nature* 149:21, 1942.
16. Baldwin BC, Wiggins TE: Action of fungicidal triazoles of the dichlobutrazol series on *Ustilago maydis*. *Pesticide Sci* 15:156–166, 1984.
17. Bertrand JC, Gilewicz M, Bazin H, Zacek M, Azoulay E: Partial purification of cytochrome P450 of *Candida tropicalis* and reconstitution of hydroxylase activity. *FEBS Lett* 105:143–145, 1979.
18. Bosterling B, Trudell JR: Association of cytochrome b_5 and cytochrome P450 reductase with cytochrome P450 in the membrane of reconstituted vesicles. *J Biol Chem* 257:4783–4787, 1982.
19. Breskvar K, Hudnik-Plevnik T: A possible role of cytochrome P450 in hydroxylation of progesterone by *Rhizopus nigricans*. *Biochem Biophys Res Commun* 74:1192–1198, 1977.
20. Cerniglia CE, Gibson DT: Oxidation of benzo[a]pyrene by the filamentous fungus *Cunninghamella elegans*. *J Biol Chem* 254:12174–12180, 1979.
21. Cerniglia CE, Gibson DT: Fungal oxidation of benzo[a]pyrene and (±)-*trans*-7,8-dihydroxy-7,8-dihydrobenzo[a]pyrene. Evidence for the formation of a benzo[a]pyrene-7,8-diol-9,10-epoxide. *J Biol Chem* 255:5159–5163, 1980.
22. Dawson JH, Andersson LA, Sono M: Spectroscopic investigation of ferric cytochrome P450-CAM ligand complexes. Identification of the ligand *trans* to cysteinate in the native enzyme. *J Biol Chem* 257:3606–3617, 1982.
23. Dawson JH, Andersson LA, Sono M: The diverse spectroscopic properties of ferrous cytochrome P450-CAM ligand complexes. *J Biol Chem* 258:13637–13645, 1983.
24. Duppel W, Lebeault JM, Coon MJ: Properties of a yeast cytochrome P450-containing enzyme system which catalyzes the hydroxylation of fatty acids, alkanes, and drugs. *Eur J Biochem* 36:583–592, 1973.
25. Dutta D, Ghosh DK, Mishra AK, Samanta TB: Induction of benzo[a]pyrene hydroxylase in *Aspergillus ochraceus* TS. Evidences of multiple forms of cytochrome P450. *Biochem Biophys Res Commun* 115:692–699, 1983.
26. Ephrussi B, Slonimski PP: Effect of oxygen on the formation of respiratory enzymes in baker's yeast. *Compt Rend* 230:685–686, 1950.
27. Ephrussi B, Slonimski PP, Perrodin G: The adaptive synthesis of cytochromes in baker's yeast. *Biochim Biophys Acta* 6:256–267, 1950.
28. Ferris JP, MacDonald LH, Patrie MA, Martin MA: Aryl hydrocarbon hydroxylase activity in the fungus *Cunninghamella bainieri*. Evidence for the presence of cytochrome P450. *Arch Biochem Biophys* 175:443–452, 1976.
29. Fink H: Classification of culture yeasts with the aid of the cytochrome spectrum. *Hoppe-Seyler's Z Physiol Chem* 210:197–219, 1932.

30. Fujii-Kuriyama Y, Mizukami Y, Kawajiri K, Sogawa K, Muramatsu M: Primary structure of a cytochrome P450: Coding nucleotide sequence of phenobarbital-inducible cytochrome P450 cDNA from rat liver. *Proc Natl Acad Sci USA* 79:2793–2797, 1982.
31. Fujita VS, Black SD, Tarr GE, Koop DR, Coon MJ: On the amino acid sequence of cytochrome P450 isozyme 4 from rabbit liver microsomes. *Proc Natl Acad Sci USA* 81:4260–4264, 1984.
32. Gallo M, Bertrand JC, Azoulay E: Participation du cytochrome P450 dans l'oxydation des alcones chez *Candida tropicalis*. *FEBS Lett* 19:45–49, 1971.
32. Ghosh DK, Dutta D, Samanta TB, Mishra AK: Microsomal benzo[a]pyrene hydroxylase in *Aspergillus ochraceus* TS. Assay and characterization of the enzyme system. *Biochem Biophys Res Commun* 113:497–505, 1983.
34. Gonzalez FJ, Nebert DW, Hardwick JP, Kasper CB: Complete cDNA and protein sequence of a pregnenolone 16α-carbonitrile-induced cytochrome P450. A representative of a new gene family. *J Biol Chem* 260:7435–7441, 1985.
35. Griffin BW, Peterson JA: *Pseudomonas putida* cytochrome P450. The effect of complexes of the ferric hemoprotein on the relaxation of solvent water protons. *J Biol Chem* 250:6445–6451, 1975.
36. Haniu M, Armes LG, Yasunobu KT, Shastry BA, Gunsalus IC: Amino acid sequence of the *Pseudomonas putida* cytochrome P450. II. Cyanogen bromide peptides, acid cleavage peptides, and the complete sequence. *J Biol Chem* 257: 12664–12671, 1982.
37. Hata S, Nishino T, Komori M, Katsuki H: Involvement of cytochrome P450 in Δ^{22}-desaturation in ergosterol biosynthesis of yeast. *Biochem Biophys Res Commun* 103:272–277, 1981.
38. Hata S, Nishino T, Katsuki H, Aoyama Y, Yoshida Y: Two species of cytochrome P450 involved in ergosterol biosynthesis of yeast. *Biochem Biophys Res Commun* 116:162–166, 1983.
39. Hatefi Y, Stiggall DL: Metal-containing flavoprotein dehydrogenases, in Boyer PD (ed): *The Enzymes*, Vol. VIII, (3rd ed). New York, Academic Press, 1976, pp 263–269.
40. Heinemann FS, Ozols J: The complete amino acid sequence of rabbit phenobarbital-induced liver microsomal cytochrome P450. *J Biol Chem* 258: 4195–4201, 1983.
41. Henry MJ, Sisler HD: Effects of miconazole and dodecylimidazole on sterol biosynthesis in *Ustilago maydis*. *Antimicrob Agents Chemother* 15:603–607, 1979.
42. Imai Y, Sato R: Substrate interaction with hydroxylase system in liver microsomes. *Biochem Biophys Res Commun* 22:620–626, 1966.
43. Imai Y, Sato R: Conversion of P450 to P420 by neutral salts and some other reagents. *Eur J Biochem* 1:419–426, 1967.
44. Imai Y, Sato R: The role of cytochrome b_5 in a reconstituted N-demethylase system containing cytochrome P450. *Biochem Biophys Res Commun* 75:420–426, 1977.
45. Ishidate K, Kawaguchi K, Tagawa K: Change in P450 content accompanying aerobic formation of mitochondria in yeast. *J Biochem* 65:385–392, 1969.
46. Ishidate K, Kawaguchi K, Tagawa K, Hagihara B: Hemoproteins in anaerobically grown yast cells. *J Biochem* 65:375–383, 1969.
47. Jayanthi CR, Madyastha P, Madyastha KM: Microsomal 11α-hydroxylation of progesterone in *Aspergillus ochraceus*. I. Characterization of the hydroxylase system. *Biochem Biophys Res Commun* 106:1262–1268, 1982.
48. Jefcoate CRE, Gaylor JL, Calabrese RL: Ligand interactions with cytochrome P450. I. Binding of primary amines. *Biochemistry* 8:3455–3463, 1969.
49. Kato T, Kawase Y: Selective inhibition of the demethylation at C-14 in ergosterol

biosynthesis by the fungicide Denmert® (S-1358). *Agr Biol Chem* 40:2379–2388, 1976.
50. Kawajiri K, Gotoh O, Sogawa K, Tagashira Y, Muramatsu M, Fujii-Kuriyama Y: Coding nucleotide sequence of 3-methylcholanthreneinducible cytochrome P450d cDNA from rat liver. *Proc Nat Acad Sci USA* 81:1649–1653, 1984.
51. Keilin D: Cytochrome, a respiratory pigment, common to animals, yeast and higher plants. *Proc Roy Soc* B98:312–339, 1925.
52. King DJ, Azari MR, Wiseman A: The induction of cytochrome P448 dependent benzo[a]pyrene hydroxylase in *Saccharomyces cerevisiae*. *Biochem Biophys Res Commun* 105:1115–1121, 1982.
53. King DJ, Azari MR, Wiseman A: Studies on the properties of highly purified cytochrome P448 and its dependent activity benzo[a]pyrene hydroxylase, from *Saccharomyces cerevisiae*. *Xenobiotica* 14:187–206, 1984.
54. Körenlampi SO, Marin E, Hänninen OP: Effect of carbon source on the accumulation of cytochrome P450 in the yeast *Saccharomyces cerevisiae*. *Biochem J* 194:407–413, 1981.
55. Kubota S, Yoshida Y, Kumaoka H: Studies on the microsomal electron-transport system of anaerobically grown yeast. IV. Purification and characterization of NADH-cytochrome b_5 reductase. *J Biochem* 81:187–195, 1977.
56. Kubota S, Yoshida Y, Kumaoka H, Furumichi A: Studies on the microsomal electron-transport system of anaerobically grown yeast. V. Purification and characterization of NADPH-cytochrome *c* reductase. *J Biochem* 81:197–205, 1977.
57. Lebeault JM, Lode ET, Coon MJ: Fatty acid and hydrocarbon hydroxylation in yeast: Role of cytochrome P450 in *Candida tropicalis*. *Biochem Biophys Res Commun* 42:413–419, 1971.
58. Lindenmayer A, Estabrook RW: Low-temperature spectral studies on the biosynthesis of cytochromes in baker's yeast. *Arch Biochem Biophys* 78:66–82, 1958.
59. Lindenmayer A, Smith L: Cytochromes and other pigments of baker's yeast grown aerobically and anaerobically. *Biochim Biophys Acta* 93:445–461, 1964.
60. Lu AYH, West SB: Multiplicity of mammarian microsomal cytochromes P450. *Pharmacol Rev* 31:277–295. 1980.
61. Marchington AF: Role of computergraphics in the design of plant protection chemicals, in *Proc 10th International Congress on Plant Protection*, 1983, pp 201–208.
62. Marichal P, Gorrens J, Vanden Bossche H: The action of itraconazole and ketoconazole on growth and sterol synthesis in *Aspergillus fumigatus* and *Aspergillus niger*. *J Med Vet Mycol* 22:13–21, 1984.
63. Matthews DE, Van Etten HD: Detoxification of the phytoalexin pisatin by a fungal cytochrome P450. *Arch Biochem Biophys* 224:494–505, 1983.
64. Mauersberger S, Matyashova RN, Müller HG, Losinov AB: Influence of the growth substrate and the oxygen concentration in the medium on the cytochrome P450 content in *Candida guilliermondii*. *Eur J Appl Microbiol Biotechnol* 9:285–294, 1980.
65. Mitropoulos KA, Gibbons GF, Reeves BEA: Lanosterol 14α-demethylase. Similarity of the enzyme system from yeast and rat liver. *Steroids* 27:821–829, 1976.
66. Morohashi K, Fujii-Kuriyama Y, Okada Y, Sogawa K, Hirose T, Inayama S, Omura T: Molecular cloning and nucleotide sequence of cDNA for mRNA of mitochondrial cytochrome P450(SCC) of bovine adrenal cortex. *Proc Natl Acad Sci USA* 81:4647–4651, 1984.
67. Müller HG, Schunck WH, Riege P, Honeck H: The alkane-hydroxylating enzyme system of the yeast *Candida guilliermondii*. *Acta Biol Med Germ* 38:345–349, 1979.

68. Müller HG, Schunck WH, Riege P, Honeck H: Cytochrome P450 of microorganisms, in Ruckpaul K, Rein H (eds): *Cytochrome P450*. Berlin, Akademie-Verlag, 1984, pp 337–369.
69. Murphy G, Vogel G, Krippahl G, Lynen F: Patulin biosynthesis: The role of mixed-function oxidases in the hydroxylation of *m*-cresol. *Eur J Biochem* 49:443–455, 1974.
70. Ohba M, Sato R, Yoshida Y, Nishino T, Katsuki H: Involvement of cytochrome P450 and a cyanide-sensitive enzyme in different steps of lanosterol demethylation by yeast microsomes. *Biochem Biophys Res Commun* 85:21–27, 1978.
71. Ohnishi T, Kawaguchi K, Hagihara B: Preparation and some properties of yeast mitochondria. *J Biol Chem* 241:1797–1806, 1966.
72. Ohnishi T, Sottocasa G, Ernster L: Current approaches to the mechanism of energy-coupling in the respiratory chain. Studies with yeast mitochondria. *Bull Soc Chim Biol* 48:1189–1203, 1966.
73. Okayasu T, Nagao M, Ishibashi T, Imai Y: Purification and partial characterization of linoleoyl-CoA desaturase from rat liver microsomes. *Arch Biochem Biophys* 206:21–28, 1981.
74. Omura T, Sato R: The carbon monoxide-binding pigment of liver microsomes. I. Evidence for its hemoprotein nature. *J Biol Chem* 239:2370–2378, 1964.
75. Omura T, Sato R: The carbon monoxide-binding pigment of liver microsomes. II. Solubilization, purification, and properties, *J Biol Chem* 239:2379–2385, 1964.
76. Omura T: Introduction: Short history of cytochrome P450, in Sato, R, Omura T (eds): *Cytochrome P450*. Tokyo, Kodansha, and New York, Academic Press, 1978, pp 1–21.
77. Ono T, Takahashi K, Odani S, Konno H, Imai Y: Purification of squalene epoxidase from rat liver microsomes. *Biochem Biophys Res Commun* 96:522–528, 1980.
78. Osumi T, Nishino T, Katsuki H: Studies on the Δ^5-desaturation in ergosterol biosynthesis in yeast. *J Biochem* 85:819–826, 1979.
79. Ragsdale, NN: Specific effects of triarimol on sterol biosynthesis in *Ustilago maydis*. *Biochim Biophys Acta* 380:81–96, 1975.
80. Riege P, Schunck WH, Honeck H, Müller HG: Cytochrome P450 from *Lodderomyces elongisporus*: Its purification and some properties of the highly purified protein. *Biochem Biophys Res Commun* 98:527–534, 1981.
81. Ryder NS, Dupont MC: Properties of a particulate squalene epoxidase from *Candida albicans*. *Biochim Biophys Acta* 794:466–471, 1984.
82. Ryder NS, Dupont MC: Inhibition of squalene epoxidase by allylamine antimycotic compounds. A comparative study of the fungal and mammalian enzymes. *Biochem J* 230:765–770, 1985.
83. Sanglard D, Käppeli O, Fiechter A: Metabolic conditions determining the composition and catalytic activity of cytochrome P450 monooxygenases in *Candida tropicalis*. *J Bacteriol* 157:297–302, 1984.
84. Sato R: Distribution and physiological functions, in Sato R, Omura T (eds): *Cytochrome P450*. Tokyo, Kodansha, and New York, Academic Press, 1978, pp 23–35.
85. Schenkman JB, Remmer H, Estabrook RW: Spectral studies of drug interaction with hepatic microsomal cytochrome. *Mol Pharmacol* 3:113–123, 1967.
86. Shafiee A, Trzaskos JM, Paik YK, Gaylor JL: Oxidative demethylation of lanosterol in cholesterol biosynthesis: Accumulation of sterol intermediates. *J Lipid Res* 27:1–10, 1986.
87. Strittmatter P, Spatz L, Corcoran D, Rogers MJ, Setlow B, Redline R: Purification and properties of rat liver microsomal stearyl coenzyme A desaturase. *Proc Natl Acad Sci USA* 71:4565–4569, 1974.
88. Tagawa K: Induction and disappearance of cytochrome P450 in yeast cells, in

Sato R, Omura T (eds): *Cytochrome P450*. Tokyo, Kodansha, and New York, Academic Press, 1978, pp 202–208.
89. Tai HH, Bloch K: Squalene epoxidase of rat liver. *J Biol Chem* 247:3767–3773, 1972.
90. Takagi M, Moriya K, Yano K: Induction of cytochrome P450 in petroleum-assimilating yeast. I. Selection of a strain and basic characterization of cytochrome P450 induction in the strain. *Cell Mol Biol* 25:363–369, 1980.
91. Takagi M, Moriya K, Yano K: Induction of cytochrome P450 in petroleum-assimilating yeast. II. Comparison of protein synthesizing activity in the cells grown on glucose and *n*-tetradecane. *Cell Mol Biol* 25:371–375, 1980.
92. Takano H, Oguri Y, Kato T: Mode of action of (E)-1-(2,4-dichlorophenyl)-4,4-dimethyl-2-(1,2,4-triazol-1-yl)-1-penten-3-ol (S-3308) in *Ustilago maydis*. *J Pestic Sci* 8:575–582, 1983.
93. Tamura Y, Yoshida Y, Sato R, Kumaoka H: Fatty acid desaturase system of yeast microsomes. Involvement of cytochrome b_5-containing electron-transport chain. *Arch Biochem Biophys* 175:284–294, 1976.
94. Trocha PJ, Jasne SJ, Sprinson DB: Novel sterols in ergosterol deficient yeast mutants. *Biochem Biophys Res Commun* 59:666–671, 1974.
95. Trocha PJ, Jasne SJ, Sprinson DB: Yeast mutants blocked in removing the methyl group of lanosterol at C-14. Separation of sterols by high-pressure liquid chromatography. *Biochemistry* 16:4721–4726, 1977.
96. Trzaskos JM, Bowen WD, Shafiee A, Fischer T, Gaylor JL: Cytochrome P450-dependent oxidation of lanosterol in cholesterol biosynthesis. Microsomal electron transport and C-32 demethylation. *J Biol Chem* 259:13402–13412, 1984.
97. Trzaskos JM, Kawata S, Gaylor JL: Microsomal enzymes of cholesterol biosynthesis. Purification of lanosterol 14α-methyl demethylase cytochrome P450 from hepatic microsomes. *J Biol Chem* 261:14651–14657, 1986.
98. Vanden Bossche H, Ruysschaert JM, Defrise-Quertain F, Willemsens G, Marichal CE, Cools W, Van Cutsem J: The interaction of miconazole and ketoconazole with lipids. *Biochem Pharmacol* 31:2609–2617, 1982.
99. Vanden Bossche H, Lauwers W, Willemsens G, Marichal P, Cornelissen F, Cools W: Molecular bases for the antimycotic and antibacterial activity of N-substituted imidazoles and triazoles: The inhibition of isoprenoid biosynthesis. *Pesticide Sci* 15:188–198, 1984.
100. Vanden Bossche H, Willemsens G, Marichal P, Cools W, Lauwers W: The molecular basis for the antifungal activities of N-substituted azole derivatives. Focus on R51 211, in Trinci APJ, Ryley JF (eds): *The Symposium of British Mycological Society, Mode of Action of Antifungal Agents*. Cambridge, Cambridge University Press, 1984, pp 321–341.
101. Vanden Bossche H: Biochemical target for antifungal azole derivatives: Hypothesis on the mode of action, in McGinnis MR (ed): *Current Topics in Medical Mycology*, Vol. 1. New York, Springer-Verlag, 1985, pp 313–351.
102. Watkinson IA, Akhtar M: The formation of an 8,14-diene system during cholesterol biosynthesis. *J Chem Soc Chem Commun* 1969:206, 1969.
103. White RE, Coon MJ: Oxygen activation by cytochrome P450. *Ann Rev Biochem* 49:315–356, 1980.
104. White RE, Coon MJ: Heme ligand replacement reactions of cytochrome P450. Characterization of the bonding atom of the axial ligand *trans* to thiolate as oxygen. *J Biol Chem* 257:3073–3083, 1982.
105. Wiseman A, Woods LFJ: Regulation of the biosynthesis of cytochrome P450 in baker's yeast. Role of cyclic AMP. *Biochim Biophys Acta* 544:615–623, 1978.
106. Woods LFJ, Wiseman A; Benzo[a]pyrene hydroxylase from *Saccharomyces cerevisiae*. Substrate binding, spectral and kinetic data. *Biochim Biophys Acta* 613:52–61, 1980.
107. Yabusaki Y, Shimizu M, Murakami H, Nakamura K, Oeda K, Ohkawa H:

Nucleotide sequence of a full-length cDNA coding for 3-methylchoranthrene-induced rat liver cytochrome P450MC. *Nucleic Acid Res* 12:2929–2938, 1984.
108. Yonetani T: Cytochrome *c* peroxidase, in Boyer PB (ed): *The Enzymes* (3rd ed) Vol. VIII. New York, Academic Press, 1976, pp 345–361.
109. Yoshida Y, Kumaoka H, Sato R: Studies on the microsomal electron-transport system of anaerobically grown yeast. I. Intracellular localization and characterization. *J Biochem* 75:1201–1210, 1974.
110. Yoshida Y, Kumaoka H, Sato R: Studies on the microsomal electron-transport system of anaerobically grown yeast. II. Purification and characterization of cytochrome b_5. *J Biochem* 75:1211–1219, 1974.
111. Yoshida Y, Kumaoka H: Studies on the microsomal electron-transport system of anaerobically grown yeast. III. Spectral characterization of cytochrome P450. *J Biochem* 78:785–794, 1975.
112. Yoshida Y, Kumaoka H: Studies on the substrate-induced spectral change of cytochrome P450 in liver microsomes. *J Biochem* 78:455–468, 1975.
113. Yoshida Y, Aoyama Y, Kumaoka H, Kubota S: A highly purified preparation of cytochrome P450 from microsomes of anaerobically grown yeast. *Biochem Biophys Res Commun* 78:1005–1010, 1977.
114. Yoshida Y, Imai Y, Hashimoto-Yutsudo C: Spectrophotometric examination of exogenous-ligand complexes of ferric cytochrome P450. Characterization of the axial ligand *trans* to thiolate in the native ferric low-spin form. *J Biochem* 91:1651–1659, 1982.
115. Yoshida Y, Tamura-Higashimaki Y, Sato R: Purification and characterization of intact cytochrome b_5 from yeast microsomes. *Arch Biochem Biophys* 220:467–476, 1983.
116. Yoshida Y, Aoyama Y: Yeast cytochrome P450 catalyzing lanosterol 14α-demethylation. I. Purification and spectral properties. *J Biol Chem* 259:1655–1660, 1984.
117. Yoshida Y: Physicochemical properties of multiple forms of cytochrome P450: A proposal for the ligand structure, in Tagashira Y, Omura T (eds): *P450 and Chemical Carcinogenesis. GANN Monograph in Cancer Research*, Vol. 30. Tokyo, Japan Scientific Societies Press, and New York, Plenum Press, 1985, pp 3–18.
118. Yoshida Y, Aoyama Y, Nishino T, Katsuki H, Maitra US, Mohan VP, Sprinson DB: Spectral properties of a novel cytochrome P450 of a *Saccharomyces cerevisiae* mutant SG1. A cytochrome P450 species having a nitrogenous ligand *trans* to thiolate. *Biochem Biophys Res Commun* 127:623–628, 1985.
119. Yoshida Y, Aoyama Y, Nishino T, Katsuki H, Maitra US, Mohan VP, Sprinson DB: Characterization of an altered cytochrome P450 from a mutant yeast, in Vereczkey L, Magyar K (eds): *Cytochrome P450, Biochemistry, Biophysics, and Induction*. Budapest, Akadémiai Kiadó, 1985, pp 439–442.
120. Yoshida Y, Aoyama Y, Takano H, Kato T: Stereoselective interaction of enantiomers of diniconazole, a fungicide, with purified $P450_{14DM}$ from yeast. *Biochem Biophys Res Commun* 137:513–519, 1986.
121. Yoshida Y, Aoyama Y: Interaction of azole fungicides with yeast cytochrome P450 which catalyzes lanosterol 14α-demethylation, in Iwata K, Vanden Bossche H (eds): *In Vitro and In Vivo Evaluation of Antifungal Agents*. Amsterdam, Elsevier, 1986, pp 123–134.
122. Yoshida Y, Aoyama Y: Interaction of azole antifungal agents with cytochrome $P450_{14DM}$ purified from *Saccharomyces cerevisiae* microsomes. *Biochem Pharmacol* 36:229–235, 1987.
123 Yoshioka H, Morohashi K, Sogawa K, Yamane M, Kominami S, Takemori S, Okada Y, Omura T, Fujii-Kuriyama Y: Structural analysis of cloned cDNA for mRNA of microsomal cytochrome P450(C21) which catalyzes steroid 21-hydroxylation in bovine adrenal cortex. *J Biol Chem* 261:4106–4109, 1986.

Index